THE RADIOLOGICAL EXAMINATION OF THE COLON

SERIES IN RADIOLOGY 3

Other volumes in this series:

1. J. Odo op den Orth, The Standard Biphasic-Contrast Examination of the Stomach and Duodenum, ISBN 90-247-2159-8.
2. Johan L. Selling and Roscoe E. Miller, Radiology of the Small Bowel: Modern Enteroclysis Technique and Atlas, ISBN 90-247-2460-0.
4. S. Forgács, Bones and Joints in Diabetes Mellitus, ISBN 90-247-2395-7.
5. Gy. Németh and H. Kuttig, Isodose Atlas for Use in Radiotherapy, ISBN 90-247-2476-7.
6. Jacques Chermet, Atlas of Phlebography of the Lower Limbs, ISBN 90-247-2525-9.

Series ISBN: 90-247-2427-9

THE RADIOLOGICAL EXAMINATION OF THE COLON

PRACTICAL DIAGNOSIS

ROSCOE E. MILLER, M.D.

Distinguished Professor and Chief of Gastrointestinal Radiology, Indiana University School of Medicine, Indianapolis, Indiana

and

JOVITAS SKUCAS, M.D.

Professor of Radiology, University of Rochester School of Medicine, Rochester, New York

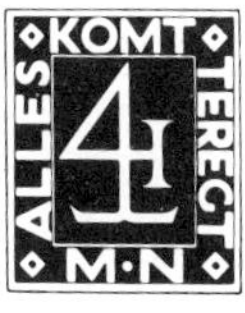

1983

MARTINUS NIJHOFF PUBLISHERS

THE HAGUE / BOSTON / LONDON

Distributors:

for the United States and Canada
Kluwer Boston, Inc.
190 Old Derby Street
Hingham, MA 02043
USA

for all other countries
Kluwer Academic Publishers Group
Distribution Center
P.O. Box 322
3300 AH Dordrecht
The Netherlands

Library of Congress Cataloging in Publication Data

Main entry under title:

The Radiological examination of the colon.

(Series in radiology ; v. 3)
Includes index.
1. Colon (Anatomy)--Radiography. 2. Colon (Anatomy)--Diseases--Diagnosis. I. Miller, Roscoe E. II. Skucas, Jovitas. III. Series.
RC804.R6R34 616.3'4 82-3593
ISBN 90-247-2666-2 AACR2

ISBN 90-247-2666-2 (this volume)
ISBN 90-247-2427-9 (series)

PRINTED IN THE NETHERLANDS

We wish to acknowledge the debt owed to our wives, Dorothy Miller and Gail Skucas, for their understanding and patience for the loss of many nights and weekends.

CONTENTS

PREFACE

The purpose of this book is to explain the current state of the art in radiological examination, interpretation, and understanding of colonic disease. The radiologic aspects of colon disease are combined here with clinical information to serve both beginners and advanced students. Major emphasis has been placed on technique for those radiologists, residents, and technologists first undertaking modern gastrointestinal radiographic techniques. The essentials of technique are stressed so that the reader obtains a clear understanding of colon disease based on sound practical information. We believe this book is a thorough and practical text of particular interest to clinical radiologists and gastroenterologists in their everyday practice, and also for teachers, residents and medical students.

Digital examination and sigmoidoscopy are the first procedures in examination of the colon. Then, the radiologic examination is the next most important procedure. Endoscopy and biopsy play a complimentary role to the radiological examination. The barium enema reveals quickly and early the overall status of the colon and it can then guide endoscopy and biopsy together with subsequent treatment. Surely, if the lesion is not detected our clinical, radiologic, endoscopic, and therapeutic skills are of no use.

This book is designed to impart an understanding of the radiological colon examination process, its performance, its diagnostic ability when done properly, and also its limitations. We believe it summarizes 'all you need to know' about radiology of the colon, but not necessarily 'all you want to know'. The latter would take several texts as long as this one. While this book is designed to be of most benefit to the team performing the radiographic examination, it should be of even greater benefit to that larger group, the nonradiologists, as an aid in interpretation and understanding of modern radiographic techniques. Another purpose of this book is to show that quality examinations can be obtained *routinely* in *any* radiologic facility – including university and community hospitals and office practices. The nonradiologic clinicians should expect similar or better quality examinations for their patients. The nonradiologists must realize that they receive the quality of radiology they deserve! If they support their radiologic colleagues with good historical and clinical information, access to adequate space, modern equipment, technical help, and proper preparation of patients, then the referring physician can expect and demand quality radiology! If under those circumstances quality is not forthcoming, the referring physician can always refer patients to someone who will produce quality work. However, the referring physician must first know what is modern, reasonable and available quality. This book is designed to supply that information. Secondly, it shows the technologist, the equipment and pharmacologic contrast manufacturers what is the current state of the art for radiological colon examinations. While there are now excellent contrast media, relaxant drugs, grids, compression devices, enema apparatus, and other equipment readily available, there is no reason to assume these things cannot be improved and examinations made even easier.

Once again we stress that the examination and diagnosis of colon diseases as illustrated in this book can be readily achieved in most facilities performing these examinations. In fact, many of the illustrations in this book were taken by beginning residents and technologists. The standards set here are only a base line and we hope that our colleagues in all branches of medicine and radiology will improve upon them. We also hope they will communicate their improvements to us.

We wish to express our sincere thanks to all those who have helped fulfill this work. This includes those residents and fellow radiologists who asked pertinent questions and stimulated further research activities.

Particular appreciation is due to our secretaries, Valerie J. Calek and Barbara J. Wiggles for their wide ranging support with the manuscript. John Groves has our thanks for the photography.

Roscoe E. Miller, M.D.
and
Jovitas Skucas, M.D.

PART I

METHODS

I.1. TECHNIQUES OF EXAMINATION

I.1.A. Noncontrast radiography

Noncontrast radiographs, often called plain films of the abdomen, can identify only those structures outlined by gas, fat, soft tissues such as muscles, liver, spleen, etc. and calcium. Still, these limitations are not meant to underrate the importance of these radiographs. Quite often they will be diagnostic or will suggest the therapy or type of examination to be performed next (Fig. A.1). At times, these radiographs will contain a contraindication to a subsequent examination. The presence of gas in certain locations will suggest an abscess, while gas in other locations will imply perforation. Gas in dilated loops of colon may signify a contraindication to an antegrade small bowel examination while such an examination may actually be indicated if gas is present only in small bowel loops. Calcifications and fat between tissue planes can likewise be a clue to underlying disease.

Gas within the colon is an excellent contrast agent. In most patients the course of the colon can be outlined by intraluminal gas. With the patient supine, fluid in the colon gravitates to the dependent portions and gas rises to fill the uppermost part of the colon. Thus, gas is present in the cecum, the transverse colon, and quite often the sigmoid and rectum. With the patient prone, gas rises into the ascending and descending colon. With the patient in a left lateral decubitus position (left side down), gas rises into the ascending colon and cecum. Contrast material residue from prior examinations can produce either confusion or can aid identification of various structures. Numerous radiopaque suppositories also may be identified as foreign objects (1).

A non-contrast radiograph can be obtained with the patient supine, prone, standing or in a decubitus position. The x-ray tube can be horizontal or vertical. Through experience it has been found that a certain combination of radiographs, obtained in a specific sequence, serves best as an initial survey for suspected intraabdominal disease. This radiographic survey, called the acute abdominal examination, is recommended for acutely ill adult patients prior to contrast studies.

With infants and children the views obtained for a 'routine' study of the abdomen vary somewhat between centers. One study found adequate consists of: anteroposterior supine, left lateral recumbent and anteroposterior erect projections (2).

The acute abdominal examination

This study is used for those patients where there is clinical suspicion of bowel perforation, bowel obstruction, ischemia, intraabdominal infection, serious trauma to the abdomen, or evaluation of a suspected intraabdominal disease process of an obscure nature. Because of the relatively low contrast structures involved, this examination should be performed at low kVp; depending upon equipment, it should be about 60–70 kVp.

For the patients who can stand, the patient is placed on the x-ray table in a left lateral decubitus position and kept in this position for approximately 10 minutes. A left lateral decubitus radiograph is then obtained; the radiograph should include the right (upper) side of the abdomen and should show the right flank sufficiently clearly without the radiologist having to bright-light it (Fig. A.2). The radiograph should be 35 × 43 cm (14 × 17 in.) in size and should be centered on the right iliac crest. Of necessity, most of the abdomen will appear white; this radiograph is designed primarily to evaluate whether a pneumoperitoneum is present. If the examination is being performed on a tilting table, with the patient still on the left side, the table is tilted into an upright position and a

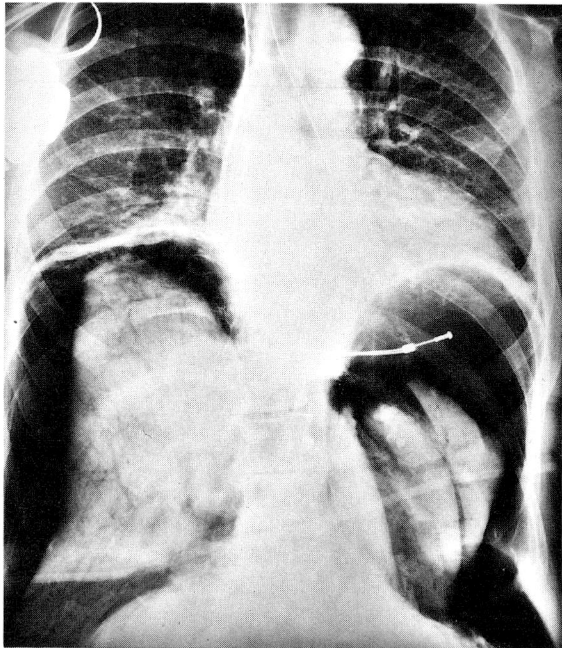

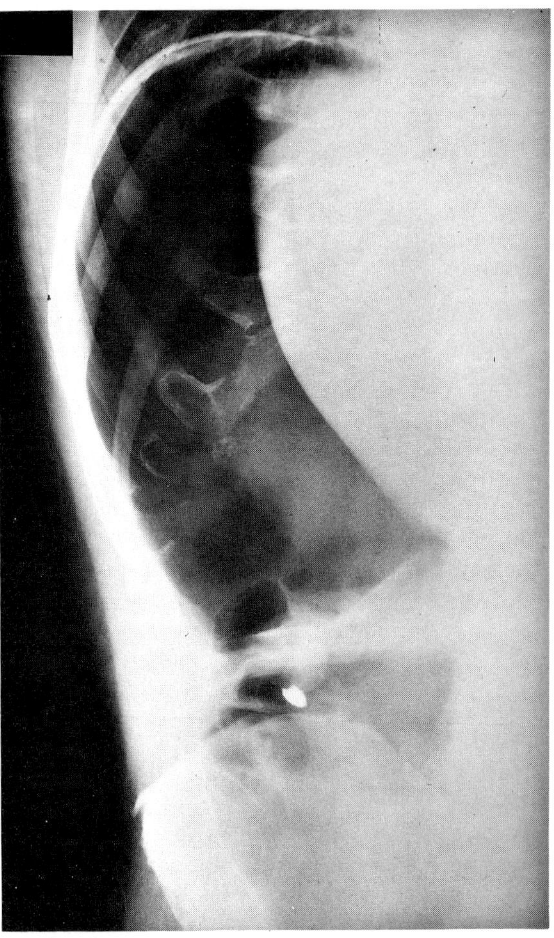

Fig. A.1. This patient has a massive pneumoperitoneum, gas within the intrahepatic portal vein radicles, elevation of both hemidiaphragms and secondary atelectasis of the lung bases. The etiology was bowel ischemia, gangrene and subsequent perforation. Obviously no further radiological examination is required nor indicated.

Fig. A.2. Left lateral decubitus radiograph reveals a massive pneumoperitoneum. In order to visualize the right flank, the dependent portion of the abdomen appears white.

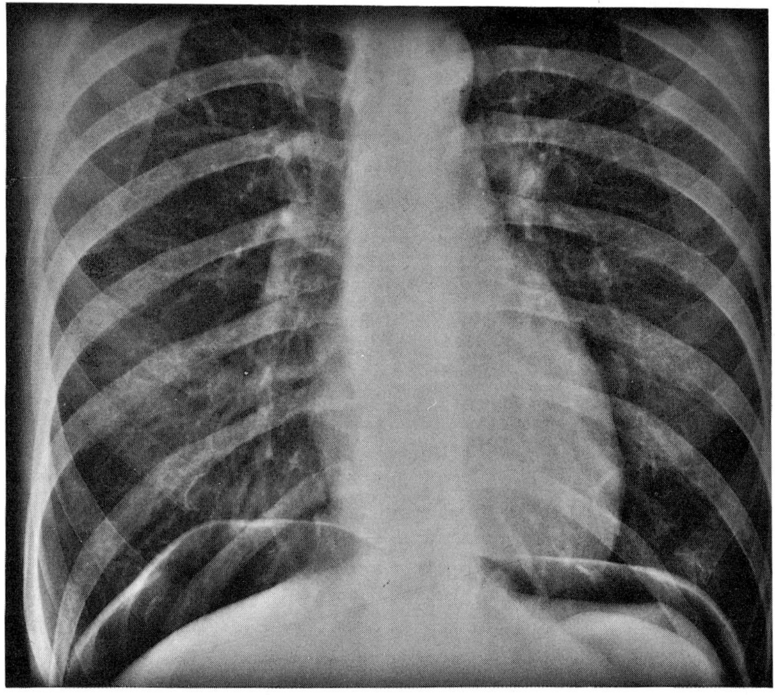

Fig. A.3. Pneumoperitoneum. The upright chest radiograph technique should be optimal for visualizing the lung fields. Of necessity, the abdomen will appear white.

posterior–anterior (PA) view of the chest is obtained (Fig. A.3). This radiograph should include the diaphragm. If a complete chest examination is also being performed at the same time, a lateral radiograph of the chest can now be obtained. The lateral radiograph likewise should include the diaphragm. Both the PA and the lateral radiographs are excellent for visualizing a small pneumoperitoneum. With the patient still upright, an upright radiograph of the abdomen is obtained, with the radiograph centered so that the lower edge of the cassette is at the symphysis pubis. The patient is then returned to a recumbent position and a single supine radiograph of the abdomen obtained, again placing the lower edge of the cassette at the symphysis pubis (Fig. A.4).

If the patient is not able to stand, the above sequence is modified as follows. The first left lateral decubitus radiograph is obtained as described above. Then a second left lateral decubitus radiograph of the entire abdomen is taken, with this second radiograph being sufficiently exposed to allow identification of gas filled loops of bowel. As a practical guide, if one quadruples the mAs of the first decubitus radiograph (which is used for detection of a pneumoperitoneum), an adequately exposed decubitus radiograph of the entire abdomen is obtained. The patient is then placed supine and supine radiographs of the chest and abdomen taken. The abdominal radiograph is centered with the lower margin of the film at the symphysis pubis.

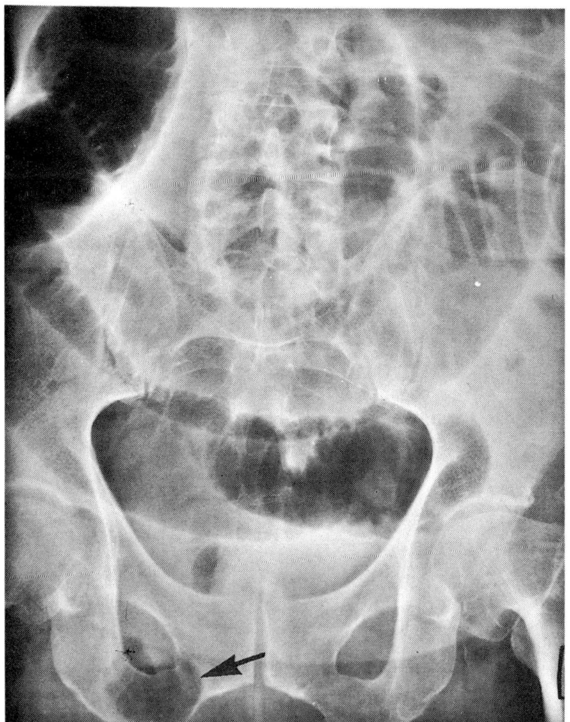

Fig. A.4. The supine radiograph, which is the last radiograph obtained in the acute abdominal examination, should include the symphysis pubis in order to detect a hernia (arrow). In obese patients two 35 × 43 cm radiographs placed crosswise may be necessary to cover the entire abdomen.

The entire examination can be speeded up by having the patient on the left side while still on a stretcher waiting to go into a radiographic room. We believe it is important to obtain the decubitus radiographs first, as outlined above. Some investigators start the radiographic examination with supine and upright radiographs and obtain additional studies later, depending upon the clinical setting and initial findings (3).

The *left* lateral decubitus position is used for two reasons; first, if there has been posterior perforation from the stomach into the lesser sac, with the patient in a left lateral decubitus position gas will percolate through the foramen of Winslow into the main peritoneal cavity and thus be identified against the uppermost right abdominal margin. Second, if one uses a *right* lateral decubitus position, free intraperitoneal gas can be confused with gas in the splenic flexure, making diagnosis difficult. Such confusion is rare with the more inferiorly placed hepatic flexure.

The right lateral decubitus view has been advocated in cases of suspected colon obstruction (4). We generally do not obtain this radiograph; if the clinical suspicion and radiological impression from the acute abdominal examination suggest colon obstruction, we proceed to a barium enema.

The upright chest radiograph should be obtained with the x-ray beam tangential with the uppermost margin of the diaphragm. If the center of the x-ray beam is too high or too low and the x-ray beam is at an oblique angle to the diaphragm, a pneumoperitoneum may be obscured. Because most upright abdominal radiographs are obtained with the x-ray beam at a considerable obliquity to the diaphragm, an upright chest radiograph is superior in detecting a small pneumoperitoneum. One should be able to identify 1 ml of gas in the peritoneal cavity (5) (Fig.

a

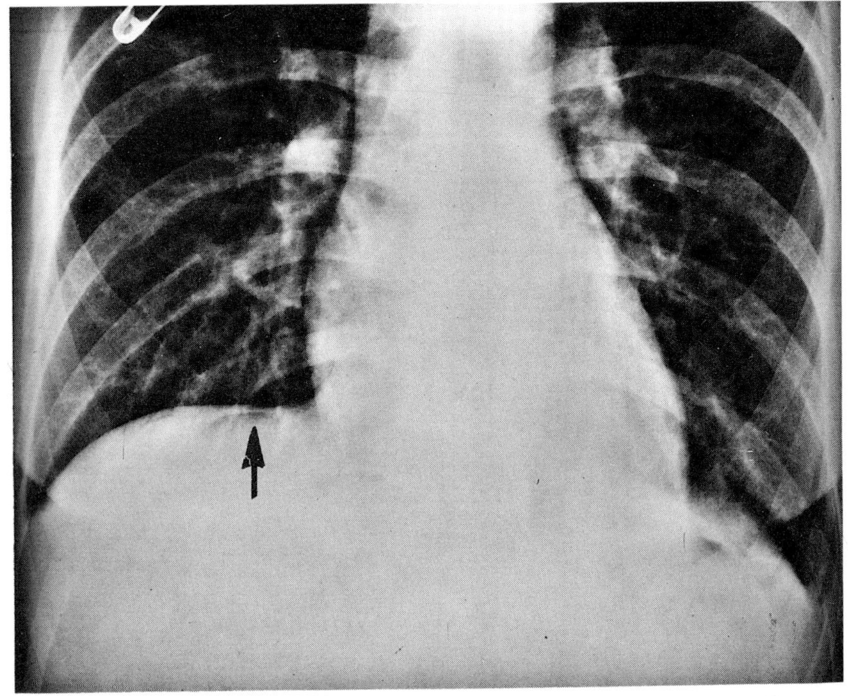

b

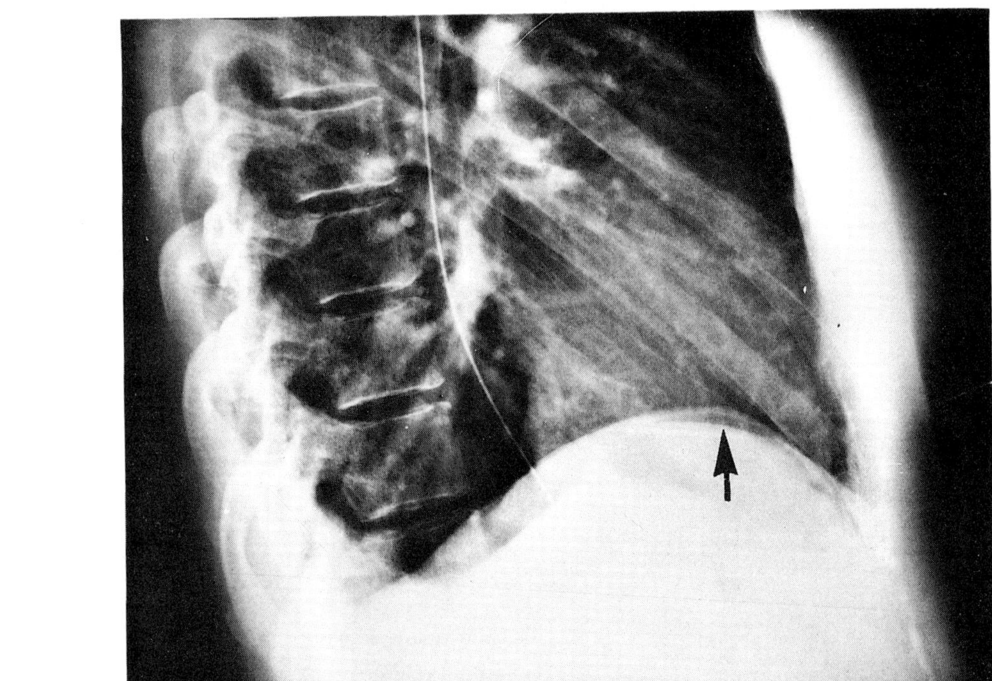

Fig. A.5. (a) Posteroanterior and (b) lateral chest radiographs. A small amount of gas is present beneath the right hemidiaphragm (arrows). The pneumoperitoneum was not detectable on upright radiographs of the abdomen. Approximately 1 ml of gas is in the peritoneal cavity.

A.5). Although it is hazardous to guess the site of perforation from the amount of pneumoperitoneum present, in general, perforation of the colon tends to result in more intraperitoneal gas than perforation in the upper gastrointestinal tract.

The chest should be studied whenever an intra-abdominal condition is suspected (6). Occasionally the patient's main problem is entirely in the chest with the abdominal complaints only secondary in nature.

The acute abdominal examination is not necessary when one is evaluating a known problem, such as a follow-up examination for the location of a ureteral calculus. A modified acute abdominal examination, however, is useful in following disorders involving bowel. As an example, with known partial bowel obstruction one should follow the degree of obstruction. It is important to obtain radiographs with a horizontal x-ray beam, because the degree of bowel distension can be difficult to judge with conventional recumbent radiographs. Occasionally bowel distension is masked by large amounts of fluid within the bowel; the true dilation can only be appreciated with horizontal x-ray beam radiographs. Similarly, bowel wall thickening is best evaluated on radiographs obtained with a horizontal x-ray beam.

References

1. Spitzer A, Caruthers SB, Stables DP: Radiopaque suppositories. Radiology 121:71–73, 1976.
2. Darling DB: Radiography of Infants and Children, 3rd edn, p 90. CC Thomas, Springfield, Ill., 1979.
3. Govoni AF, Whalen JP: The acute abdomen. In: Teplick JG, Haskin ME (eds) Surgical Radiology, Vol I, pp. 169–247. WB Saunders, Philadelphia, 1981.
4. Frimann-Dahl J: The acute abdomen. In: Margulis AR, Burhenne HJ (eds) Alimentary Tract Roentgenology, 2nd edn, Vol 1, p 173. CV Mosby, Saint Louis, 1973.
5. Miller RE: The radiological evaluation of intraperitoneal gas (pneumoperitoneum). Crit Rev Clin Radiol 4:61–85, 1973.
6. Freimanis AK, Nelson SW: The chest roentgenogram in the diagnosis of acute abdominal disease. Radiol Clin North Am 2:3–20, 1964.

I.1.B. The single-contrast barium enema

The first known colon examination using a radiopaque contrast enema was performed by Schüle in 1904, with the contrast agent being bismuth subnitrate (1). Several years later the advantages of barium sulfate led to the almost universal acceptance of this contrast medium as the ideal agent in the study of the colon. Eventually the double-contrast examination was added, using barium sulfate and air as the two contrast agents, and this combination remains currently the ideal in the radiographic study of the colon.

For many years the single-contrast barium enema had been the accepted method of studying the colon. Although the number of full column barium enemas being performed now is difficult to estimate, in 1963 it was believed that approximately 2.5 million were performed in the United States annually (2). Currently, for most indications a double-contrast examination is preferable, yet the single-contrast barium enema is useful in certain situations. Our indications for performing a full-column barium enema are:

1. If the acute abdominal examination suggests colon obstruction, a single-contrast barium enema is performed to locate the site of obstruction. Laxatives are obviously contraindicated in such a situation (Fig. B.1).
2. If a lesion in the distal small bowel is suspected and a reflux small bowel examination is being performed, the appropriate radiographs of the

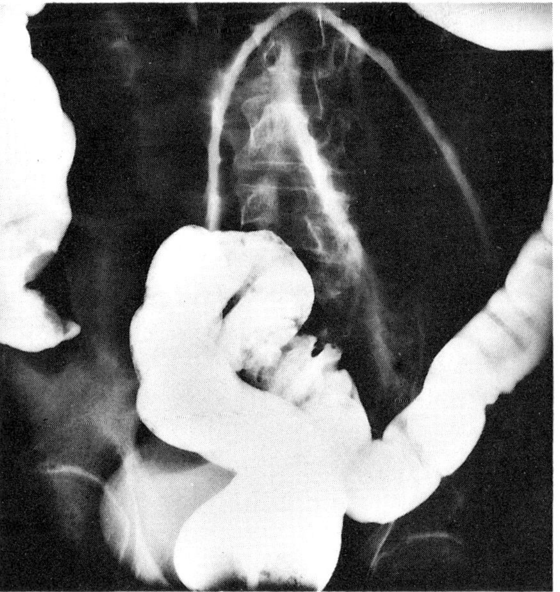

Fig. B.1. The acute abdominal examination revealed obstruction either in the distal small bowel or the proximal colon. A single-contrast barium enema, performed on an unprepared colon, reveals obstruction at the ileocecal valve. Retained stool did not interfere with the examination. An adenocarcinoma arising from the ileocecal valve was resected.

colon are obtained while filling the colon with barium sulfate. Barium is then refluxed to the area of interest in the small bowel (Fig. B.2).

3. If a volvulus or intussusception is suspected from the acute abdominal examination and an attempt at reduction is made, a full-column barium enema is performed.

It should be kept in mind by both the radiologist and referring physician that such an emergency examination simply pinpoints the site of obstruction; very little can be said about the probability of other lesions being present in the colon (Fig. B.3).

As part of the double-contrast barium enema the patient must be able to lie prone. Therefore, if a patient cannot lie in the prone position (such as patients with recent abdominal surgery), a single-contrast barium enema must be performed.

One should avoid proctoscopic examination immediately prior to a single-contrast barium enema, because often large amounts of air are introduced into the colon, resulting in numerous gas bubbles on the subsequent barium enema. Sometimes a cleansing tap water enema can eliminate most of this air.

As in the double-contrast examination, the most important and indispensable condition for the effectiveness of a full-column barium enema is that the colon must be clean (3). Otherwise, not only will lesions be missed but there will also be a significant number of false positive examinations (4).

Even with the low density barium used with the single-contrast examinations, one has to use a relatively high kilovoltage technique in order to 'see through' the barium. Gianturco, in particular, has been a strong advocate of the high kilovoltage technique (5, 6). Because the low density barium sulfate suspension used for full-column enemas flows readily, one should avoid squeezing the enema bag; such an action can increase the intraluminal colon pressure considerably. The air–fluid level in the enema bag should be no higher than 1 m above the table top. If the barium flows too fast one can always lower the enema bag.

The sequence of filming during a single-column barium enema is reversed from that of a double-contrast study. One places the patient in appropriate positions and obtains spot radiographs while barium is being introduced. After the entire colon is filled, overhead radiographs are obtained.

There are probably as many different techniques of performing a single-contrast barium enema as there are radiologists. Most radiologists follow the head of the barium column with fluoroscopy, interrupt the addition of barium during spot radiography, and use a variety of devices to achieve adequate compression. Some radiologists advocate that a scout radiograph be obtained prior to the barium enema. This radiograph serves several purposes: it allows the radiologist to inspect the entire abdomen for any unusual calcifications or collections of gas, it allows a judgment regarding the cleanliness of the colon, and it aids the radiographic technologist in establishing an exposure technique for the subsequent barium enema. Because of the last reason, the scout radiograph should be obtained using the same kVp as the subsequent barium study, realizing that low contrast objects may be poorly seen with such a technique. If the studies are being performed with automatic exposure termination, the scout radiograph does not help establish technique and thus can be obtained at a lower kVp.

A common technique is as follows. First, screening fluoroscopy of the chest and abdomen is performed. Then, with the patient in the LPO position (with respect to the table), barium is added until the sigmoid distends sufficiently, at which time a LPO radiograph is obtained. The optimal degree of obliquity varies from patient to patient and is established fluoroscopically. The barium is then shut off and the patient rotated towards the right into an RAO position and another oblique radiograph of the sigmoid obtained. These views are 180° apart and help differentiate between polyps and air bubbles. The patient is then rotated supine and flow of barium continued. Palpation with a lead glove helps separate any overlying loops of colon. If a filling defect is seen, palpation allows, at times, differentiation between a polyp, moveable stool or air bubble. As the flow of barium reaches the splenic flexure the patient is turned to the right (RPO) and a radiograph of the splenic flexure is obtained. The degree of obliquity is such that the flexure is fully unraveled. That portion of the transverse colon which is inferior to the rib cage is then palpated as the patient is again turned supine. When barium begins to distend the hepatic flexure the patient is turned towards the left (LPO) suf-

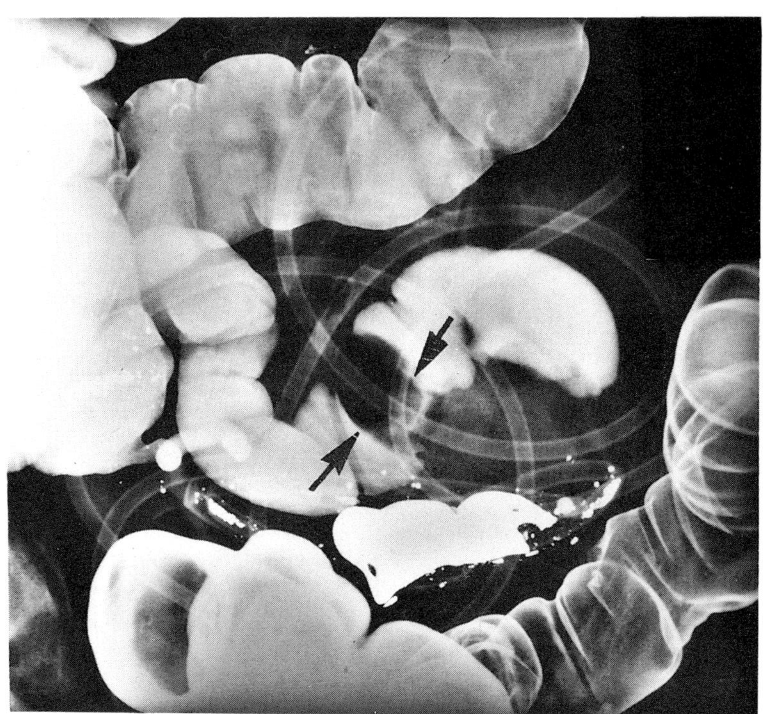

Fig. B.2. Reflux small bowel examination in a patient with distal small bowel obstruction. A circumferential 'napkin-ring' lesion is present in the ileum (arrows), the result of metastatic ovarian cystadenocarcinoma. After the colon was filled with barium sulfate, saline was used to push the barium proximally into the small bowel (8). A portion of the colon has a double-contrast appearance, but in this case instead of air, saline is the second contrast agent.

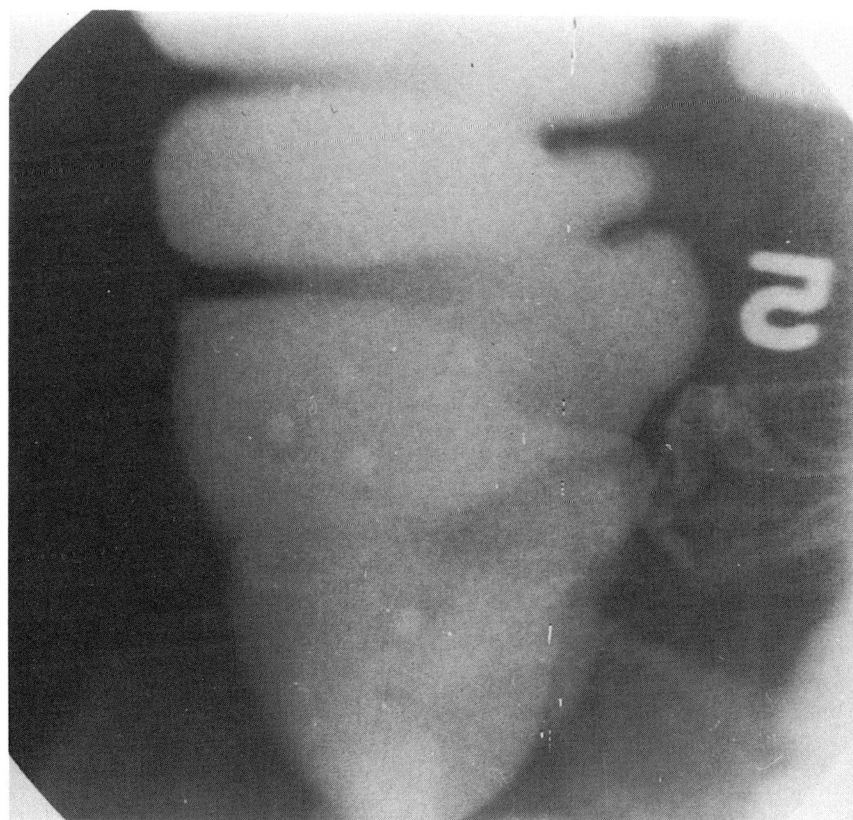

Fig. B.3. One centimeter polyethylene balls with a 'B-B' embedded in the center were swallowed by a volunteer. A full-column barium enema was later performed. Radiographs were obtained at 150 kVp, using 70 mm filming, a high ratio grid, collimation, and compression. The contrast medium was 15% weight/volume barium sulfate. Without the central 'B-B' markers these 1 cm tumors probably would not be seen. (From Miller (9); copyright, Year Book Medical Publishers, 1975.)

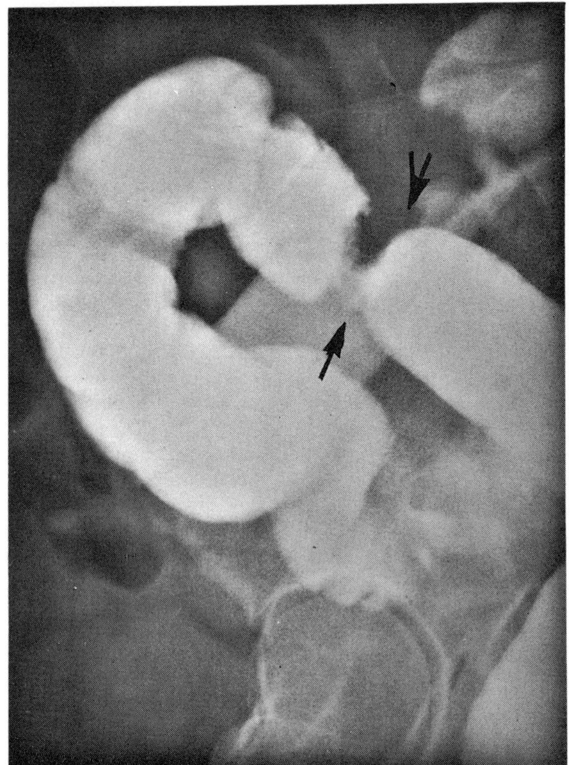

a

Fig. B.4. (a) A narrowed segment (arrows) is present in the sigmoid colon. (b) Another patient showed two narrow segments (arrows) in the ascending and transverse portions of the colon. These segments were present on all radiographs in the examinations. In neither patient was glucagon used. In both examinations the radiologists concluded that a carcinoma was present; in fact, in the second patient it was believed that there were two synchronous carcinomata. Both patients underwent a laparotomy with no abnormality seen. Follow-up double-contrast barium enemas in both patients were normal.

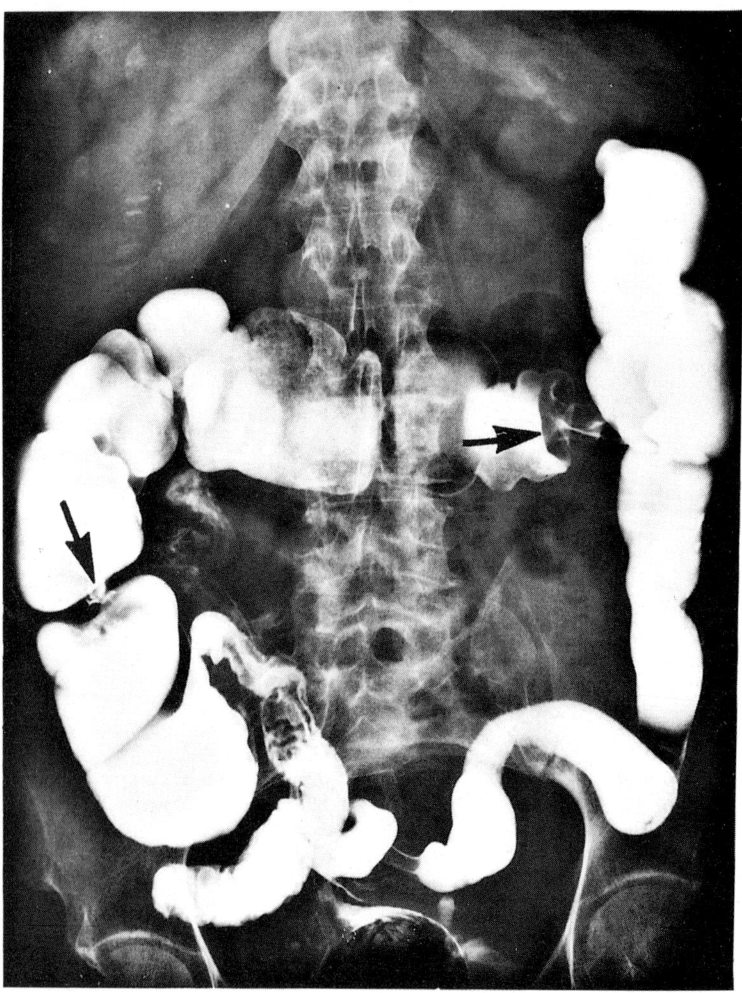

b

ficiently to unravel this flexure and another spot radiograph obtained. When the cecum fills sufficiently, the flow of barium is stopped and spot radiographs of the cecum obtained with the patient in an appropriate oblique position. It is useful to compress the cecum during radiography. The first part of the examination is now complete; the patient is turned prone and posterior–anterior, angled sigmoid, both oblique and lateral rectal radiographs are obtained with the overhead x-ray tube. If only a single undertable x-ray tube is available, the technologist can take these same radiographs using fluoroscopic control for positioning. Many radiologists add additional views, depending upon their past experience and training. A standard set of overhead radiographs simply represents a base line examination, with additional radiographs being obtained depending upon the suspicion of a lesion in a particular area.

By tradition glucagon has not been used with single-contrast barium enemas. If, however, during the examination there is difficulty distending any area, glucagon can be of considerable help (Fig. B.4).

With a full column barium enema one usually tries to avoid filling the terminal ileum during the initial stage of the examination, because barium in the ileum can hide a lesion in the overlapping sigmoid colon. However, one must eventually establish that the cecum has been filled, because a cecal carcinoma with intussusception can be missed entirely by assuming that the patient has a short right colon when in reality one has only filled to the ascending colon. To establish definitely that the entire colon is filled one must either:

1. reflux into the terminal ileum and thus identify the cecum,
2. reflux into the appendix, or
3. definitely identify the ileocecal valve.

The last criterion is the least accurate because at times a lesion can mimic the valve.

Depending upon the type of x-ray generator and grid available, 110–120 kVp probably is optimal for the single-contrast barium enema, although some radiologists are using up to 150 kVp. The barium column should be compressed to the maximum using a lead glove and a non-opaque compression device, such as a large wooden spoon. Compression decreases the thickness of the barium column and allows smaller lesions to be seen (Fig. B.5). Unfortunately, compression is difficult beneath the ribs and in portions of the pelvis. Overlapping loops of sigmoid can hide a lesion; a 'see-through' effect is difficult to achieve with two overlapping loops (Fig. B.6).

After completion of the overhead radiographs a supine 35 × 43 cm postevacuation radiograph is obtained. If one is suspecting a colovesical or colovaginal fistula and none was demonstrated on the barium-filled radiographs, a postevacuation lateral rectal radiograph may show the fistula. Occasionally if there was no reflux through the ileocecal valve during the initial portion of the examination, the postevacuation radiograph will show barium reflux into the ileum. Because there is usually little barium left within the colon, the technologist should use a lower kVp.

It should be emphasized that a single-contrast barium enema should not be performed at the same

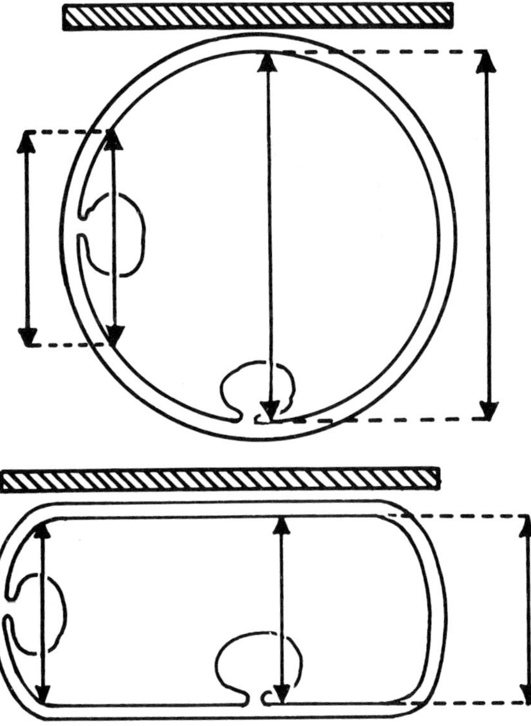

Fig. B.5. (a) Schematic diagram of two tumors in the colon. The x-ray beam penetrates through much less barium when the tumor is radiographed near the edge of the barium column rather than in the center. (b) With compression both tumors will be seen about equally well because the x-ray beam now penetrates approximately the same amount of barium suspension for both tumors. (From Miller (9); copyright, Year Book Medical Publishers, 1975.)

a

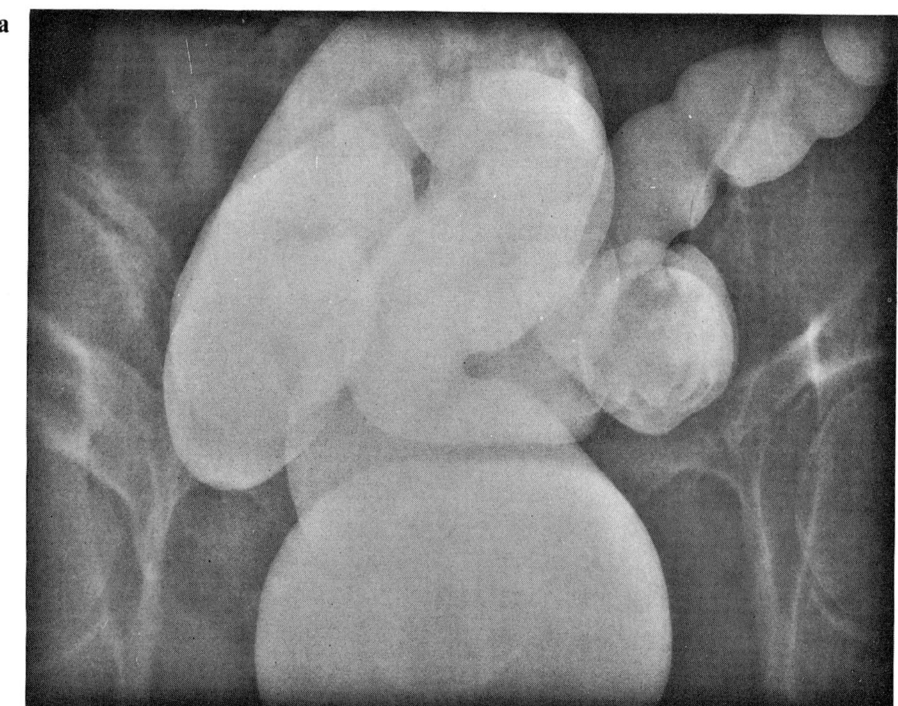

b

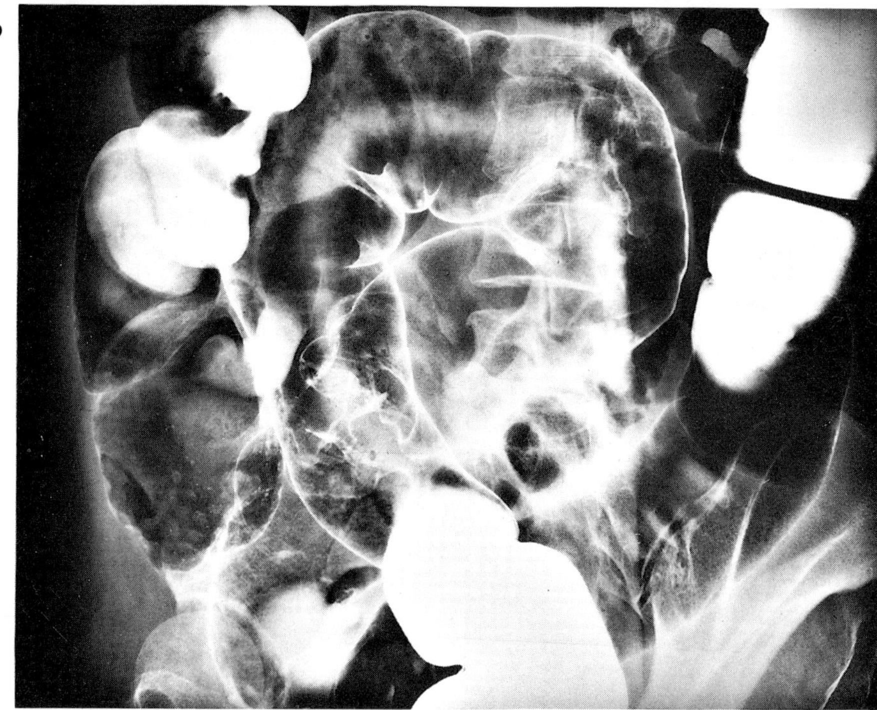

Fig. B.6. (a) Overlapping loops of sigmoid colon made it impossible to see the lesion. Oblique radiographs likewise were of no help. (b) A double-contrast examination reveals the carcinoma (arrows). Although the two loops of sigmoid still overlap, the 'see-through' effect allows identification of the cancer.

time as a double-contrast enema. The barium sulfate suspensions used for the full-column examination do not coat the mucosa well and they are simply used to fill the colon lumen with an opaque contrast medium. As an example, if after evacuation of a single-contrast barium enema one simply adds air, the result is a poorly coated air distended colon showing few if any details. Lesions are readily missed using such an approach.

If an attempt at therapeutic reduction of a volvulus or intussusception is being considered, several clinical criteria should be kept in mind; if there is clinical evidence of peritonitis, most radiologists would consider that as a contraindication to a barium enema. Similarly, bowel obstruction should be viewed with suspicion because there may be an ischemic incarcerated lesion present. In such a situation, it appears that either a water-soluble contrast enema or surgical consultation would be more appropriate although some investigators still favor a barium enema (7).

An attempt at therapeutic reduction of an intussusception in an infant should be performed with the infant sedated. The infant's abdomen should not be palpated. Like all single-contrast barium enemas, the enema bag should not be squeezed, because the resultant excessive intracolonic pressure can result in perforation. Once the barium column reaches the intussusception, continuous pressure begins to outline the 'coil-spring' appearance and, in most cases, starts to reduce the intussusception. If the entire colic portion of the intussusception is reduced, enough reflux into the distal ileum should be obtained to ensure that there is no ileoileal intussusception.

Occasionally, if the attempted reduction does not succeed initially, a postevacuation radiograph will show some reduction of the intussusception. A second attempt at reduction may be more successful than the first, and most radiologists recommend at least two attempts at reduction of an intussusception before admitting defeat.

References

1. Schüle A: Über die Sondierung und Radiographie des Dickdarms. Arch Verdauungskrankheiten 10:111–118, 1904.
2. Thomas SF: All speed and no control. AJR 89:889–890, 1963.
3. Margulis AJ: Is double-contrast examination of the colon the only acceptable radiographic examination? Radiology 119:741–742, 1976.
4. Knutson CO, Williams HC, Max MH: Detection of intracolonic lesion by barium contrást enema. The importance of adequate colon preparation to diagnostic accuracy. JAMA 242:2206–2208, 1979.
5. Gianturco C: High-voltage technique in the diagnosis of polypoid growths of the colon. Radiology 55:27–29, 1950.
6. Gianturco C, Miller GA: Routine search for colonic polyps by high-voltage radiography. Radiology 60:496–499, 1953.
7. Nordshus T, Swensen T: Barium enema in pediatric intussusception. A review of 108 cases. ROEFO 131:42–46, 1979.
8. Miller RE: Reflux examination of the small bowel. Radiol Clin North Am 7:175–184, 1969.
9. Miller RE: Examination of the colon. Curr Probl Radiol 5:2–40, 1975.

I.1.C. Water-soluble contrast enema

Although the water-soluble iodinated contrast agents, first suggested for use in the gastrointestinal tract in 1955 (1), did enjoy some early popularity, their hyperosmolarity has been shown to result in varying degrees of dehydration. In addition, they have a saline laxative effect and low radiographic contrast. As a result, these contrast agents are not often used for most gastrointestinal tract examinations. Currently, their primary use is when there is clinical or radiological suspicion of acute perforation. Thus, a patient with peritonitis suspected to be caused by colon perforation should *not* be studied with barium. If any diagnostic enema is required at all, the iodinated water-soluble contrast media should be employed. Similarly, a patient with suspected acute diverticulitis or other acute inflammatory condition should be studied with the water-soluble media; there is an increased risk of colon perforation in these patients, with the perforation being either into the peritoneal cavity or into an abscess. Other indications for a water-soluble contrast enema include suspected perforated carcinoma, suspected acute ischemia, recent postoperative study of an anastamosis, extensive prior radiation, in the study of long-term defunctionalized loops of bowel, or any other condition where the integrity of the colon is in doubt. As an example, if a patient has had a transverse colostomy for several years, and one is interested in the integrity of the distal colon, the initial examination of the distal loop of bowel should be performed with a water-soluble agent. Simple distention of such a disused segment can result in perforation.

Similarly, if a patient has had a colostomy followed by radiation therapy, with the disused segment of colon being included within the therapy ports, we start with a water-soluble contrast enema even if that part of the colon has been by-passed only for several months.

Children with suspected Hirschsprung's disease or meconium plug syndrome are probably best studied with a water-soluble contrast agent. Similarly, children with intussusception who are believed to be prone to perforation should be studied with a water-soluble agent (2). This latter group of patients includes those who are very ill and those suspected of intestinal obstruction.

Patients with uncomplicated colon obstruction are routinely studied with barium sulfate. Although there is a possibility of barium inspissation proximal to a stricture, use of fluoroscopy together with common sense make this danger more theoretical than real. Barium sulfate allows better delineation of the obstruction and helps evaluate the etiology of an obstruction.

The greatest danger of colon perforation is during the acute episode of a disease. Once a disease such as diverticulitis has stabilized and the patient has been under adequate medical therapy, there is little danger of perforation because the inflammation is generally sufficiently well walled off. Thus, in a patient with suspected diverticulitis we use the water-soluble contrast media only if the colon examination must be performed during the acute attack.

With suspected internal fistulae, such as seen with regional enteritis, barium sulfate is the recommended contrast medium. Likewise, with a suspected vesicocolic fistula we generally use barium sulfate once the acute phase of the disease has passed.

Although there are several commercially available iodinated water-soluble contrast media, in the United States, two of the diatrizoate compounds have achieved greater acceptance than the rest. These two are: Gastrografin, which is a flavored variety of sodium and meglumine diatrizoate, and Oral Hypaque, which consists of sodium diatrizoate together with a flavoring agent. There is some absorption from the gastrointestinal tract and occasionally one visualizes contrast being excreted by the kidneys even in the absence of any gastrointestinal perforation.

We generally prepare both of these contrast media into a 1000 ml enema. With Gastrografin, which comes in 120 ml bottles and contains approximately 37% bound iodine, we generally use two bottles and dilute these with tap water to a total volume of 1000 ml. With these dilutions Gastrografin still is hyperosmolar. The radiographic contrast, however, is still less than can be achieved with barium sulfate. As a result, the radiographic filming technique should be adjusted accordingly by using a lower kilovoltage (kVp). Empirically, we generally use approximately 10 kVp less as compared to a full-column barium study.

Water soluble enemas have been used extensively in pediatric patients with meconium ileus, meconium plug syndrome, and in patients with cystic fibrosis and intestinal obstruction (3–5). The reasons advocated for using these agents rather than barium sulfate are that barium may become inspissated and thus lead to further problems, the amount of fluid in the bowel is increased with the water soluble agents because of their hypertonic effect, and finally the water soluble agents produce a 'wetting' effect. Although several earlier publications mention extensive acute inflammation of the colon with the use of some of the water-soluble agents (6, 7), these reports were subsequently disproven (8). This latter study found that neither Gastrografin nor its major components produced any significant biological changes in the colon, except when an excessive volume of undiluted Gastrografin was used.

One of the complications of these agents is dehydration due to their hyperosmolarity. It has therefore been recommended that in the neonate patient an isotonic dilution be used and that the contrast agent be introduced in a controlled volume only. An essentially isotonic solution of Gastrografin can be obtained by using one part Gatrografin and five parts of water.

These contrast agents should be used with caution if an obstruction is encountered in the colon because they are hypertonic even when moderately diluted; if a significant amount of the contrast is allowed to flow proximal to an obstruction there can be further fluid drawn into an already distended loop of bowel, the pressure increased further, and result in perforation (9).

Gastrografin contains several components, the most important one in relieving obstruction probably being polysorbate-80 (Tween-80). This surface wetting agent is not significantly absorbed from the bowel. A solution of Tween-80, when introduced into a meconium obstruction, tends to relieve the obstruction (10, 11). A 10% solution of Tween-80 produced no histological abnormalities in the colon mucosa (8).

Although children with meconium ileus and meconium plug syndrome are probably best studied using a water-soluble contrast agent and fluoroscopic control, adults with cystic fibrosis and obstruction probably are best treated with an enema containing Tween-80 only. The Tween-80 enema can be performed either in the Radiology Department or in the patient rooms.

Amipaque (metrizamide) is a nonionic contrast agent which, at an approximate concentration of 170 mg of iodine/ml, is isotonic with blood. Amipaque thus overcomes the major limitation of Gastrografin in the gastrointestinal tract, namely, Gastrografin's hyperosmolar effect. As a result, with Amipaque there is less fluid drawn into the bowel and the resultant radiographic contrast tends to be higher. Amipaque is almost nonabsorbable from the gastrointestinal tract; probably less iodine is absorbed from Amipaque than from a corresponding dose of Gastrografin (12). In addition, although diarrhea is frequent after the ingestion of Gastrografin, there is little effect after Amipaque.

Ideally, Amipaque should be the contrast material of choice in those examinations where a water soluble agent is required; unfortunately the very high cost of Amipaque at present prohibits its general application for such use. Hopefully, in the future the price will decrease.

References

1. Canada WJ: Use of Urokon (sodium-3-acetylamino-2,4,6-triiodobenzoate) in roentgen study of the gastrointestinal tract. Radiology 64:867–873, 1955.
2. Armstrong EA, Dunbar JS, Graviss ER, Martin L, Rosenkrantz J: Intussusception complicated by distal perforation of the colon. Radiology 136:77–81, 1980.
3. Huang NN, Denning CR: Drugs used for late intestinal complications. In: Guide to Drug Therapy in Patients with Cystic Fibrosis, pp 91–94. The National Cystic Fibrosis Research Foundation, 1974.
4. Noblett HR: Treatment of uncomplicated meconium ileus by Gastrografin enema: a preliminary report. J Ped Surg 4:190–197, 1969.
5. Wagget J, Bishop HC, Koop CE: Experience with Gastrografin enema in the treatment of meconium ileus. J Ped Surg 5:649–654, 1970.
6. Lutzger LG, Factor SM: Effects of some water-soluble contrast media on the colonic mucosa. Radiology 118:545–548, 1976.
7. Leonidas JC, Burry VF, Fellows RA, Beatty EC: Possible adverse effect of methylglucamine diatrizoate compounds on the bowel of newborn infants with meconium ileus. Radiology 121:693–696, 1976.
8. Wood BP, Katzberg RW, Ryan DH, Karch FE: Diatrizoate enemas: facts and fallacies of colonic toxicity. Radiology 126:441–444, 1978.
9. Steltzer SE, Jones B: Cecal perforation associated with Gastrografin enema. AJR 130:997–998, 1978.
10. Dey DL: The surgical treatment of meconium ileus. Med J Austral 50:179–180, 1963.
11. McPartlin JF, Dickson JAS, Swain VAJ: The use of Gastrografin in the relief of residual and late bowel obstruction in cystic fibrosis. Br J Surg 60:707–710, 1973.
12. Johansen JG: Assessment of a non-ionic contrast medium (Amipaque) in the gastrointestinal tract. Invest Radiol 13:523–527, 1978.

I.1.D. Antegrade study of the colon

Although most radiologists prefer to study the colon through a retrograde enema, some have advocated an antegrade study using a 'colonic cocktail' (1). Such an examination consists of giving a contrast agent orally and approximately 4 hours later insufflating air through the rectum, resulting in a double-contrast examination of the colon. If barium sulfate USP is given orally, by the time it reaches the colon the suspension has dried out and there is relatively poor coating and poor definition of detail. Therefore, it has been suggested that the cocktail consist of barium sulfate, sorbitol, and an iodinated water-soluble contrast agent in a 43% w/w suspension (1). Sorbitol is used in the barium mixture as a stabilizing agent so that the barium sulfate would not flocculate. Sorbitol also tends to accelerate small bowel transit time. Fast transit is also achieved by adding a water-soluble iodinated contrast medium to the barium sulfate suspension.

We have not had experience with this method. The route of administration and complexity involved do not seem to offer any advantage over a conventional double-contrast barium enema.

Others have advocated examination only of the right colon using oral barium sulfate followed by rectally insufflated air (2). This technique is not new; oral barium and rectal air had already been described in 1961 (3), yet the technique has few advocates today.

We believe that in the average patient oral examination of the colon is a rather limited examination and cannot be compared to a conventional double-contrast study. Most authors have used the oral examination only for evaluation of the cecum and ascending colon. They had compared this examination against a full column barium enema. We believe that a double-contrast barium enema is far superior to any of these techniques.

In the occasional patient where a barium enema cannot be performed or leads to an incomplete study, an antegrade study of the colon is an alternative available and, for the right side of the colon, may be worth attempting. The other option available is colonoscopy.

References

1. Pochaczevsky R: Oral examination of the colon. 'The colonic cocktail'. AJR 121:318–325, 1974.
2. Kellett MJ, Zboralske FF, Margulis AR: Peroral pneumocolon examination of the ileocecal region. Gastrointest Radiol 1:361–365, 1977.
3. Heitzman ER, Berne AS: Roentgen examination of the cecum and proximal ascending colon with ingested barium. Radiology 76:415–420, 1961.

I.1.E. Colonoscopy

a. Introduction

The fiberoptic colonoscope has become readily available only since 1970. As with most other newer techniques, after some initial experience most investigators develop a relatively high success rate in reaching the cecum. Right colon polypectomy has been developed since 1971 (1, 2), with many of the developments originating in Japan. Colonoscopy in the pediatric age group can be readily performed (3, 4).

The available flexible fiberoptic colonoscopes vary in length and diameter. Illumination is usually provided by a high-intensity light source such as a xenon lamp, with the light being carried to the tip of the colonoscope through thin glass fibers. Remote control allows the tip of the colonoscope to be flexed in all four directions, similar to that of a steerable angiographic catheter. A hollow lumen allows the colonoscopist to use a biopsy forceps, a brush for cytology, or a snare for removal of pedunculated polyps. A channel provides for suction or insufflation of air or fluid. There are provisions for photography of the visualized image.

Among the tools developed for the study of the gastrointestinal tract, the 60 cm flexible short colonoscope results in low risk and high yield in experienced hands and is extremely useful in examination and biopsy of the distal colon and rectum (5, 6). Some physicians maintain that an examination of the rectosigmoid should be a part of every physical examination in patients above the age of 40 years and in those patients where there are any complaints referable to the colon.

Initially there was considerable competition between colonoscopy and barium enema. Yet these two studies do not compete but complement each other. If the findings on colonoscopy and barium enema conflict, then either one or both examinations should be repeated. Similarly, even if both examinations are negative in the face of clinical or laboratory evidence of colon disease, then a repeat examination should be performed. By using both examinations wisely the number of missed lesions can be kept to a minimum.

The current indications for colonoscopy include:

1. Polypectomy of known polyps.
2. Biopsy of a known lesion to determine its composition.
3. An equivocal double-contrast barium enema.
4. Clinical evidence of colon disease in the face of a 'normal' double-contrast barium enema.
5. A primary evaluation of the colon in suspected disease in those centers where double-contrast barium enemas are not available.
6. Surveillance for early cancers or dysplasia in patients with long-standing ulcerative colitis or recurrent polyposis.

Some clinicians advocate performing a barium enema before colonoscopy (7, 8). We agree that a double-contrast barium enema should precede colonoscopy. The error rate during a subsequent colonoscopic examination can be reduced significantly if a double-contrast enema is used as a guide for colonoscopy (9). Thus colonoscopy should remain a secondary examination in those institutions where an adequate double-contrast barium enema examination is performed routinely in the investigation of colon disease. Colonoscopy can then be used to biopsy, perform polypectomy, or clarify incompletely identified areas on the barium enema. The time required to perform colonoscopy and the expense of the examination are considerably greater than that of a barium enema (10).

Colonoscopic biopsy of inflamed areas may reveal the mild inflammatory changes associated with nonspecific proctitis, while even a technically excellent barium enema can be normal in these patients. In addition, polyps less than 1.0 cm in diameter, superficial ulcers, and vascular malformations are more readily seen with colonoscopy.

Colonoscopy tends to be emphasized in those institutions where the gastroenterologists tend to be aggressive or where gastrointestinal radiology is weak and vice versa. Unfortunately, both disciplines are debased if colonoscopy is invoked because of poor radiographic technique (11). Lesions have been missed by both methods. It is our impression that colonoscopy as the primary colon examination is more frequently performed if no double-contrast barium enema facilities are available.

The success rate in reaching the cecum depends upon the experience of the colonoscopist. On the average, the rate is approximately 60% (12), with variations being 40% (13) to 80% (14) (Fig. E.1). An incomplete examination obviously can miss a colon lesion. In these patients the colonoscopist must provide a clear report stating that only a limited examination had been performed, rather than state or even imply that the colon is 'normal'. An endoscopic examination that fails to visualize the cecum is no better than a poor barium enema contrast study (15).

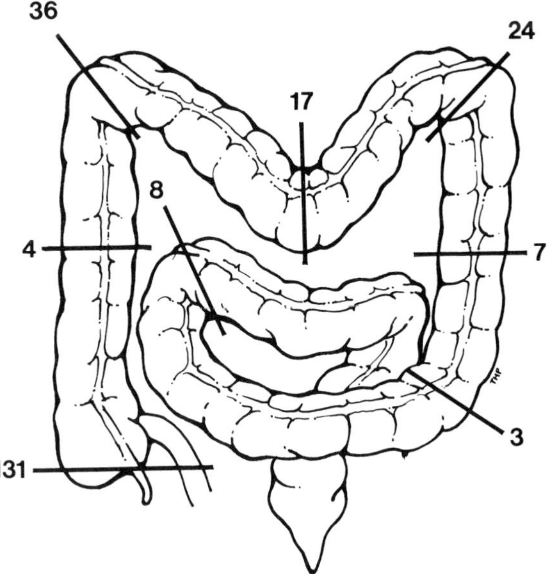

Fig. E.1. Sites of termination of 230 colonoscopies. (Adapted from Gelfand et al. (12).)

Further technical advances are to be expected in colonoscopy. Some colonoscopists can visualize the terminal ileum. A colonoscopic appendectomy on an intussuscepted appendix has been reported (16).

b. Advantages

Colonoscopy is an excellent instrument for biopsy. Some colonoscopists also rely on the gross appearance of a lesion. A graphic description of a lesion by the colonoscopist or photographs taken during colonoscopy allow the colonoscopist to make certain gross predictions based on the statistical incidence of various lesions. Even a pedunculated polyp, however, can be either a benign adenoma or cancer; this differentiation cannot be made visually and only the pathologist can tell the difference. In general, a diagnostic impression reached only by visual colonoscopic observation is fraught with danger and the lesion should either end up with the pathologist or else multiple biopsies should be obtained if diffuse disease is suspected. The value of a colonoscopic biopsy varies with the resultant pathologic finding. If a biopsy reveals a carcinoma, the biopsy obviously is diagnostic. If, however, a biopsy is negative in the face of other convincing evidence that the lesion may be a carcinoma, then a negative biopsy simply tends to confuse the picture. With diffuse colonic disease a biopsy can be nonspecific with the pathologist simply reporting inflammation being present. In particular, with the various colitides a biopsy may show inflammation without identifying the specific disease entity. If a lesion appears such that subsequent surgery is warranted, a barium enema should be obtained, if it has not yet been performed, in order to localize the lesion within the colon and search for other possible lesions.

Although false positive reports of small polyps do occur with a barium enema, such false positive examples are rare with colonoscopy. In the face of severe diverticular disease a barium enema may not reveal a polyp; if colonoscopy through such a diseased area is possible, the polyp may be identified.

c. Limitations

Considerable training and experience is required to perform colonoscopy properly, more than is necessary to perform a double-contrast barium enema adequately. In addition, colonoscopy takes longer to perform than a barium enema and in most places colonoscopy is more expensive; colonoscopy may cost three or more times as much as a barium enema. More medication is required for colonoscopy and as a result the patient recovery time is longer.

Distance measurements during colonoscopy can be misleading; telescoping of the colon around the colonoscope may falsely show a lesion at other than its actual location (17).

Colon redundancy makes pancolonoscopy difficult if not impossible (Fig. E.2). It is difficult to advance the colonoscope through a redundant colon (Fig. E.3). Whenever large diverticula are encountered, there is the possibility of advancing the colonoscope into the diverticulum in the mistaken belief that that is the colon lumen with resultant rupture. Whenever difficult colonoscopy is expected, fluoroscopic guidance is helpful.

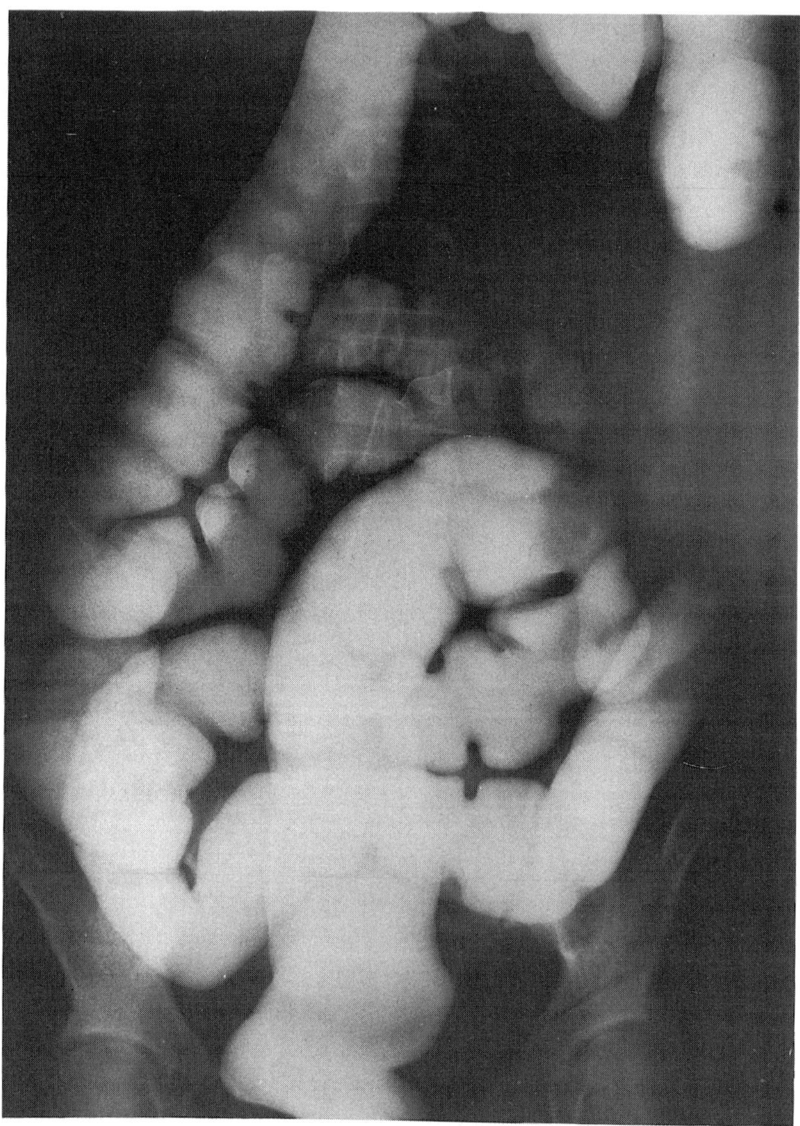

Fig. E.2. A redundant colon such as this one makes complete colonoscopy very difficult.

Since the colonoscope cannot make very sharp bends, lesions located along the proximal concave side of a bend of the colon can be missed (18, 19). We have collected 94 cases through 1981, where colonoscopy missed a polyp which was subsequently detected by radiology (18). In all of these patients the colonoscopist was at or beyond the lesion, yet failed to identify the tumor (Fig. E.4). Most of the missed lesions were at 'blind' areas, located at the valves of Houston, in the sigmoid colon, at the flexures, or in the cecum (Fig. E.5). Thus a 'normal' colonoscopy report should be interpreted with full knowledge of the limitations of the procedure.

A further limitation of colonoscopy is the inability to examine areas proximal to a stricture due to adhesions, inflammation, or tumor (Fig. E.6). Since there is an increased incidence of synchronous colon cancers, the colonoscopic finding of a rectal or sigmoid carcinoma and the inability to pass the colonoscope proximal to the lesion can miss other lesions. We believe that in such a situation, if there are no contraindications and a barium enema has not yet been performed, one should perform a barium enema to exclude other lesions.

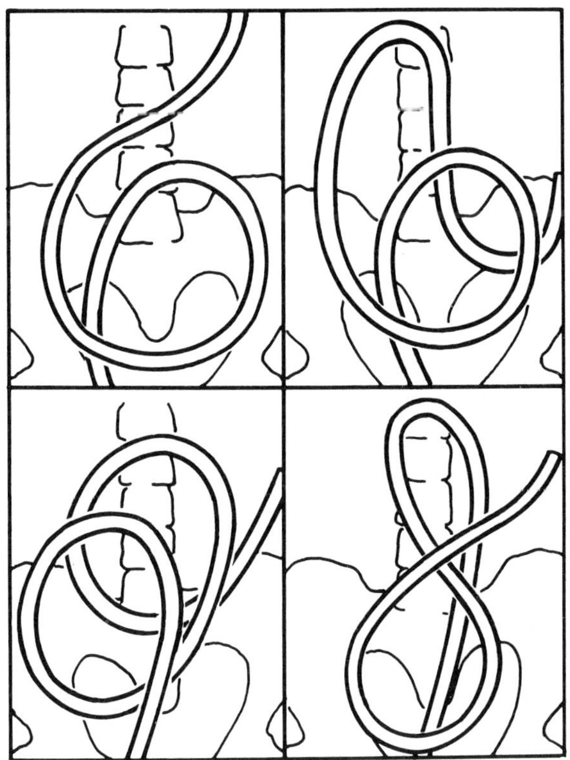

Fig. E.3. Colonoscope configurations making further advance difficult.

Colonoscopy can be difficult, and at times impossible, in the presence of massive colon bleeding or in those patients with marked constipation. Quite often blood or retained stool results in an unsatisfactory examination due to obstruction of the colonoscopic lens. A limitation likewise exists for a barium enema, where blood clots and stool may mimic large tumors.

In patients with clinically suspected obstruction an emergency single-contrast barium enema can be performed on the unprepared colon simply to diagnose or exclude obstruction. Barium may flow around blood clots or stool and identify an obstruction.

If an intussusception is suspected, a barium enema can be not only diagnostic but also therapeutic. We are not aware of colonoscopic reduction of colon intussusception.

The post-operative colon can have considerable surgical distortion and a barium enema may not distinguish between surgical deformity and possible recurrent tumor. Here, colonoscopy with biopsy is an excellent tool and may help identify mucosal lesions. However, it must be realized that those tumors extrinsic or intramural in location and not involving the mucosa are missed by colonoscopy, with the overlying mucosa appearing normal. A barium enema may be helpful in these patients since tumor involvement of the colon wall may be detected by the radiographic examination. Computerized tomography (CT) is being used more and more by us in the follow-up of these patients with suspected recurrent tumors. Although present-day CT is relatively insensitive in detecting small mucosal lesions, CT is an excellent tool for bones and soft tissues and can detect extrinsic spread of tumor. In addition, a CT study may show distal metastases to the liver or lymph nodes.

d. Complications

The incidence of complications can be kept to a minimum with careful selection of patients and awareness of the risks involved, yet the complication rate is higher than that of a barium enema, with the incidence of colon perforation during colonoscopy depending upon the expertise of the

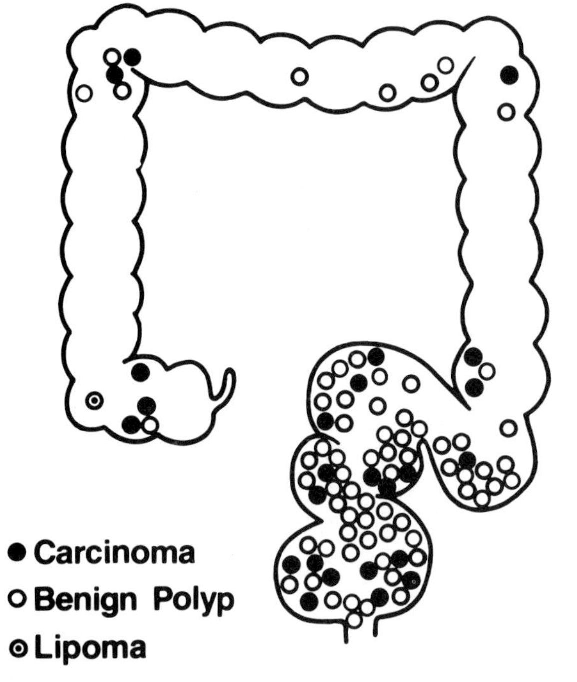

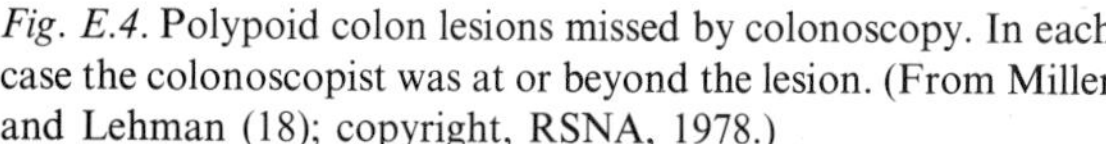
Fig. E.4. Polypoid colon lesions missed by colonoscopy. In each case the colonoscopist was at or beyond the lesion. (From Miller and Lehman (18); copyright, RSNA, 1978.)

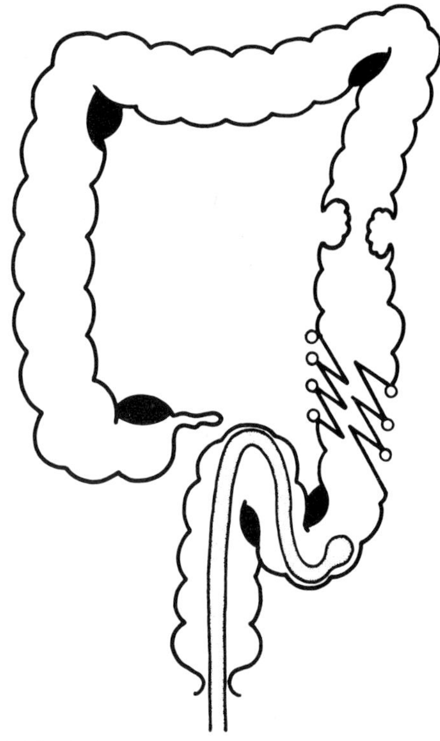
Fig. E.5. The dark areas show sites where colonoscopic visualization is difficult due to acute angulation. (From Miller and Lehman (17); copyright, AMA, 1976.)

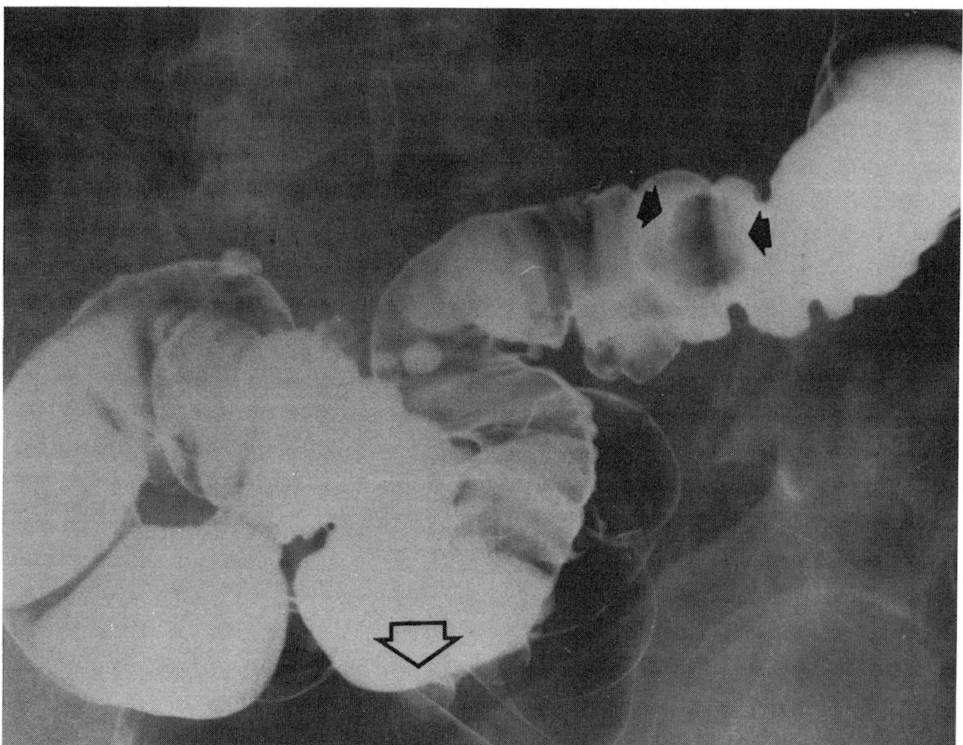
Fig. E.6. A sigmoid polyp (closed arrows) could not be reached by the colonoscope because of adhesions from prior diverticular disease (open arrow).

examiner. The most common complication of colonoscopy is perforation, with a 0.2–0.9% rate being reported (20–24). Diastatic serosal laceration may occur even when no mucosal changes are appreciated during colonoscopy (25, 26). Bacteremia and retroperitoneal emphysema (27) are other complications encountered during colonoscopy. The major complication of polypectomy is hemorrhage, with a 1–2% incidence reported (21, 24).

Sigmoidoscopy, whether accompanied by a biopsy or not, can also result in perforation (28). A barium enema performed shortly after may complete a perforation, leading to barium spillage into the peritoneal cavity. Since biopsies are generally performed in an area where disease is suspected, any underlying disease may add to weakening of the colon wall. Likewise, there may be colo-rectal perforation following a biopsy (29, 30).

Most colon perforations become evident almost immediately. Quite often the patient will have severe pain during the episode of rupture. An acute abdominal examination should reveal the perforation. Occasionally, the patient will exhibit signs of perforation only hours later, with the initial symptoms possibly being masked by medication. Extraperitoneal perforation may become apparent only after some delay (31). The perforation may be unrecognized until a subsequent barium enema, leading to barium spillage either into the peritoneal cavity or the extraperitoneal tissues (32). It has been recommended that at least ten days (33) to two weeks (34) elapse between a colorectal biopsy and a subsequent barium enema, although there are divergent opinions between the surgeons who perform biopsies and radiologists who perform barium enemas (35). An interval of time allows any possible colon damage to heal.

Colonoscopy can result in a 'benign' pneumoperitoneum (36) or pneumatosis intestinalis (37). A pneumoperitoneum probably represents a localized perforation without significant peritoneal soiling. The treatment of either of these findings after colonoscopy should be individualized. Just like an extraperitoneal perforation during a barium enema, such a patient may be treated successfully with medical management or the patient may require surgical intervention.

A rare complication is explosion during colonoscopic polypectomy (38). It is believed that mannitol degradation into hydrogen and methane is responsible and, if mannitol is used for bowel preparation, oral antibiotics or insufflation of carbon dioxide should be administered to prevent such an explosion (39).

Colonoscopy is contraindicated in patients with suspected toxic megacolon, nonviable bowel, acute diverticulitis, peritonitis, or perforation. Similar contraindications exist for a barium enema.

References

1. Deyhle P, Seuberth K, Jenny S, Demling L: Endoscopic polypectomy in the proximal colon. Endoscopy 3:103–105, 1971.
2. Shinya H, Wolff WI: Therapeutic applications of colonofiberoscopy: polypectomy via the colonoscope [Abstr.]. Gastroenterology 60:830, 1971.
3. Plucnar BJ: Colonoscopy in infancy and childhood with special regard to patient preparation and examination technique. Endoscopy 13:14–18, 1981.
4. O'Connor JJ: Colonoscopy in children. Am J Surg 141:344–345, 1981.
5. Winawer SJ, Leidner SD, Boyle C, Kurtz RC: Comparison of flexible sigmoidoscopy with other diagnostic techniques in the diagnosis of rectocolon neoplasia. Dig Dis Sci 24:277–281, 1979.
6. Carter HG: Short flexible fiberoptic colonoscopy in routine office examinations. Dis Colon Rectum 24:17–19, 1981.
7. Williams CB, Hunt RH, Loose H, Riddell RH, Sakai Y, Swarbrick ET: Colonoscopy in the management of colon polyps. Br J Surg 61:673–682, 1974.
8. Winawer SJ, Sherlock P, Schottenfeld D, Miller DG: Screening for colon cancer. Gastroenterology 70:783–789, 1976.
9. Thoeni RF, Menuck L: Comparison of barium enema and colonoscopy in the detection of small colonic polyps. Radiology 124:631–635, 1977.
10. Teague RH, Manning AP, Thornton JR, Salmon PR, Read AE: Colonoscopy for investigation of unexplained rectal bleeding. Lancet 1:1350–1351, 1978.
11. Williams C, Teague R: Progress report—colonoscopy. Gut 14:990–1003, 1973.
12. Gelfand DW, Wu WC, Ott DJ: The extent of successful colonoscopy: its implication for the radiologist. Gastrointest Radiol 4:75–78, 1979.
13. Knoepp LF Jr, McCulloch JH: Colonoscopy in the diagnosis of unexplained rectal bleeding. Dis Colon Rectum 21:590–593, 1978.
14. Knutson CO, Max MH: Value of colonoscopy in patients with rectal blood loss unexplained by rigid proctosigmoidoscopy and barium contrast enema examinations. Am J Surg 139:84–87, 1980.
15. Knutson CO, Max MH: Diagnostic and therapeutic colonoscopy. A critical review of 662 examinations. Arch Surg 114:430–435, 1979.
16. Wirtschafter SK, Kaufman H: Endoscopic appendectomy. Gastrointest Endosc 22:173–174, 1976.
17. Miller RE, Lehman G: The barium enema. Is it obsolete? JAMA 235:2842–2844, 1976.
18. Miller RE, Lehman G: Polypoid colonic lesions undetected by endoscopy. Radiology 129:295–297, 1978.

19. Laufer I, Smith NCW, Mullens JE: The radiological demonstration of colorectal polyps undetected by endoscopy. Gastroenterology 70:167–170, 1976.
20. Berci G, Panish JF, Schapiro M, Corlin R: Complications of colonoscopy and polypectomy. Gastroenterology 67:584–585, 1974.
21. Rogers BHG, Silvis SE, Nebel OT, Sugawa C, Mandelstam P: Complications of flexible fiberoptic colonoscopy and polypectomy. Gastrointest Endosc 22:73–77, 1975.
22. Meyers MA, Ghahremani GG: Complications of gastrointestinal fiberoptic endoscopy. Gastrointest Radiol 2:273–280, 1977.
23. Geenen JE, Schmitt MG Jr., Hogan WJ: Complications of colonoscopy [Abstr.]. Gastrointest Endosc 20:179–180, 1974.
24. Overholt BF: Colonoscopy — a review. Gastroenterology 68:1308–1320, 1975.
25. Livstone EM, Cohen GM, Troncale FJ, Touloukian RJ: Diastatic serosal lacerations: an unrecognized complication of colonoscopy. Gastroenterology 67:1245–1247, 1974.
26. Wu TK: Occult injuries during colonoscopy. Measurement of forces required to injure the colon and report of cases. Gastrointest Endosc 24:236–238, 1978.
27. Lezak MB, Goldhamer M: Retroperitoneal emphysema after colonoscopy. Gastroenterology 66:118–120, 1974.
28. Kiser JL, Spratt JS Jr, Johnson CA: Colon perforations occuring during sigmoidoscopic examinations and barium enemas. Mo Med 65:969–974, 1968.
29. McDonald CC, Rowe RJ: Retrorectal fistula secondary to barium-abscess granuloma: report of a case. Dis Colon Rectum 19:71–73, 1976.
30. Thorbjarnarson B: Iatrogenic and related perforations of the large bowel. Arch Surg 84:608–614, 1962.
31. Reinhardt K: Retropneumoperitoneum und pneumomediastinum im Anschlus an eine Rektoskopie. ROEFO 131:50–53, 1979.
32. Hemley SD, Kanick V: Perforation of the rectum: a complication of barium enema following rectal biopsy. Am J Dig Dis 8:882–884, 1963.
33. Bartram CI: Radiology in the current assessment of ulcerative colitis. Gastrointest Radiol 1:383–392, 1977.
34. Amberg JR: Complications of colon radiography. Gastrointest Endosc 26 (Suppl):15S–17S, 1980.
35. Mullin HJ: Timing of barium enema studies following sigmoidoscopy [Letter]. JAMA 241:941, 1979.
36. Taylor R, Weakley FL, Sullivan BH Jr: Non-operative management of colonoscopic perforation with pneumoperitoneum. Gastrointest Endosc 24:124–125, 1978.
37. Meyers MA, Ghahremani GG, Clements JL Jr, Goodman K: Pneumatosis intestinalis. Gastrointest Radiol 2:91–105, 1977.
38. Bigard M-A, Gaucher P, Lassalle C: Fatal colonic explosion during colonoscopic polypectomy. Gastroenterology 77:1307–1310, 1979.
39. Taylor EW, Bentley S, Youngs D, Keighley MRB: Bowel preparation and the safety of colonoscopic polypectomy. Gastroenterology 81:1–4, 1981.

I.1.F. Miscellaneous techniques

a. Angiography

While arteriography is not a substitute for other colon examinations, vascular lesions, especially if they are small and intramural, lend themselves to angiographic study. Angiography is not used often in the investigation of colon cancers. Patients with major colonic bleeding are best studied by arteriography to establish the site of bleeding. Therapeutic embolization or vasoactive drug infusion can be performed and surgery either postponed or avoided completely.

When investigating an unknown bleeding site, some angiographers first study the inferior mesenteric artery and subsequently study the superior mesenteric artery. If the procedure is reversed, contrast excreted in the bladder may obscure the rectosigmoid area, making identification of a bleeding site difficult. Or, the patient can simply void after the superior mesenteric artery study.

A description of the various angiographic techniques employed is beyond the scope of this publication. Several angiographic textbooks are available.

The normal vascular anatomy and angiographic appearance of various lesions are described in the appropriate sections.

b. Computer tomography

Computer tomography (CT) of the abdomen has been of value primarily in the solid structures such as the liver, spleen, pancreas and other extraperitoneal organs. Most of the initial studies did not mention any application for hollow viscera.

Considerable improvement is necessary in computer tomography before intraluminal diseases can be evaluated adequately. The main problem is the relatively poor spatial resolution even with the modern computed tomographic units. The faster scanners gradually becoming available reveal a marked improvement in efficacy as compared to the older generation slow scanners (1) and future application to the colon will undoubtedly increase. Further advances, such as sequential angiographic CT scanning, may aid tumor evaluation and possibly eliminate some catheter angiography (2).

Although intraluminal masses today are still best demonstrated by the double contrast examination, CT has been of value in evaluating both intramural masses and serosal involvement (3) (Fig. F.1). At times a large tumor is detected incidentally when CT is performed for other purposes (4). CT can recognize tumors 2 cm in diameter (5, 6). If a lesion is demonstrated by barium enema, CT can show whether there is extraluminal extension. Invasion of the pararectal fat can be suspected when the fat planes are obliterated. CT can be of value if the question arises as to whether an intramural mass originates in the colon or represents extramural invasion. Although computer tomography can provide information regarding tissue density, outside of extreme ranges normal tissue and tumor cannot be readily differentiated. Yet, such lesions as mesenteric cysts or lipomas can be suggested by CT because of their lower CT numbers. An abscess has a mottled gas-filled appearance with poorly defined borders (Fig. F.2).

The colon can be best evaluated if it is distended with a contrast enema. Distending the colon and outlining its intramural portion aids in identifying the surrounding anatomical landmarks. A dilute diatrizoate solution (approximately 2% solution) is being used, although a specially formulated low density barium sulfate has been proposed (7) and such products are available from several manufacturers.

Most of the current applications have been in the rectum and sigmoid. Not only primary intramural lesions but also gynecological tumors with secondary spread to the rectosigmoid can be evaluated. If necessary, CT can be an aid in percutaneous biopsy (8). Some have proposed preoperative CT of rectal carcinoma to help evaluate local spread and aid subsequent therapy (6, 9).

Liver and bone metastases, hydronephrosis, and adenopathy can be studied readily with computer tomography (Fig. F.3). Although other radiographic examinations may show any one abnormality, it is believed that CT, overall, delineates more abnormalities than any one other diagnostic test (10).

CT should not be the primary means of investigating colon lesions, but as a supplemental examination it aids diagnosis in some diseases.

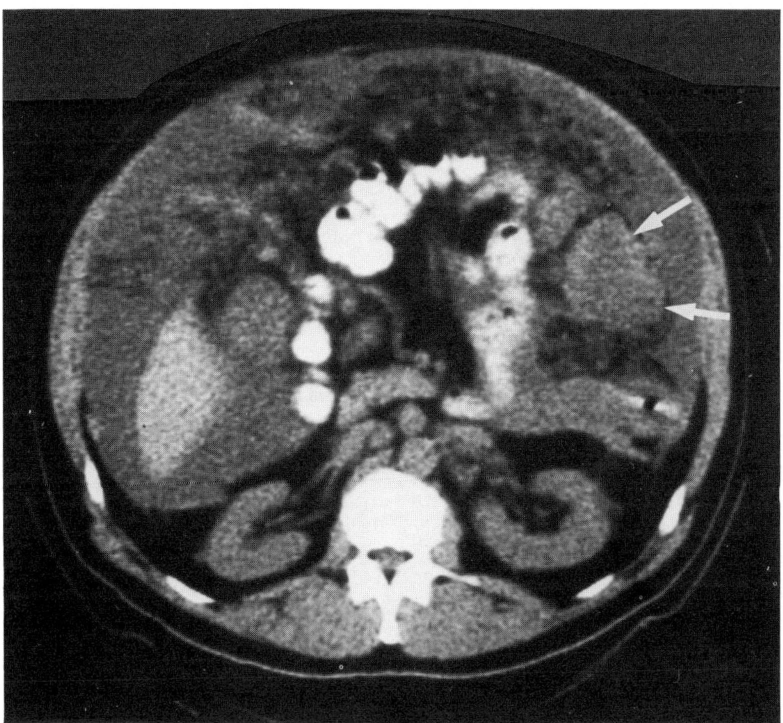

Fig. F.1. CT scan through the mid-abdomen revealed a large tumor extending along the left flank (arrows). Massive ascites is also present. A barium enema showed extensive serosal metastases involving the descending colon.

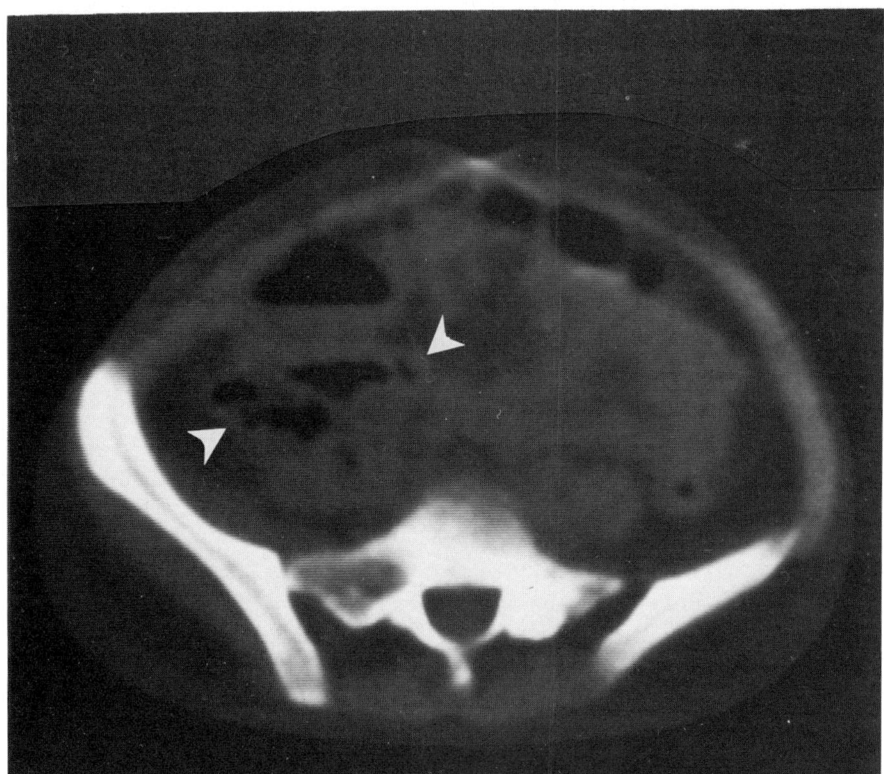

Fig. F.2. A poorly marginated mass with central collections of gas is present in the right lower quadrant (arrowheads). The mass was a tubo-ovarian abscess. An abscess secondary to regional enteritis or appendicitis can have a similar appearance.

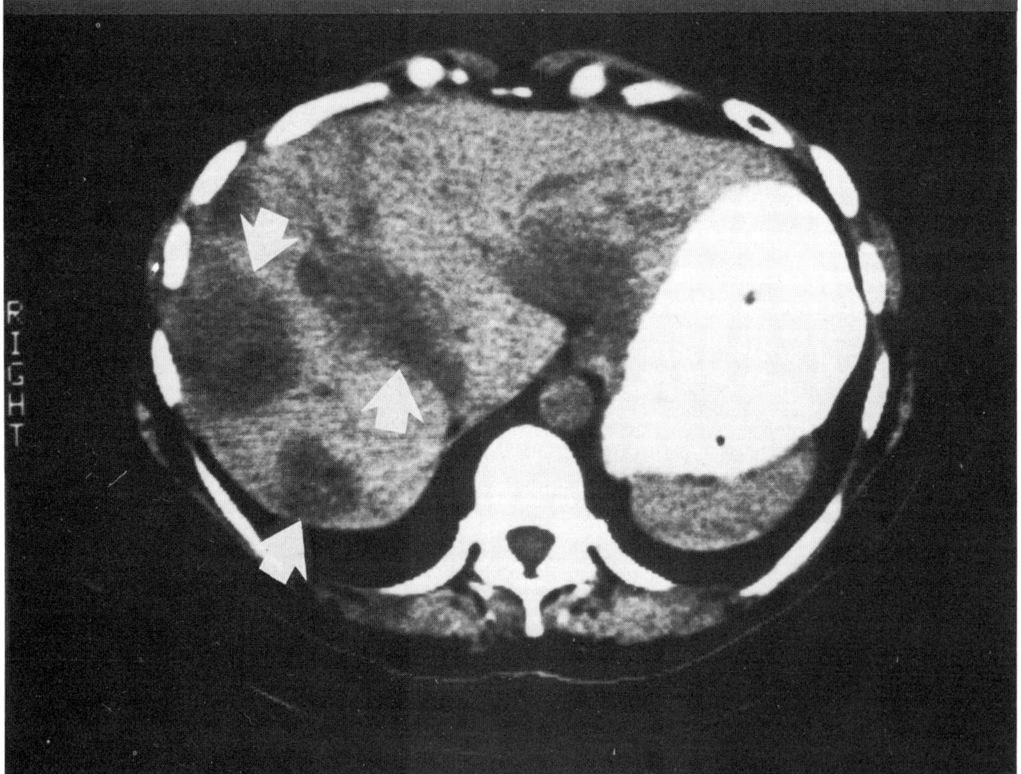

a

Fig. F.3. (a) CT scan of the liver reveals multiple liver metastases (arrowheads). The patient had a primary colon poorly differentiated adenocarcinoma. (b) CT scan of the chest obtained at the same time revealed several lung metastases. The one shown is in the right lower lobe (arrowhead). (c) Chest radiograph at the time of the CT scan was normal. Only 13 months later could the pulmonary metastases be seen on a chest radiograph (arrows), illustrating the considerably earlier detectability of metastases by CT.

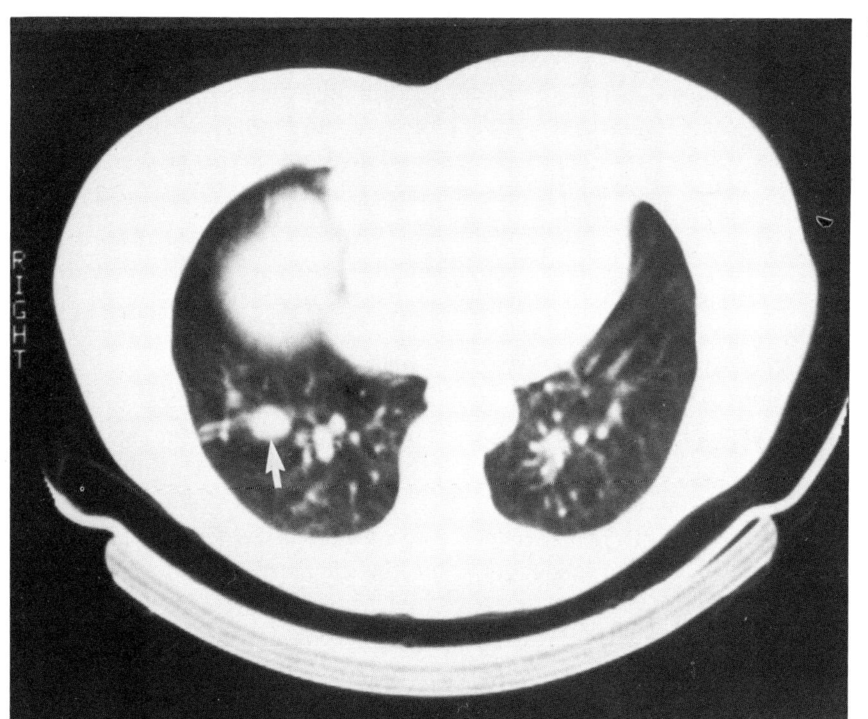

b

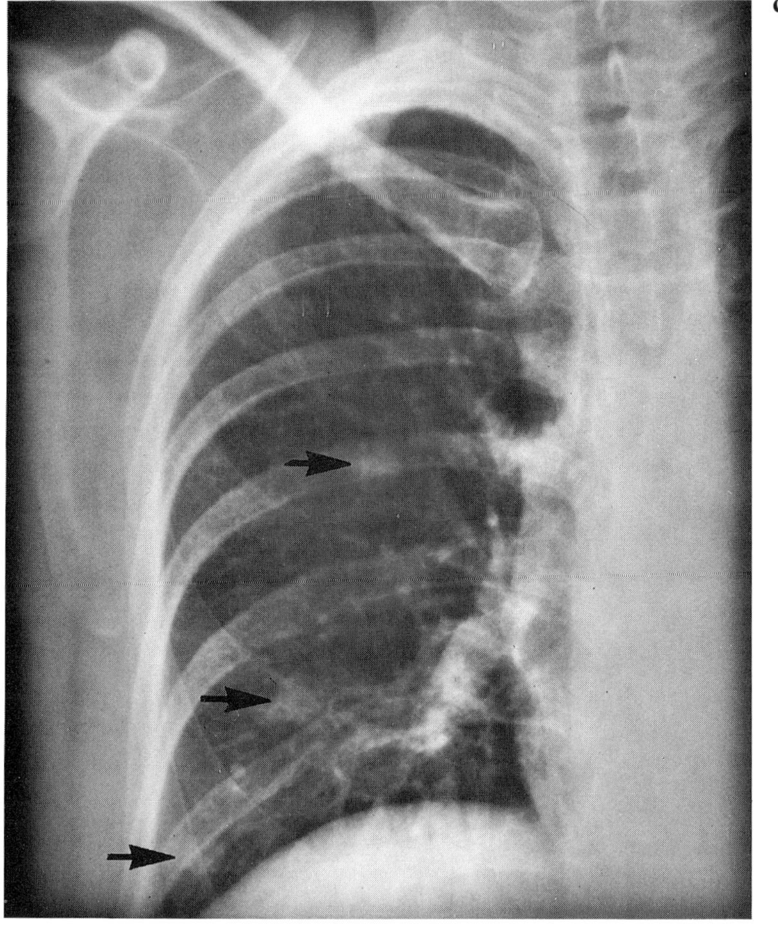

c

Whether one should routinely obtain computed tomography of the liver in patients who have carcinoma demonstrated on a barium enema is not clear; the resultant efficacy of such an examination has not been adequately studied.

c. Nuclear medicine

The use of gallium-67 citrate for tumor localization is a relatively new development with the first such observation being by chance (11). Why gallium localizes in tumors is not known; gallium is found in the lysosomes within the cytoplasm of tumor cells. Gallium is also found in some normal cells (12). Unfortunately not all colon tumors show gallium uptake, with uptake being highest in poorly differentiated tumors (13). Varying amounts of gallium are found throughout the gut, leading to problems of interpretation. Laxatives or enemas prior to a scan are helpful. There can be considerable variation in the retention rate between patients.

A normal gallium scan does not rule out a colon carcinoma. The future of gallium scanning for colon cancers may be primarily in the search for metastases. Additional experience is necessary before this diagnostic modality can be readily accepted.

A positive gallium scan is seen with an abscess and in surgical wounds (Fig. F.4). Caution is thus necessary in interpreting these scans. The extent of ulcerative colitis correlates with the regional uptake of gallium (14). The scans may revert to normal during periods of remission.

Technetium-99m-sulfur colloid is a promising agent in the evaluation of gastrointestinal bleeding (15). ^{99m}Tc-SC can detect hemorrhage at slower rates than detected during angiography (16, 17). However, because the colloid is cleared by the body's reticuloendothelial system, bleeding will be seen only if the patient is actively bleeding during the time that the tracer remains in the blood (Fig. F.5). Thus, intermittent bleeding can be missed. ^{99m}Tc-labeled red blood cells remain in the blood for prolonged periods of time and numerous scans can be made to detect intermittent bleeding (18, 19). Heat treated ^{99m}Tc-labeled red blood cells appear to be rather sensitive, with gastrointestinal bleeding as low as 0.12 ml/min being detected (20).

Skeletal metastases can be evaluated with technetium diphosphonate as the contrast agent. Unfortunately, there are numerous normal and benign conditions that can produce a positive scan and, as a result, the scan should not be interpreted without corresponding radiographs (21). The scan is highly sensitive but of rather low specificity. However, the bone scan is more sensitive than skeletal radiographs and when used together with radiographs can yield considerable useful data.

d. Ultrasonography

Ultrasonography was initially applied to the solid organs; its application to the colon and related structures is only now slowly being appreciated. Artifacts from retained gas both within the small bowel and colon are the major limitations of ultrasonography in the abdomen.

At present ultrasonography is an ancillary modality in study of the colon and should not replace conventional examinations. Although there are reports of ultrasonography showing large colon cancers (22–24), a barium enema remains the primary examination for these lesions. A typical appearance of a primary or metastatic carcinoma is a 'bull's-eye' pattern consisting of a concentric or eccentric sonolucent rim (25). When the metastases are small they will appear lucent throughout (Fig. F.6). Ultrasonography may be useful in an evaluation of sarcomata, where a large mass with sonographic signs of central necrosis suggests the possibility of a sarcoma (26).

Ultrasonography has a limited role in study of the colitides. It can help identify and define the extent of an abdominal or pelvic abscess or phlegmon due to diverticulitis, appendicitis, enterocolitis, or prior surgery (27) (Fig. F.7). An intra-abdominal abscess can be suggested by ultrasound because of its characteristic appearance (28). The abscess appears as a sonolucent mass with thick irregular margins. Usually there are few internal echoes although an occasional abscess may appear solid. Acoustic shadowing is an inconsistent finding. A gas-containing abscess may appear as an echo dense mass because of a 'microbubble' effect (28). Ultrasonography can define ascites, hematoma and lymphoceles (29).

Ultrasonography should be performed prior to any barium studies, because residual barium sulfate produces artifacts. Residual barium of several days duration, however, may allow ultrasound to penetrate through the barium-filled mass (30). Although residual gas within the bowel does render ultrasonography of the colon and the adjacent structures difficult if not impossible, colon distension with a water enema can outline the colon and distinguish it from adjacent structures (31). Pretreatment with simethicone also appears to improve visualization (32).

The application of ultrasound to the colon is still in its infancy. Hopefully, newer advances and new modalities will enhance the ultrasonographic study of bowel disease.

References

1. Robbins AH, Pugatch RD, Gerzof SG, Faling LJ, Johnson WC, Spira R, Gale DR: Further observations on the medical efficacy of computed tomography of the chest and abdomen. Radiology 137:719–725, 1980.
2. Tada S, Fukuda K, Aoyagi Y, Harada J: CT of abdominal malignancies: dynamic approach. AJR 135:455–461, 1980.
3. Kressel HY, Callan PW, Montagne J-P, Korobkin M, Goldberg HI, Moss AA, Arger PH, Margulis AR: Computed tomographic evaluation of disorders affecting the alimentary tract. Radiology 129:451–455, 1978.
4. Hildell J, Nyman U, Rosengren J-E: Lymphoma of the colon detected by CT. Br J Radiol 54:144–146, 1981.
5. Zaunbauer W, Haertel M, Fuchs WA: Computed tomography in carcinoma of the rectum. Gastrointest Radiol 6:79–84, 1981.

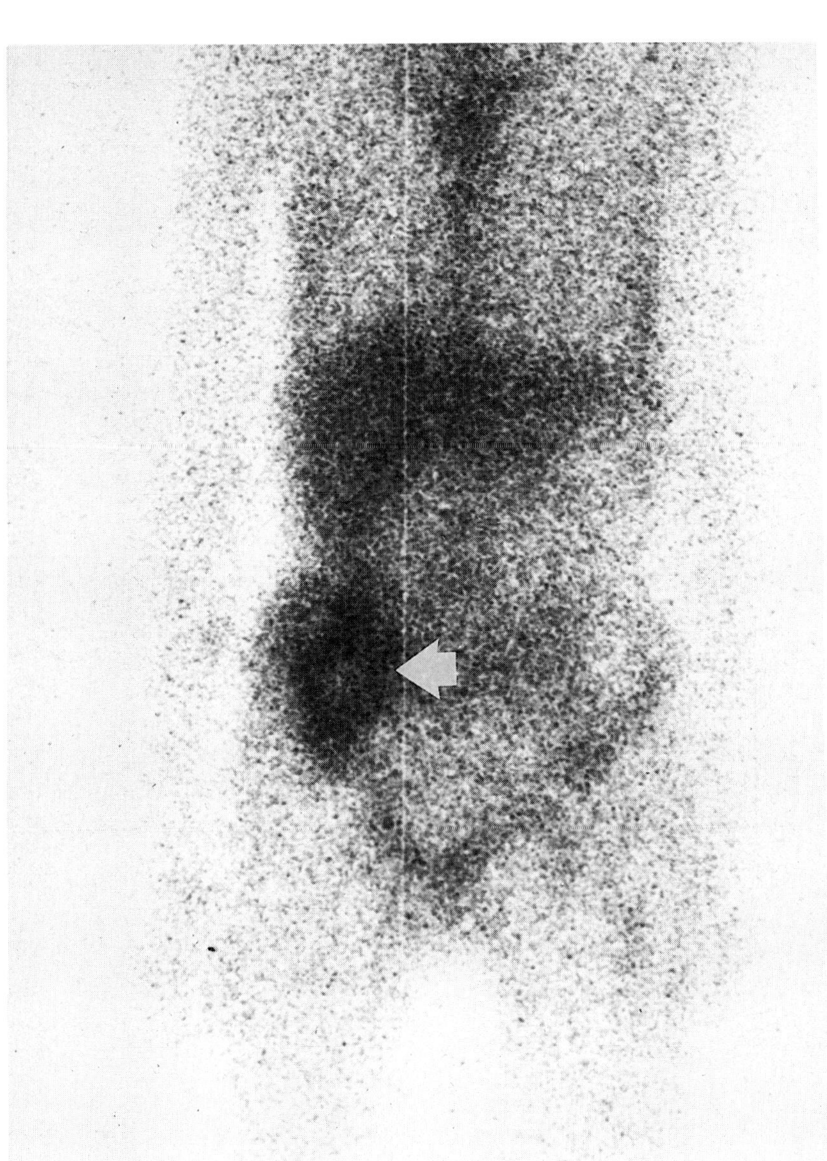

Fig. F.4. Anterior scan 24 hours after ^{67}Ga shows marked uptake in the right lower quadrant (arrowhead). A peri-appendiceal abscess was subsequently drained. (Courtesy of Dr. R. O'Mara, University of Rochester Medical Center.)

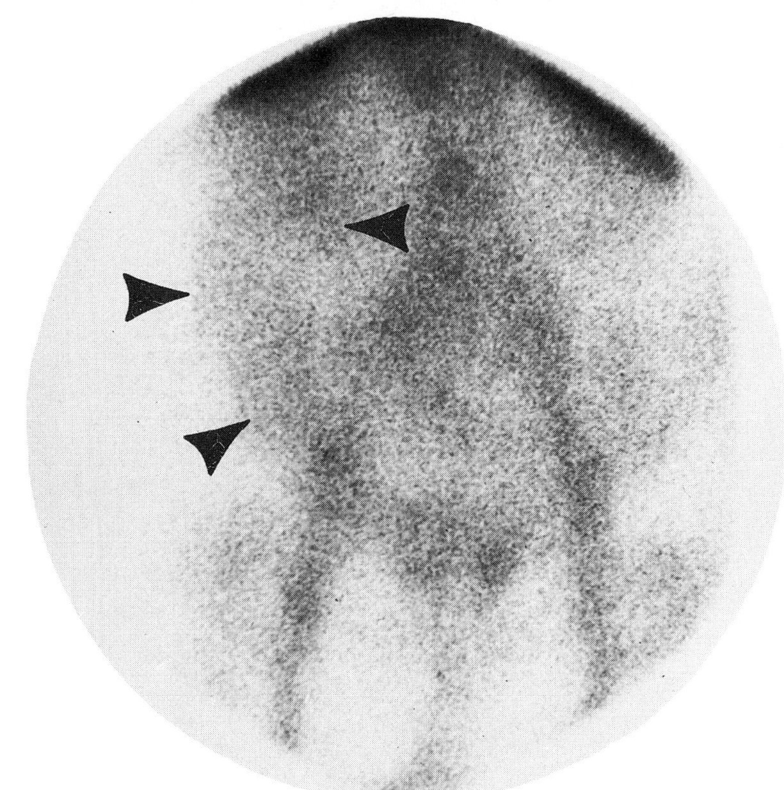

Fig. F.5. ^{99m}Tc-SC scan one hour after injection. Considerable uptake is present in the right colon (arrowheads). The patient presented with Henoch-Schoenlein purpura. (Courtesy of Dr. R. O'Mara, University of Rochester Medical Center.)

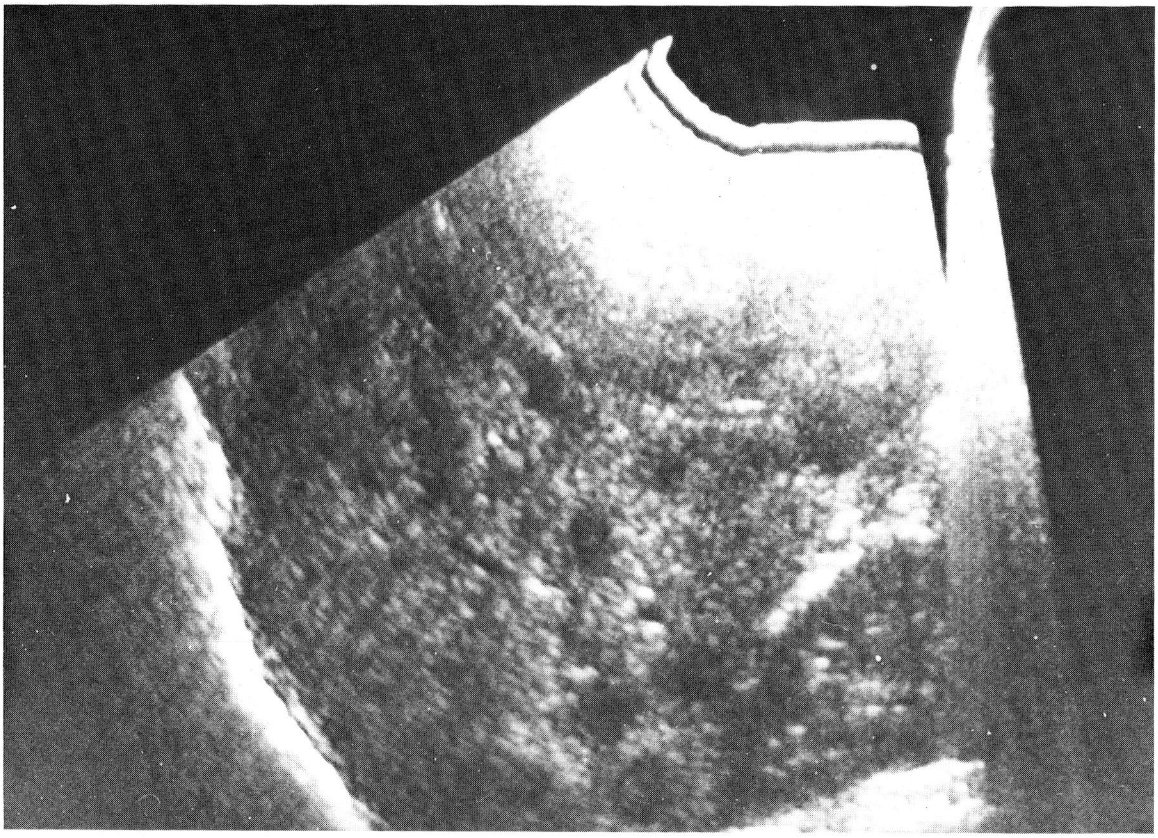

Fig. F.6. Multiple liver metastases present as lucent inhomogeneous masses scattered throughout the liver. (Courtesy of Dr. P. Wilson, University of Rochester Medical Center.)

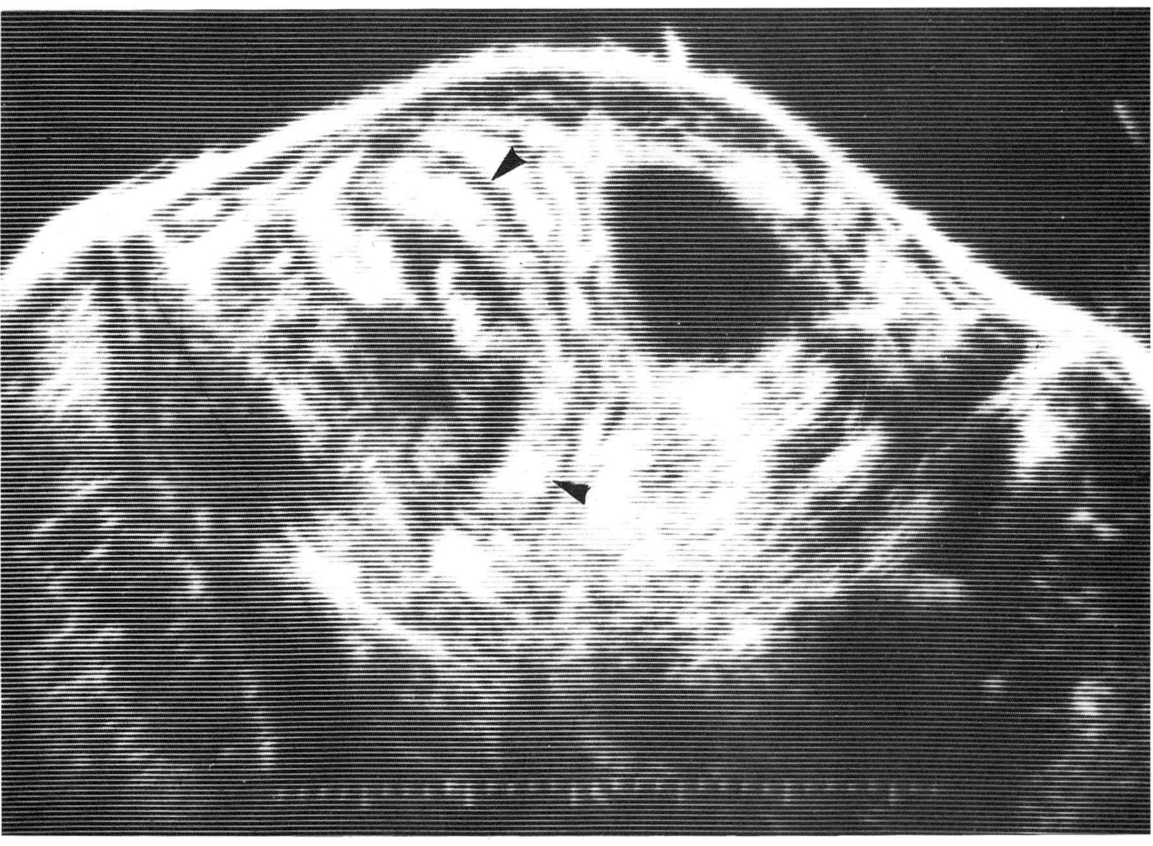

Fig. F.7. Right lower quadrant phlegmon in a patient with regional enteritis involving the distal ileum (arrowheads). Several loops of bowel are caught in the phlegmon. (Courtesy of Dr. P. Wilson, University of Rochester Medical Center.)

6. Dixon AK, Fry IK, Morson BC, Nicholls RJ, Mason AY: Pre-operative computed tomography of carcinoma of the rectum. Br J Radiol 54:655–659, 1981.
7. Hatfield KD, Segal SD, Tait K: Barium sulfate for abdominal computer assisted tomography. J Comput Assist Tomogr 4:570, 1980.
8. Zelas P, Haaga JR, Lavery IC, Fazio VW: The diagnosis by percutaneous biopsy with computed tomography of a recurrence of carcinoma of the rectum in the pelvis. Surg Gynecol Obstet 151:525–527, 1980.
9. Thoeni RF, Moss AA, Schnyder P, Margulis AR: Detection and staging of primary rectal and rectosigmoid cancer by computed tomography. Radiology 141:135–138, 1981.
10. Mayes GB, Zornoza J: Computed tomography of colon carcinoma. AJR 135:43–46, 1980.
11. Edwards CL, Hayes RL: Tumor scanning with ^{67}Ga citrate. J Nucl Med 10:103–105, 1969.
12. Hayes RL, Edwards CL: New applications of tumour-localizing radiopharmaceuticals. In: Medical Radioisotope Scintigraphy, Vol II, pp 531–552, International Atomic Energy Agency, Vienna, 1973.
13. Nash AG, Dance DR, McCready VR, Griffiths JD: Uptake of gallium-67 in colonic and rectal tumours. Br Med J 3:508–510, 1972.
14. Jones B, Abbruzzese AA, Hill TC, Adelstein SJ: Gallium-67-citrate scintigraphy in ulcerative colitis. Gastrointest Radiol 5:267–272, 1980.
15. Barry JW, Engle CV: Detection of hemorrhage in a patient with cecal varices using ^{99m}Tc-sulfur colloid. Radiology 129:489–490, 1978.
16. Alavi A, Dann RW, Baum S, Biery DN: Scintigraphic detection of acute gastrointestinal bleeding. Radiology 124:753–756, 1977.
17. Alavi A, Ring EJ: Localization of gastrointestinal bleeding: superiority of ^{99m}Tc sulfur colloid compared with angiography. AJR 137:741–748, 1981.
18. Smith RK, Arterburn JG: The advantages of delayed imaging and radiographic correlation in scintigraphic localization of gastrointestinal bleeding. Radiology 139:471–472, 1981.
19. Winzelberg GG, Froelich JW, McKusick KA, Waltman AC, Greenfield AJ, Athanasoulis CA, Strauss HW: Radionuclide localization of lower gastrointestinal hemorrhage. Radiology 139:465–469, 1981.
20. Som P, Oster ZH, Atkins HL, Goldman AG, Sacker DF, Harold WH, Fairchild RG, Richards P, Brill AB: Detection of gastrointestinal blood loss with ^{99m}Tc-labeled heat-treated red blood cells. Radiology 138:207–209, 1981.
21. O'Mara RE: Nuclear techniques in skeletal neoplastic disease. In: Radiographic and Other Biophysical Methods in Tumor Diagnosis, pp 153–165. Clinical Conference on Cancer, 1973. Year Book Medical Publishers, Chicago, 1975.
22. Kremer H, Lohmoeller G, Zollner N: Primary ultrasonic detection of a double carcinoma of the colon. Radiology 124:481–482, 1977.

23. Peterson LR, Cooperberg PL: Ultrasound demonstration of lesions of the gastrointestinal tract. Gastrointest Radiol 3:303–306, 1978.
24. Gooding GAW: Ultrasonography of the cecum. Gastrointest Radiology 6:243–246, 1981.
25. Morgan CL, Trought WS, Oddson TA, Clark WM, Rice RP: Ultrasound patterns of disorders affecting the gastrointestinal tract. Radiology 135:129–135, 1980.
26. Bree RL, Green B: The gray scale sonographic appearance of intraabdominal mesenchymal sarcomas. Radiology 128:193–197, 1978.
27. Taylor KJW, Sullivan DC, Wasson JFMcI, Rosenfield AT: Ultrasound and gallium for the diagnosis of abdominal and pelvic abscesses. Gastrointest Radiol 3:281–286, 1978.
28. Kressel HY, Filly RA: Ultrasonographic appearance of gas-containing abscesses in the abdomen. AJR 130:71–73, 1978.
29. Doust BD, Thompson R: Ultrasonography of abdominal fluid collections. Gastrointest Radiol 3:273–279, 1978.
30. Sarti DA, Lazere A: Reexamination of the deleterious effects of gastrointestinal contrast material on abdominal echography. Radiology 126:231–232, 1978.
31. Rubin C, Kurtz AB, Goldberg BB: Water enema: a new ultrasound technique in defining pelvic anatomy. J Clin Ultrasound 6:28–33, 1978.
32. Sommer G, Filly RA, Laing FC: Use of simethicone as a patient preparation for abdominal sonography. Radiology 125:219–221, 1977.

I.2. THE DOUBLE-CONTRAST BARIUM ENEMA

I.2.A. Introduction

Since the initial description of a double-contrast barium enema by Fischer in 1923 (1), there have been numerous improvements in contrast media, equipment, technique, and interpretation. More recently Welin popularized the procedure (2). The examination can be performed in a single phase by simply instilling a barium sulfate suspension followed immediately by air. In the two-stage method, the colon is first filled with barium, the patient is then sent to the bathroom, and afterwards air is added to distend the barium-coated colon until a double-contrast effect has been achieved. We and others have modified the two-stage method into a single stage by filling the colon with barium to the splenic flexure, draining barium from the rectum, and finally adding enough air until the cecum is filled with both barium and air and the colon is distended.

The double-contrast method takes longer to perform than a single contrast enema. As a result, if the barium sulfate suspension being used has a tendency towards early flocculation, considerable artifacts can be produced. A disadvantage of the single stage method is that often barium pooling occurs throughout the colon and as a result multiple radiographs in different projections are necessary in order to obtain double-contrast views of the entire colon and rectum. We find that by limiting the amount of barium to 350–400 ml, the average double-contrast examination reveals less barium pooling and is less expensive than if larger amounts of contrast were to be used.

The barium enema remains the primary method of examining the colon and terminal ileum. Unfortunately, the barium enema is one of the most poorly performed and most misunderstood examinations in radiology. It is not unusual for the radiologist to obtain several radiographs of the barium filled colon and then conclude that no lesion is seen. At times, the radiologist tries to cover himself by stating in the consultation that the colon has been inadequately prepared, no *gross* abnormality is seen, or that there is excessive redundancy in the colon and thus cannot be evaluated completely (3). Many lesions are missed because of poor preparation, poor technique or inadequate attention to detail. With an adequate double-contrast barium enema the only errors should be errors of interpretation. Such purely perceptive errors were found to represent approximately 50% of all missed cancers (4). Ninety percent of the missed cancers were visible in retrospect. The most common perceptive error was failure to recognize the lesion, although it was seen in retrospect. The technical reasons for missing a cancer included excessive barium, poor distension, poor coating, wrong film exposure or too much ileal reflux obscuring a portion of the colon (4). In only one out of the 31 patients where a cancer was missed did the examination appear adequate but the cancer could still not be seen even in retrospect. Thus, a technically adequate and well examined double-contrast barium enema is a very accurate examination.

A radiologist performs a disservice not only to the radiological profession, but also to the patient and the patient's referring physician when he or she performs a technically inadequate examination. A poor barium enema is worse than no barium enema at all! Quite often the referring physician translates the radiologist's report of 'no gross lesion' or 'poor preparation' to mean that the barium enema is normal, leading to a false sense of security both by the patient and the referring physician.

The radiologist *must* assume full responsibility for the preparation, performance, and interpretation of barium enema examinations. No portion of this responsibility can be delegated to others. Likewise, we insist that no patient leave until all of the radiographs are reviewed by the radiologists involved in the study and a diagnosis is made. If there is any suspicion or an area is incompletely visualized, the radiologist can take additional radiographs to either confirm or exclude a lesion.

Some physicians have raised the objection that a double-contrast barium enema leads to more patient discomfort, extra time, and can miss lesions (5). Most of these objections can be countered by using a barium sulfate preparation which coats the mucosa readily and does not flocculate, proper patient preparation, films obtained in a rational sequence, and unraveling all of the loops of the colon. The double-contrast examination does take additional effort; however, the results are clearly worthwhile.

The indications for a barium enema are poorly defined. Some clinicians develop a keen sense for suspecting bowel disease. To the authors, one indication for a barium enema is a statement by a competent referring physician that 'I feel strongly that there is a lesion in the colon'. Generally, the physician is right. If barium enemas were to be performed *only* for significant indicators of disease (such as bleeding, palpable mass, etc.) it is estimated that only 13% of all examinations would be eliminated (6). Unfortunately, use of such well-defined criteria would also miss 10% of patients with disease (6).

References

1. Fischer AW: Über eine neue röntgenologische Untersuchungsmethode des Dickdarms: Kombination von Kontrasteinlauf und Luftaufblähung. Klin Wschr 2:1595–1598, 1923.
2. Welin S, Welin G: The Double Contrast Examination of the Colon. Experiences with the Welin Modification. Georg Thieme Verlag, Stuttgart, 1976.
3. Rogers CW: Radiology's stepchild — the colon. JAMA 216:1855–1856, 1971.
4. Kelvin Gardiner R, Vas W, Stevenson GW: Colorectal carcinoma missed on double contrast barium enema study: a problem in perception. AJR 137:307–313, 1981.
5. Pantone AM, Berlin L: Air-contrast examination of the colon. An entity of the past. Am J Dig Dis 12:110–112, 1967.
6. Gerson DE, Lewicki AM, McNeil BJ, Abrams HL, Korngold E: The barium enema: evidence for proper utilization. Radiology 130:297–301, 1979.

I.2.B. Equipment

a. Introduction

The vast majority of gastrointestinal radiography performed in the United States utilizes image intensified fluoroscopy with automatic collimation and either a small format camera or spot filming. Although direct viewing of a fluoroscopic screen, without image intensification, is used in some parts of the world, such an arrangement is rare in the United States. Whether one views the final images on a television monitor or a mirror system depends on the preferences of the radiologist and the type of practice. In a private group without a radiology residency, a mirror system probably would suffice. Most teaching programs use television monitoring, because then not only the instructor but also residents and other students can observe the fluoroscopic examination. In a resident teaching situation we have found it also useful to have an additional central television monitor outside of the fluoroscopy room, where the instructor can monitor the examinations being performed by a resident (Fig. B.1).

b. Room design

Although most installations are already designed and built and the radiologist has little choice about room size, a new installation requires careful and detailed planning to ensure that the gastrointestinal section is adequately designed for efficient operation. Ideally, the cassette pass boxes in the radiographic rooms should be located close to the darkroom, or an independent film loading system should be used. The film processor feeding from the darkroom should be located adjacent to the area where the examinations are being viewed and interpreted.

A typical layout which works reasonably well is known in Fig. B.2. Four fluoroscopic rooms feed a centrally located darkroom. A single film processor is adequate to handle the work load. The films are taken from the processor and placed on one of two adjacent viewing alternators. We have found that with 10 to 20 examinations each day, two alternators help reduce congestion and are a considerable convenience not only to the radiologists but also to the referring clinicians when they come to

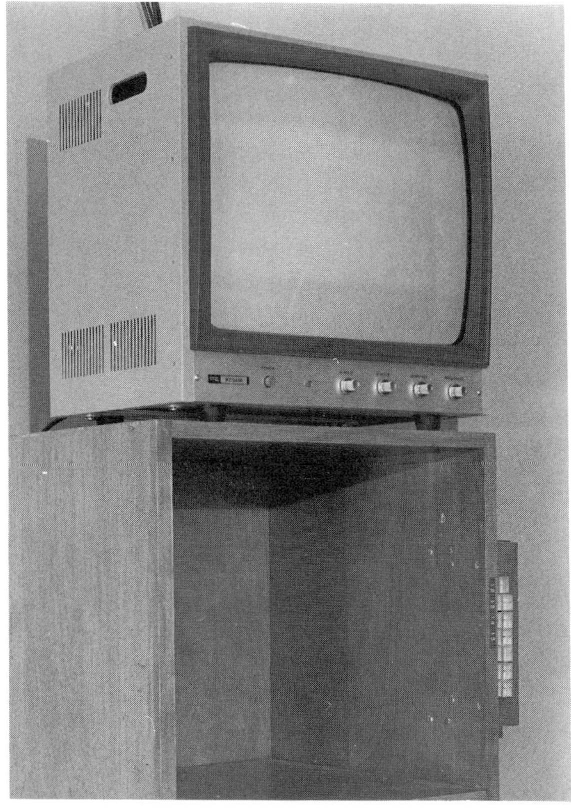

Fig. B.1. A TV monitor in a central reading area allows supervision of several ongoing examinations. Similarly, interested clinicians can observe an examination without having to be in the fluoroscopic room. Although a separate monitor for each fluoroscopic room would be ideal, a single monitor with facilities for switching between several rooms has been found adequate.

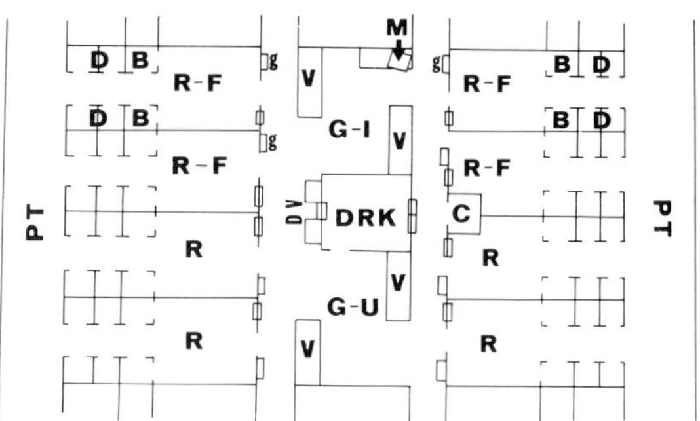

Fig. B.2. Schematic of typical gastrointestinal (G-I) and genitourological (G-U) radiology sections. There are four radiographic/fluoroscopic (R-F) rooms and four radiographic (R) rooms. Thus gastrointestinal radiography requiring no fluoroscopy can be performed in the adjacent radiographic rooms while genitourologic examinations requiring fluoroscopy are performed in the fluoroscopic rooms. One central darkroom (DRK) uses two developers (DV) and the radiographs are viewed on two multipanel viewers (V) in each area. Although ideally the inpatients can be separated from the outpatients by the two patient (PT) waiting areas, for most efficient use of the rooms some mixing of the two groups of patients is necessary. Each room has four dressing booths (D) and two bathrooms (B). The room generators (g) are placed in the technologist's corridors. Supervision of patient flow for both sections is from a separate control room (C). A TV monitor (M) is in the central reading area.

view examinations on their patients.

c. Generator

Theoretically one should use the largest size x-ray generator possible in order to decrease patient motion. Until several years ago such an approach was practical and was being used routinely. With the introduction of fast screen–film combinations, however, the choice of generator size has become more complex.

The primary purpose of a generator is to insure that a maximum number of x-ray photons are generated within a small area on the anode of the x-ray tube. The real limitation to the generator is the x-ray tube anode size. Over the years there have been numerous engineering advances in x-ray tube design, but probably only limited further improvement in the x-ray photon density will be achieved in the future. Currently even with extremely fast anode rotation, a portion of the anode glows red hot during x-ray production.

X-ray photons are produced at any one time from an area on the anode which is several mm^2. Such an x-ray focal spot size is still finite; because there is an inherent built-in magnification in most abdominal radiography, it is necessary that geometric unsharpness be present in the resultant image. This finite and often significant geometric unsharpness limits the clinically resolvable object size; in general, the *practical* limit of x-ray resolution in every day radiography is approximately two times the size of the effective anode focal spot (1).

If a radiologist is using a large x-ray focal spot together with a large capacity generator, the major image degradation is due to geometric unsharpness of the finite size x-ray focal spot (2). Such a system is not being used to its most optimum advantage and a judicious compromise, which is discussed below, can improve the system considerably.

If one installs par speed screens and uses XRP or similar speed film (referred to as a 1 × par speed system), then in many radiology departments a number of films produced each day will have significant motion unsharpness. In these installations motion unsharpness is by far the major factor in image degradation. As a rough guide, with a 1× par speed system one has to use at least a nominal focal spot of approximately 1.0 mm or greater in order to achieve the output necessary to minimize motion unsharpness (although the actual focal spot size of an x-ray tube is considerably greater than that of the 'nominal rating', most x-ray tubes sold are based on this nominal rating). A typical installation uses a 1.2 mm nominal focal spot x-ray tube and 100 kW generator. A three phase system, although more costly to install initially, helps decrease exposure time further (3). Such a system should be able to deliver 600 to 800 mA at approximately 100 to 140 kVp, resulting in a typical abdominal exposure time of several hundred milliseconds. Using such a system, if one simply substitutes a smaller focal spot the exposure times are prolonged and significant motion unsharpness will be present due to the inherent lower rating of the smaller focal spot. If, on the other hand, the generator and x-ray tube are kept the same but the par speed screen–film combination is changed to a 2× par speed system, there should be little visible motion unsharpness. Thus, motion unsharpness in high contrast high kVp gastrointestinal radiography can be reduced significantly with a 2× par speed screen–film combination if one uses a relatively 'large' focal spot.

We have found that an optimal practical system consists of a 0.6 mm nominal focal spot x-ray tube, approximately 400 mA generator output, and a 4× par speed screen–film system. Used on the average patient such a system tends to result in geometric unsharpness being essentially of equal magnitude to motion unsharpness.

A focal spot smaller than 0.6 mm, coupled with faster screen–film combinations, may offer significant improvement in image quality in the future. Due to the inherently high mottle characteristics of the extremely fast screen–film combinations, however, these systems so far have had rather limited acceptance by gastrointestinal radiologists. A small focal spot may make magnification radiography of the gastrointestinal tract feasible. Such a system might be combined either with very fast screen–film combinations or possibly some other new imaging modality.

d. Screen-film

The least image unsharpness results when motion unsharpness, geometric unsharpness, and screen–film unsharpness are of the same relative magnitude. To our knowledge, no conclusive study measuring all of these parameters has been evaluated in gastrointestinal radiology.

With the introduction of rare-earth screens, speeds of approximately 4 to 16 times par can be readily achieved. With these faster screens motion unsharpness is even less apparent and the major limitation in resolution is the finite size of the x-ray focal spot and its resultant geometric unsharpness.

We believe that there is no place today for a radiologist to install a par speed screen–film system in gastrointestinal radiography. Although a 2× par speed system does result in essentially eliminating most patient motion, a 4× par speed system is even better and appears to give optimum flexibility while minimizing geometric and motion unsharpness (2).

If a radiologist wants to increase the speed of a system, either a faster screen, a faster film, or a combination of the two can be used. If the radiologist simply substitutes a suitable faster film but keeps the same screens, the resultant faster system will exhibit an increase in radiographic mottle. If, on the other hand, the radiologist substitutes faster screens but keeps the same film, the resultant faster system will have more unsharpness and less radiographic mottle. The analogy does not apply if one substitutes screens containing a different phosphor material. In general, if a system has unacceptably high mottle, slower film but faster screens should be used. If, on the other hand, the system has unacceptable sharpness, then slower screens and a faster film should be substituted. Using an extreme example, there are very fast 16× par speed screen–film systems available. These systems have a very prominent and annoying mottle and are not sharp. The radiologist can arrive at a useful and workable system by simply lowering speed both with the screens and the film until both mottle and sharpness are acceptable. We have found that a 4× par system having relatively fast screens and slow film is generally acceptable to most of our radiologists. Substitution of a faster film simply results in an increased mottle and it is believed that some loss of diagnostic information is present, especially of low contrast objects. Undoubtedly the future introduction of new phosphor materials will result in faster and sharper systems.

e. Tables

Until recently, most x-ray manufacturers tended to recommend curved rather than flat table tops. The reason for such a recommendation was that with a curved table top the patient is located slightly closer to the undertable cassette and with overhead filming there is less geometric unsharpness. With a large x-ray focal spot the difference in geometric unsharpness between a curved and a flat table top can be considerable. Unfortunately, a curved table makes it considerably more difficult to move the patient. In addition, with the patient centered in the middle of a curved table, decubitus views cut off the recumbent portion of the colon and result in unacceptable studies.

If a 4 × par speed screen–film combination together with a small x-ray focal spot are used, geometric unsharpness due to patient positioning is considerably smaller. Currently we insist that all of the x-ray tables installed in our departments have flat surfaces. The Toshiba Gyroscope remote control table allows infinite remote positioning of the patient and is an exception to the rule of a flat table top.

The conversion of table tops and cassettes to carbon fiber material should be considered. Some equipment manufacturers are beginning to provide carbon fiber table tops as standard equipment. Carbon fiber interspace grids also appear promising.

Generally table tilting 90° one way and 15° the other way is adequate for gastrointestinal radiology. However, if myelography is also performed in the same room, then a 90° –90° tilting table should be installed.

Whether a front loading spot film device or a backloader is installed depends on the preference of the radiologist. Some manufacturers have provision for both. Many radiologists prefer a backloader since they believe that such a unit is faster and results in shorter examination times. Most technologists who have to load the cassettes, however, tend to have an intense dislike of backloaders. The eventual choice depends upon room size, location of the x-ray table, accessibility to the back of the table, and personal preference. Such units as the Gyroscope, with a multifilm magazine, eliminate most of these problems.

f. Grids

A considerable amount of scatter radiation is present at the relatively high kVp being used in abdominal radiography. Low ratio grids simply result in grey-appearing radiographs. Years ago low ratio grids were necessary to keep exposure times within tolerable limits. After the fast screen–film combinations became available, this problem no longer exists. We believe that at least 12:1 linear or 6:1 criss-cross grids should be installed. Whether one installs reciprocating or stationary grids is a personal preference. Current stationary grids, consisting of four line-pairs per millimeter, are barely visible on close inspection. The reciprocating mechanism may itself introduce artifacts, especially at the extremely short exposure times necessary when rare-earth screens are used. For overhead filming it is necessary to use a linear rather than a criss-cross grid, with the grid lines oriented parallel to the table; angled views of the sigmoid would not be possible with a criss-cross grid because of grid cut-off.

It should be emphasized that if the anode-to-film distance for a vertical x-ray beam routinely is 100 cm, then all angled views must be obtained with the x-ray tube 100 cm vertically above the plane of the film; this means that the anode-to-film distance for these angled views will be greater than 100 cm. Such an arrangement is necessary to prevent grid cut-off (4).

Because of the inherent design of the equipment in spot filming, the x-ray beam is always perpendicular to the cassette and one is not limited to a linear grid. With most conventional tables the tube-to-film distance can vary considerably during an examination and a high latitude grid is necessary. A 6:1 criss-cross grid gives the latitude of a 6:1 linear grid yet has the clean-up of a 12:1 linear grid. A 12:1 linear grid cannot be readily installed in the spot filming mechanism in most tables because of near-table and far-table grid cut-off. In most spot-filming installations the highest ratio grid which can be used practically is 8:1. An 8:1 criss-cross grid allows use of higher kVp than usual. A grid ratio limitation does not apply, of course, for those installations where the x-ray tube-to-film distance is always fixed. A typical such latter example is the Siemens Orbiscop, where the x-ray tube and the cassette holder are mechanically fixed at a 100 cm distance.

Although x-ray equipment manufacturers have been slow to adopt a criss-cross grid arrangement for the fluoroscopic spot film device, such a design has been described by us several years ago and is currently available from some manufacturers (5). We use a 6:1 linear grid for fluoroscopy and an additional 6:1 linear grid, oriented 90° to the first grid, moves into place (i.e. a 6:1 criss-cross grid) for spot filming (Fig. B.3).

With a large x-ray generator and fast screen–film combinations, the usual single 8:1 linear grid generally provided by some manufacturers for spot and camera filming should be replaced with a duplex grid as described above, or if such an installation is not feasible, a 6:1 fixed criss-cross grid should be installed. Although the resultant fluoroscopic image does suffer somewhat with a fixed criss-cross grid, there is marked improvement in the resultant film quality.

g. Lateral decubitus x-ray tube

We have found that the most valuable views in a barium enema are the two lateral decubitus views. Unfortunately, in the average radiology installation, the decubitus views are obtained simply by tilting the overhead tube horizontally, positioning an x-ray cassette alongside the patient, and manually lining up the geometry of the system. A low ratio grid must be used due to the 'portable' nature of such a system. The low ratio grid results in excessive scatter radiation, while a high ratio grid is difficult to use because of positioning latitude limitations. Due to the press of time in the middle of a barium enema examination the technologist tends not to measure the anode-to-film distance accurately. Such a portable approach prevents even a good technologist from routinely obtaining high quality radiographs (6). The resultant films tend to be grey, poorly centered, show grid cut-off, and exhibit considerable variation in density from one study to another.

The above limitations of decubitus filming can be overcome if a permanently mounted decubitus x-ray tube is installed. This tube, which can be a previously discarded tube from other use, is permanently mounted horizontally on the wall, with the x-ray beam centered slightly above the horizontal table. The alignment is such that a cassette holder mounted on the side of the table, opposite the x-ray tube, is always aligned with the tube whenever the table is horizontal. Depending upon the type of table, the cassette holder may be either permanently attached to the table or it may be removable between examinations (7) (Fig. B.4). The cassette holder can be readily constructed locally or it can be designed by the x-ray company installing the equipment. With the table horizontal, such an installation has a fixed alignment and the technologist can readily establish technique charts. Since the x-ray tube is fixed and cannot be angulated, criss-cross grids should be employed. We have found a 6:1 criss-cross grid satisfactory for most installation has a fixed alignment and the technologist can readily establish technique charts. Since

When patients lie on their side the soft tissue of the abdomen gravitates towards the dependent side. Most decubitus views thus result in an image where the upper part of the abdomen is overexposed and the lower part underexposed. A solution to this density variation is simply to add a compensating aluminum wedge filter into the x-ray beam. The filter consists of a triangular bar of aluminum permanently mounted on the front of the decubitus x-ray tube collimator. It covers the upper one-half of the x-ray beam (Fig. B.5). The thickest part of the triangular filter, measuring approximately 14 mm in thickness, is located so that an x-ray beam passing through this portion would be close to the upper edge of a horizontally placed 35 × 43 cm cassette. The thinnest part of the filter is located in the middle of the collimator so that an x-ray beam passing through this part would be in the middle of the x-ray film and close to the patient's midline. There is thus no filter for the bottom one-half of the radiograph. The filter starts at the patient's midline and increases linearly in thickness. Such a filter results in an essentially equal film density between the uppermost portion and the most dependent portion of the abdomen.

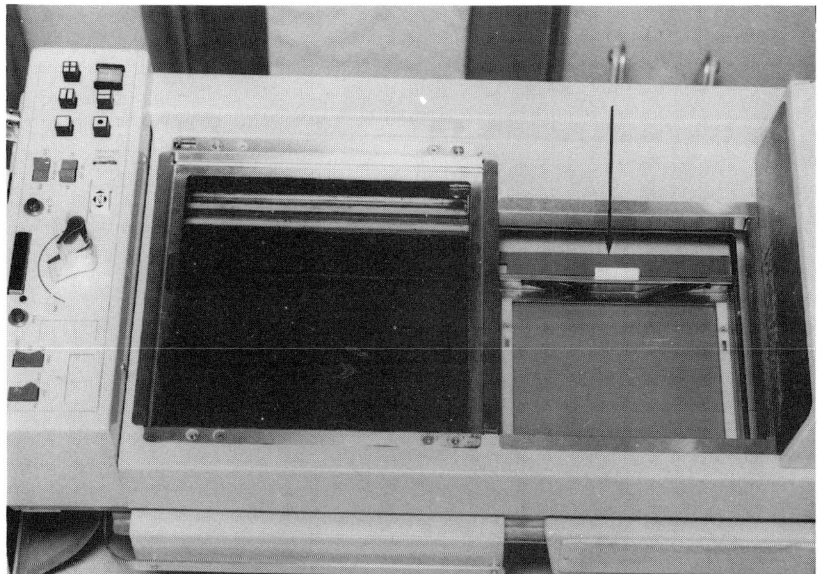

a

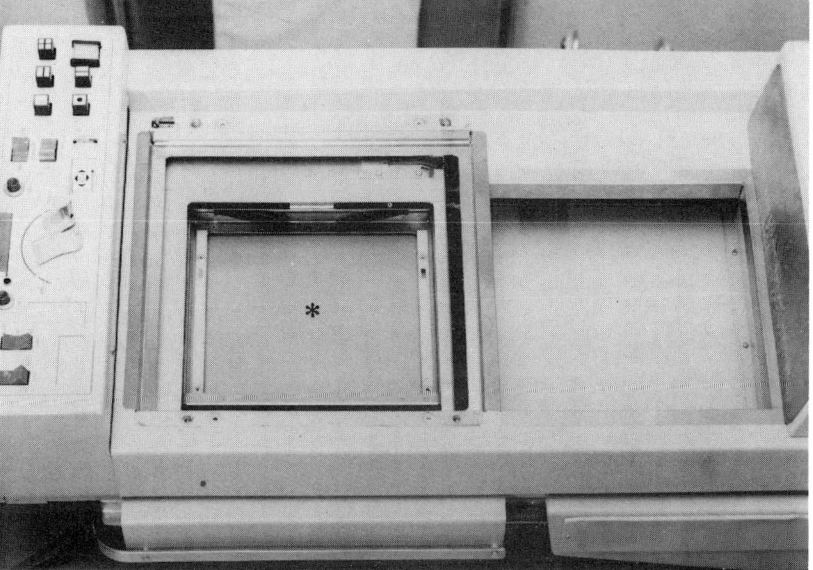

b

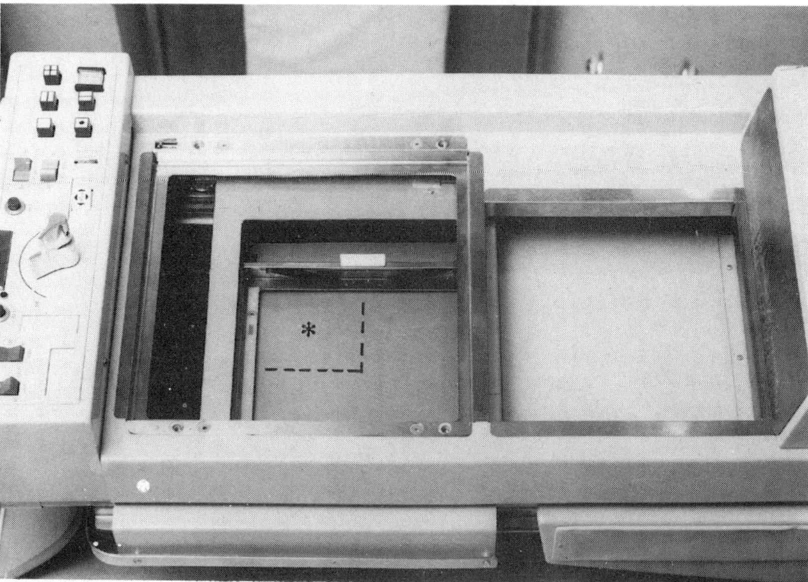

c

Fig. B.3. (a) The additional 6:1 linear grid (arrow) is mounted below the cassette carriage. The image intensifier has been removed for illustration purposes. (b) In a one-on-one filming mode, the grid and the cassette are both centered to the x-ray beam; the center of the x-ray beam is marked with a star. (c) In a four-on-one filming mode, the grid is still centered to the x-ray beam, while the cassette has been positioned in its appropriate place for the first exposure. The center of the collimated x-ray beam is marked with a star. (From Skucas and Gorski (5); copyright, RSNA 1975.)

h. X-ray recording cameras

There are 70, 90 and 105 mm recording cameras on the market. Some of the manufacturers claim that these cameras are equal, if not superior, to conventional filming.

We have compared the image quality of conventional spot filming with 105 mm filming (8). Using a par speed screen–film combination for conventional filming, it was found that the 105 mm system resulted in inferior images when cooperative patients were studied. It was only with uncooperative patients and relatively obese patients that the 105 mm films tended to be superior. With 4 × par speed screen–film systems it is expected that conventional spot filming is even more superior. Especially in the colon, we believe that the larger

a

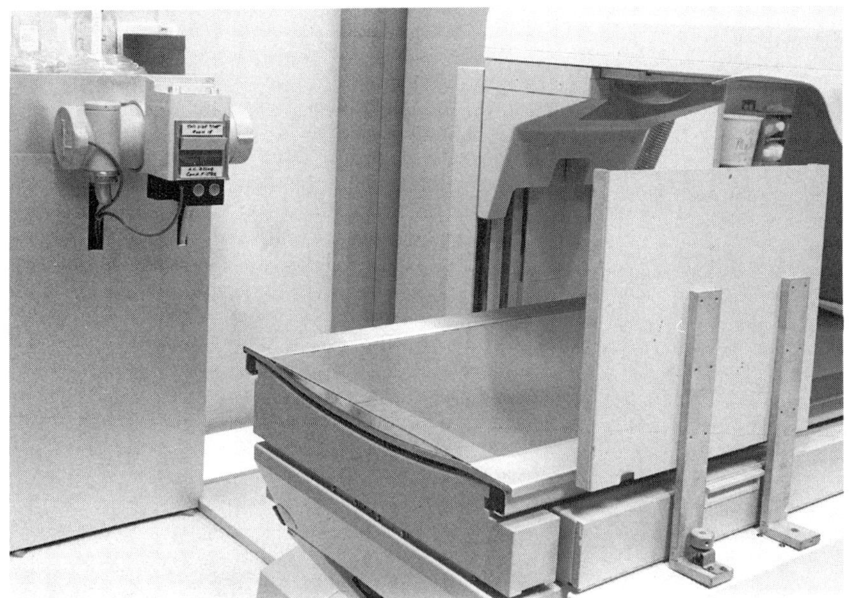

b

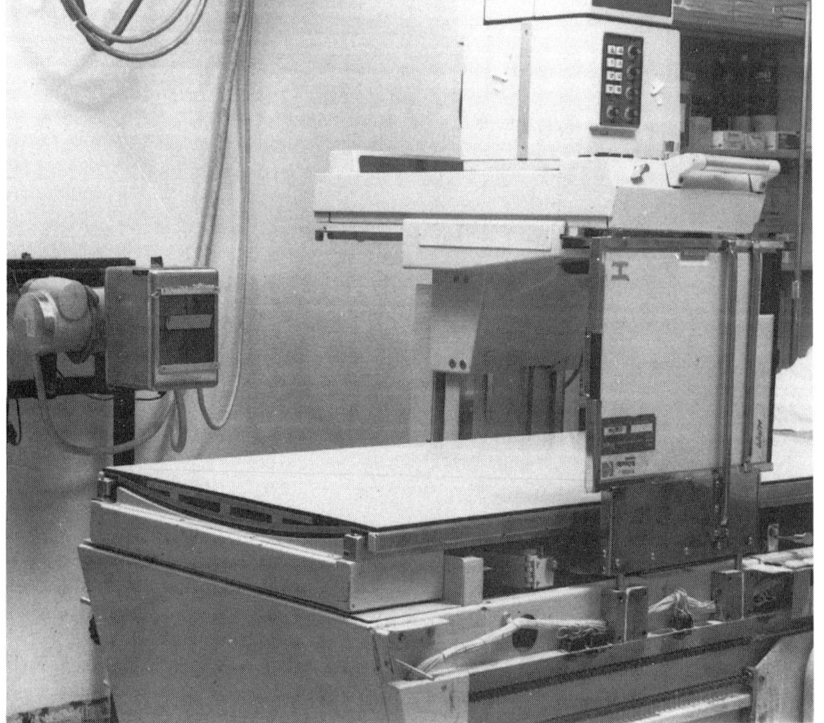

Fig. B.4. (a) Removable decubitus cassette holder. Pegs in the holder fit into holes drilled in the side of the x-ray table. The cassette holder is permanently aligned to the wall-mounted x-ray tube whenever the table is horizontal. The patient can be positioned by longitudinal movement of the table top. (b) Another type decubitus cassette holder. The table front cover has been removed to show method of attachment. (c) Still another type of cassette holder. When not used, the cassette holder pivots downward out of the way.

c

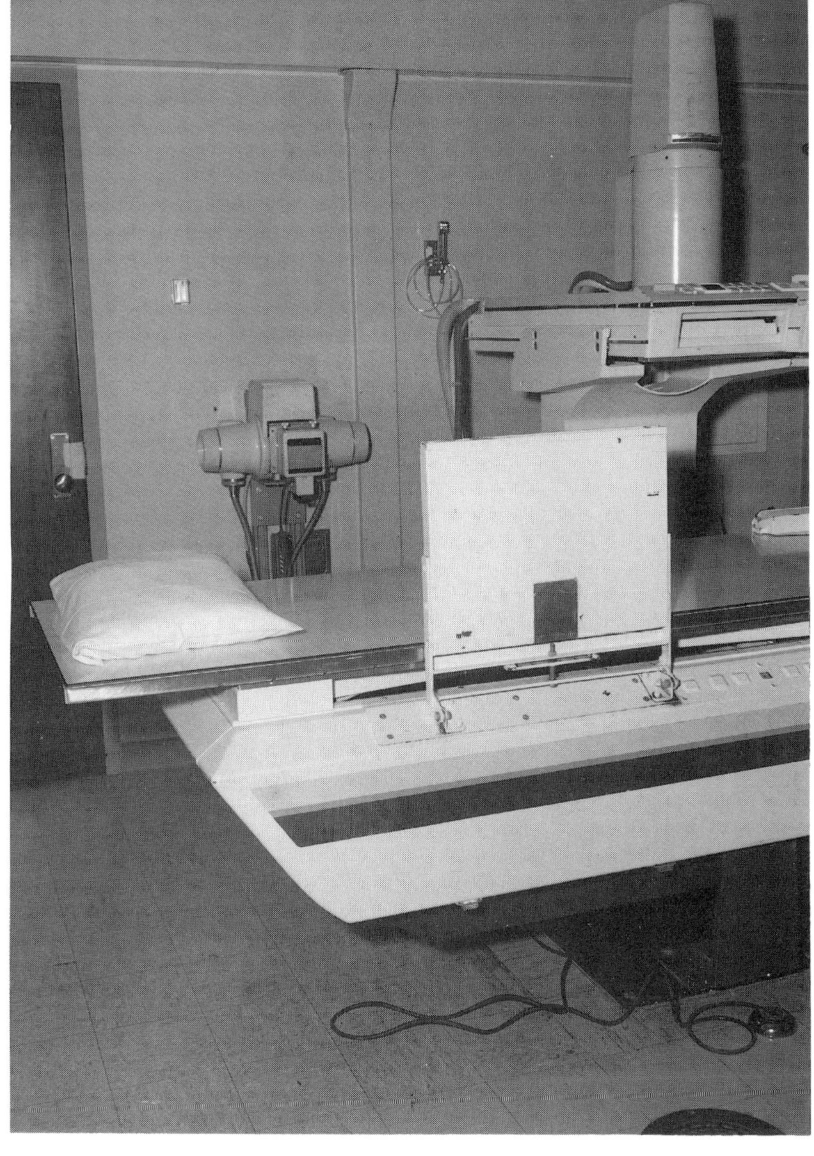

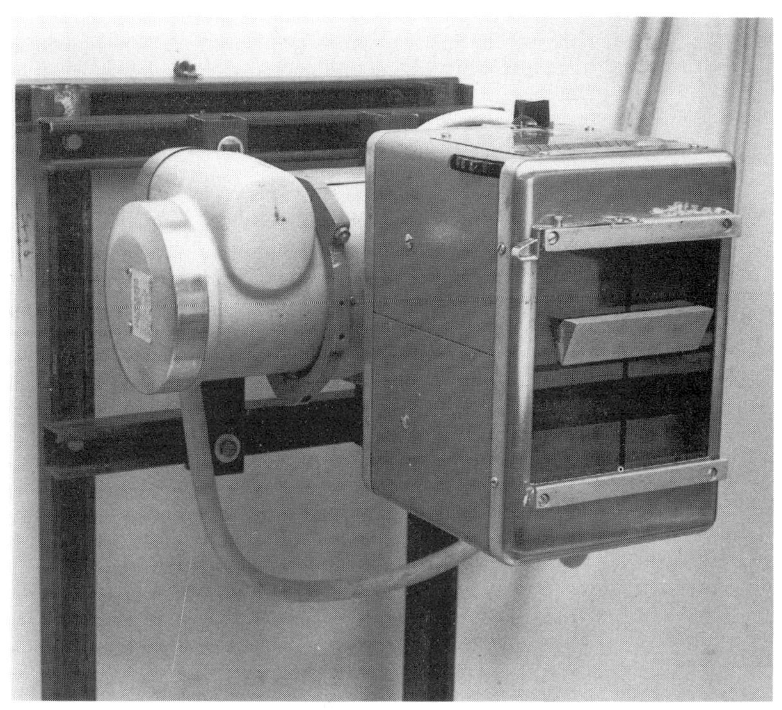

Fig. B.5. Compensating filter mounted on the collimator housing. The filter covers the upper half of an average size patient's body. The thickest portion of the filter covers the uppermost part of the abdomen, which generally has the least thickness. An over-all view of such an installation is shown in Fig. B.4.(b).

format spot films are an advantage. They not only give a better image quality but also provide easier orientation for the radiologist and the referring clinician who must view the resultant radiographs.

Cost can no longer be considered an advantage of 105 mm filming. With the worldwide increase in the cost of silver and the resultant film price fluctuations, the price of film for a single 105 mm exposure is in the same range as the price of film for a single four-on-one spot film exposure.

References

1. Brinker RA, Skucas J: Radiology Special Procedure Room, p. 104. University Park Press, Baltimore, 1973.
2. Skucas J, Gorski J: Application of modern intensifying screens in diagnostic radiology. Med Radiogr Photogr 56:25–36, 1980.
3. Brinker RA, Skucas J: Radiology Special Procedure Room, p. 31. University Park Press, Baltimore, 1973.
4. Christensen EE, Bull KW, Dowdey JE: Grid cutoff with oblique radiographic techniques. Radiology 111:473–474, 1974.
5. Skucas J, Gorski J: New grid design for a fluoroscopic spot film device. Radiology 115:732–733, 1975.
6. DeLacey G, Wignall B, Ambrose J, Baylis K, Bridges C: The double contrast barium enema: improvements to lateral decubitus views including the use of a wedge filter. Clin Radiol 29:197–199, 1978.
7. Miller RE: Simple apparatus for decubitus films with horizontal beam. Radiology 97:682–683, 1970.
8. Skucas J, Gorski J: Comparison of the image quality of 105 mm film with conventional film. Radiology 118:437–443, 1976.

I.2.C. Contrast agents

The type of barium sulfate suspension to be used depends on the type of examination performed and the patient's condition. With a single-contrast barium enema one uses a relatively low density (between 12 and 20% weight to volume) barium sulfate suspension. The aim is to achieve a 'see through' capability bu using a low density barium suspension (1). Ideally one would like to use an even lower density suspension; however, barium sulfate suspensions at low densities tend to settle out rather quickly and one may miss lesions located in the nondependent part of the colon. Unfortunately a low density barium suspension makes fluoroscopic visualization more difficult.

Several good commercial products are on the market designed for single-contrast barium enema examinations.

For double-contrast barium examinations the choice of contrast medium is more critical. A compromise of the various barium suspension characteristics is generally adopted. The barium sulfate suspension should have a relatively high density yet also have low viscosity. The resultant mucosal coating should be sufficiently thick to be readily visible on the radiographs and should form a uniform film on the mucosa without cracking or flaking, thus producing few artifacts. The barium sulfate should remain in suspension, without settling, for considerable periods of time. The final suspension should not foam in order to prevent confusing gas bubbles. Finally, the suspension must be nontoxic.

The same barium sulfate concentration cannot be used for both the double-contrast and the single-contrast barium enema. The double-contrast suspensions are considerably more dense and if used for a single-contrast examination would simply result in the entire colon lumen appearing completely white. Likewise, if the low-density barium used for single-contrast examinations is used for a double-contrast barium enema, the poor coating generally results in an inadequate examination (Fig. C.1).

The factors involved in the basic properties, processing conditions, mixing, testing, and resultant mucosal coating of various barium sulfate suspensions have been previously described by us (2).

Until several years ago, one had to buy barium sulfate in a dried powder form in bulk and mix the resultant suspension prior to use. Currently, several pharmaceutical companies have prepackaged products available specifically designed for double-contrast examination of the colon. Some of these products consist of dry barium sulfate powder in prepackaged enema bags and one needs only to add the required amount of water. This method is not quite accurate because the collapsible bags can be compressed and the liquid added may vary, even though the level is apparently the same.

The addition of arbitrary amounts of water introduces other variable factors to the prepackaged dry formulations. Water hardness, suspended impurities in the water, and soluble agents vary considerably from region to region (3). These factors all have a profound effect upon subsequent barium coating. Although the manufacturers caution that the enema bag should be shaken until all

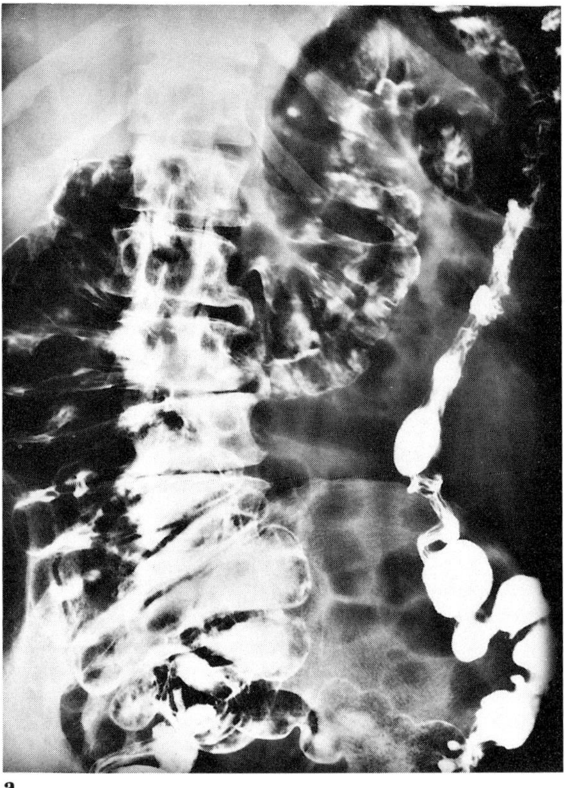

a

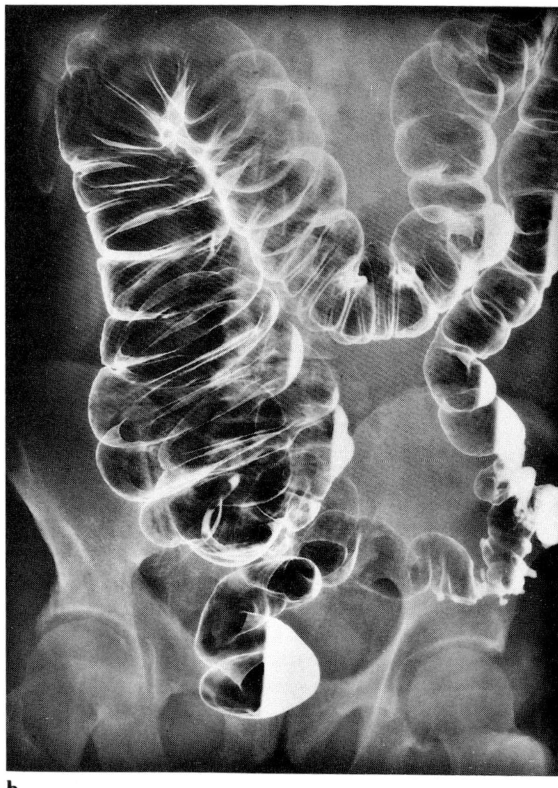

b

Fig. C.1. (a) A single-contrast barium enema was performed, the barium drained and air instilled. The low-density barium suspension resulted in very poor coating. (b) The patient underwent a double-contrast examination using the correct density barium suspension. Marked improvement in coating is evident.

of the barium sulfate is in suspension, full suspension is achieved only after prolonged and vigorous shaking and quite often this is not done. Whether the enema is performed immediately after mixing or whether the suspension is allowed to stand overnight will also influence the subsequent coating quality.

There can be variation in quality if one buys the barium sulfate as a dry powder in bulk containers, stores the containers for varying lengths of time and then subsequently mixes the suspension as needed. Extreme standardization is necessary and only a trial and error approach will give the radiologist the best coating properties possible. When preparing a suspension from the dry powder, one should measure the barium by weight and not by volume; in bulk storage, barium sulfate tends to settle and becomes more compact at the bottom of the container. As a result, an equal volume taken from the bottom will contain more barium sulfate than that taken from the top (4). Whether one mixes simply by shaking the bag, uses a large volume low speed blender (which are available in many hosital pharmacies), or uses a small volume high shear blender will also influence the resultant coating.

Almost all commercially available barium sulfate preparations have additives present which are adsorbed on the barium sulfate crystal surface. These additives are generally not listed on the container. A wide variety of such substances are used by the pharmaceutical manufacturers to influence the various coating properties of their suspensions (5). Some of these substances are organic, long molecular chains adherent to the barium sulfate crystals. The high speed blenders, in particular, tend to tear apart these long chains. A high speed blender can thus produce different coating properties depending on machine speed during blending and length of blending. In addition, some freshly suspended barium mixtures must be 'aged' for several days to achieve optimal coating. Obviously, standardization of the overall procedure is all-important to achieve reproducible results.

Other products are already in a liquid suspension

and one simply shakes the jug and pours the desired amount into an enema bag. The desired amount should be measured each time. We do this by pouring the suspension into a common glass household measuring cup that has a thin line marked with fingernail polish at the 350 ml level.

Theoretically, within this latter group, there should not be any variation in the coating properties of different batches, yet practically, one occasionally does encounter considerable variation. The storage conditions, especially if the product has been allowed to freeze, together with the length of time in storage, may influence resultant colon coating. These problems should be solved in the future by the pharmaceutical companies.

It is not unusual to see a drop of barium hanging from the superior surface of the colon (6). Such a barium stalactite can be readily identified on both vertical and horizontal x-ray beam radiography (Fig. C.2). The *en face* appearance is that of a dense and circular drop of barium. This phenomenon often is transient.

If the thickness of the barium coating is insufficient, generally a higher specific gravity or a more viscous product will improve coating, although a too viscous medium will flow poorly

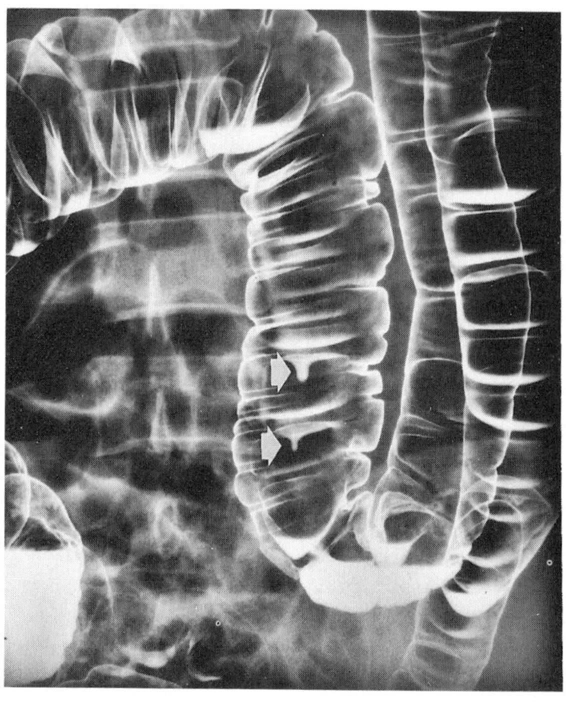

a

Fig. C.2. (b) Barium stalactite (arrowhead). In several seconds the drop of barium fell into the dependently located pool of barium. This phenomenon is due to the relatively high viscosity of the barium suspension. (a) Another patient with two barium stalactites (arrowheads).

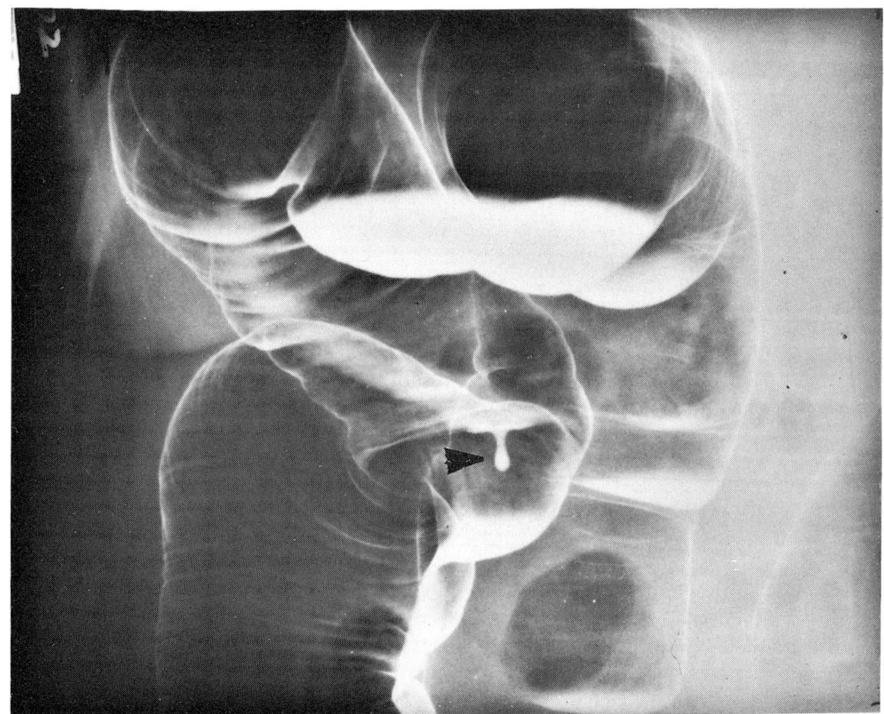

b

through the enema tubing and will tend to clump and coat unevenly (Fig. C.3). Precipitation and flaking of the barium coating can be due to several causes. Some commercial products are simply not suited for double-contrast colon use and result in gross artifacts; other products precipitate only if excess mucus is present. If there is an excessive delay between barium addition and subsequent radiography, most barium suspensions will begin to dry out and flake. Initially, the appearance is that of small filling defects mimicking lymphonodular hyperplasia (Fig. C.4). Eventually there is a coarse checkerboard pattern (Fig. C.5). Obviously, the better commercial products will not begin to flake within the length of time required to complete an examination, a factor of importance if delays are encountered because trainees are performing the examinations. The tendency to flake appears to be reduced if the barium sulfate contrast medium is suspended in 0.4% saline rather than water (7). If the saline is increased to 0.9% the result is a 'wet' coating and a loss in diagnostic quality (7).

As a general rule, it should be realized that the prepackaged liquid preparations cost the most per volume bought, but with accurate measurement may cost less per examination. Barium bought in bulk and mixed locally may appear to have the least cost per examination. However, the suspension that is discarded, the technician time for mixing, repeated examinations and poor results may easily make the dry type of barium the most expensive. We have reduced our barium costs for double-contrast examinations by accurate measurement of the final liquid suspensions and by using only 350 ml. However, the ultimate factor in the choice of product should be the resultant examination's quality and not the cost.

A clinical test evaluating several barium sulfate products and using independent observers has been published (8). Unfortunately, the field of barium sulfate formulation is changing constantly and each year one sees new and usually better products available.

Although a purely clinical comparison of several suspensions may not be a truly scientific study, the radiologist has few other options. A comparison of viscosity, density or even the coating properties on an artificial medium in vitro may bear little re-

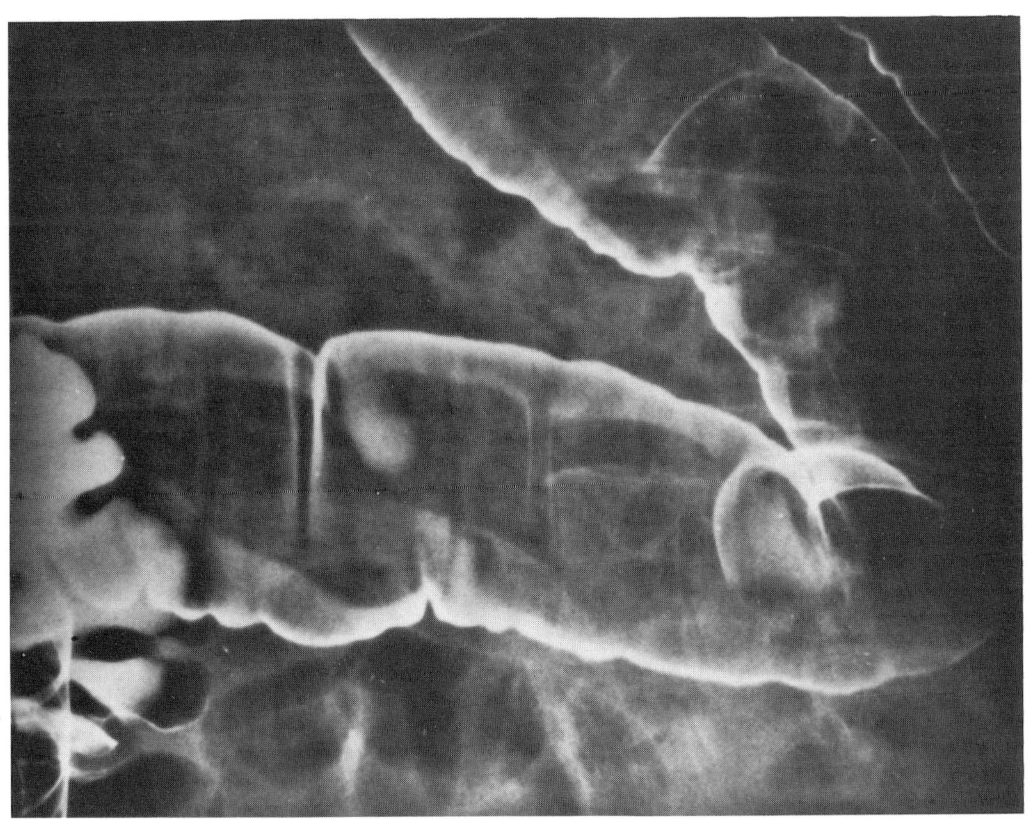

*Fig. C.3.***a.** For legend see page 44.

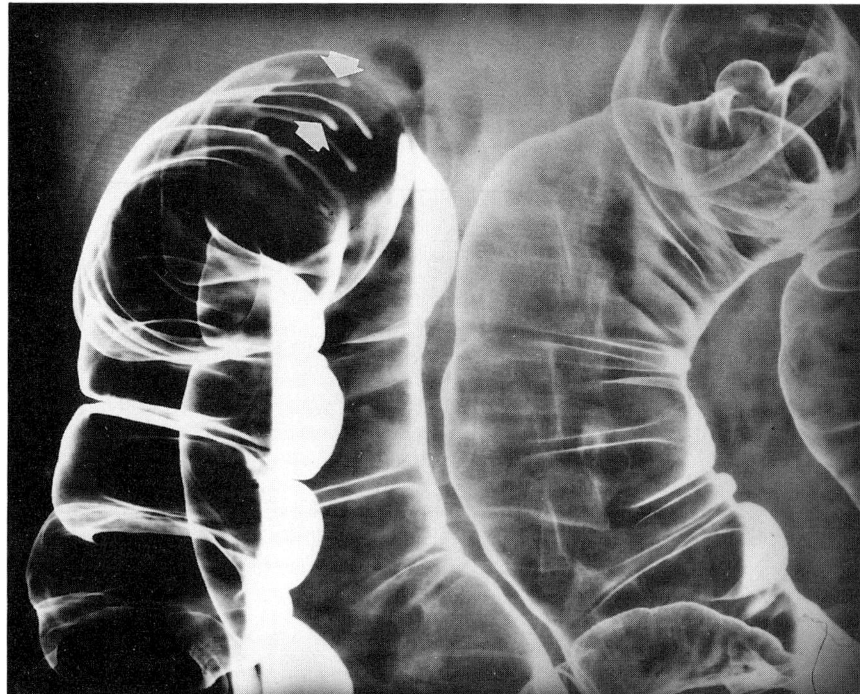

*Fig. C.3.***b.**

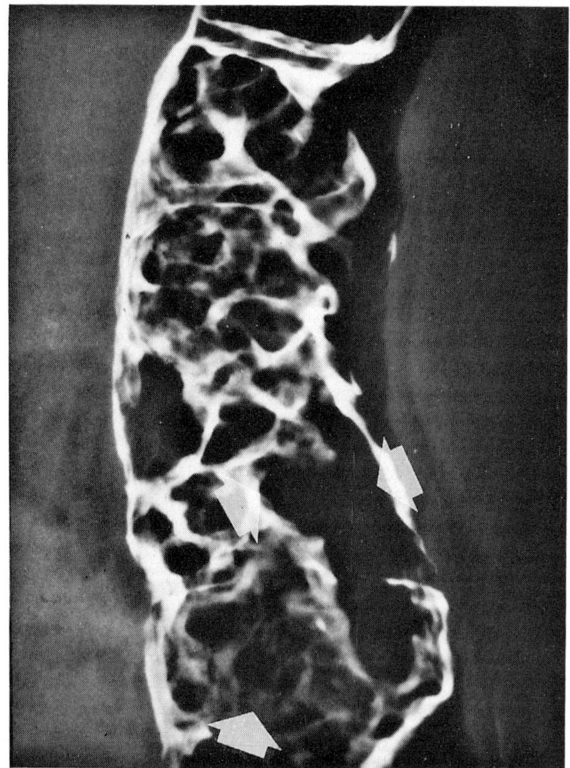

c

Fig. C.3. (a) Uneven barium coating. The barium thickness varies considerably from one area to another. (b) Flow artifacts. Several streaks of barium are flowing down the wall of the colon (arrowheads) In this case simply rotating the patient will result in a more homogeneous coating. (c) A too viscous barium suspension resulted in very poor coating. Portions of the colon were simply not coated at all (arrowheads). Rotating the patient will not result in any significant improvement.

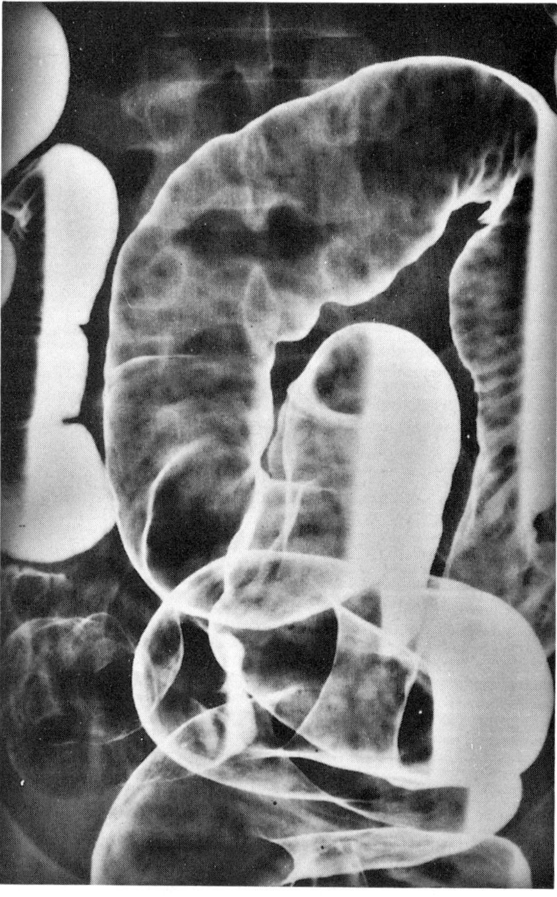

Fig. C.4. Early barium flaking. There is an uneven coating throughout the sigmoid colon.

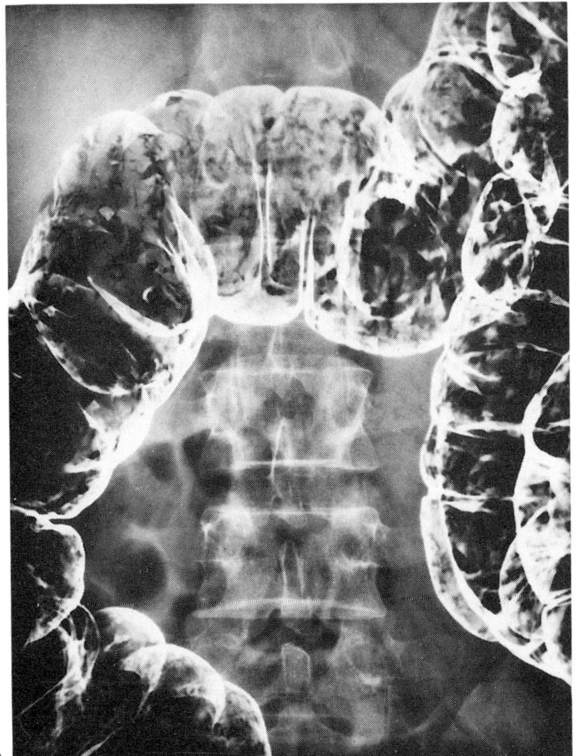

a

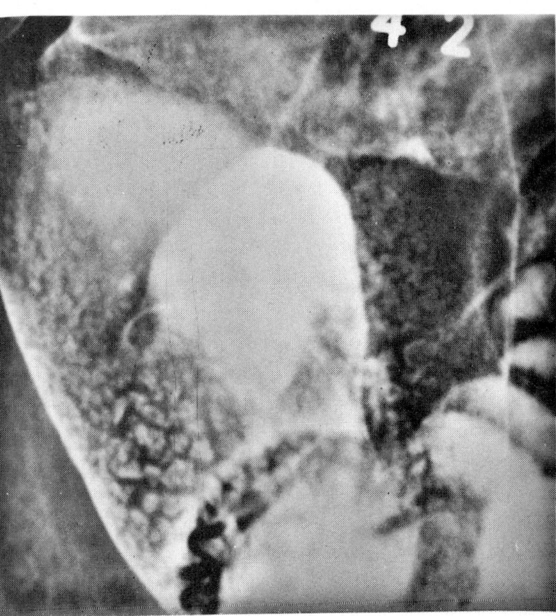

b

Fig. C.5. (a) Barium flaking. The barium suspension is beginning to dry out and results in a coarse pattern. (b) More severe flaking. Such a coating results in a useless study.

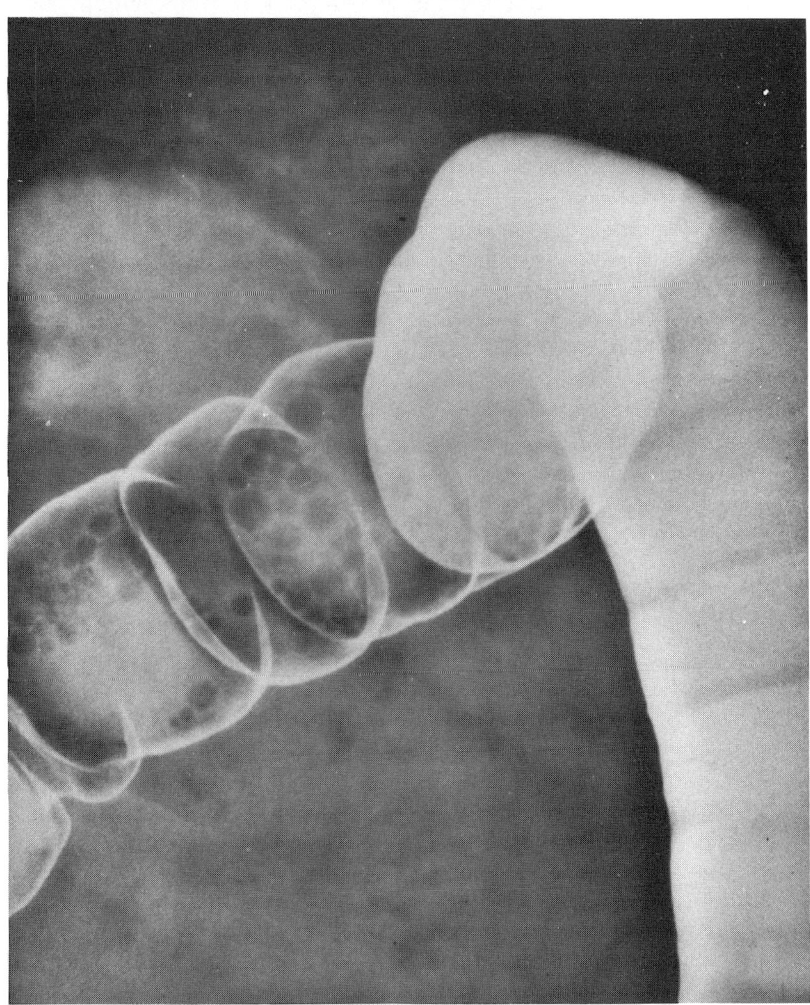

Fig. C.6. Air bubbles in transverse colon. Bubble artifacts can be readily eliminated by adding an anti-foam agent, such as simethicone, to the barium sulfate suspension.

semblance to coating of the colon in vivo. Likewise, animal models have not been fully acceptable, due primarily to variability of the results.

A radiologist beginning to perform double-contrast examinations should start with one of the currently available prepackaged liquid mixtures designed specifically for this purpose. A comparison of several such products should allow a determination of which one is optimal in that particular practice.

When comparing two different barium products, it is important that no change be made either in routine, equipment, or exposure factors. Since an examination may occasionally result in either exceptionally good or poor coating, numerous examinations are necessary to adequately compare any two products. If a particular mixture results in too many annoying air bubbles (Fig. C.6), 1–2 ml of simethicone added to the suspension usually eliminates the problem.

Overall, we find the liquid commercial barium media optimal. The processor of liquid media is forced to control these factors because an unsatisfactory product will be returned.

References

1. Potter RM: Dilute contrast media in diagnosis of lesions of the colon. Radiology 60:500–505, 1953.
2. Miller RE, Skucas J: Radiographic Contrast Agents. University Park Press, Baltimore, 1977.
3. Miller RE, Skucas J: Clinical application of barium sulfate. In: Miller RE, Skucas J (eds) Radiographic Contrast Agents, pp 94–96. University Park Press, Baltimore, 1977.
4. Ibid., p 69.
5. Ibid., pp 54–55
6. Op den Orth JO, Ploem S: The stalactite phenomenon in double contrast studies of the stomach. Radiology 117:523–525, 1975.
7. De Carvalho A, Madsen B: Prevention of crackle in double contrast examinations of the colon. Acta Radiol (Diagn.) 22:63–66, 1981.
8. Miller RE, Skucas J: Clinical application of barium sulfate. In: Miller RE, Skucas J (eds) Radiographic Contrast Agents, pp 143–167. University Park Press, Baltimore, 1977.

I.2.D. Patient preparation

a. Introduction

Regardless of what type of colon examination is being performed, adequate cleansing of the colon is by far *the* most important factor in achieving good results. The colon *must* be clean. Aside from the occasional examination where only the site of obstruction is being sought, a clean colon is necessary for an adequate examination. Fecal matter can simulate polyps and vice versa (Fig. D.1). In fact, a common reason for missing colon polyps is that the radiologist assumes that a defect seen on the barium enema represents retained stool (1, 2) (Fig. D.2). A dim view should be taken of an examination where there is retained fecal material and the radiologist leaves the choice of whether to repeat the examination or not up to the referring clinician.

Diet, various laxatives, and enemas are used for successful colon cleansing.

There are several philosophies to achieving a clean colon. Relatively weak cathartics can be given over a period of several days, or one can give strong cathartics and achieve a clean colon within 12–18 hours. Both methods are effective in their end result. In most patients we prefer a rather vigorous preparation over an 18 hour period.

Obviously, patients with suspected obstruction should not be given any laxatives. These patients are best studied unprepared with a single-contrast barium enema. Likewise, patients with colitis should receive cathartics tailored to the extent and severity of the disease. It should be apparent that any cathartic or enema is contraindicated for patients with toxic megacolon. Some advocate an 'instant' double-contrast barium enema on an unprepared colon in patients with inflammatory disease (3) (Fig. D.3). We have not had any experience with this method. We currently recommend that patients with active disease be studied after mild preparation of the colon. Those patients with significant diarrhea can generally be cleansed by a clear liquid diet followed by a cleansing enema while patients with less active disease may require a partial dose of a saline cathartic such as magnesium citrate. Patients with little or no active disease may require a full preparation. If in doubt, it is safer to give the patient a weaker preparation, and if the colon is not clean the next day, the preparation can be either repeated or increased in strength. Debilitated patients should likewise be evaluated and prepared individually.

Most cathartics do not work well if the patient is

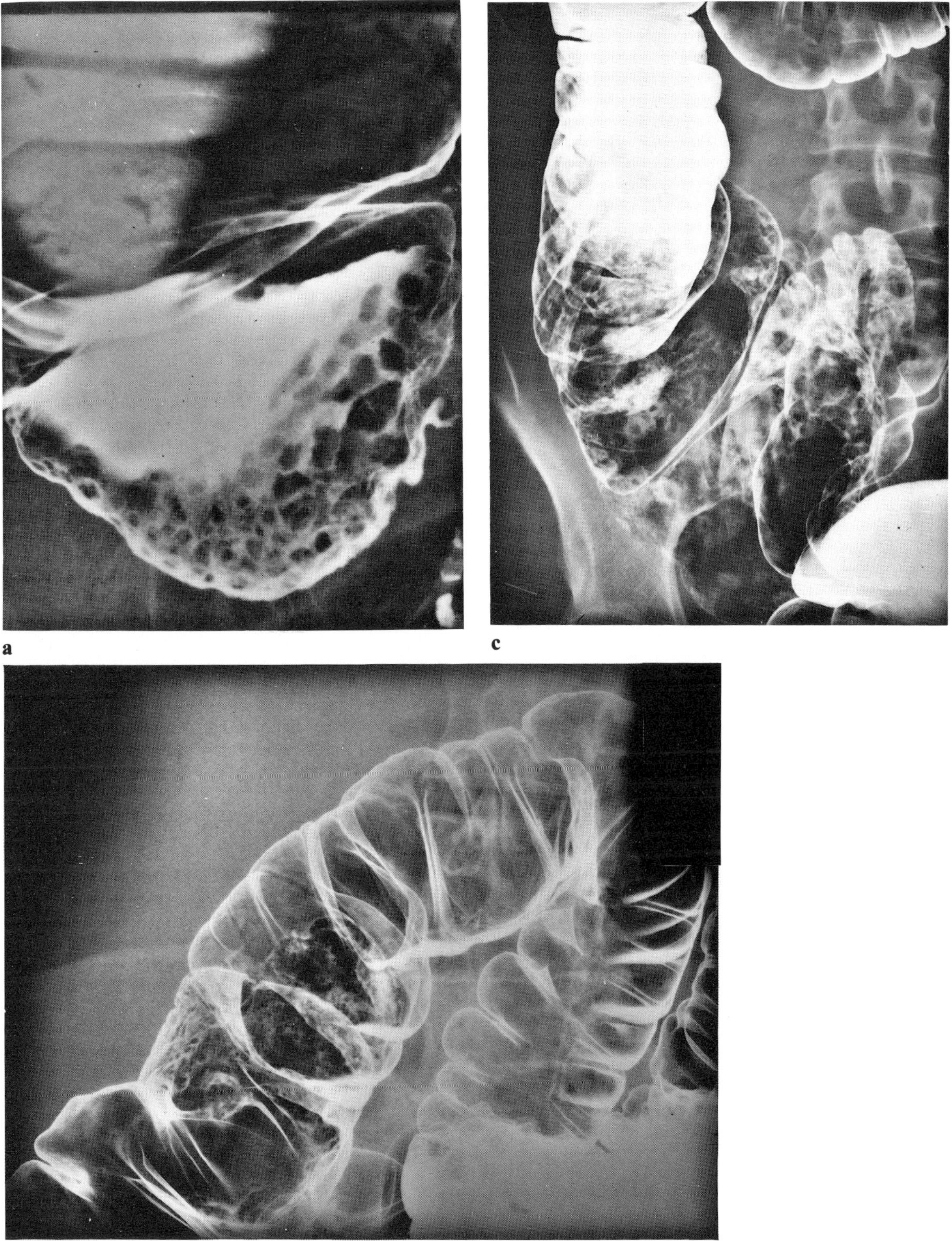

Fig. D.1. (a) Retained stool in cecum. Any of these defects could represent a neoplasm. Inflammatory polyps can also have a similar appearance. (b) An irregular mass is present in the ascending colon. Grossly it appears that the mass is infiltrating the colon wall. Subsequent examination showed this area to be normal. (c) Stool in right colon. A similar pattern was present during several examinations and the patient was initially diagnosed as having regional enteritis.

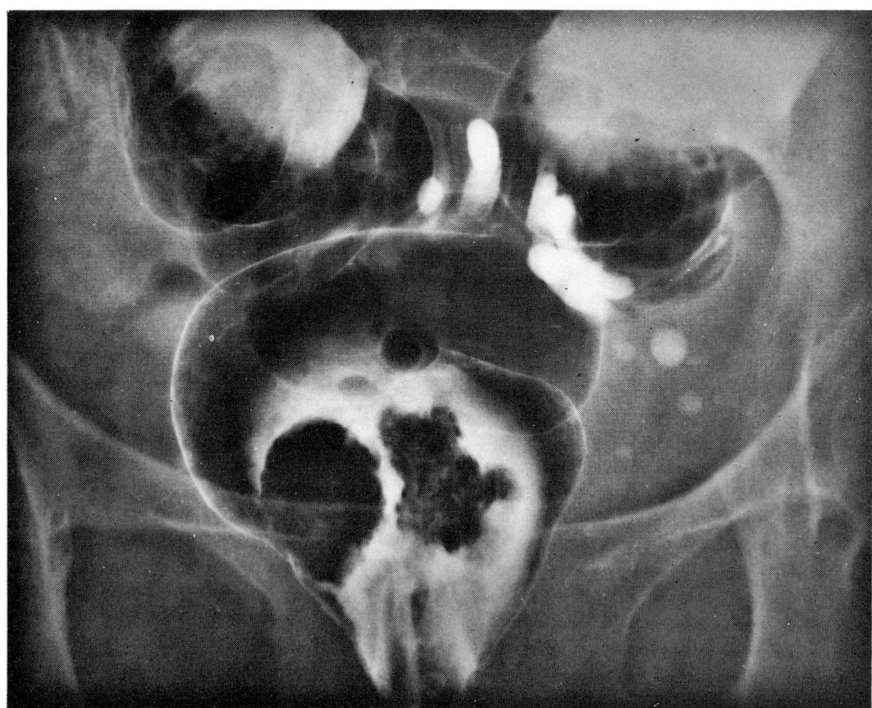

Fig. D.2. Stool appears to be present around the enema tip. In reality, this was an infiltrating rectal adenocarcinoma.

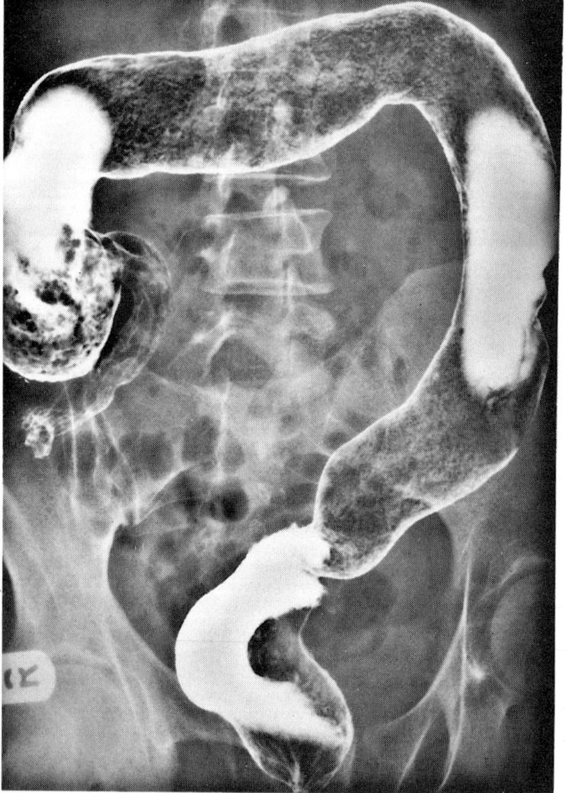

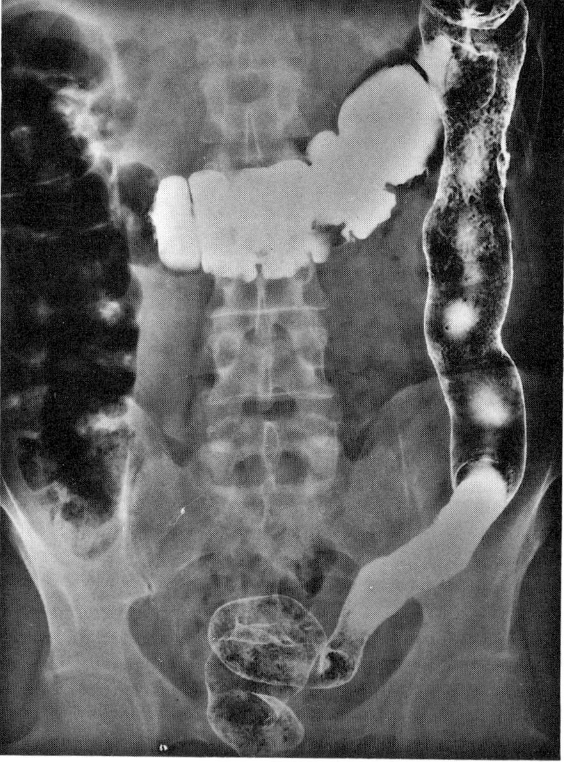

Fig. D.3. Two examples of an 'instant' double-contrast enema on an unprepared colon. (a) There is relatively good visualization of the extent of colitis. Retained stool is present in the cecum. (b) The right colon was not filled in this patient. Colitis involving the left colon is well seen. (Courtesy of Dr. Clyve Bartrum, St. Mark's Hospital, London, England.)

dehydrated and hydration plays a large part in cleaning out the colon (4–6) (Fig. D.4). The importance of adequate hydration cannot be overestimated; a glass of clear liquid every hour for four to six hours during the afternoon previous to the examination gives an optimal result. Although such a regimen works well in most patients, caution is urged in patients with congestive heart failure. With these patients it is probably best to proceed slowly.

The most common technique of cleansing the colon involves giving various laxatives orally together with oral fluids. Another method consists of numerous tap water enemas, although it is of little value in cleaning out the entire colon. A combination of hydration, oral laxatives, and total colonic lavage currently appears to be the optimum method in achieving a clean colon (6). A further aid in obtaining a clean colon is to give the patient written instructions on the importance of a clean colon and how to achieve it. We furnish printed instructions for the patient and supply copies to each nursing station and out-patient appointment area.

b. Laxatives

The normal intestine absorbs water and electrolytes, while laxatives induce the intestine to secrete water and electrolytes. The laxatives used to achieve a clean colon include stimulants, saline cathartics, lubricants, and wetting agents.

Stimulants include castor oil and the anthraquinone group of cathartics, such as senna fruit extract or cascara. The latter act primarily in the colon. Similarly, the stimulant bisacodyl induces peristalsis in the colon through the perisympathetic nervous system.

The saline cathartics are osmotically active; it has been postulated that these hypertonic solutions draw fluid into the intestine and the additional fluid then induces emptying, although this theory is controversial. Common agents in this group are magnesium citrate and magnesium sulfate.

Lubricants and wetting agents are rarely used by radiologists in cleansing the colon for radiography. They are sometimes useful after a barium enema to prevent constipation.

Bisacodyl. Some investigators use bisacodyl exclusively for cleansing the colon (7). Bisacodyl (Dulcolax) is a poorly absorbable stimulant laxative acting on both the distal small bowel and the colon (8). It increases colon tonicity and causes the colon to contract (7). The oral enteric coated tablets should be swallowed whole to prevent gastric irritation. Milk and antacids may release some of this laxative in the stomach, producing gastric irritation, and thus should be avoided. The suppositories should be used with care in patients with anal fistulas. Tenesmus may result with use of the suppository. After oral administration, evacuation occurs 6–10 hours later. The suppository generally is effective within one hour. The usual oral and suppository dose is 10 mg.

Cascara and senna agents. Both of these drugs contain anthraquinone derivatives and are stimulant laxatives acting directly on the colon. The action is induced both by the drug's glycoside reaching the colon directly through the intestine and through the bloodstream. These agents have

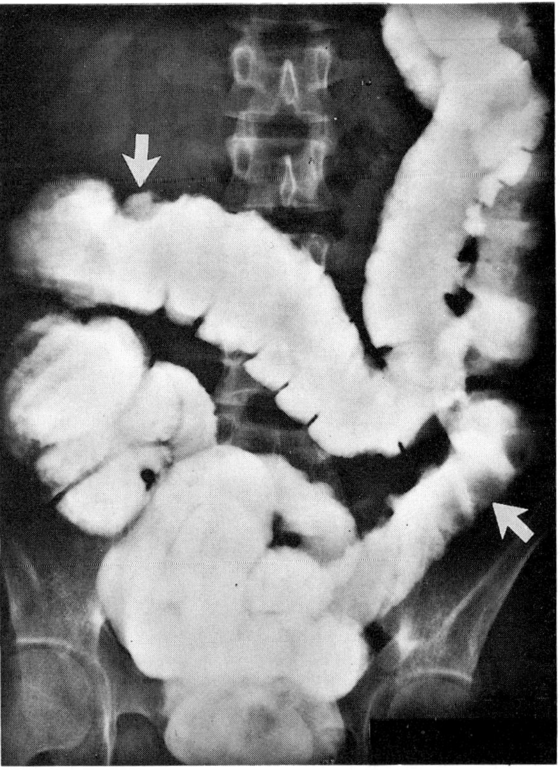

Fig. D.4. Although this patient did receive laxatives, he was not hydrated. Retained stool mimics sessile tumors or bowel wall edema (arrows). Subsequent examination revealed a normal colon.

little effect on the small bowel, with both agents inducing hyperperistalsis in the colon, presumably through Auerbach's plexus. Both cascara and senna result in brown or red urine, depending upon the degree of acidification.

Senna is more potent than cascara. Senna is available in tablets, syrup, granules and as a suppository. A standardized extract of senna fruit (X-Prep Liquid) is available in a 75 ml bottle; this particular preparation contains 50 g of sugar per bottle. The senna products appear to be more acceptable to patients than castor oil (9).

Castor oil. Castor oil is a strong agent which is classified as a stimulant. It is inactive in the stomach, but like any other fat it results in delayed gastric emptying and thus should be given on an empty stomach. Some castor oil is absorbed from the intestine. Other vegetable oils, such as olive oil, also exert a stimulant cathartic action. Castor oil in the small bowel liberates ricinoleic acid, which apparently inhibits fluid reabsorption and results in excessive intraluminal fluid. There is also a direct stimulating action on the smooth muscle of the bowel.

It is believed that the primary site of action for castor oil is in the distal small bowel and the proximal part of the colon. Its action is accentuated if the patient is well hydrated. An emulsion of castor oil (Neoloid) is available and is said to have better patient acceptance because of its better taste. The dosage of the emulsion must be doubled because of the large amount of water contained. The taste of castor oil is improved if it is chilled or taken with a cold carbonated beverage. The dose for an average patient is 60 ml.

Saline cathartics. There are several such products available on the market, with magnesium citrate and magnesium sulfate being typical examples. Diarrhea results several hours after ingestion. These cathartics should be used with caution in patients with renal failure, although normal kidneys can excrete the small amount absorbed. The magnesium salts should not be used with neomycin, while the laxative sodium salts should be used with caution in patients with cardiac failure.

The dose varies between the various saline cathartics. Magnesium citrate is effective in an oral dose of 150-200 ml.

c. Preparation for barium enema

Aside from certain emergency situations, the colon must be well prepared. Currently we are using a combination of diet, several laxatives and colon lavage to achieve relatively good results. Adequate oral and written instructions to the patient help increase patient compliance for the preparation (10).

We recommend a low residue diet or clear liquids for breakfast and lunch on the day prior to the examination and follow this by two laxatives; we prefer 60 ml of castor oil at approximately 1 p.m., followed by 75 ml of liquid X-Prep at approximately 4 p.m. Because castor oil works primarily in the distal small bowel and the right side of the colon, while X-Prep acts in the distal portion of the colon, there is a synnergistic effect. In addition, during this time we also recommend large volumes of clear fluids orally. A 240 ml glass of clear liquid per hour for four to six hours seems to work well.

If the barium enema is to be performed the next morning, the patient should not take anything by mouth after midnight. Even coffee the morning of the examination may result in sufficient spillage from the ilium into the right side of the colon to render the subsequent examination uninterpretable. Such heightened postprandial activity is due to an ileocolic reflex (11).

When the patient presents for the barium enema examination the next morning, a 2000 ml tap water enema should be given at least 30 minutes prior to the barium enema. A one hour delay is even better. The above regimen should be satisfactory in the majority of patients.

Those patients who cannot tolerate castor oil can substitute 300 ml of magnesium citrate orally. All of the laxatives are better accepted by the patient if they are ingested cold.

In our experience, castor oil alone, combined with a cleansing enema, does not clean out the colon well. Some radiologists have had satisfactory results with castor oil and a clear liquid diet for 24–28 hours (12). Others have found bisacodyl and magnesium citrate superior to castor oil and phosphate enema (13). One investigator found that bisacodyl by itself produced adequate results (14). Another study comparing three different bowel cleansing regimens, consisting of a) magnesium citrate and senna extract, b) magnesium citrate and castor oil, and c) castor oil and senna extract found that the regimen consisting of magnesium citrate and senna extract yielded the best overall results (15). The combination of magnesium citrate and castor oil was least effective in bowel cleansing. Yet this study in geriatric patients yielded acceptable results in only 65% of the patients and the authors subsequently tried a two day preparation. Bowel preparation with oral senna extract (X-Prep) resulted in better diagnostic quality than oral mannitol, although mannitol is considered a stronger purgative (16).

The colon can be cleansed by giving relatively mild cathartics for 2–3 days, together with a liquid diet, followed by colonic lavage. It is our contention, however, that a single concentrated preparation the afternoon before the barium enema examination is better accepted by the average patient than a milder preparation extended over several days. In addition, by giving laxatives in the afternoon rather than in the evening, the colon is essentially clean late in the evening and most patients can obtain a night's rest prior to the barium enema. Undoubtedly many other regimens in cleansing the colon are being used. If any method does clean out the colon in 95% of the patients, it is worthwhile keeping and is useful; otherwise, a better method must be sought.

If the colon must be cleansed fast, whole gut irrigation should be considered (17). The entire gastrointestinal tract can be flushed out readily within a matter of hours. The irrigant solution recommended for total bowel lavage has a pH between 8.2 and 8.3 and contains 6.14 g of sodium chloride, 0.75 g of potassium chloride, 2.94 g of sodium bicarbonate and distilled water to a total volume of 1000 ml. The patient can either drink the solution or it can be instilled via a gastric tube. Although initially we waited 30–40 minutes between the bowel lavage and subsequent examination, a longer period of time would allow even more fluid to drain out, resulting in even less retained colonic fluid. However, since the conventional colon preparation as used by us has been found to be successful in 95% of the patient population (18), we do not believe nor do we advocate that whole gut irrigation should supplant conventional methods. In fact, because of retained fluid whole gut irrigation is not as effective as a conventional cathartic method in preparing the colon for double-contrast barium enema examinations (19) (Fig. D.5).

There is always a possibility of overloading the body circulatory system with fluids ingested orally. Thus, until more data are available, patients who have a compromised cardiovascular status or impaired renal function probably should not be studied with a total whole-gut irrigation method. Obviously, neither this method nor any other cleansing method should be used in patients with suspected bowel obstruction.

Both bisacodyl (7) and bisacodyl tannex (Clysodrast) (12) have been advocated as being useful when added to the tap water enema. Since these agents are stimulants, they should help stimulate colon evacuation. We performed a double-blind study by adding Clysodrast to the tap water enema in 50 patients and using a control group of 50 patients with no added Clysodrast. The resultant barium

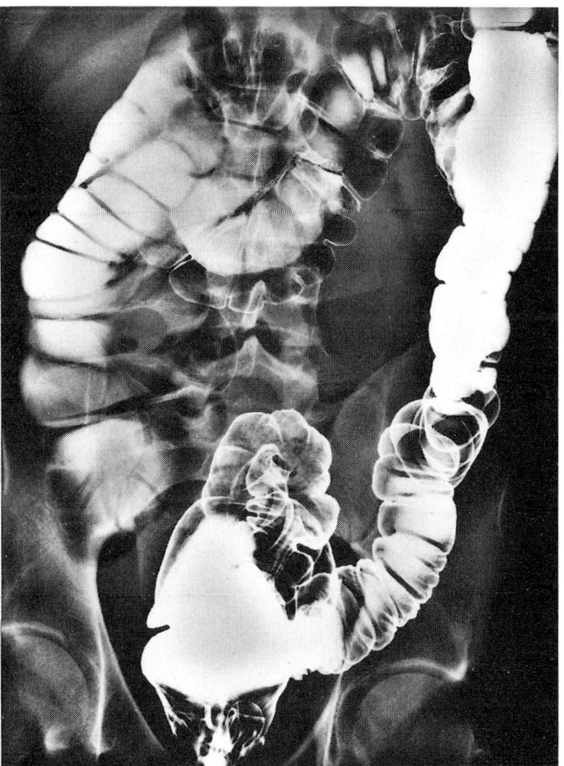

Fig. D.5. Whole gut irrigation was performed on this volunteer. The patient was on a regular diet and had not received any laxatives. This barium enema was performed two hours after the start of the gut irrigation. Although the colon has been cleansed of stool, liquid from the irrigation limits visualization of the right colon.

enema examinations were then analyzed for the amount of stool retained, the amount of colon spasm present, and the degree of mucosal visualization. Overall, the addition of Clysodrast to the cleansing enema did not improve the results (the only exception was in the 60 to 70 age group; however, there were only nine patients within this age group and the results may not be significant). As a result, we are not routinely using Clysodrast in the tap water enema, although some investigators still use it (12).

The chief action of tannic acid is that of a deflocculating agent. Its effect is more apparent with USP barium sulfate and least effective with the modern barium sulfate products designed specially for double-contrast examination (20). Thus, tannic acid can make a *poor* barium product look better.

d. Cleansing enema

The cleansing enema, whose function is misunderstood and which is generally relegated to the newest, lowest and most uninformed employee on the hospital staff, is one of the most important tools of cleaning out the colon. Not only do nurses' aides not know how to give colon lavage but the same also applies to interns, residents and practicing physicians. Because the cleansing enema is part of the barium enema, the radiologist involved in the procedure must take full responsibility. The importance of this cleansing enema cannot be overemphasized (21–24). One *must* have a clean colon. Because the referring physician is not performing the examination, he cannot be held responsible for cleaning the colon. Delegation of this responsibility is not possible and the radiologist must assume complete responsibility for the entire examination. He should determine whether the patient needs a barium enema in the first place. As a general rule, if the patient's symptoms indicate the need for a barium enema, then the patient should certainly have a cleansing enema. Obviously, if there is suspected perforation of the colon a completely different approach should be taken.

If there are poor results the radiologist must take appropriate action with the person giving the tap water enema. If the tap water enema is left to the hospital nursing staff, the radiologist performing the barium enema has little control over the end result. Ideally, the tap water enema should be performed in the Radiology Department under the direct supervision of the radiologist. Such an approach requires a considerable commitment of time, space and personnel both by radiology and by the hospital administration.

Although the cleansing enema can be given on the x-ray table, it is more convenient and does not tie up an x-ray room if a special room equipped with a toilet is used. A dressing booth adjacent to a toilet can be converted into an enema room. The room dimensions must be sufficient to accept a small stretcher or table. A foam rubber mattress can be cut to shape and covered with a plastic sheet.

One viable alternative is to have an aide, directly under the radiologist's supervision, perform the cleansing enema on hospitalized patients directly in the patient's room. The radiologist still maintains control over the procedure; in addition, an adequate time interval between the cleansing enema and subsequent barium enema can be ensured.

An order of 'enemas until clear' is worthless. This simply means that a tap water enema is given with water running in and out until the rectum is clear. Although such a procedure may clean a rectum, it is worthless as far as cleaning out the right side of the colon is concerned. In addition, the rectum is sore and irritable. One carefully performed tap water enema is a far better approach. In the average adult, a tap water enema of approximately 2000 ml at or near body temperature should be given (6). The tap water enema bag should not be raised suddenly above the patient; the height of the water in the enema bag above the level of the patient's colon will determine the resultant pressure with which water will flow. The patient is more comfortable if the enema bag is first at the level of the patient and then is gradually raised until a one meter level is achieved. The enema bag should not be raised more than one meter above the patient. We start the tap water enema with the patient lying with the left side down. After approximately 500 ml of water has been instilled, the patient is instructed to lie prone. This maneuver helps fill the transverse colon. After running in approximately 1 to 1.5 liters, the patient is turned onto the right side so gravity can aid in filling the cecum. At this point, the enema bag is raised to its full one meter height to help fill the cecum. Immediately after, the enema bag is lowered and as much fluid drained out as possible. The patient then goes to the toilet. At least 30 minutes should elapse before the barium enema is performed, and the patient encouraged to evacuate as much as possible, because retained fluid can dilute the barium suspensions and hide lesions. Some recommend an interval of several hours between the cleansing enema and the barium enema (25).

The average colon can hold a 2000 ml tap water enema readily. When the tap water enema is first started, the patient may have a feeling of fullness or cramps as soon as the rectum distends. Deep breathing provides subjective relief. If the patient is having discomfort, the enema tubing should *not* be clamped, but rather the enema bag should be lowered to the level of the patient. Closing of the enema tubing during a period of spasm will simply increase intracolonic pressure (26), the patient will experience pain and may not be able to retain the enema. When the spasm clears, the enema bag can again gradually be raised up to a maximum of 1 m above the colon.

A tap water enema is not without complication. Most solutions produce varying degrees of mucosal irritation. Water intoxication is a real problem in the very young and very old. The dilutional hyponatremia may result in weakness, shock, convulsions, or coma. Patients with megacolon can have prolonged water retention with resultant increased absorption. Potassium is lost during a tap water enema and hypokalemia may result, especially in patients taking antihypertensive or diuretic agents who already have decreased potassium levels. Excess fluid retention may worsen congestive heart failure. Fortunately, complications are rare in the average patient.

Some patients with steatorrhea may have a radiographic colon appearance similar to that seen in inflammatory bowel disease, even after a conventional bowel preparation. It is believed that this irregular appearance is due to 'fat encrustation' due to excessive fat in the stool (27). Generally, further preparation reveals the true nature of the condition.

References

1. Eyler WR: Colon preparation. In: Detection of Colon Lesions, p 108. 1st Standardization Conference, 1969. American College of Radiology, Chicago, 1973.
2. Saunders CG, MacEwen DW: Delay in diagnosis of colonic cancer — a continuing challenge. Radiology 101:207–208, 1971.
3. Thomas BM: The instant enema in inflammatory disease of the colon. Clin Radiol 30:165–173, 1979.
4. Barner MR: How to get a clean colon — with less effort. Radiology 91:948–949, 1968.
5. Irwin GAL, Shields JE, Wolff W: Clearer roentgenographic visualization of the colon. A study of a conveniently packaged kit for preparing the colon, and its effect on electrolyte balance. Gastroenterology 67:47–50, 1974.
6. Miller RE: The cleansing enema. Radiology 117:483–485, 1975.
7. Cobben JJ: The use of bisacodyl and the application of molecularly dispersed bisacodyl (dissolved in polyethylene glycol) in the cleansing enema and in the radiological contrast medium in the examination of the colon. Medicamundi 13:76–88, 1969.
8. Donowitz M: Current concepts of laxative action: mechanisms by which laxatives increase stool water. J Clin Gastroenterol 1:77–84, 1979.
9. Cargill A, Hately W: Preparation of the colon prior to radiology — a comparison of the effectiveness of castor oil, Dulcodos and X-Prep liquid. Br J Radiol 51:910–912, 1978.
10. Fordham SD: Increasing patient compliance in preparing for barium enema examination: AJR 133:913–915, 1979.
11. Misiewicz JJ: Colonic motility. Gut 16:311–314, 1975.
12. Laufer I: Double Contrast Gastrointestinal Radiology with Endoscopic Correlation, p 496. W.B. Saunders, Philadelphia, 1979.
13. Dodds WJ, Scanlon GT, Shaw DK, Stewart ET, Youker JE, Metter GE: An evaluation of colon cleansing regimens. AJR 128:57–59, 1977.
14. Kaye J, Solomon A, Lazar SJ: Further experience with dulcolax in barium enema examinations. Med Proc (Johannesb) 12:111–117, 1966.
15. Casal GL, Martinex LO, Silberman MR: Preparation of the colon for barium enema. Gastrointest Endosc 26 (Suppl.):5S–6S, 1980.
16. Lee JR, Hares MM, Keighley MRB: A randomised trial to investigate X-Prep, oral mannitol, and colonic washout for double-contrast barium enema. Clin Radiol 32:591–594, 1981.
17. Skucas J, Cutcliff W, Fischer HW: Whole-gut irrigation as a means of cleaning the colon. Radiology 121:303–305, 1976.
18. Miller RE: The clean colon. Gastroenterology 70:289–290, 1976.
19. Bakran A, Bradley JA, Bresnihan E, Lintott D, Simpkins KC, Goligher JC, Hill GL: Whole gut irrigation. An inadequate preparation for double contrast barium enema examination. Gastroenterology 73:28–30, 1977.
20. Miller RE, Skucas J: Radiographic Contrast Agents, pp 29–30. University Park Press, Baltimore, 1977.
21. Miller RE, Brahme F: The clarity of good technic. Am J Dig Dis 12:418–420, 1967.
22. Rogers CW: Radiology's stepchild — the colon. JAMA 216:1855–1856, 1971.
23. Welin S: Modern trends in diagnostic roentgenology of the colon. The Mackenzie Davidson Memorial Lecture. Br J Radiol 31:453–464, 1958.
24. Welin S: Results of the Malmö technique of colon examination. JAMA 199:369–371, 1967.
25. Diglas S, Garbsch H: Über die Verwendung eines Kontaktlaxans zur Vorbereitung und als Kontrastmittelzusatz für Irrigoskopien. Wien Z Inn Med 43:30–37, 1962.
26. Noveroske RJ: Intracolonic pressures during barium enema examination. AJR 91:852–863, 1964.
27. Quigley EMM, Mills PR, Cole TP, Girdwood T, Scott-

Harden WG, Watkinson G: The fat-encrusted colon. A radiological abnormality of colonic mucosa occurring in patients with steatorrhoea. Scand J Gastroenterol 15:841–848, 1980.

I.2.E. Pharmacological agents

By tradition most radiologists do not use any pharmacological agents to aid in colon relaxation when performing a single-contrast barium enema. This is because the radiologist depends considerably upon postevacuation films. Early in the development of the double-contrast barium enema it was found that there was better colon relaxation and less spasm if a hypotonic agent was used. There is also less dependence upon postevacuation films.

Pharmacological agents first came into use in the performance of hypotonic duodenograms in 1944 (1). Morphine was used initially as the hypotonic agent but because of unsatisfactory results several other agents replaced morphine, with many of the early investigators recommending an intramuscular (IM) anticholinergic agent, propantheline bromide (Pro-Banthine) (2–4). Propantheline, similar to other anticholinergic agents, decreases motor activity in the colon and also reduces the gastrocolic reflex.

Unfortunately, the dose of Pro-Banthine required to induce intestinal hypotonia is such that most of these patients develop a variety of side effects (5). Although most of these side effects are transient reactions, life threatening complications, such as massive gastric dilation, have also been reported (6). Some have suggested that if Pro-Banthine is to be used, 5–10 mg be given intravenously (IV) to avoid the larger doses necessary with an intramuscular injection (7). Although hypotonia can be induced satisfactorily with such doses, the side effects are still significant. In one study, use of IV Pro-Banthine resulted in over 80% of patients developing tachycardia, 12% de-

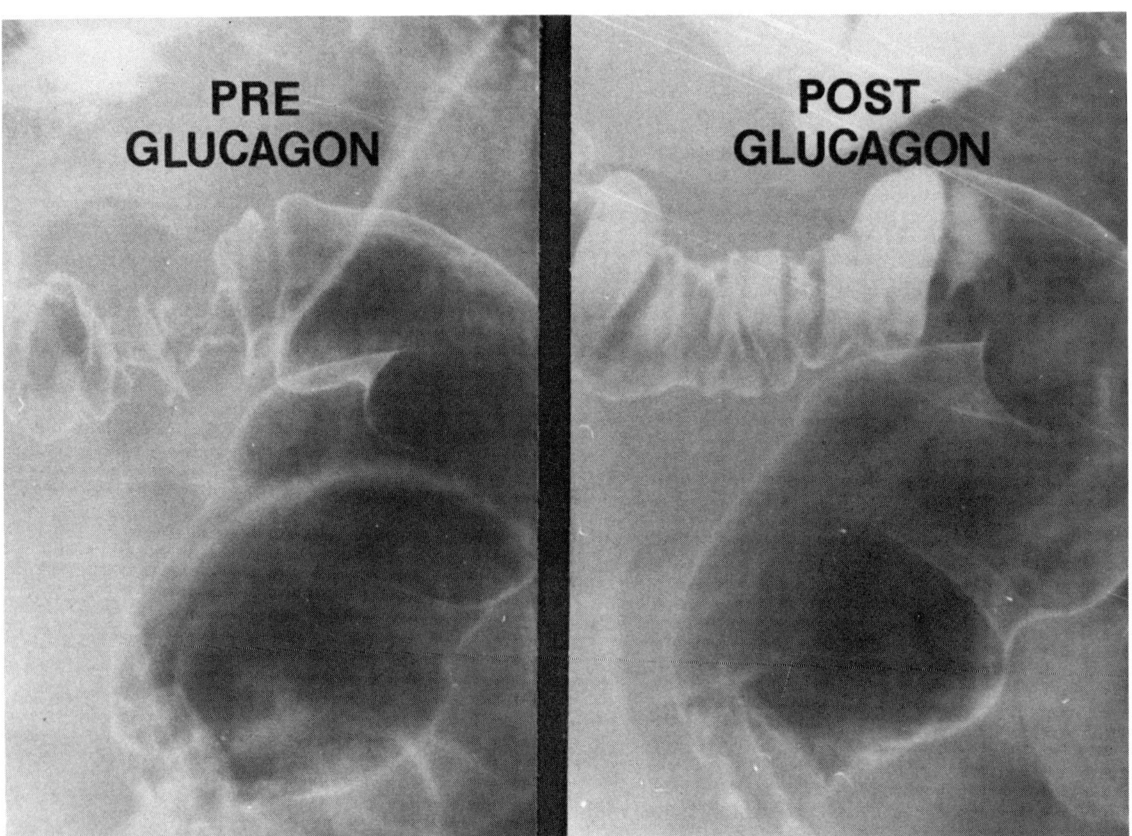

Fig. E.1. Initially a narrowed segment was encountered in the sigmoid. Is it a cancer, benign stricture, or simply spasm? After glucagon the sigmoid distends fully revealing no lesion; the narrowing was thus due to spasm.

veloping urinary retention with half of these requiring catheterization, and 4% having visual blurring (7). Pro-Banthine is contraindicated in patients with glaucoma, prostatism, or cardiovascular disease. At present the anticholinergic drugs should be used sparingly since safer and much shorter acting hypotonic agents are available.

While studying the effect of glucagon on the gallbladder (8), it was found that duodenal hypotonia was induced whenever glucagon was injected. The usefulness of glucagon as a formal hypotonic agent in hypotonic duodenography was subsequently confirmed (9). A double-blind cross-over study in normal volunteers then showed that glucagon was significantly better than either propantheline or atropine in the hypotonic examination of the stomach, duodenal bulb, and duodenal sweep (10). The encouraging results in the duodenum led us to compare glucagon against atropine in the colon (11). The number and intensity of side effects encountered were much lower with glucagon than with atropine (11).

The patient is more comfortable, the colon more relaxed, and interpretation of the examination is easier when glucagon is used as a hypotonic agent (Fig. E.1). Generally, the examination can be completed faster and patient discomfort due to spasm abolished. At times, spasm prevents filling of the colon; glucagon not only helps distend the spastic segment but may also allow visualization of any underlying disease (Fig. E.2).

One to two milligrams glucagon IM results in

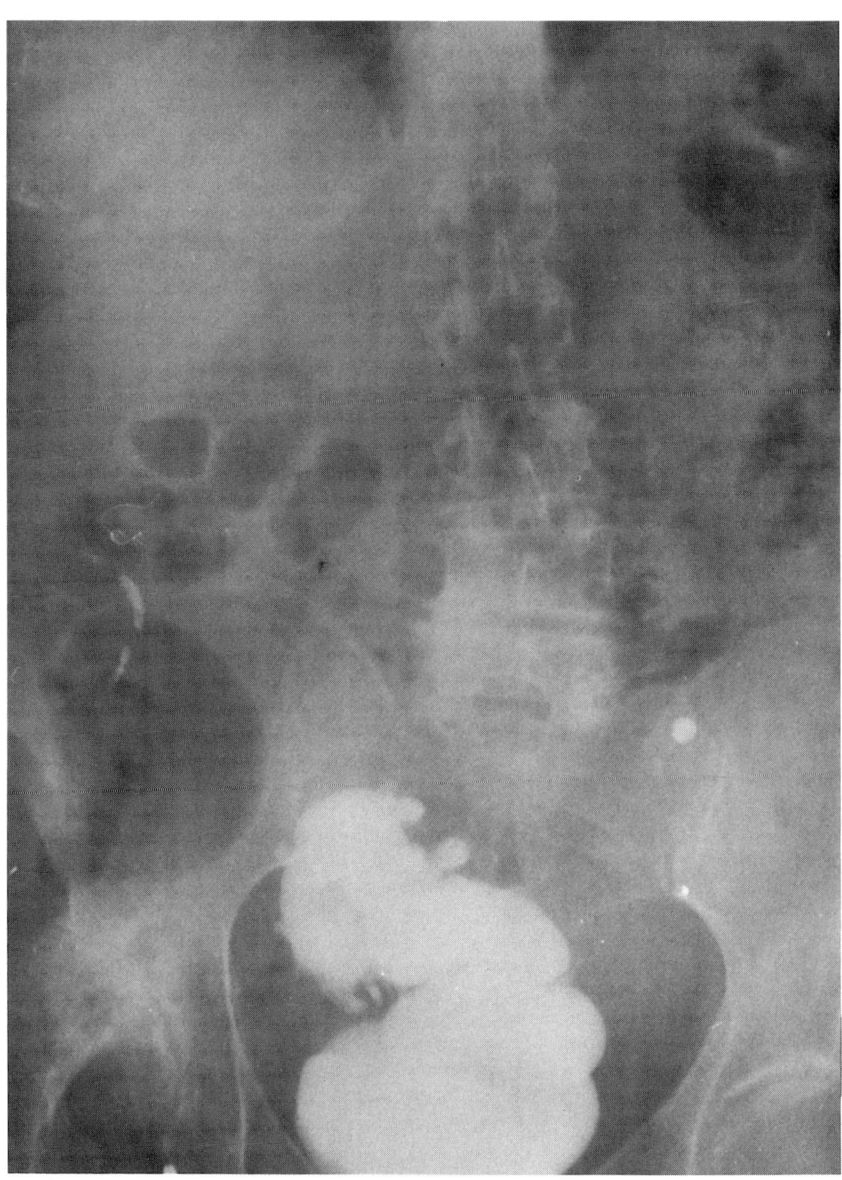

*Fig. E.2.***a.** For legend see page 57.

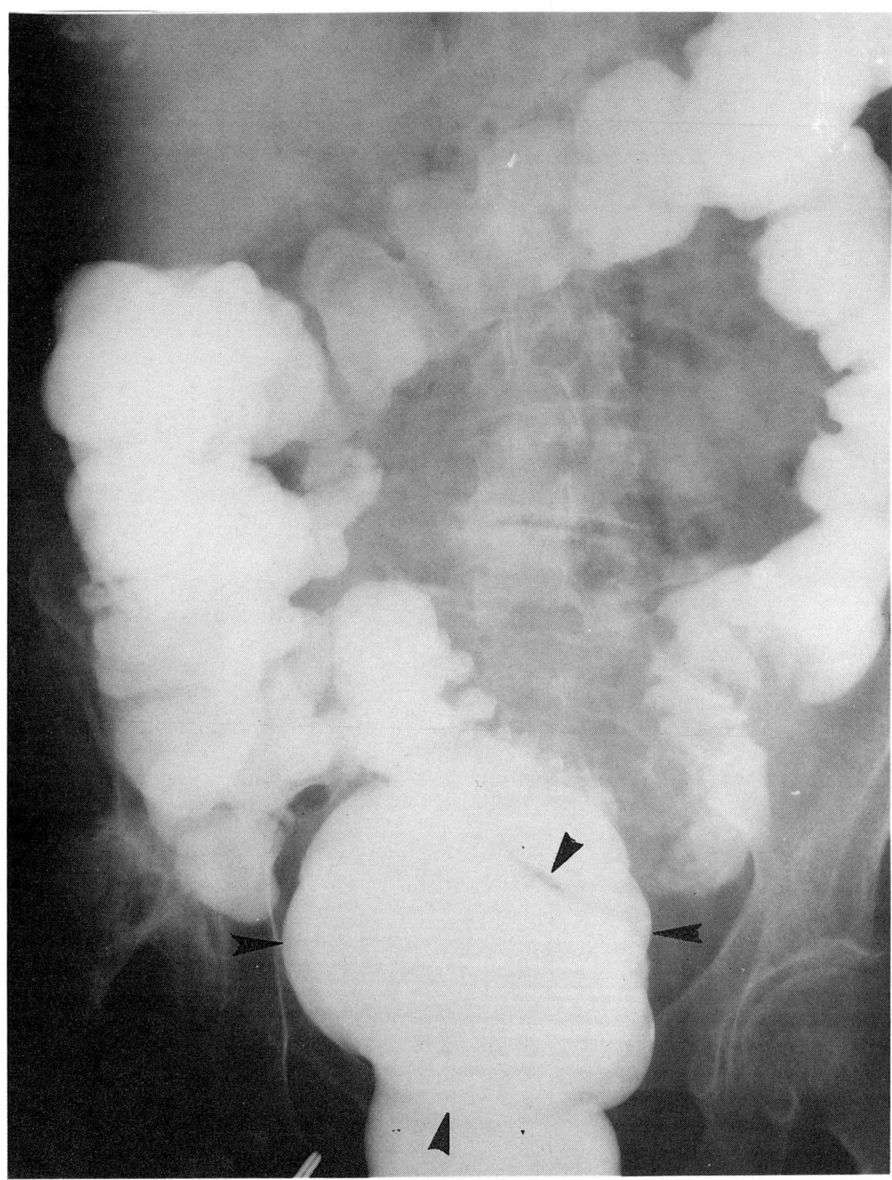

*Fig. E.2.***b.**

colon hypotonia beginning approximately 5 minutes after injection and lasting for approximately 30 minutes. 0.5 mg glucagon intravenously (IV) has essentially the same hypotonic effect; however, the onset is almost immediate and the effect wears off in approximately 10–15 minutes (12). Oral glucagon is ineffective. Due to the high cost of glucagon, we prefer giving 0.25 – 0.50 mg IV rather than the larger dose intramuscularly.

Glucagon is a crystal polypeptide having a molecular weight of 3485 (13). It is composed of 29 amino acid residues. The commercial preparation, available both from beef and pork pancreatic tissue, has the same amino acid sequence as is found in humans. The hormone originates in the pancreas and is produced by the alpha cells in the islands of Langerhans.

Glucagon is considered a stress hormone (12, 14), having widespread function (Table E.1). Stress induced in experimental animals results in endogenous release of glucagon. Glucagon inhibits gastric acid secretion (15). In normal individuals the administration of glucagon increases the total white blood cell count, primarily due to an increase in neutrophiles and bands and there is an associated decrease in lymphocytes. Such changes are similar

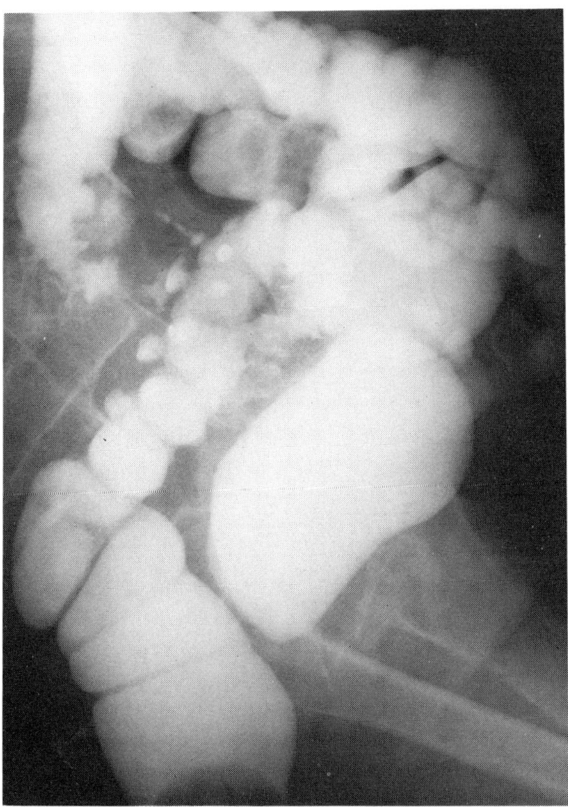

*Fig. E.2.***c.**

Fig. E.2. (a) Initial attempt at a barium enema is unsuccessful, with no filling proximal to the sigmoid. (b) After glucagon, spasm is diminished and the entire colon fills. In addition, a pelvic structure fills (arrowheads) which on the lateral view (c) is seen to be the bladder. The patient had chronic diverticulitis with a colovesical fistula.

to those encountered in normal individuals undergoing a stressful situation (16). Glucagon does not affect the pulse rate or blood pressure (16, 17). The side effects with glucagon are minimal and are not much greater than placebo (16). There are fewer side effects with a 2 mg intramuscular (IM) dose of glucagon as compared to a 1 mg IM dose of atropine sulfate, or a 30 mg IM dose of propantheline bromide (10).

Although it is theoretically possible to develop a sensitivity to glucagon, we have not seen any reactions. If patients with an insulinoma are given glucagon, they may exhibit hypoglycemia due to an insulin releasing effect (18, 19). Similarly, glucagon should be used with caution in patients with suspected pheochromocytoma where it can produce a hypertensive response (20), although glucagon has

Table E.1. Pharmacological action of glucagon (adapted from (25)).

Gastrointestinal hypotonia
Relaxation of gallbladder
Decreased mucosal blood flow
Decreased gastric acid production
Increased cardiac output
Bronchodilation
Increased insulin release
Increase in bile flow

been recommended as a provocation test for suspected pheochromocytoma (21). Phentolamine mesylate (Regitine®) should be available to control a hypertensive attack in the rare patient with an unsuspected pheochromocytoma. A dose of 5 mg may be tried to control the hypertension.

Glucagon has been proposed as a pharmacological aid in helping reduce ileocolic intussusception, especially in children (22, 23). The effect is probably due to its hypotonic action although further work is necessary to prove this advantage.

Other hormones inhibiting intestinal motility are secretin, pancreatic polypeptide, and VIP (vasoactive intestinal peptide); currently they have little practical use in gastrointestinal radiology. Hormones stimulating the gastrointestinal tract, such as cholecystokinin and motilin, are occasionally used as small bowel stimulants to speed up a small bowel examination. Cholecystokinin may stimulate segmental colon contractions (24).

References

1. Porcher P: La stase duodénale provoquée. Procédé simple, rapide et fidèle, d'améliorer la visibilité radiologique et les détails de l'image du bulbe ulcéreux. Arch Mal App Dig 33:24–26, 1944.
2. Baum M, Howe CT: Hypotonic duodenography in the diagnosis of carcinoma of the pancreas and its further use when combined with percutaneous cholangiography and pancreatic scintiscanning. Am J Surg 115:519–525, 1968.
3. Bilbao MK, Rösch J, Frische LH, Dotter CT: Hypotonic duodenography in the diagnosis of pancreatic disease. Semin Roentgenol 3:280–287, 1968.
4. Bilbao MK, Frische LH, Dotter CT, Rösch J: Hypotonic duodenography. Radiology 89:438–443, 1967.
5. Goldstein HM, Zboralske FF: Tubeless hypotonic duodenography. JAMA 210:2086–2088, 1969.
6. Gelfand DW, Moskowitz M: Massive gastric dilatation complicating hypotonic duodenography. Radiology 97:637–639, 1970.
7. Merlo RB, Stone M, Baugus P, Martin M: The use of Pro-Banthine to induce gastrointestinal hypotonia. Radiology 127:61–62, 1978.

8. Chernish SM, Miller RE, Rosenak BD, Scholz NE: Effect of glucagon on size of visualized human gall bladder before and after fat meal. Gastroenterology 62:1218–1226, 1972.
9. Chernish SM, Miller RE, Rosenak BD, Scholz NE: Hypotonic duodenography with the use of glucagon. Gastroenterology 63:392–398, 1972.
10. Miller RE, Chernish SM, Skucas J, Rosenak BD, Rodda BE: Hypotonic roentgenology with glucagon. AJR 121:264–275, 1974.
11. Miller RE, Chernish SM, Skucas J, Rosenak BD, Rodda BE: Hypotonic colon examination with glucagon. Radiology 113:555–562, 1974.
12. Miller RE, Chernish SM, Brunelle RL: Gastrointestinal radiography with glucagon. Gastrointest Radiol 4:1–10, 1979.
13. Bromer W: Glucagon: Chemistry and action. Fortschr Chem Org Naturst 28:429–452, 1970.
14. Bloom SR: Glucagon, a stress hormone. Postgrad Med J 49:607–611, 1973.
15. Christiansen J: Pancreatic glucagon and gastric acid secretion. Scand J Gastroenterol 15:257–258, 1980.
16. Chernish SM, Davidson JA, Brunelle RL, Miller RE, Rosenak BD: Response of normal subjects to a single 2-milligram dose of glucagon administered intramuscularly. Arch Int Pharmacodyn Ther 218:312–327, 1975.
17. Harned RK, Stelling CB, Williams S, Wolf GL: Glucagon and barium enema examinations: a controlled clinical trial. AJR 126:981–984, 1976.
18. Lawrence AM: Glucagon. Annu Rev Med 20:207–222, 1969.
19. Lawrence AM: Glucagon in medicine: new ideas for an old hormone. Med Clin North Am 54:183–190, 1970.
20. Gomez-Pan A, Blesa Malpica G, Arnao R, Oriol Bosch A: Glucagon as a drug. In: Picazo J. (ed) Glucagon in Gastroenterology, p 12. University Park Press, Baltimore, 1979.
21. Lawrence AM, Forland M: Glucagon provocative test for pheochromocytoma. J Lab Clin Med 64:878, 1964.
22. Fisher JK, Germann DR: Glucagon-aided reduction of intussusception. Radiology 122:197–198, 1977.
23. Hoy GR, Dunbar D, Boles ET: The use of glucagon in the diagnosis and management of ileocolic intussusception. J Pediatr Surg 12:939–944, 1977.
24. Harvey RF, Read AE: Effect of cholecystokinin on colonic motility and symptoms in patients with the irritable-bowel syndrome. Lancet 1:1–3, 1973.
25. Meeroff JC, Jorgens J, Isenberg JI: The effect of glucagon on barium-enema examination. Radiology 115:5–7, 1975.

I.2.F. Technique

a. Introduction

Because most commercial barium sulfate preparations suitable for double-contrast examination have a high viscosity, relatively large bore enema tubing must be used to ensure adequate flow. At least 1.25 cm (1/2 in.) internal diameter tubing should be used (1), although if less viscous products are developed in the future a 1.0 cm diameter may be sufficient. The rate of flow through a tube is determined, in part, by Poiseuille's law:

$$Q = \frac{\pi \, Pr^4}{8 \, nl}$$

where Q = flow rate of material (in ml/sec),
P = pressure (dynes/cm^3),
r = radius of tubing (cm),
n = viscosity coefficient of material (poises),
l = length of tubing (cm).

Although all of these factors determine the flow rate, obviously the radius of the tubing has the major effect. Thus, wide bore tubing should be used with relatively viscous contrast media. The tubing length should be as short as possible yet still be convenient to use; 90 to 100 cm length is fully adequate. The barium suspension can be instilled by simply squeezing the enema bag. Although one should not squeeze the enema bag while performing a single-contrast barium enema, the high viscosity of the denser barium suspensions used for double-contrast examinations acts as a safety factor preventing high intracolonic pressures.

Some radiologists have adopted a 'calking gun' type of mechanism to aid in the instillation of the barium suspension. Others use a reversible roller pump to squeeze the tubing (2). Still others use a 60 ml syringe to add the barium (3). Multiple barium filled syringes are necessary with this latter method.

A digital rectal examination should precede the barium enema. The rectal examination allows determination of sphincter tone, helps predict possible incontinence, may detect low-lying lesions, and reduces trauma for the subsequently inserted enema tip (4, 5). We find it easiest to insert the enema tip with the patient in a left lateral position with either both hips and knees flexed in a knee–chest position or the left leg straight and the right leg flexed. Enema tube angulation is determined from the preceding digital rectal examination. Deep, slow respiration by the patient, together with having the patient 'bear down,' sometimes helps. Gradual pressure, applied gently, is probably the most important factor in patient comfort.

Many different types of enema tips are available for the performance of a barium enema. For a double-contrast enema a separate conduit for adding air is necessary, with the tip of this conduit extending beyond the enema tip (6). Such an enema tip allows ready introduction of barium, drainage of barium from the rectum, and subsequent addition of air without introducing any excess barium.

A balloon can help a patient to retain the enema. For most patients a balloon is not necessary; it simply adds to patient discomfort and can possibly lead to rectal perforation. As a general rule, we do not blow up the balloon in patients less than 50 years of age unless it appears that there may be difficulty retaining the enema. Rectal incontinence correlates well with sphincter tone. Little leakage should occur in those patients with good sphincter tone (7). We do not inflate the balloon in any patient unless we are able to visualize the rectum fluoroscopically and ensure that there is not a lesion present.

In the examination of infants and children soft rubber enema tips are recommended (8). An inflated Foley balloon may obscure a portion of the rectum.

Electrical stimulation of the anal sphincter has been used as an aid to barium retention (9). A significant reduction in examination failure rate was achieved. We have not had any experience with such a unit.

b. Barium addition

In the average patient the barium suspension is added until it has reached the splenic flexture. Throughout this time the patient is kept prone or in a left decubitus position. If the examination involves a patient who has difficulty turning, we add extra barium because the additional barium aids in the subsequent filling of the cecum without having to turn the patient as much as usual. If a patient has had a prior hemicolectomy, barium added only to the mid-descending colon generally suffices for subsequent filling of the entire colon.

The average patient requires approximately 350 ml of the barium sulfate suspension, although there is variation among patients. The exact amount of barium added is not important; what is important is that each individual patient have enough barium to obtain a technically satisfactory examination. The disadvantage of using too much barium is that subsequently one may not be able to obtain *double-contrast* views of the entire colon. With too much barium a greater effort will be necessary to ensure that the entire colon is covered with double-contrast views and that a small lesion does not remain buried in a barium pool.

c. Drainage

Adequate barium drainage and subsequent air insufflation is mandatory in evaluation of the rectum. If the rectum is not drained adequately, excessive residual barium can hide lesions. Many studies have shown that both benign and malignant lesions of the rectum have been missed by competent examiners using other diagnostic methods, yet these lesions can be readily identified on double-contrast examinations.

Adequate rectal drainage can be achieved simply by keeping the patient prone and placing the enema bag below table top level, thus allowing drainage by gravity (10). In the prone position almost all of the barium in the rectum can be readily drained, while if the patient is supine the enema tip is located above the barium pooling along the posterior wall of the rectum (Fig. F.1). Tilting the table slightly so that the patient's head is up and depressing the enema tip will aid barium drainage (Fig. F.2). Sometimes by slowly adding air through the enema tip one can increase the rate of drainage and thus speed up the examination. If the enema tip is inserted too far, adequate drainage may not be possible. Adequate positioning using fluoroscopic visualization will aid drainage.

Barium in the rectum can be drained into the sigmoid if the patient is placed into a steep Trendelenburg position, a maneuver used in Japan, where the strapped-in patient is turned almost upside down.

If one attempts to drain the rectum but there are no returns, there probably is a kink either in the tubing or at the junction of the tubing and the enema bag.

d. Air insufflation

Air insufflation adds little to patient discomfort if bowel relaxation has been achieved with a hypotonic agent. After the rectum has been drained of barium, air is gradually insufflated until air can readily be identified at the splenic flexure. Both during drainage and during the initial air insufflation the patient is kept prone. Thus, the anteriorly located transverse colon fills with barium

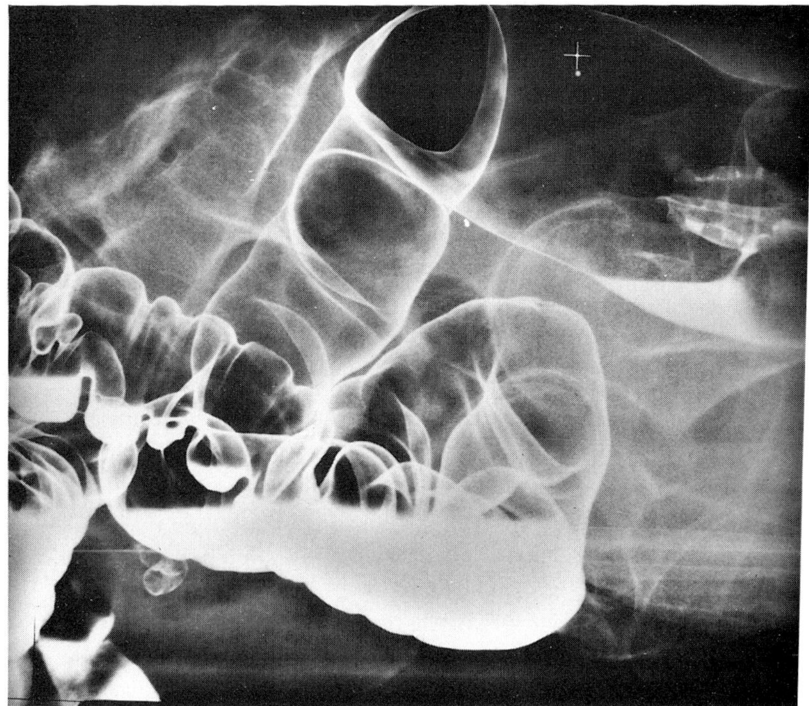

a

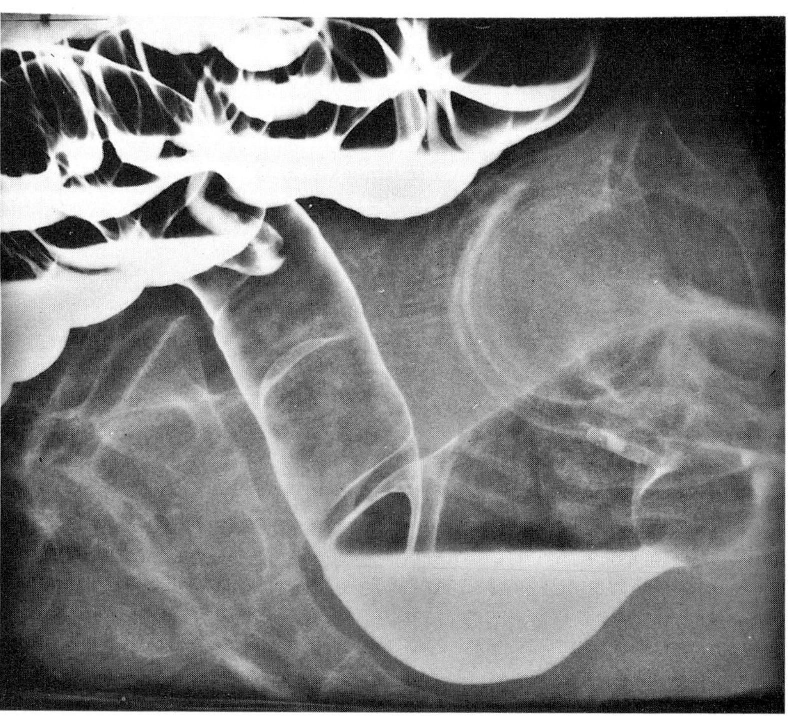

b

Fig. F.1. (a) With the patient prone barium drain from the rectum by gravity. (b) If the patient is turned supine, barium pools along the posterior rectal wall and drainage by gravity does not occur.

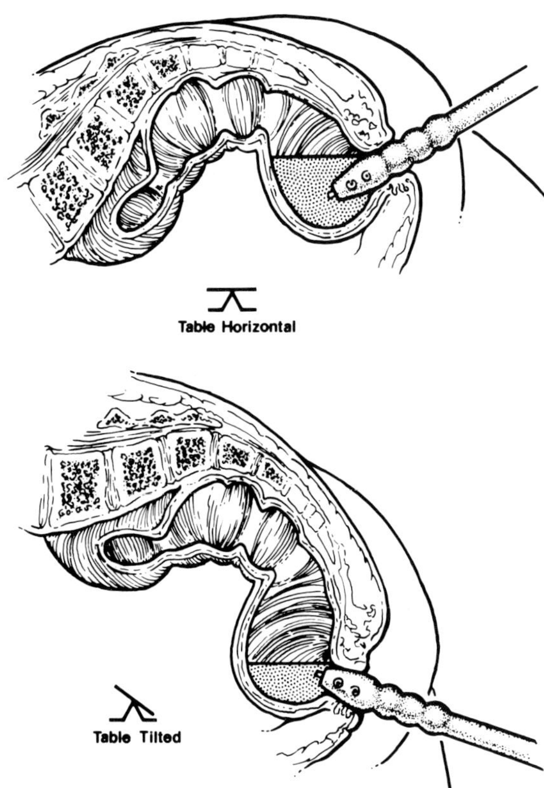

Fig. F.2. With the patient prone it is not possible to drain the rectum completely. If the patient is tilted feet down and the enema tip depressed, more barium can be drained out. (From Miller and Peterson (10); copyright, RSNA, 1978.)

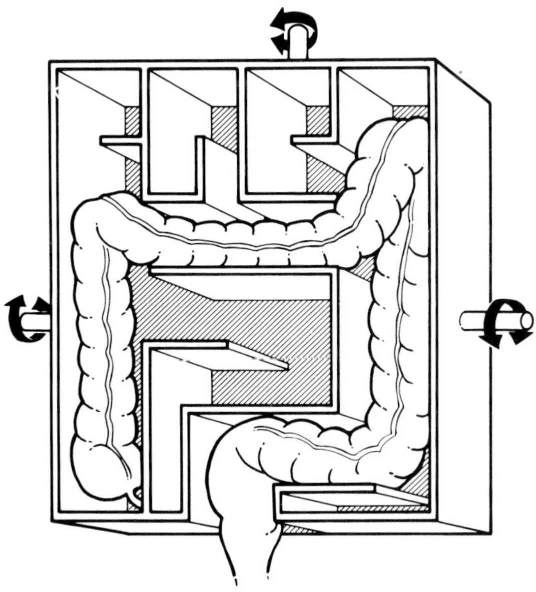

Fig. F.3. By selective tilting and turning of the patient, barium will flow by gravity into the proximal part of the colon, similar to a ball in a maze. (From Miller (11); copyright ARRS, 1979.)

both because of gravity and because of the pressure exerted by air in the distal part of the colon. If one continues adding air with the patient prone, air will percolate through the barium in the dependent part of the transverse colon and fill the right colon. The result will be a single contrast study of the right colon. Instead, after air has reached the splenic flexure, the patient is turned on the right side. Further addition of air will now result in barium flowing proximally into the right colon (Fig. F.3). In most patients, simply by turning them on the right side is enough to fill the entire colon. Patients with a redundant colon may need to be turned supine or even into an LPO position to fill the ascending colon. Occasionally, if there is enough barium in the ascending colon but none in the cecum, the patient can be stood up, although in most patients tilting the table upright is not necessary and simply wastes time. It is not necessary to coat the entire cecum at this time, since subsequent patient positioning during filming will produce sufficient coating.

In the double-contrast examination barium flows 'downhill' and will flow into a desired loop if that loop is placed dependent in relationship to the barium (Fig. F.4). Thus, one must know the anatomical relationship of the colon to the surrounding structures and must use this knowledge during fluoroscopy to position the patient such that the entire colon is eventually filled (Fig. F.5). If, during the filling phase, one cannot tell where the

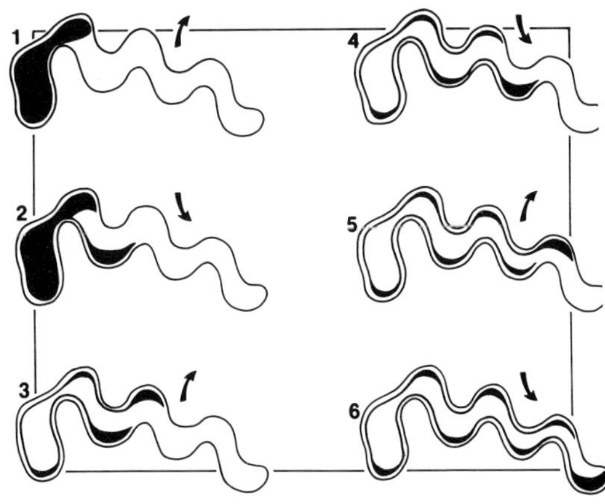

Fig. F.4. Barium flows downhill. By positioning the patient with the appropriate side down (arrows), the contrast agent (black) can be made to flow proximally in the colon.

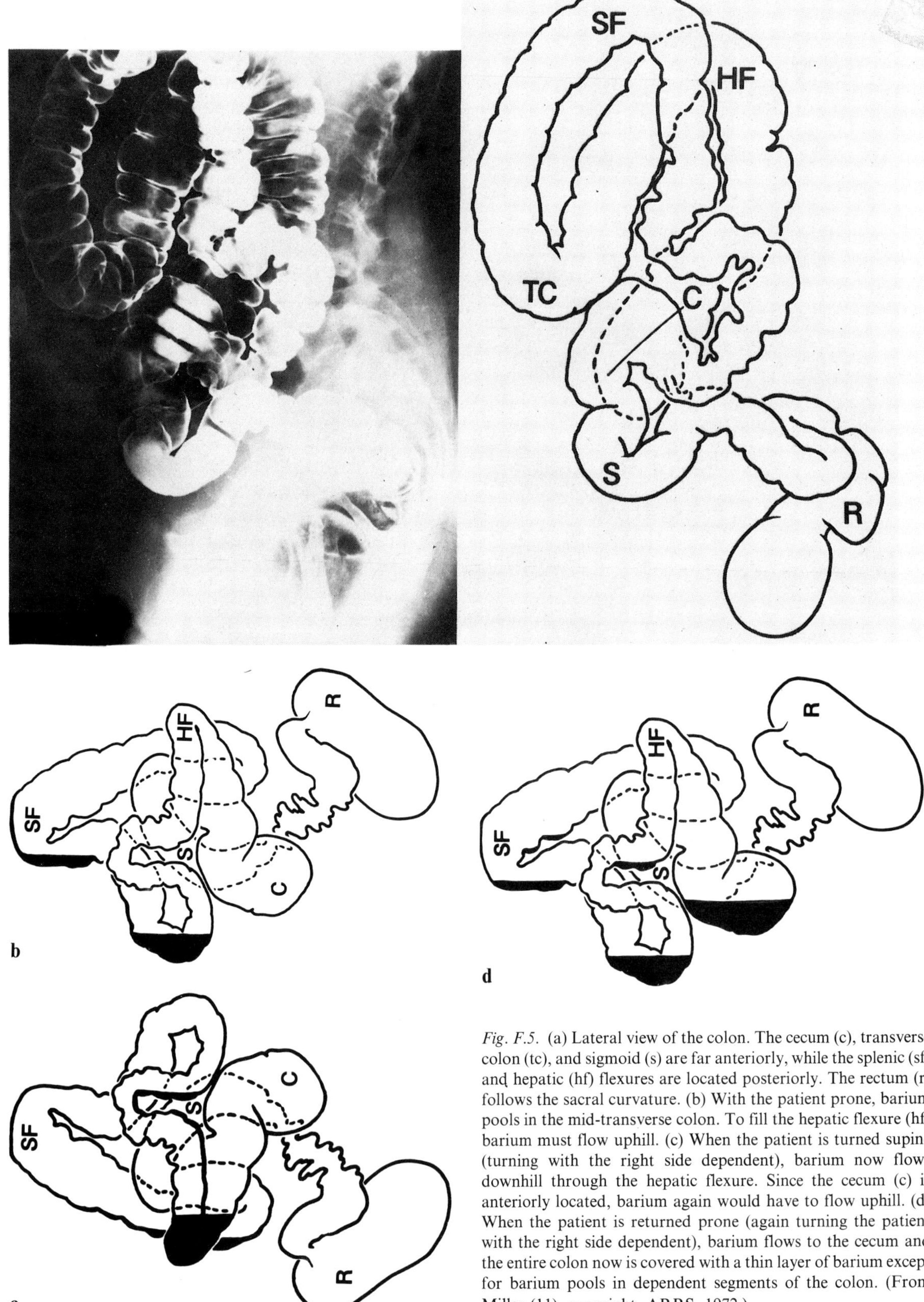

Fig. F.5. (a) Lateral view of the colon. The cecum (c), transverse colon (tc), and sigmoid (s) are far anteriorly, while the splenic (sf) and hepatic (hf) flexures are located posteriorly. The rectum (r) follows the sacral curvature. (b) With the patient prone, barium pools in the mid-transverse colon. To fill the hepatic flexure (hf) barium must flow uphill. (c) When the patient is turned supine (turning with the right side dependent), barium now flows downhill through the hepatic flexure. Since the cecum (c) is anteriorly located, barium again would have to flow uphill. (d) When the patient is returned prone (again turning the patient with the right side dependent), barium flows to the cecum and the entire colon now is covered with a thin layer of barium except for barium pools in dependent segments of the colon. (From Miller (11), copyright, ARRS, 1972.)

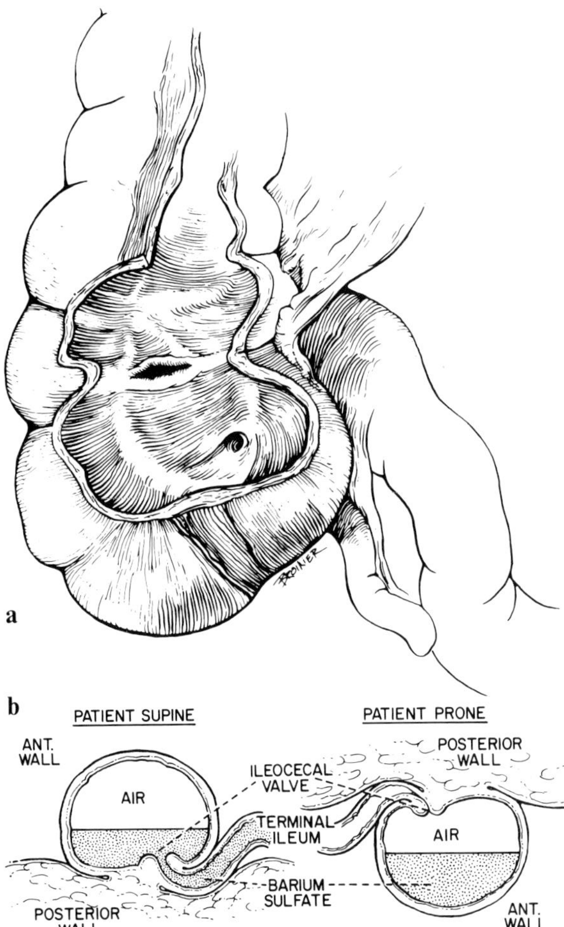

Fig. F.6. (a) Dissection of the right colon, which has been opened anteriorly, reveals the usual posteriorily placed ileocecal valve. The appendix likewise inserted posteriorly. (b) A cross-section of the cecum reveals that with the patient supine (left), barium is adjacent to the ileocecal valve and there is reflux of barium into the terminal ileum. If the patient is kept prone whenever there is barium in the cecum (right), only air will reflux into the ileum. (From Miller (11); copyright, ARRS, 1979.)

head of the barium column is, the patient is turned either prone or supine. In either position the fluoroscopist can generally identify the head of the barium column and proceed accordingly.

Care should be used to avoid refluxing barium into the terminal ileum. The distal ileum quite often overlies the sigmoid colon and a lesion in the sigmoid can be obscured by the barium-filled ileum. Since in most patients the ileocecal valve is located posteriorly and medially, barium reflux can be avoided if the patient is *not* turned supine or towards the left side anytime there is barium present alongside the ileocecal valve (Fig. F.6). With the patient prone or right side down, air is adjacent to

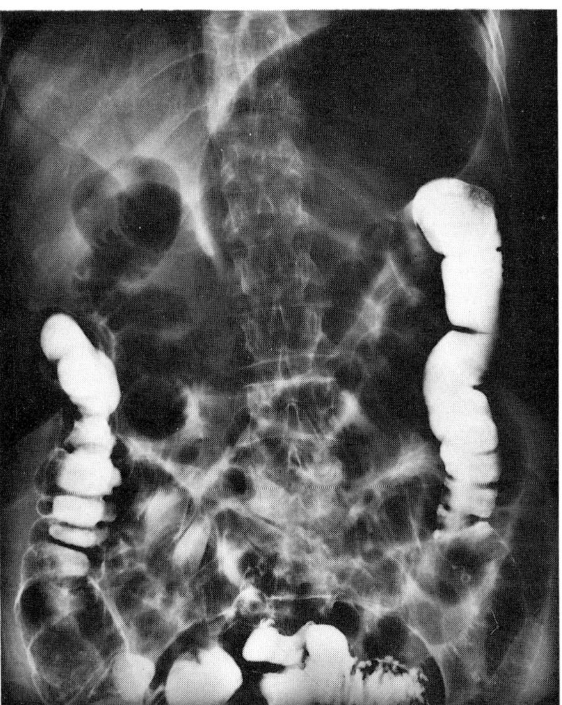

Fig. F.7. This patient had a very incompetent ileocecal valve and considerable residual spasm throughout the colon. To help distend the colon, air was added intermittently during radiography. Although all of the barium is still in the colon, air has not only refluxed into the small bowel but has also distended the stomach.

the valve and can reflux freely. An incompetent ileocecal valve acts as a safety valve preventing undue pressures from building up in the colon. Obviously, refluxed air in the small bowel does not obscure the sigmoid (Fig. F.7).

If the patient has been turned supine or stood up, the rectum should again be checked fluoroscopically to make sure that excess barium has not drained from the sigmoid into the rectum. If necessary, with the patient prone, any residual barium can again be drained simply by placing the enema bag in a dependent position and releasing the clamp on the enema tube (10). The patient is left in a prone position for the first overhead film.

If there is air proximal to the barium column, simple patient positioning may not be adequate to advance the barium. Such so-called 'air block' is generally due to insufficient colon dilatation and resultant 'kinking' of the colon (11). In such a situation the colon can be readily filled simply by adequate colon distension (Fig. F.8). Distension straightens out the various sharp angulations and 'kinks' in the colon.

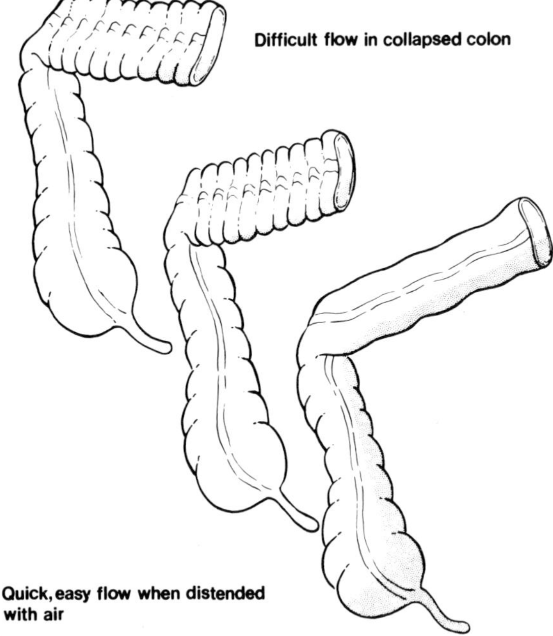

Fig. F.8. Barium does not flow readily in a collapsed colon. Inflation of the colon smooths out obstructions and permits easier flow.

Miller and Maglinte have recently described a simplified 'Seven-Pump Method' for double-contrast colon examination (12).

The '7 pump' method ensures adequate amounts of barium in the right side using less time, barium, and radiation. Three hundred to 400 ml of barium is first instilled in the rectum. Each step then takes seven full squeezes or pumps on a sphygmomanometer bulb for introducing air in seven different positions. These positions are: a) 7 pumps, prone position; b) 7 pumps, left lateral position; c) 7 pumps, left anterior oblique position; d) 7 pumps, prone position; e) 7 pumps, right anterior oblique position; f) 7 pumps, right lateral position; and g) 7 pumps, supine position. After brief fluoroscopy steps 'a' and 'b' are repeated before filming. Occasionally additional air and patient positioning under fluoroscopy are necessary to ensure optimal distribution and coating of the barium. This technique is based on the usual anatomical positions of the various colon segments, the role of gravity and time in each position. All steps can be performed first without fluoroscopy to reduce radiation and shorten examination time. Only a final fluoroscopic check is needed to find the 10% of patients who need additional maneuvers to place barium in the cecum.

This method has reduced examination time, cost, and patient radiation. It can be performed either by the skilled radiologist, the resident in training, or a skilled technologist.

References

1. Miller RE: Faster-flow enema equipment. Radiology 123:229–230, 1977.
2. Berney JW: Reversible barium pumps for air contrast barium-enema examinations. Radiology 136:789, 1980.
3. Hogan MT, Antico DA, Pollak C: A simple method of barium administration for double-contrast enemas. Radiology 123:230, 1977.
4. Dodds WJ, Stewart ET, Nelson JA: Rectal balloon catheters and the barium enema examination. Gastrointest Radiol 5:277–284, 1980.
5. Stewart ET, Dodds WJ, Nelson JA: The value of digital rectal examination before barium enema. Radiology 137:567, 1980.
6. Peterson GH, Miller RE: The barium enema: a reassessment looking toward perfection. Radiology 128:315–320, 1978.
7. Stewart ET, Dodds WJ: Predictability of rectal incontinence on barium enema examination. AJR 132:197–200, 1979.
8. Kirks DR, Kane PE, Taybi H: Pediatric enema tip. Radiology 118:232, 1976.
9. Clark K, Rowan D: Electrical stimulation for anal sphincter control in barium enema examinations: an extended trial. AJR 127:429–431, 1976.
10. Miller RE, Peterson GH: Drainage of the rectum: a simple maneuver to improve the accuracy of colon examinations. Radiology 128:506–507, 1978.
11. Miller RE: Solution for the 'air block' problem during fluoroscopy. AJR 132:1020–1021, 1979.
12. Miller RE, Maglinte DDT: Barium pneumocolon: technologist-performed '7 pump' method. AJR 131, 1230–1232, 1982.

I.2.G. Radiography

a. Introduction

It is believed by some that a well performed double-contrast barium enema is by far the most accurate method of detecting colon lesions. The radiographs obtained should be designed so that the entire colon can be readily visualized not only in the average patient, but also in that patient who has a redundant colon. Unfortunately, residual barium can pool in the colon and as a result multiple views in different projections are necessary in order to clear various parts of the colon. Animal studies have suggested that at least ten or more projections are necessary for adequate coverage of the entire colon (1). Gravity has, by far, the greatest effect on the flow of barium. Views 180° apart are necessary to visualize the entire colon adequately.

About half of the medical centers obtain a preliminary (scout) radiograph of the abdomen (2). Some have found that this preliminary radiograph does not affect the overall diagnostic accuracy of the examination (3), while others believe it is cost effective and contributes to the patient's care (4). Currently, we do not obtain a preliminary radiograph, unless it is determined beforehand that the radiograph may be useful to answer some specific question.

b. Rectum

Although some radiologists have questioned whether a lateral rectal view is routinely necessary, both we and others (5) believe that this view should be part of every examination. Fistulas to adjacent anteriorly located structures, disease involving the pre-sacral space, invasion of the pouch of Douglas, and the anterior and posterior walls of the rectum can best be evaluated with this view (Fig. G.1). If barium has been adequately drained from the rectum, a PA (or AP with an undertable tube) radiograph of the rectum, together with a right lateral radiograph, will adequately visualize the rectum in a majority of patients. It is important that the *right* lateral, rather than the left lateral, view be obtained, since with the latter, the ileocecal valve is placed in a dependent position and barium can reflux into the terminal ileum, overlap the sigmoid and obscure a lesion.

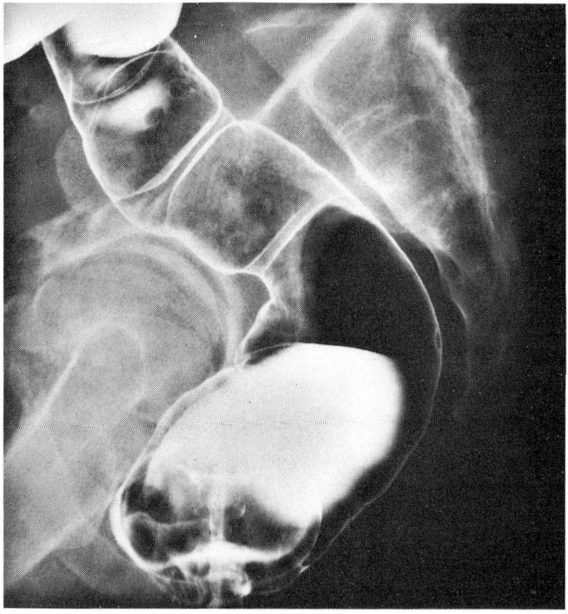

Fig. G.1. Normal lateral rectal radiograph. Both the anterior and posterior rectal wall can be evaluated on this radiograph. Widening of the presacral space, metastasis to the pouch of Douglas, or local invasion by gynecological tumors are usually first identified on this radiograph.

The angled view of the sigmoid causes foreshortening of the rectum, obscuring a lesion (Fig. G.2). The LAO and the RAO projections quite often are satisfactory for portions of the rectum (Fig. G.3). The supine position is least satisfactory since almost always some barium drains into the rectum and obscures a portion of it.

Although a prone cross-table radiograph of the rectum has been found satisfactory by some (6), we found the right lateral radiograph superior to the prone cross-table lateral radiograph in approximately 65% of patients (7). The reason is because some barium pools in the distal rectum when the patient is prone. Although the same amount of barium is present with the patient in the right lateral position, this barium is spread out over a larger area and thus the barium cover is thinner.

Both decubitus radiographs are excellent for visualizing the rectum; sometimes these are the only radiographs where the entire rectum is clearly seen. Because the decubitus views also provide excellent visualization of the rest of the colon, these two radiographs should be included in every examination.

With adequate rectal drainage, good colon distension, and a cooperative patient the enema tip can often be removed before the overhead radiographs are obtained. Without the enema tip even the most distal end of the rectum can be adequately evaluated (Fig. G.4).

c. Sigmoid colon

In 1929, Chassard and Lapiné (8) described a new position of the pelvic outlet for use in pelvimetry. This view was introduced into the United States in 1951 by Rapp for a study of the pelvic contents (9). Ettinger and Elkin, in 1954, applied this view to the sigmoid colon (10) and subquently many radiologists adopted the Chassard-Lapiné view as part of their barium enema technique. This radiograph is taken with the patient sitting on the edge of the table and bending forward until the symphysis pubis and the ischial tuberosities are horizontal. In effect, the patient bends forward as far as possible

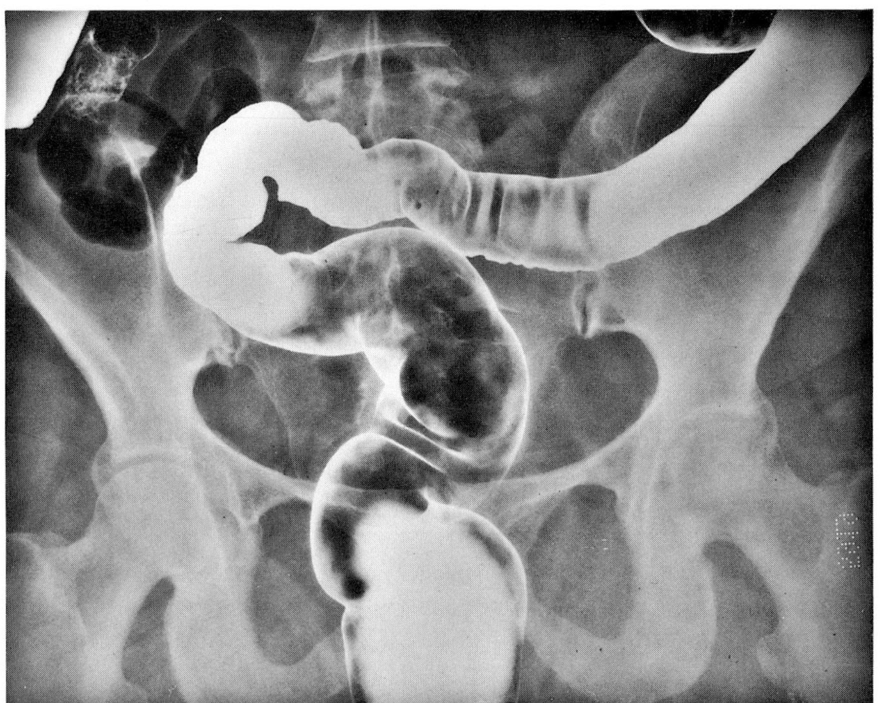

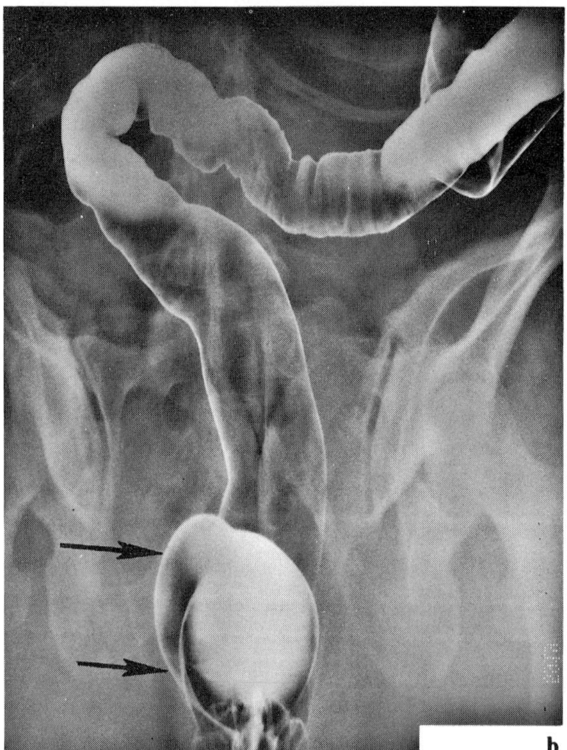

Fig. G.2. (a) **Prone posteroanterior radiograph** of the rectosigmoid reveals a larger segment of the rectum than (b) the angled-prone radiograph. The latter is excellent in unraveling a redundant sigmoid and visualizing the proximal portion of the rectum, but the distal rectum is markedly foreshortened and distorted (arrows).

and a vertical x-ray beam is centered over the pelvis. A foot-stool aids in assuring patient security. Although such a view is useful in evaluating the pelvis and the sigmoid colon, having patients assume this sitting position routinely with an enema tip in place and the colon distended can lead to problems. Also, not all patients can cooperate enough to assume this position during the barium enema. We have abandoned the routine use of this view and have adopted the angled view of the sigmoid instead as described by Dysart and Stewart (11). This angled view, obtained with the patient prone and the x-ray tube angled 35° caudad, elongates and uncoils the sigmoid (12). Initially, this view was believed valuable only in an occasional patient (11); however, many radiologists are now using this view routinely. This radiograph can be obtained either by having the patient prone with the x-ray tube angled 30–35° caudad or the patient can be supine and the x-ray tube is angled 30–35° cephalad (Fig. G.5 a,b). If there is barium pooling in the sigmoid, turning the patient from the prone position into the supine position will generally clear these areas.

The 30–35° x-ray tube angulation is a compromise. If the x-ray tube is angled 15° there often is insufficient separation of the sigmoid loops. If the x-ray tube is angled 45° there is excellent separation

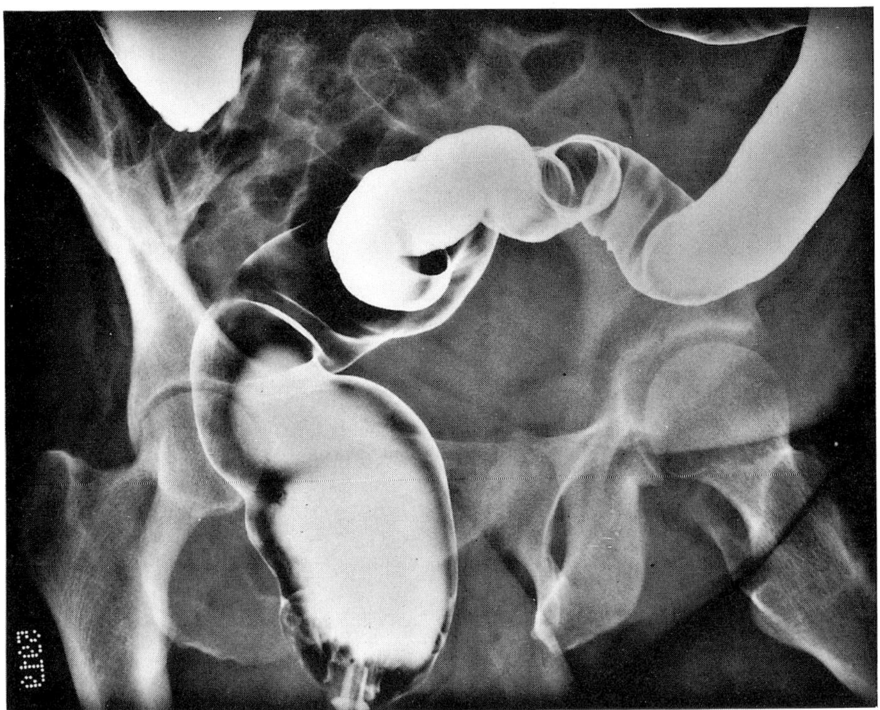

a

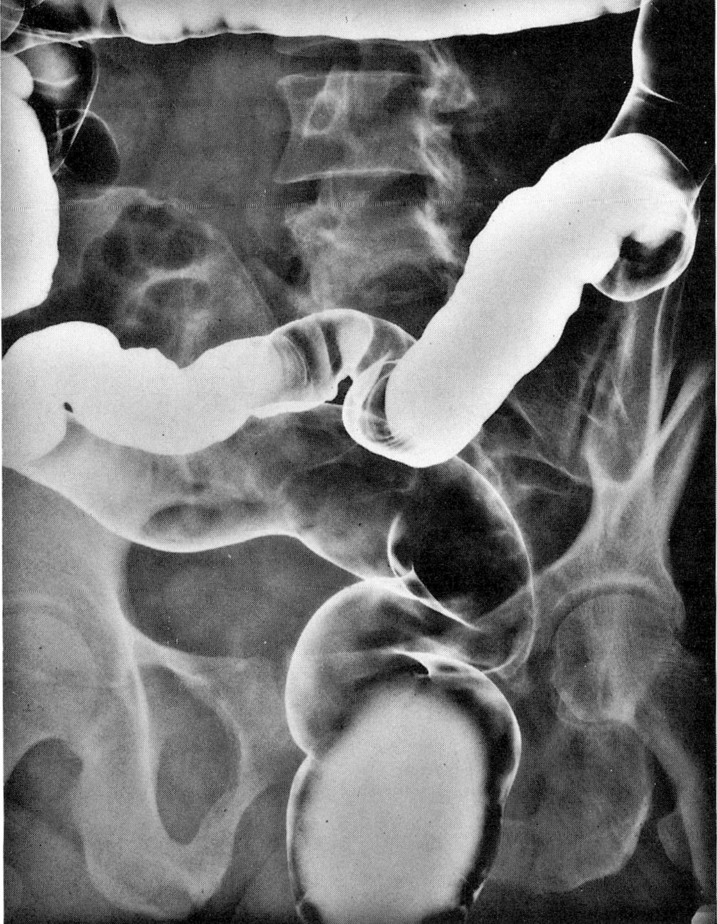

b

Fig. G.3. (a) The right anterior oblique (RAO) and (b) left anterior oblique positions allow visualization of different portions of the rectum and sigmoid.

of the sigmoid loops; but unfortunately at such steep obliquity there are positioning difficulties for the technologist and excessive scatter radiation, resulting in films of inferior quality.

If the x-ray tube is angled 30° caudad and, in addition, the patient is turned 15° into an RAO projection there is further separation of the sigmoid loops. Such an 'angled-oblique' view combines the advantages of vertical separation of the sigmoid obtained with the angled view and horizontal separation obtained with the oblique view (13, 14) (Fig. G.5c). The disadvantages are an increase in scatter radiation resulting in some loss of contrast and somewhat greater positioning difficulties for the technologist. Overall, we believe that such a projection is by far the best for visualizing the sigmoid and we routinely include this projection in every examination. A similar projection can be obtained by having the patient in an LPO position and angling the x-ray tube 30–35° cranially (Fig. G.5d). Because the prone and supine angled-oblique projections are 180° apart, they are complimentary (7). A portion of the sigmoid may be obscured in one radiograph but should be visible on the other (Fig. G.6).

These projections are useful primarily for the sigmoid because the remainder of the colon is considerably distorted due to the angulation. The angled-oblique radiograph tends to separate the sigmoid away from other loops of bowel. If there has been inadvertent reflux of barium into the terminal ileum, the angled-oblique projections tend to separate the overlapping small bowel from the sigmoid colon. Oblique views are also sometimes helpful in unraveling any overlapping sigmoid loops (15, 16) (Fig. G.3). A lateral view may likewise uncoil redundant sigmoid loops. On some occasions an upright lateral view of the sigmoid is useful for evaluating the most cephalic portion of the sigmoid loop (17). The PA and both lateral

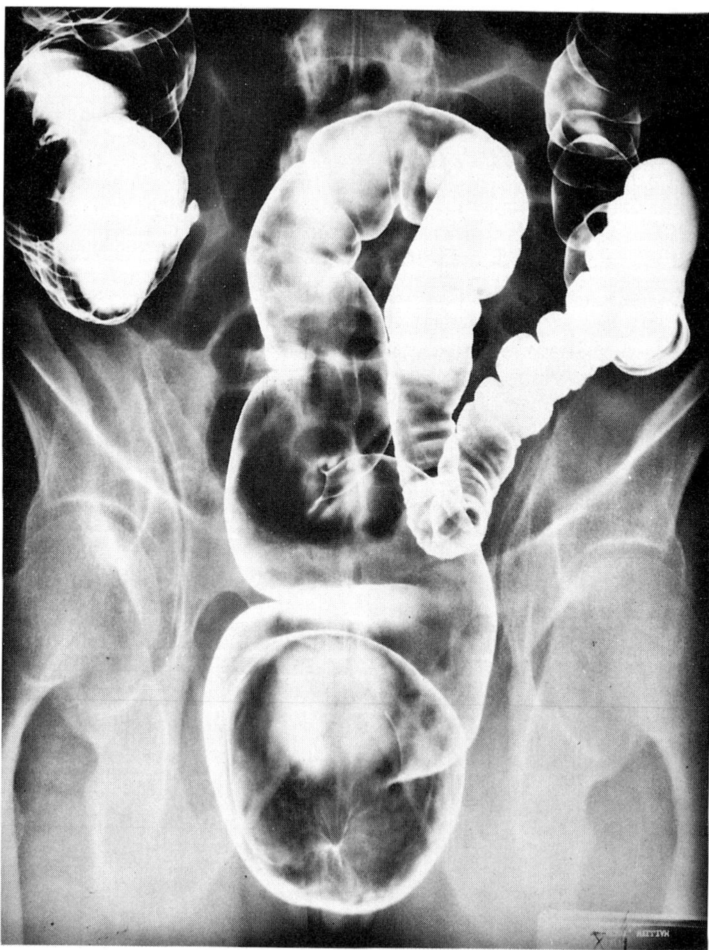

Fig. G.4. The enema tip was removed before the overhead radiographs were obtained. As a result, the entire rectosigmoid is clearly seen.

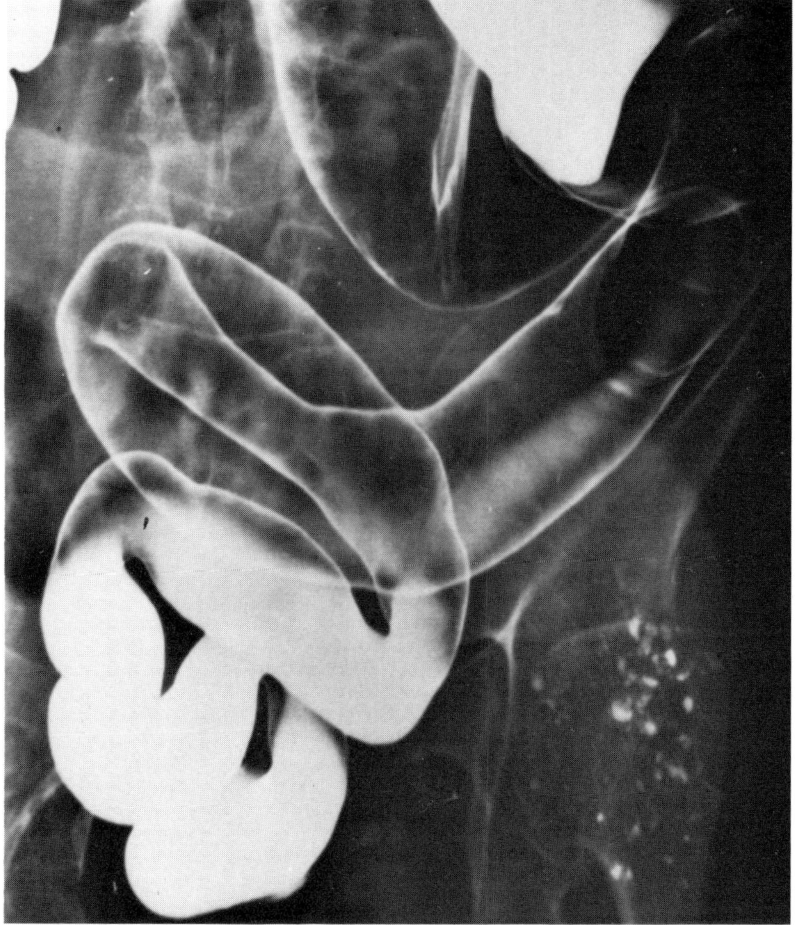

a

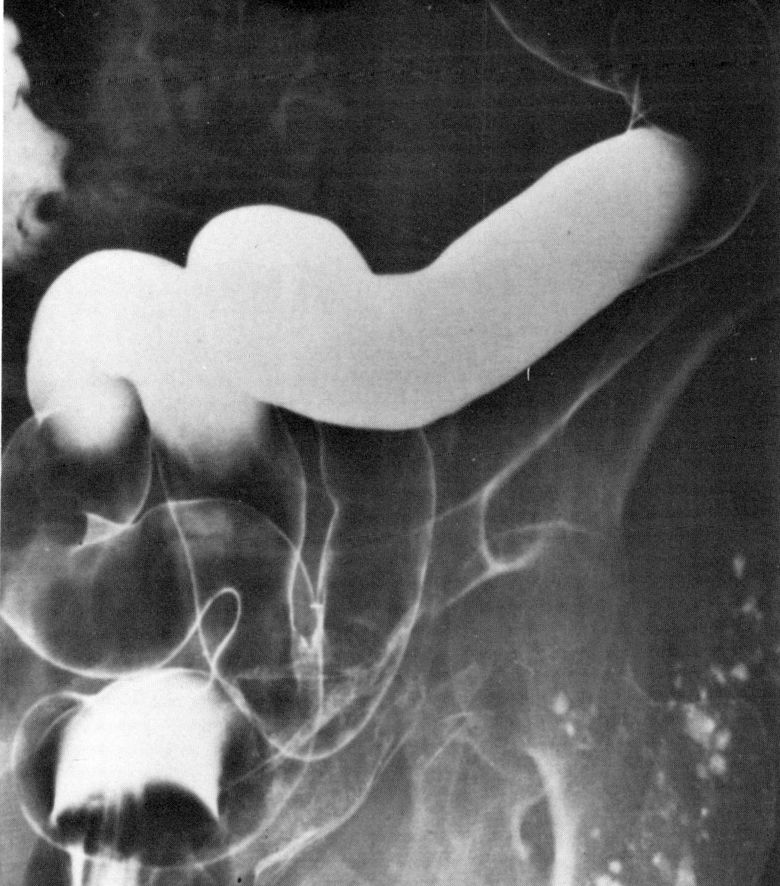

b

Fig. G.5. For legend see page 71.

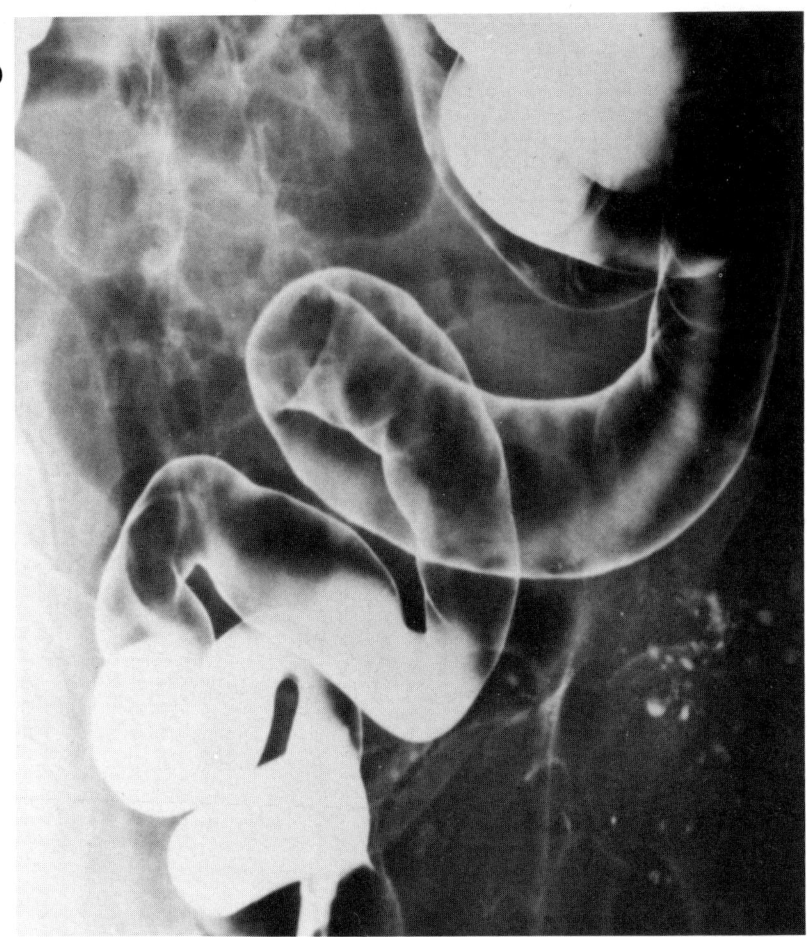

c

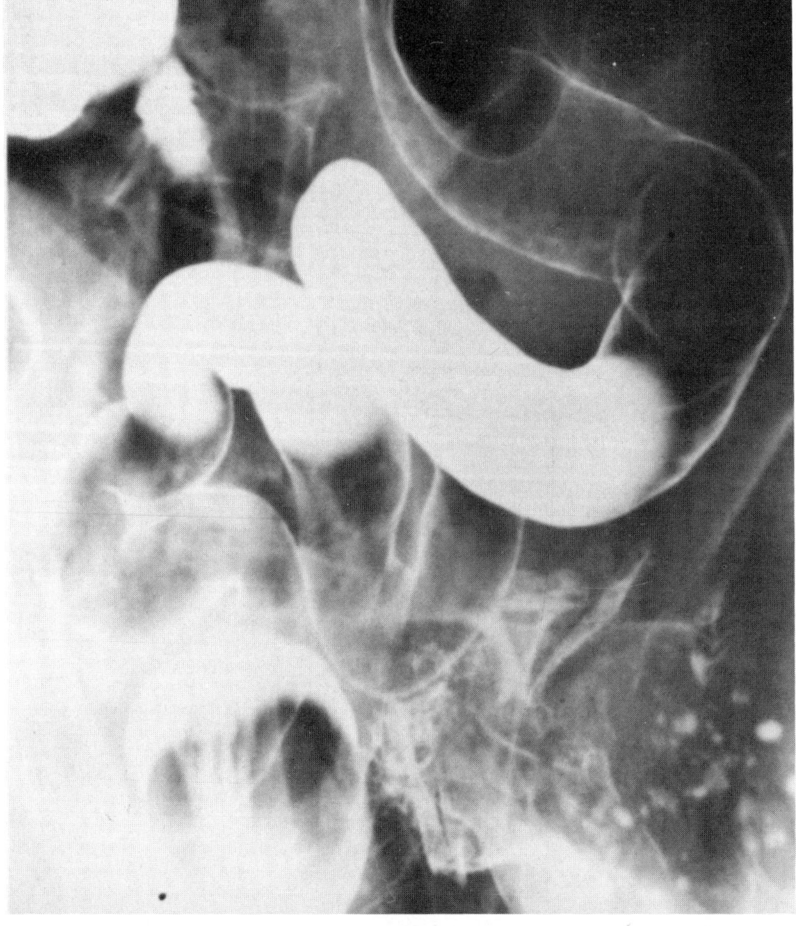

d

Fig. G.5.

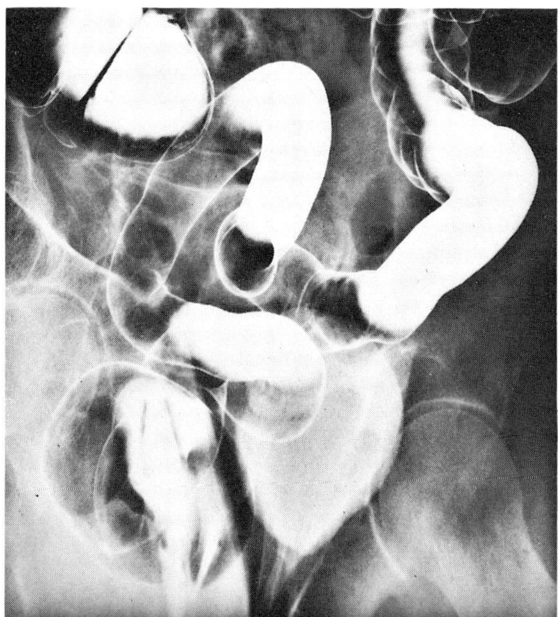

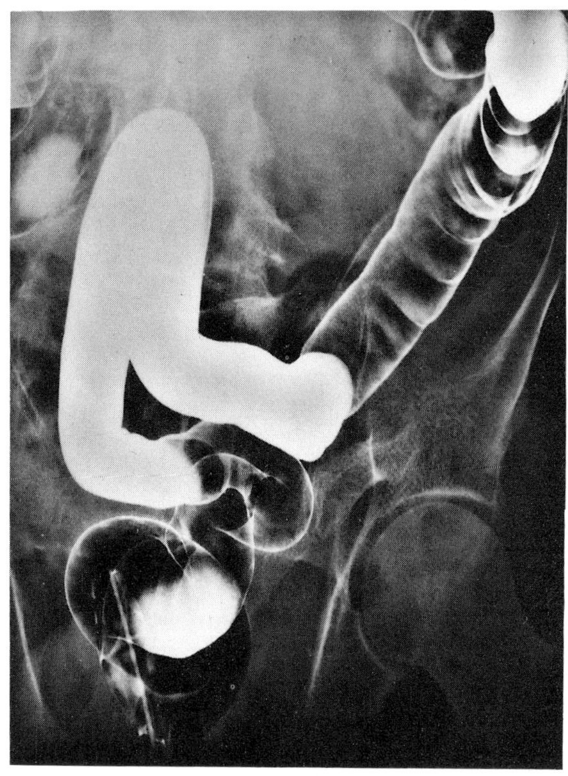

Fig. G.6. (a) The prone 15° RAO–35° x-ray tube angulation ('prone angled-oblique') radiograph shows barium pooling in several loops of bowel. (b) The supine 15° radiograph shows that most of the previously barium-filled loops now are seen in double-contrast.

decubitus views also add to the visualization of the sigmoid and should be obtained routinely.

Occasionally a redundant sigmoid is best studied with the bladder distended and the sigmoid thus elevated and 'unraveled' (15, 18). The bladder can be distended by two methods; the patient can ingest a considerable amount of clear fluids beforehand, or the bladder can be catheterized and enough fluid instilled to produce adequate distension. Both of these methods have their disadvantages and probably should be used very infrequently.

d. Descending colon

The left colon is best seen on the right lateral decubitus and right posterior oblique (RPO) radiographs. In the right lateral decubitus position the left colon tends to distend and is essentially free of barium pooling, aside from barium trapped within haustra. Similarly, in the right posterior oblique (RPO) position the left colon is uppermost in position and tends to distend. The RPO radiograph should be centered so that the splenic flexture is included. Approximately a 20° obliquity appears adequate for most patients (Fig. G.7); a steeper obliquity tends to superimpose the right and left portions of the colon, making interpretation more difficult. The right lateral decubitus view is also of importance in visualizing the rectum and sigmoid and it should be centered so that the bottom of the radiograph includes the entire rectum. Both of these radiographs should be obtained after the right lateral rectal radiograph, because with both of these radiographs additional barium drains into the rectum and obscures adequate visualization of the rectosigmoid.

Fig. G.5. An illustration of how patient positioning aids in unraveling the colon. (a) P–A prone view with the x-ray tube angled 35° caudad. (b) A–P supine view with the x-ray tube angled 35° cephalad. (a) and (b) are complementary views 180° apart. (c) The patient has been obliqued into a 15° RAO position (with respect to the table) and the x-ray tube is angled 35° caudad.The sigmoid colon is slightly more unraveled. (d) 15° LPO position and 35° cephalad tube angulation. (c) and (d) are complementary views 180° apart. In general, the angled x-ray views with the patient obliqued 15° tend to be superior to the non-obliqued views (either PA or AP). Technically, however, the angled oblique views are more difficult to obtain. (From Peterson and Miller (7); Copyright; RSNA, 1978.)

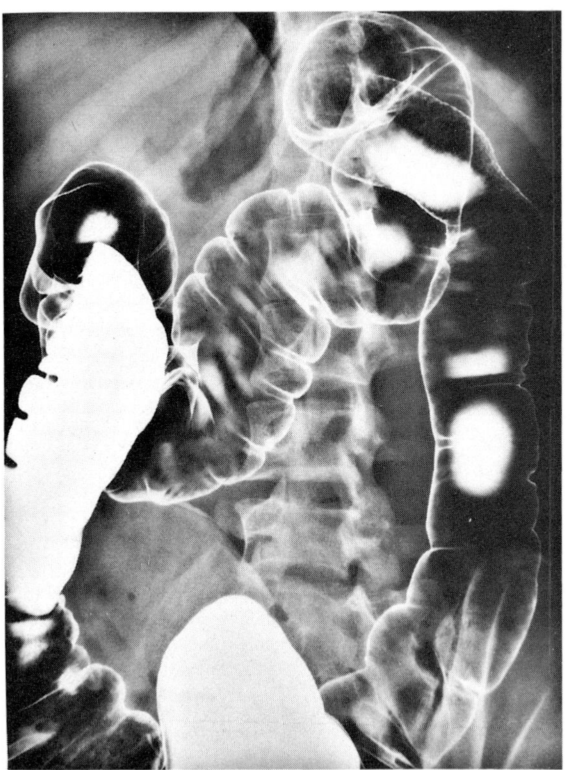

e. Transverse colon

In any well-controlled barium enema examination the transverse colon and both flexures are usually the easiest parts to study. The best views of these areas are taken with the patient erect. Both flexures can be radiographed on appropriate spot films with the patient erect and obliqued just enough to open up the flexures. Although ideally an overhead large format radiograph should be obtained with the patient erect, not all fluoroscopic installations have such a capability.

Because the transverse colon lies far anterior and is quite mobile, with the patient in the upright position the mid-transverse colon can fall into the pelvis. Barium both proximal and distal to this segment then drains into the most dependent loop, obscuring a portion of the transverse colon. Thus, to visualize this area a supine radiograph of the abdomen should be obtained, with centering so that

Fig. G.7. Right posterior oblique (RPO) radiograph showing the splenic flexure and descending colon.

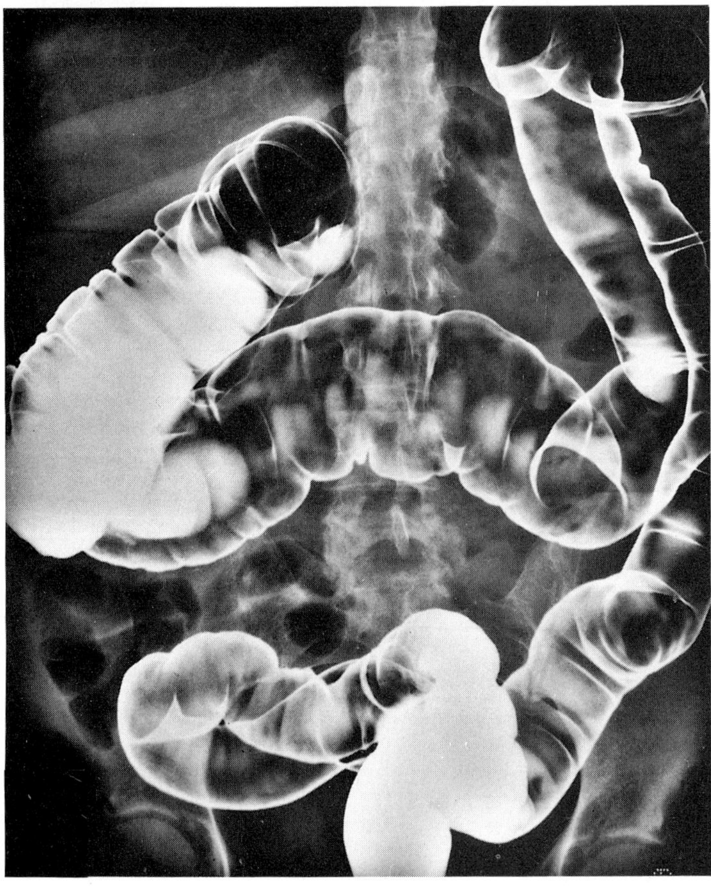

Fig. G.8. Supine antero-posterior radiograph of the transverse colon. In obese patients the cassette should be placed cross-wise.

both flexures are included on the radiograph (Fig. G.8). Also, the two decubitus radiographs usually cover the transverse colon. If there is an extra redundant loop in the proximal transverse colon, the left posterior oblique (LPO) position can be of value. This radiograph is best obtained with the patient in a 45° oblique position (7) (Fig. G.9). If for some reason there is too much barium within the transverse colon, the patient can be turned briefly on the left side just before this radiograph is obtained.

f. Ascending colon

The ascending colon and cecum are usually well seen on the left lateral decubitus radiograph. However, this radiograph does not cover the medial portion of the cecum because there often is a considerable amount of retained barium in the right colon. The right lateral decubitus radiograph, however, usually covers the medial side of the cecum (Fig. G.10). The most important factor in visualizing the right colon is to have the right amount of barium present. With too much barium, an inadequate double-contrast examination results. If there is not enough barium and the mucosa is not coated adequately, a lesion may be missed.

The ascending colon is usually well seen on the LPO radiograph; unfortunately, on this radiograph the cecum is quite often overlapped by the sigmoid. An upright spot radiograph of the ascending colon can be helpful.

We usually obtain several spot radiographs of the cecum with the patient in various LPO projections, using fluoroscopic guidance for optimal positioning (Fig. F.11). These radiographs are obtained before the patient is stood up, thus minimizing excessive amounts of barium in the cecum. If there is too much barium in the cecum, turning the patient into a left lateral decubitus or even an LAO projection can drain some barium from the cecum. Having the patient in the Trendelenberg position also helps, although some fluoroscopic tables are not adapted for adequate Trendelenberg tilting.

g. Terminal ileum

A double-contrast examination of the terminal ileum can be readily performed in the vast majority of patients. If evaluation of distal ileum is deemed necessary, it is helpful to add more barium than usual into the right colon. Because the ileo-cecal valve is generally posterior and medial in the wall of the right colon, it is usually sufficient to simply have

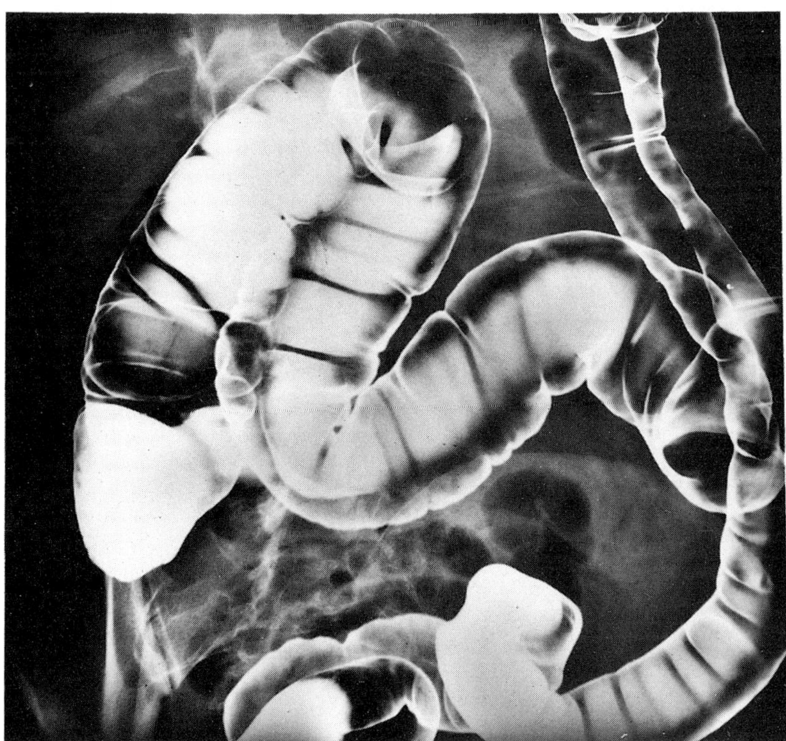

Fig. G.9. 45° left posterior oblique (LPO) projection. The radiograph is centered so that the entire hepatic flexure is included.

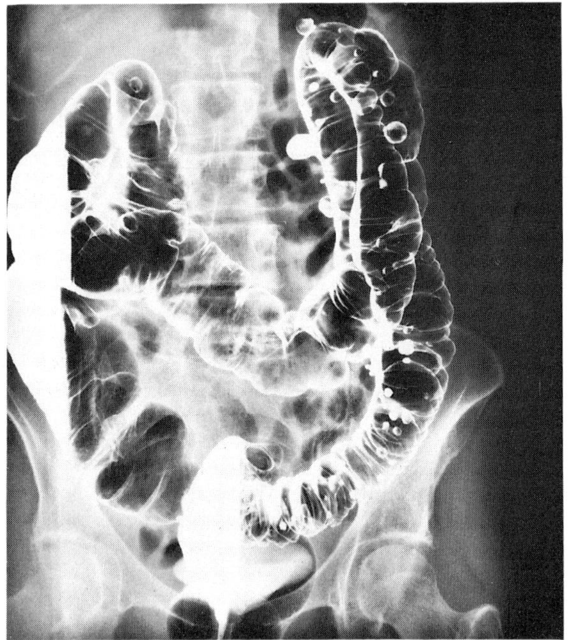

a

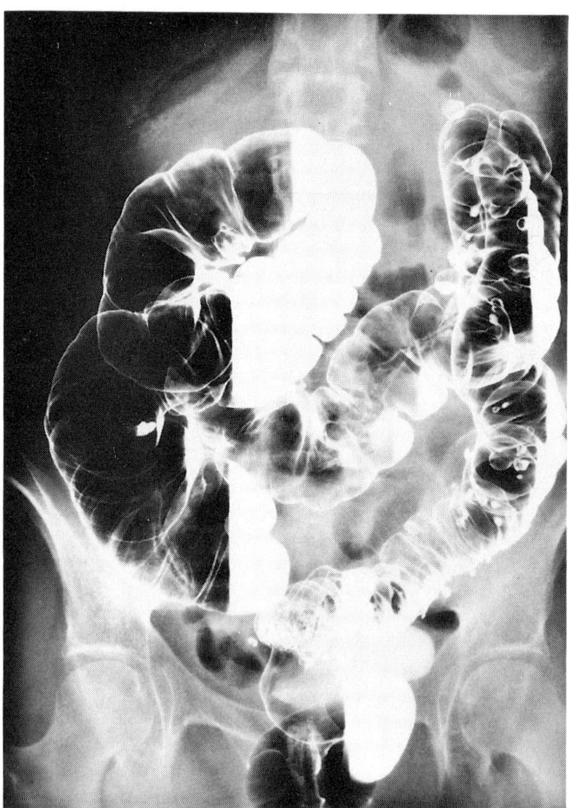

b

Fig. G.10. (a) Right lateral decubitus radiograph. (b) Left lateral decubitus radiograph. These two radiographs are the most diagnostic and most important in the entire examination. A larger portion of the colon is visualized on these two radiographs than on any other. They should be centered so that the rectum is included. The descending colon may be collapsed on the left lateral decubitus radiograph but the opposite decubitus radiograph should open this segment.

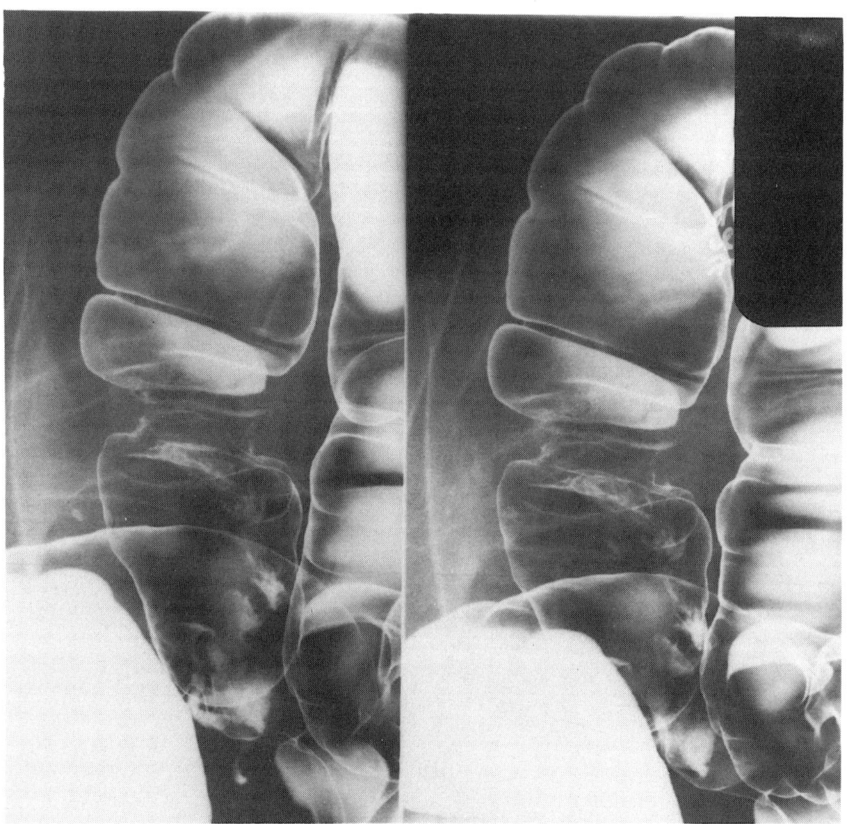

Fig. G.11. 2-on-1 radiograph of the cecum. These two views of the cecum are generally obtained in slightly different projections. At this point in the examination, reflux of barium into the terminal ileum is generally present and a double-contrast evaluation of the terminal ileum is possible.

barium adjacent to the valve for reflux to occur. If there is still no reflux into the terminal ileum after the overhead radiographs have been obtained, massaging the right colon can help relax the valve and induce spillage into the terminal ileum. If necessary, additional air added at this time helps push extra barium into the ileum.

h. Sequence of filming

The above-described radiographs cannot be obtained in a random or haphazard manner; if this were done, there would be considerable variation in the overall quality of examinations.

When the radiologist completes the initial part of the examination by filling the colon with barium and air, the patient should be in a prone position and any excess barium in the rectum should be drained out. Colon distension is double-checked fluoroscopically. The technologist then obtains a prone radiograph, using a vertical x-ray beam centered so the rectum is at the bottom of the radiograph. Such centering can be achieved by placing the lowest part of the cassette approximately 2 or 3 cm below the gluteal folds.

Next, the angled sigmoid view should be obtained. This can either be a straight angled sigmoid (with the x-ray tube angled 30° caudad) or an angled-oblique view (with the patient obliqued into a 15° RAO position in addition to angling the tube 30° caudad). The x-ray tube, however, must still be kept at 100 cm above the plane of the cassette in order to prevent grid cut-off (19). For the angled-oblique radiograph, both legs of the patient should be kept extended; if the right thigh is flexed, as taught by some, the additional soft tissues of the right hip will be superimposed over the pelvis, adding to scatter degradation.

If the prone oblique radiographs (RAO and LAO) are being obtained, the technologist next centers the x-ray beam vertically and places the bottom of the cassette at the gluteal folds. In the average patient these two views probably can be eliminated unless there is a specific interest in the areas covered.

The patient is then placed in the right lateral position and a 24 × 30 cm (10 × 12 in.) radiograph of the rectum obtained. A 35 × 43 cm (14 × 17 in.) radiograph is rarely useful for this view because of marked bowel superimposition; in fact, the large film simply adds considerable scatter radiation and results in image degradation.

The patient is then turned into a 20° RPO position and the cassette is centered so that the upper edge of the cassette is superior to the splenic flexure. The x-ray beam is centered slightly towards the left of midline. This view is primarily for the splenic flexure and descending colon and thus the cassette should not be turned cross-wise even with an obese patient, because that would only obscure a part of the descending colon.

The patient then lies supine and an A–P radiograph is obtained with a vertical x-ray beam and the cassette centered over the flexures and transverse colon. In obese patients, the cassette is turned transversely for this view in order to visualize both flexures on the same radiograph.

The patient is then turned further into a 45° LPO position and a radiograph of the hepatic flexure and the right colon obtained. Here the film is centered towards the right side of the patient in order to include the hepatic flexure. The cassette should not be turned transversely because quite often the rectum and portions of sigmoid are also included.

If the installation permits, the patient is then placed in a 15° LPO position, the x-ray tube angled 35° cranially, and a supine angled-oblique view obtained. This angled-oblique radiograph is 180° rotated from the standard prone angled-oblique radiograph obtained earlier in the examination. Thus areas which were filled with barium on the prone angled-oblique view are now seen in double-contrast.

The patient is then turned into a right lateral decubitus position and a horizontal x-ray beam is used to obtain the decubitus view. The bottom of the cassette is centered at the gluteal folds so that the rectosigmoid is included on this radiograph. Lastly, the patient is turned into a left lateral decubitus position with similar centering and a corresponding radiograph obtained. If there has been no prior reflux of barium into the terminal ileum reflux generally results with the patient in this position.

While the technologist is obtaining the above radiographs, the radiologist can either be performing another examination or monitoring the radiographs as they are being developed. We generally do not wait for the last decubitus radiographs to be developed but as soon as the technologist is finished with the overhead radiographs we obtain a 2-on-1 spot compression radiograph of the cecum with the patient in an LPO position. The degree of obliquity depends on the relative position of the cecum. If the sigmoid had been insufficiently visualized on the initial overhead radiograph, a spot radiograph with the patient in an LPO position is now obtained (Fig. G.12).

The x-ray table is then brought upright and radiographs of the flexures and mid-transverse colon are obtained with the patient upright (Fig. G.13). The degree of obliquity required for the flexures varies depending on the patient's anatomy.

The x-ray table is then lowered, the patient turned on the left side, the enema tubing unclamped and barium and air drained back into the enema bag. If there was any question about adequate visualization of the rectum, the rectal balloon can be deflated, the enema tubing clamped, enough air added to distend the rectum, and then the enema tube removed and double-contrast radiographs of the rectum obtained.

At this point the radiologist examines all of the films to determine if all parts of the colon have been adequately studied and whether additional radiographs are necessary. Only after inspecting all of the radiographs should the patient leave the department.

Although the above description appears complicated, the sequence of steps is quite logical and most beginning radiology residents and technologists master the sequence within several days.

A postevacuation radiograph is of considerable importance in a full column barium enema; we are not sure whether a similar useful function is served with a double-contrast enema. Several years ago we stopped obtaining postevacuation radiographs *routinely* after a double-contrast enema and currently reserve this option only for selected patients where a view of the collapsed colon would be useful, such as reflux into unfilled loops of small bowel, suspected fistula, or evaluation of adjacent structures.

A summary of the views we currently recommend for adequate study of the colon is outlined in Table G.1. Although a large lesion can be seen readily on many views of the colon, we believe that an adequate examination in the majority of patients re-

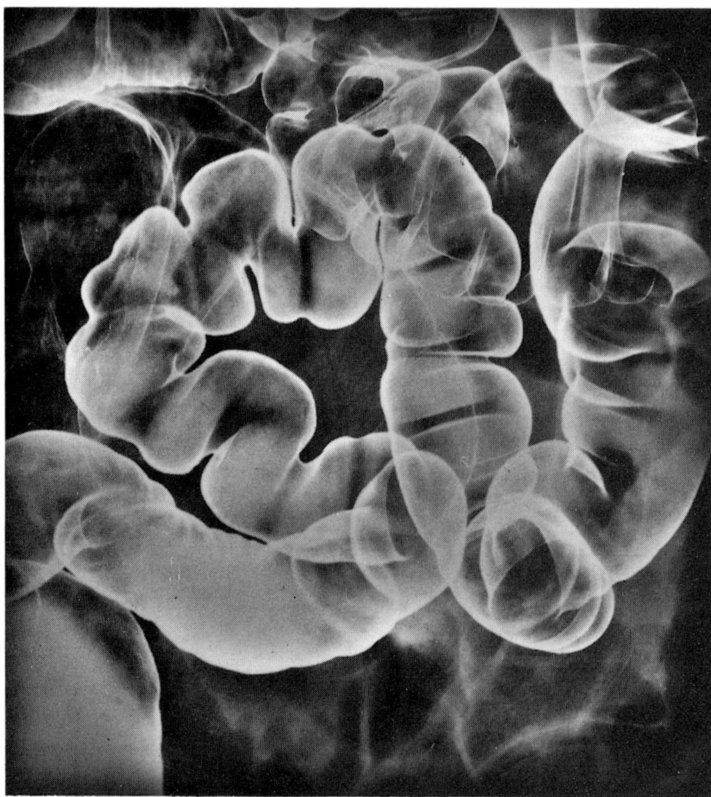

Fig. G.12. Spot radiograph of the sigmoid colon obtained at the end of the examination to clear a suspicious area seen on previous radiographs. Fluoroscopy was used to obtain the desired obliquity.

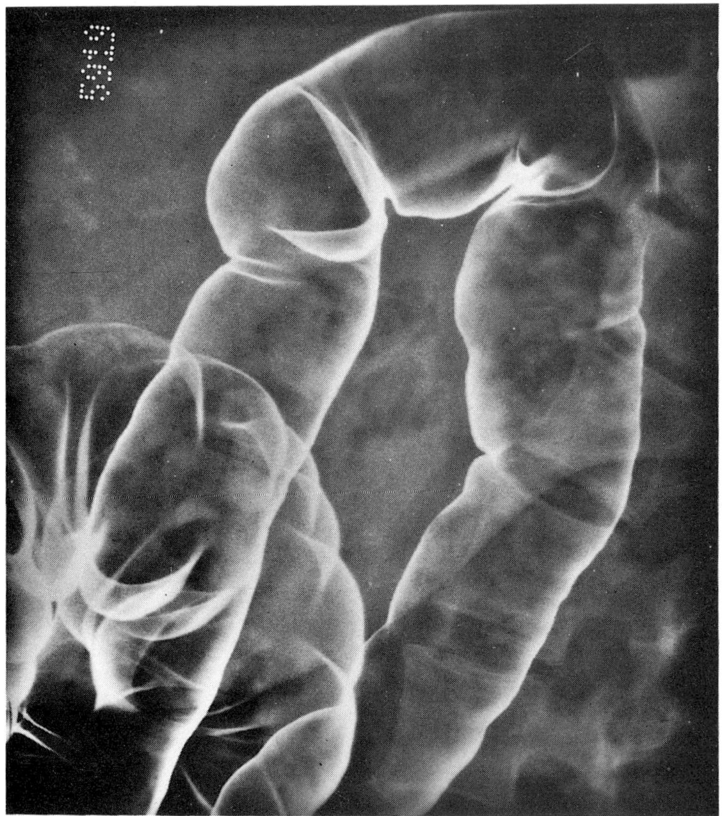

a

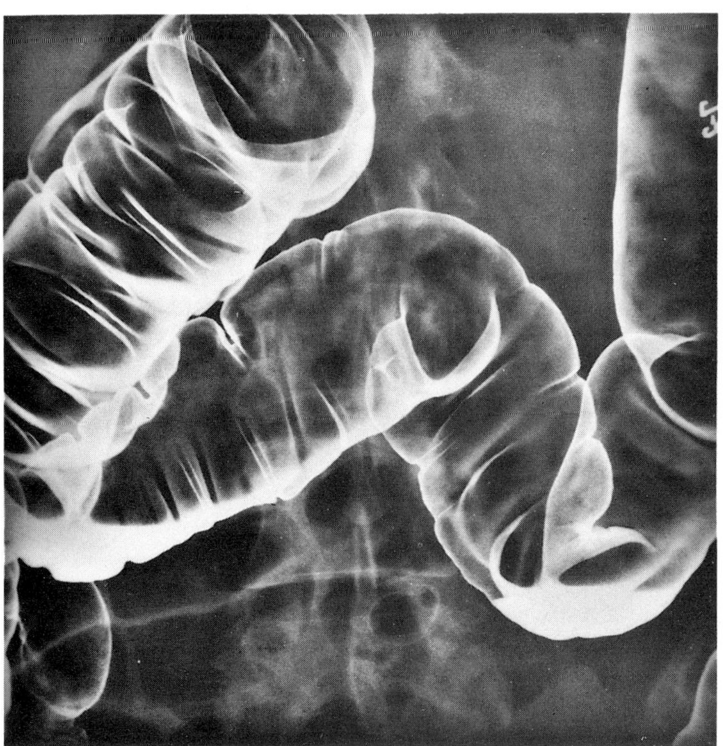

b

Fig. G.13. Upright spot radiographs. (a) Splenic flexure. The patient is in a RPO position. The obliquity is such that the flexure is 'unwound'. (b) Mid-transverse colon. The patient is flat against the x-ray table. (c) Hepatic flexure. In order to 'unwind' the flexure the patient had to be turned into a steep LPO position. Although the hepatic flexure is superimposed upon a portion of the left colon, the double-contrast allows adequate evaluation.

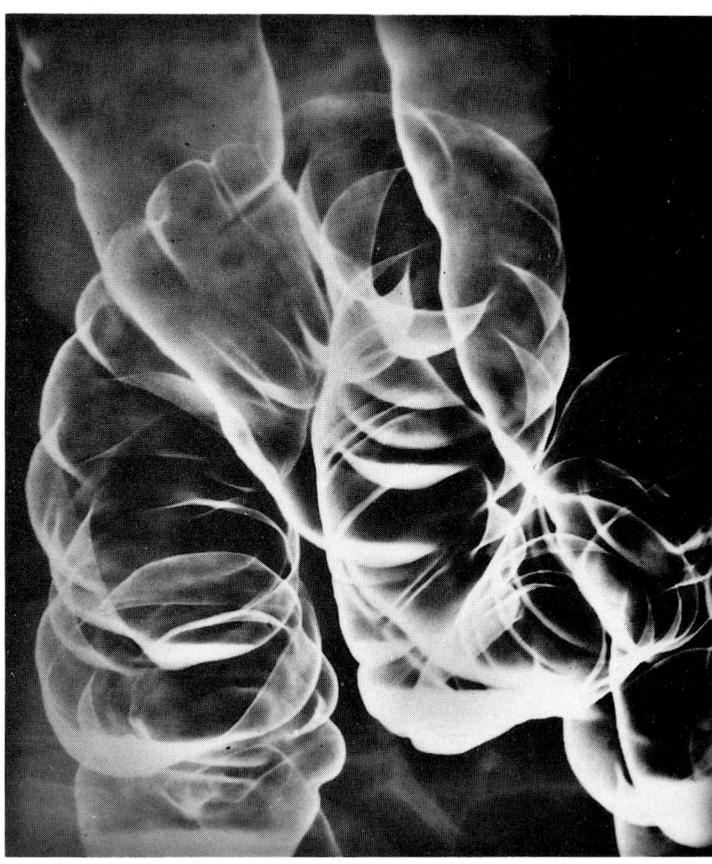

*Fig. G.13.***c.**

Table G.1. Recommended sequence of radiographs obtained.

Sequence	Patient position	X-ray tube angulation	X-ray beam orientation	Film size	Film centering
1	Prone	None	Vertical	35 × 43 cm	Must include rectum
2 (a)	Prone	30° caudad	Oblique	35 × 43	Must include rectum
(b)	15° RAO	30° caudad	Oblique	35 × 43	Must include rectum
3	R. lateral	None	Vertical	24 × 30	Rectum
4	20° RPO	None	Vertical	35 × 43	Must include splenic flexure
5	Supine	None	Vertical	35 × 43	Must include both flexures
6	45° LPO	None	Vertical	35 × 43	Must include hepatic flexure
7	15° LPO	30° cranial	Oblique	35 × 43	Must include recto-sigmoid
8	R. lat.	None	Horizontal	35 × 43	Must include rectum
9	L. lat.	None	Horizontal	35 × 43	Must include rectum
10	LPO	None	Vertical	Spot-film	Cecum
11	Upright LPO	None	Horizontal	Spot-film	Hepatic flexure
12	Upright straight	None	Horizontal	Spot-film	Transverse colon
13	Upright RPO	None	Horizontal	Spot-film	Splenic flexure

Notes:

1. If the prone oblique radiographs are being obtained they should be taken prior to the right lateral radiograph (#3).
2. Usually either the angled (#2a) or the angled-oblique radiograph (#2b) is obtained. Occasionally with a very redundant sigmoid both are helpful.
3. Quite often the supine radiograph (#5) can be omitted, because the transverse colon is covered later by spot-radiographs.
4. If necessary, additional views of the rectum can be obtained last.

quires at least eight overhead radiographs and at least four spot radiographs. With colon redundancy, even more radiographs are obviously necessary. This number of radiographs is less than what we had been advocating in the past (20, 21). We believe that if the number of radiographs is cut back significantly, a number of early lesions will be missed. The proposed procedure is a modification of Welin's two stage technique and results in a considerably shorter one stage method. Other investigators, especially in Europe, cut back the number of radiographs obtained even further (22).

References

1. Rosengren J-E, Lindström CG: Experimental colonic tumors in the rat. II. Double contrast examination and microscopy. Acta Radiol 19:465–478, 1977.
2. Thoeni RF, Margulis AR: The state of radiographic technique in the examination of the colon: a survey. Radiology 127:317–323, 1978.
3. Eisenberg RL, Hedgcock MW: Preliminary radiograph for barium enema examination: is it necessary? AJR 136:115–116, 1981.
4. Harned RK, Wolf GL, Williams SM: Preliminary abdominal films for gastrointestinal examinations: how efficacious? Gastrointest Radiol 5:343–347, 1980.
5. Teplick SK, Stark P, Clark RE, Metz JR, Shapiro JH: The retrorectal space. Clin Radiol 29:177–184, 1978.
6. Niizuma S, Kobayashi S: Rectosigmoid double contrast examination in the prone position with a horizontal beam. AJR 128:519–520, 1977.
7. Peterson GH, Miller RE: The barium enema: a reassessment looking toward perfection. Radiology 128:315–320, 1978.
8. Chassard M, Lapiné M: Étude radiographique de l'arcade pubienne chez la femme enceinte; une nouvelle méthode d'appréciation du diamètre bi-ischiatique. J Radiol Electrol 7:113–124, 1923.
9. Rapp G: A position of value in studying the pelvis and its contents. South Med J 44:95–99, 1951.
10. Ettinger A, Elkin M: Study of the sigmoid by special roentgenographic views. AJR 72:199–208, 1954.
11. Dysart D, Stewart HR: Special angled roentgenography for lesions of the rectosigmoid. AJR 96:285–291, 1966.
12. Wener L: The angle prone projection: its value in diagnosis of low-lying lesions. AJR 110:393–398, 1970.
13. Perl T, Goldman W: Unraveling the tangled sigmoid: routine angulation of the tube in the detection of occult lesions. AJR 110:399–405, 1970.
14. Brown RC, Cohen WN: A new projection for demonstrating the sigmoid colon. J Can Assoc Radiol 21:27–30, 1970.
15. Fletcher GH: An improved method of visualization of the sigmoid. AJR 59:750–752, 1948.
16. Stewart WH, Illick HE: A method of more clearly visualizing lesions of the sigmoid. AJR 28:379–384, 1932.
17. Wolf A: Das Rektum und das untere Zigmoid. Fortschr Geb Roentgenstr 42:358–363, 1930.
18. Billing L: Zur Technik der Kontrastuntersuchung des Colon sigmoideum. Acta Radiol 25:418–422, 1944.
19. Christensen EE, Bull KW, Dowdey JE: Grid cutoff with oblique radiographic techniques. Radiology 111:473–474, 1974.
20. Miller RE: Examination of the colon. Curr Prob Radiol 5(2):3–40, 1975.
21. Miller RE: Die vollständige Colonuntersuchung. Radiologe 15:410–420, 1975.
22. Dihlmann W: Die ökonomisch-standardisierte Kontraströntgenuntersuchung des Kolons beim Erwachsenen. Deutsch Med Wochenschr 105:1138–1141, 1980.

I.2.H. Colostomy enema

Encountered occasionally is a patient with extensive pelvic malignancy and secondary colon involvement where the distal colon and rectum have been resected. If these patients subsequently develop signs and symptoms referrable to the remaining portion of the colon, a barium enema must be performed through the colostomy. Likewise, those patients who have had partial distal colonic resection, due to colon malignancy or other reasons, need follow-up examination of the remaining portion of the colon on a serial basis.

In the future the need for a permanent colostomy should decrease; rectal stapling now allows the surgeon to successfully anastomose bowel even if the resection margin is in the mid-rectum.

The radiographic appearance after partial colon resection reflects the residual anatomy. It is extremely helpful to know the particular resection and anastomosis performed beforehand; the subsequent examination can then be tailored accordingly (1). The same radiographic criteria apply to these patients whether a single-contrast or a double-contrast examination is performed, although a double-contrast examination discloses far more detail. The shorter the length of the residual colon, the easier it is to perform a double-contrast barium enema. During the double-contrast examination barium in the colon flows primarily by gravity; therefore, throughout most of the examination the patient should lie on the right side. When a sufficient amount of barium has reached the right side of the colon, the patient is turned slightly prone or the table is elevated to aid filling the cecum.

The greatest difficulty in performing *any* barium enema on a patient with a colostomy is to ensure an adequate seal at the stoma. The simplest method is to use a Foley balloon catheter, with the balloon blown up beforehand to its maximum diameter.

The protruding catheter tip is then inserted into the colostomy stoma and the patient holds the balloon pressed tightly against the stoma. If the patient has a descending or transverse colostomy, we generally have the patient use their left hand to hold the balloon in place; the subsequent radiographs will contain an image of the overlying right arm if the right hand is used.

It should be emphasized that a balloon should not be inflated inside a colostomy. Invariably at the stoma there is fibrosis and scarring resulting in poor distensibility. In addition, occasionally one encounters a patient with acute disease, such as regional enteritis, involving the residual colon up to the stoma. In either case, a balloon inflated inside the stoma can readily perforate and lead to peritonitis.

The fact that such a simple method as a balloon catheter is not always successful is attested by the many mechanical devices available on the market for the performance of a colostomy enema. These devices include mechanical 'plugs', specially developed catheters, and externally applied suction cups. Some radiologists have found the patient's own irrigation device (2) or a stoma irrigation bag (3) adequate for the barium enema. A colostomy enema tip can be adapted to a Miller double-contrast barium enema tip (Fig. H.1). An alternative method is to use a large, soft, rubber catheter containing several side holes, with the catheter being inserted through an infant feeding nipple which has its tip cut off (4). The catheter should slide freely through the nipple, yet the junction should still be tight enough to provide a seal with little leakage. With the patient either lying down or sitting up the catheter is inserted into the colostomy stoma. The feeding nipple is then pushed down against the stoma and the patient is asked to hold the nipple tight against the stoma to prevent spillage. Some radiologists prefer a right-angle tube rather than a straight catheter; a collar held tightly against the skin prevents leakage (5). Others have devised large solid cylinders, using vacuum to hold the appliance in place (6).

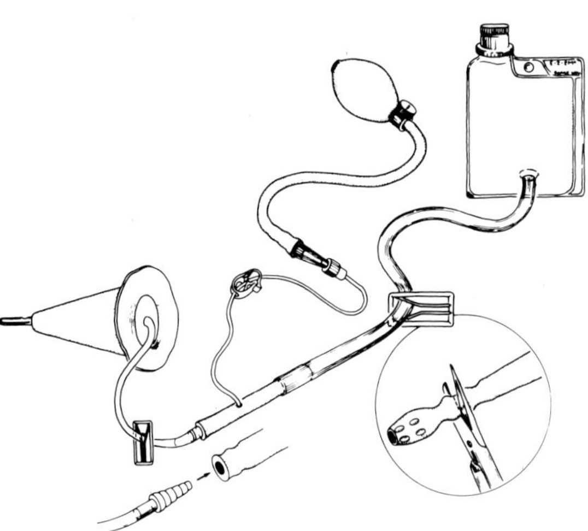

Fig. H.1. Double-contrast barium enema through a colostomy can be performed by cutting off the end of the Miller air tip and connecting a colostomy tip. Barium can be instilled through the large bore tubing while air is added through the smaller caliber tubing.

A double-contrast barium enema in a patient with a colostomy should result in approximately one-half of the remaining colon being filled with barium. Because the patient is supine or on the right side, generally it is not feasible to drain out any significant amount of barium. We start adding air after the colon has been half-filled with barium, using a sphygmomanometer bulb attached to the catheter through a large bore needle. Air is initially added with the patient lying on the right side and in this position air will force barium into the most dependent portion of the colon, which is the cecum (Fig. H.2). If the cecum does not fill readily with the patient on the right side, the patient should be turned into an RAO position and the cecum will usually fill. Ideally, the prone position is best for filling the cecum, although this position is difficult for patients with a colostomy.

The radiographs obtained depend upon the length and tortuosity of the residual colon. If the patient has had a descending colostomy, we routinely obtain supine, RPO, LPO, and right lateral decubitus overhead films. Although a left lateral decubitus radiograph would also be very useful, turning the patient on the left side at this point is an invitation to barium spillage on the table. Following the right lateral decubitus radiograph, the patient is stood up and oblique radiographs of both flexures and the transverse colon are obtained. Views of the cecum can be taken either before or after standing the patient up, depending upon the amount of barium present. As an aid in gauging colon evacuation, a post-drainage radiograph is at times useful.

Barium study through an ileostomy can be performed in a similar manner to that described above. Generally the patient can insert the catheter into the stoma more easily than the radiologist, since most patients are usually quite adept at irrigating the stoma. Although a double-contrast barium enema is also readily performed through an ileostomy, if long segments of the small bowel must be studied we prefer a single-contrast retrograde enema, since when using the latter procedure the latter procedure the patient simply lies supine and contrast flows proximally solely by gravity.

The colon segment distal to a double-barreled colostomy must also be studied occasionally. This distal segment is best approached through the rectum rather than through the stoma (mucous fistula). Such a retrograde approach allows more distension and results in better visualization of the anatomy. An exception is when the retrograde approach reveals complete obstruction. If knowledge of the proximal extent of the obstruction is desired, then contrast instilled through the mucous fistula will outline the proximal margin of the obstruction. Although barium sulfate can probably be used safely in a mucous fistula, we generally use one of the water soluble iodinated contrast agents. Our reasoning, although only theoretical, is that barium proximal to an obstruction may inspissate since water is absorbed even from an unused colon segment. Such inspissation should not occur with the water soluble agents.

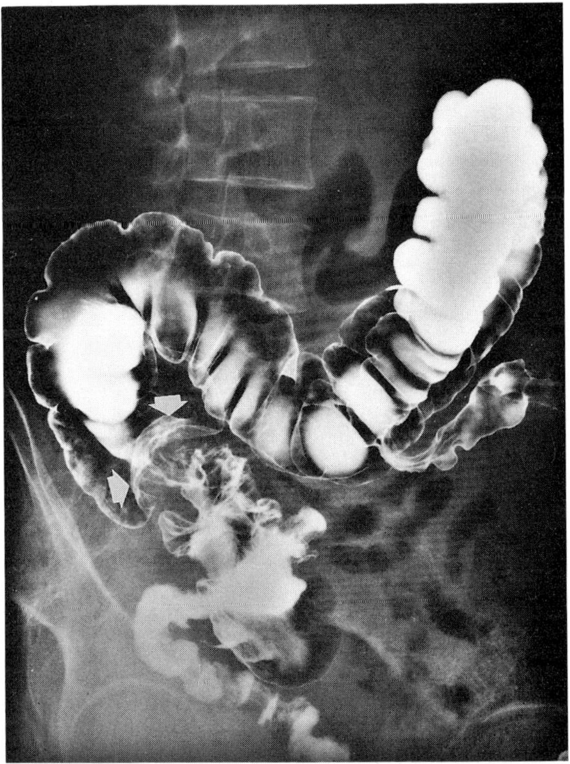

Fig. H.2. Barium enema through a descending colostomy. Through appropriate positioning the entire colon and terminal ileum have been filled. There is a circumferential carcinoma in the ascending colon (arrowheads). The patient previously had rectosigmoid resection for a carcinoma and now has developed a metachronous cancer.

References

1. Nahum H, Fékété F, Margulis AR: Radiology of the Postoperative Digestive Tract, pp 75–89. Masson, New York, 1979.
2. Burhenne HJ: Technique of colostomy examination. Radiology 97:183–185, 1970.
3. Bartow JH, Rao BR: Simplified barium enema examination via colostomy. AJR 135:1302–1303, 1980.
4. Goldstein HM, Miller MH: Air contrast colon examination in patients with colostomies. AJR 127:607–610, 1976.
5. Chabouis CF, Mordy M, Desoutter P: Sonde pour lavement baryte en double contraste chez les colostomies. J Radiol 62:275–276, 1981.
6. Sarashina H, Ozaki A, Fukao K, Takase Y, Todoroki T, Nagoshi K, Ohshima M, Kawakita I, Iwasaki Y: A new device for barium-enema examination following colostomy. Radiology 133:241–242, 1979.

I.2.I. Complications

a. Introduction

Although a barium enema is a very safe examination having a high diagnostic yield, complications do occur even in the best of hands (1). Some of the complications which occurred in the past, however, may have been prevented if the radiologist had paid closer attention to the indication for the examination, the clinical condition of the patient, and more meticulous attention to the technical detail during performance of the examination. Some radiologists are lulled into a false sense of security because they encounter relatively few complications. Yet these complications may leave the patient permanently crippled for life or lead to death (2).

The incidence of perforation is difficult to gauge; it has ranged from one in 2250 (3) to as few as one in 12,000 studies (4). The reported series may be biased through patient selection and any one report may not reflect the incidence accurately.

The barium sulfate used in commercial preparations has a low solubility and is generally considered 'safe'. Inadvertent substitution of soluble barium salts for the essentially insoluble barium sulfate should not occur, yet there still are occasional reports, often from Third World countries, of such substitutions (5). Poisoning with soluble barium salts has included such compounds as barium sulfide (6), barium carbonate (7), barium polysulfide (8), and barium chloride (9). These patients may present with hypokalemia, profound muscle weakness, and they may develop hypertension unresponsive to phentolamine (10). There is an intracellular movement of potassium resulting in an increased erythrocyte potassium level (10). Sulfhemoglobin may be found (8). Respiratory acidosis may develop if the respiratory muscles become involved. Death can result even with the ingestion of small amounts of an inappropriate substance. Therapy should consist of adequate intravenous potassium replacement, vigorous diuresis, and if the patient requires, assisted ventilation.

Barium impaction is a possibility in patients with chronic constipation or if large amounts of barium are instilled proximal to a stenosis. These patients must thus be individualized and the examination terminated as soon as the diagnosis is obtained, without adding excessive amounts of barium proximal to a stricture. Currently, most commercial barium sulfate products used contain carboxymethylcellulose and other suspending agents, and do not dry out readily, thus presenting a decreased danger of impaction. Although a few radiologists still routinely recommend a mild laxative after a barium enema (11), most do not.

At times there is massive reflux into the small bowel. Reflux into the stomach with vomiting and aspiration can occur. Small bowel reflux, however, is of no significance; in fact, the reflux small bowel examination is specifically designed to reflux most or even all of the small bowel (12, 13) (Fig. I.1).

A complication may be due to an error in technique or to underlying disease, such as anal fissure, ulcer, cryptitis, tumor, or one of the colitides. Some complications may be preventable while others are not. Complications, together with ways of preventing them, are best discussed by considering each type and the factors which cause them separately.

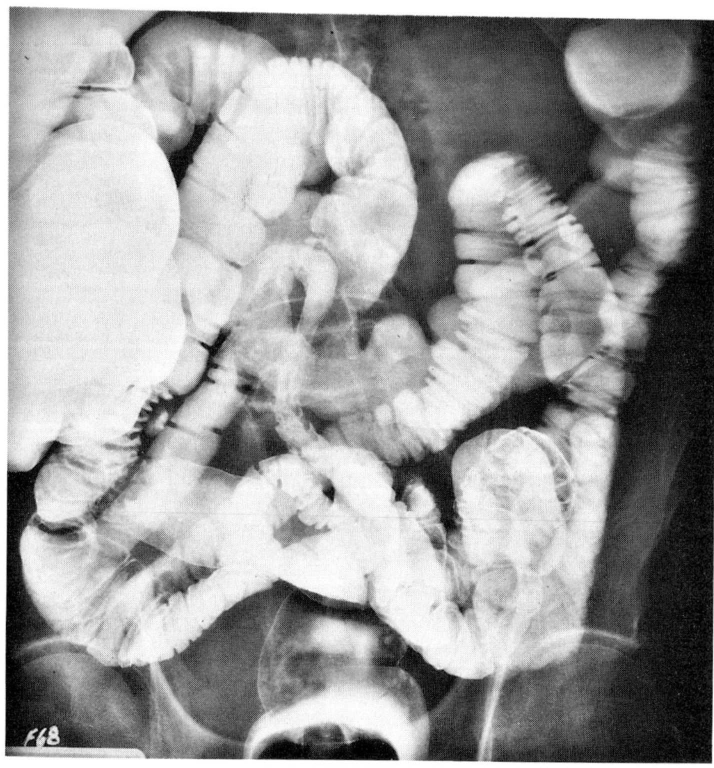

Fig. I.1. Reflux small bowel examination. After adding 2000 ml of barium sulfate, saline was used to reflux barium into the small bowel, resulting in a 'see-through' effect in the colon.

b. Enema tip trauma

The enema tip being used for a barium enema examination or for a tap water enema may lacerate or perforate through the rectum (14, 15), with many of these perforations being along the anterior wall of the rectum. One survey found *extraperitoneal* perforation in 1 out of 40,000 examinations (4). Since these complications are rarely reported they are probably considerably more common than the literature suggests. Some perforations, especially those that are extraperitoneal, may not result in immediate symptoms, with symptoms in some patients appearing only later and after the addition of barium (16). One cannot always count on the patient to complain about a perforation since the rectum above the pectinate line is rather insensitive to pain. Even an experienced fluoroscopist can miss the perforation initially and instill large volumes of barium sulfate into the peritoneal cavity (17).

The trauma can vary from mucosal abrasion, submucosal tear, to complete transmural perforation, with perforations below the peritoneal reflection generally resulting in barium being deposited in the perirectal soft tissues. The lateral view of the rectum, in particular, is best for identifying these extraperitoneal perforations. A rectal laceration, if not recognized and treated, can result in an ischiorectal abscess (18). Barium in the soft tissues surrounding the rectum initially leads to an inflammatory reaction, eventually resulting in fibroblastic proliferation, multinucleated giant cells with refringent intracytoplasmic barium sulfate crystals and extensive fibrosis (16, 19). Such extravasation can lead to indurated, ulcerated rectal masses resembling a carcinoma (20). Some of the barium sulfate may enter lymphatic channels. We are not aware of any documented carcinoma arising at the site of barium granuloma formation. In some patients such an inflammatory reaction and granuloma formation may eventually result in ureteric obstruction (21, 22). The appearance of prior extraperitoneal perforation and barium granuloma perforation can be confusing (23). A biopsy should be diagnostic. Even minute amounts of barium sulfate deposited in the colon wall should be identified by the pathologist because of the crystal shape. The crystals are anisotropic in polarized light.

If the enema tube is incorrectly located in the vagina and barium is instilled, there may be vaginal rupture and intravasation of barium (4). Vaginal rupture is generally because of overinflation of a balloon. Fortunately, rupture is rare, with most instances of incorrectly placed enema tubes resulting simply in an outline of the vagina (Fig. I.2).

c. Perforation due to balloon

A balloon catheter is quite often used to help a patient retain the enema. Some radiologists adopt a cavalier attitude and inflate the balloon without even utilizing fluoroscopic control as guidance. Others allow the technologist to insert the enema tip and inflate the balloon catheter. Fortunately, both of these groups are small, with most radiologists preferring not to inflate the balloon catheter at all, or, if necessary, to inflate the balloon only after some barium has been instilled and then use fluoroscopic guidance (24). Pressure on a syringe does not indicate volume accurately (25); besides, an identical volume cannot possibly be used in all patients. The routine inflation of a balloon in all

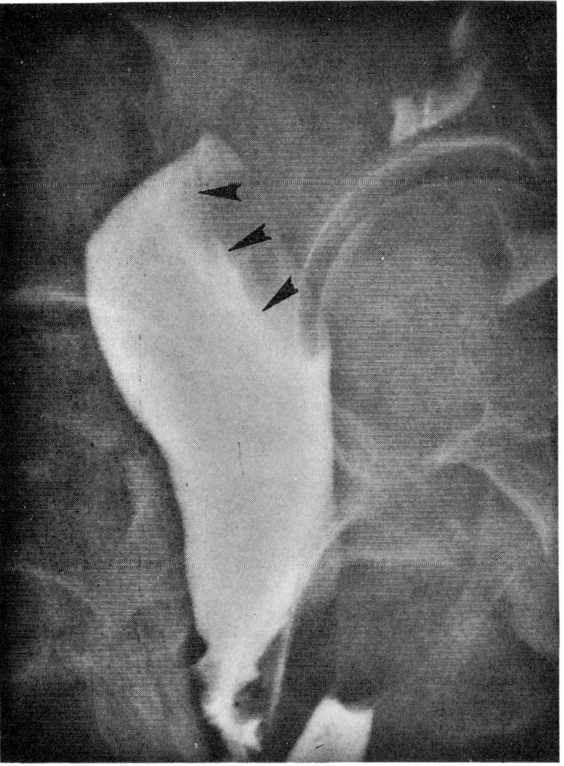

Fig. I.2. Incorrectly placed enema tip in vagina. The cervix presents as a soft tissue mass indenting the superior aspect of the vagina (arrowheads). In this patient the balloon was not inflated, incorrect placement of the enema tip recognized, and no sequellae seen.

patients is bound to increase risk of perforation. Likewise, an inflated balloon may hide a rectal tear or lesion (26). The rectal balloon should be positioned low in the rectum against the anal sphincter.

Colon rupture is associated with balloon overinflation (25). Since most balloons are close to the tip of the catheter, the perforations are generally extraperitoneal, although perforation can occur into the peritoneal cavity at the anteriorly located pouch of Douglas (27). In one series, almost 50% of the colon perforations occurred with the use of a balloon catheter (15). Sometimes the perforation is seen only on the post-evacuation radiographs after the balloon has been deflated and removed; in such instances the inflated balloon may have helped block the perforation, with spillage occurring only after deflation (26) (Fig. I.3).

Extraperitoneal emphysema can occur after extraperitoneal perforation. It is often not known if the perforation resulted from enema tip trauma, an overdistended balloon, underlying bowel disease, or a combination of factors. Although the gas may be reabsorbed leaving few if any sequelae, the nature of the injury is similar to perforation and subsequent barium spillage. Extraperitoneal perforation of the rectosigmoid during a double-contrast barium enema may result not only in air in the extraperitoneal tissues, but also in air tracking into the chest producing pneumomediastinum (28). The emphysema may extend into the neck (29). In some patients follow-up sigmoidoscopy has been normal, with no site of perforation being identified.

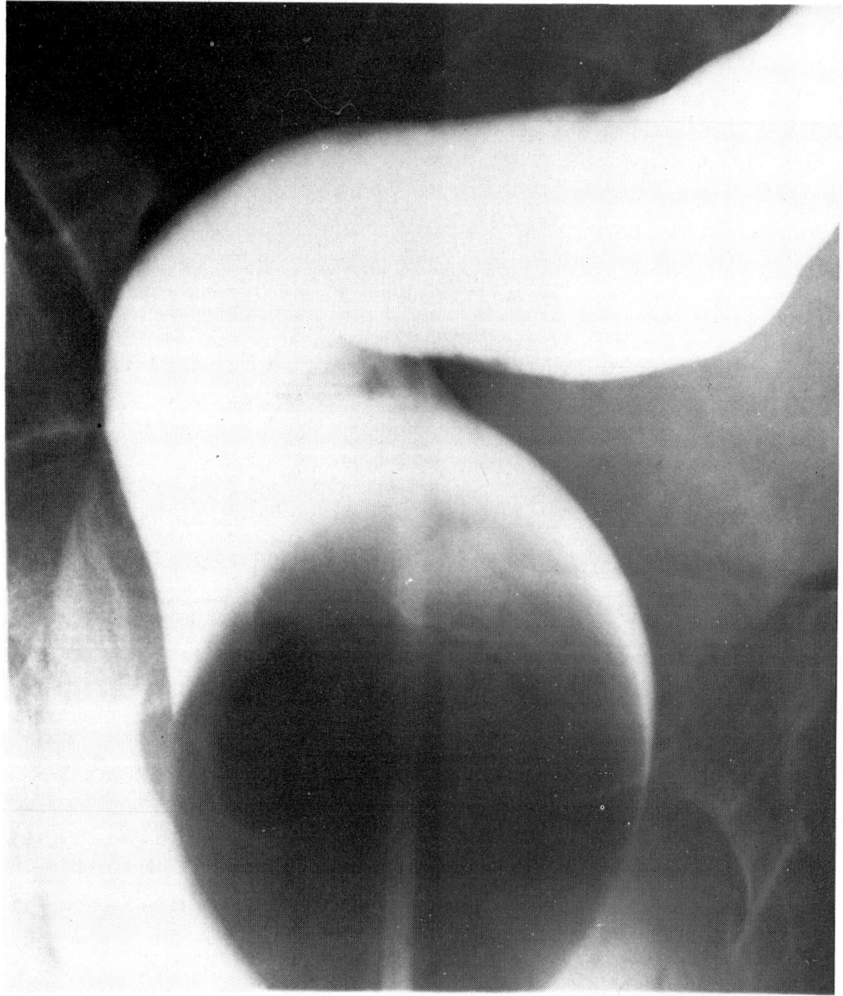

Fig. I.3. Rectal tear with an inflated balloon. (a) With the balloon inflated no tear can be identified. (b) After removal of the enema tip there is extraperitoneal extravasation through a tear. (Courtesy of Drs. W.J. Dodds et al. (26) copyright 1980, Springer-Verlag.)

d. Perforation due to increased pressure

The pressure required to rupture the colon is difficult to measure. In human cadavers cecal rupture occurred at 81 mm Hg, while sigmoid rupture required 169 mm Hg (30), yet rupture can occur throughout the colon (2). Perforation has been reported in diseased colons, especially in a setting of inflammatory disease, even when apparently nonexcessive pressures are used (31, 32) (Fig. I.4). Some of these perforations are readily recognized during fluoroscopy after the initial addition of barium while others first become apparent only after evaluation of the subsequent radiographs (33). Rarely, a spontaneous perforation may occur proximally through nondiseased bowel (Fig. I.5).

A disused colon segment distal to a colostomy is especially prone to perforation. If there has been radiation therapy to the pelvis or if the distal colon segment has been disused for a considerable length of time, extreme caution must be used (Figs. I.6 and I.7). If in doubt, a water soluble contrast agent should be considered.

Although it has been inferred that a *double-contrast* barium enema may be more dangerous than a *single-contrast* enema (34), there is no convincing evidence that this is true. Perforation associated with any enema is probably related to increased pressure rather than the type of contrast material being used. While the double contrast barium enema may spill air into the peritoneal cavity (35), extraperitoneal structures, or the portal vein, a single contrast barium enema in a similar situation would result in barium peritonitis or barium emboli in the liver and an obviously graver prognosis (Fig. I.8).

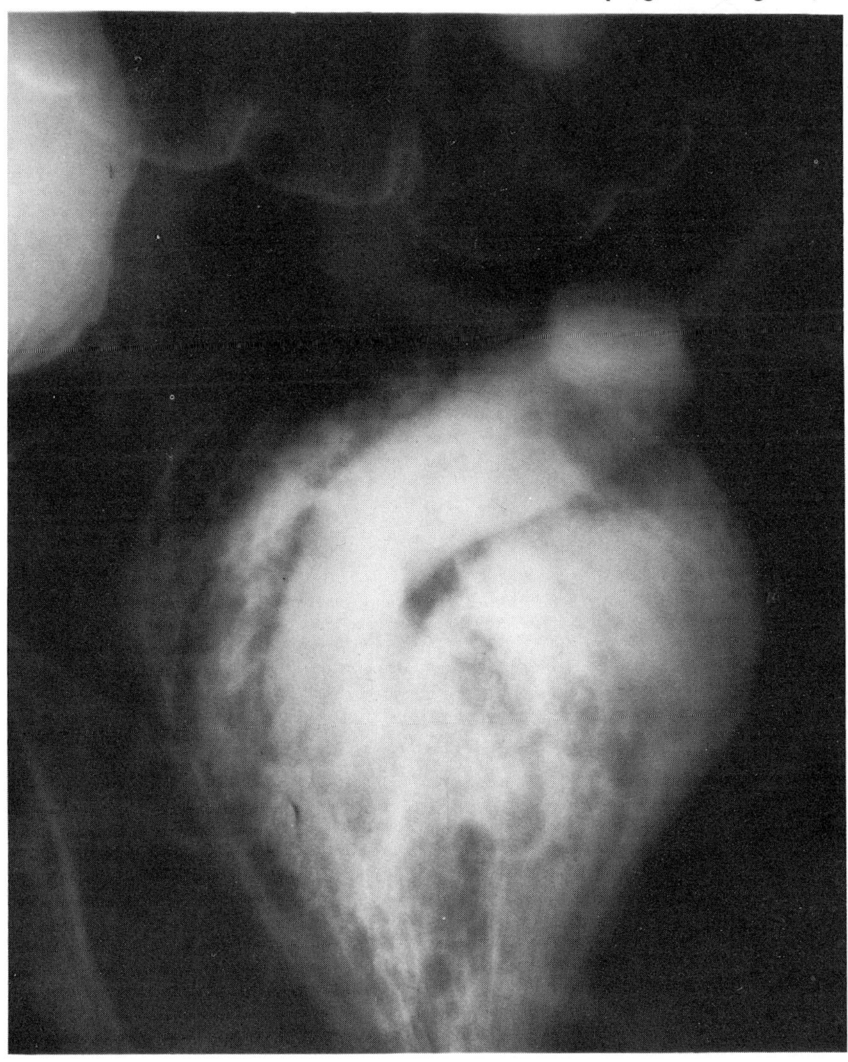

*Fig. I.3.***b.**

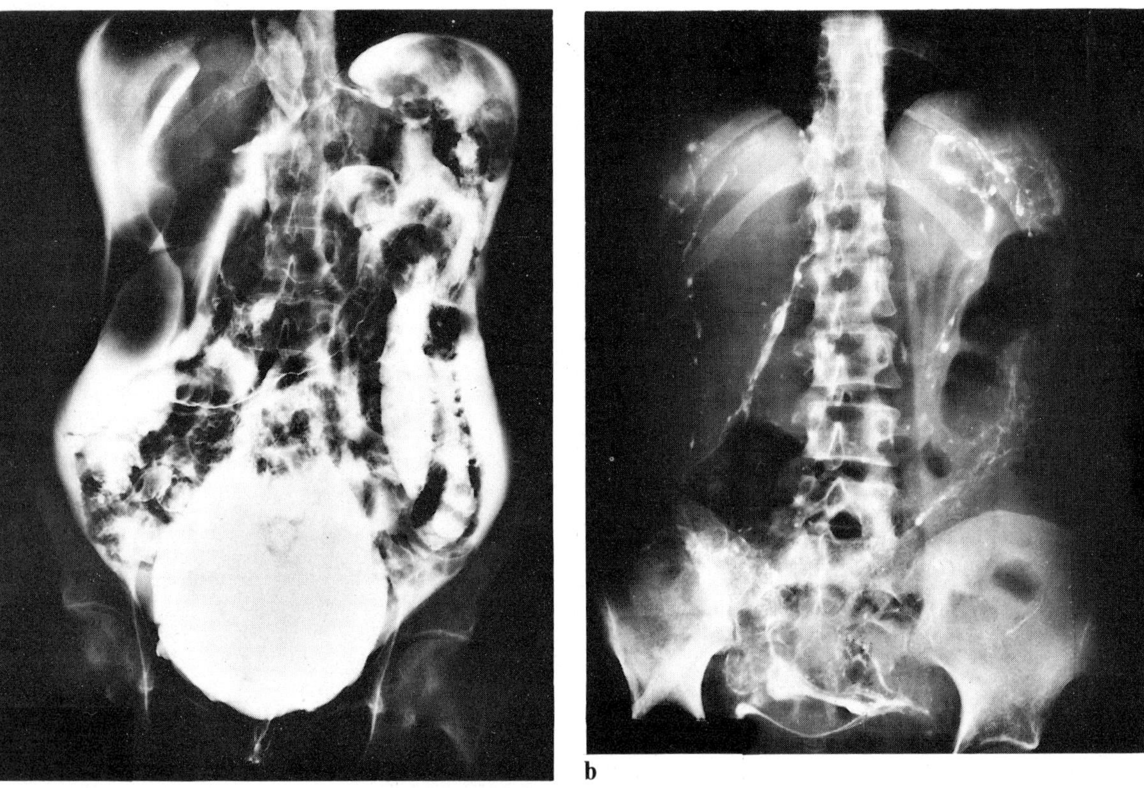

Fig. I.4. Barium peritonitis. The patient had regional enteritis for at least five years, with the disease limited to the distal ileum and right colon. (a) Massive spillage of barium occurred into the peritoneal cavity when the patient was turned over prone. Cecal perforation was found at surgery. (b) After surgery residual barium is adherent in the peritoneal cavity.

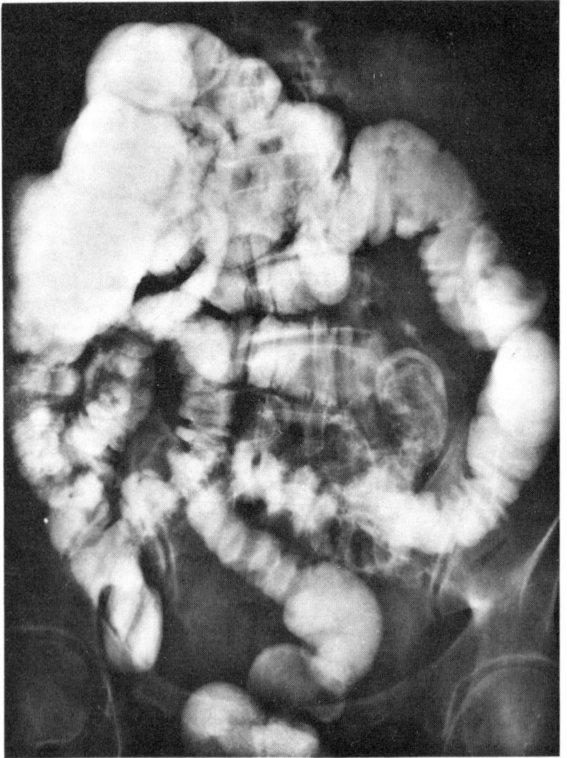

Fig. I.5. Spontaneous bowel perforation. (a) A single-contrast barium enema with considerable reflux of the ileum showed no spill. Glucagon was not used. (b) Barium peritonitis was seen only on the post-evacuation radiograph. Subsequent surgery revealed a perforation in the terminal ileum. (c) Six months later residual barium is still present in the peritoneal cavity.

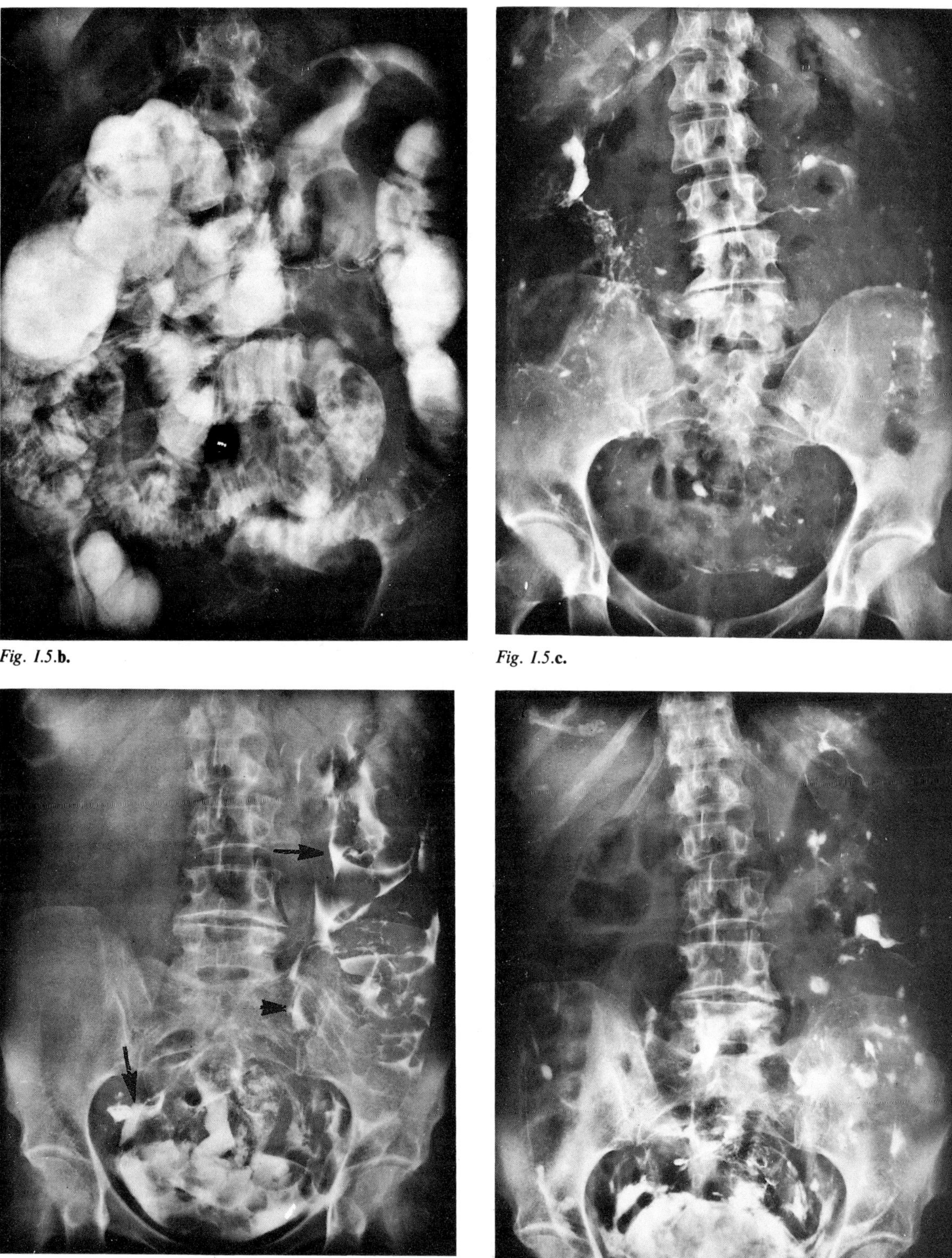

*Fig. I.5.***b.**

*Fig. I.5.***c.**

a

b

Fig. I.6. Barium peritonitis. The patient had a diverting colostomy and radiation therapy to the pelvis three years previously. (a) After instilling barium through the rectum, radiographs revealed spill into the peritoneal cavity (arrows). (b) Residual contrast in the peritoneal cavity.

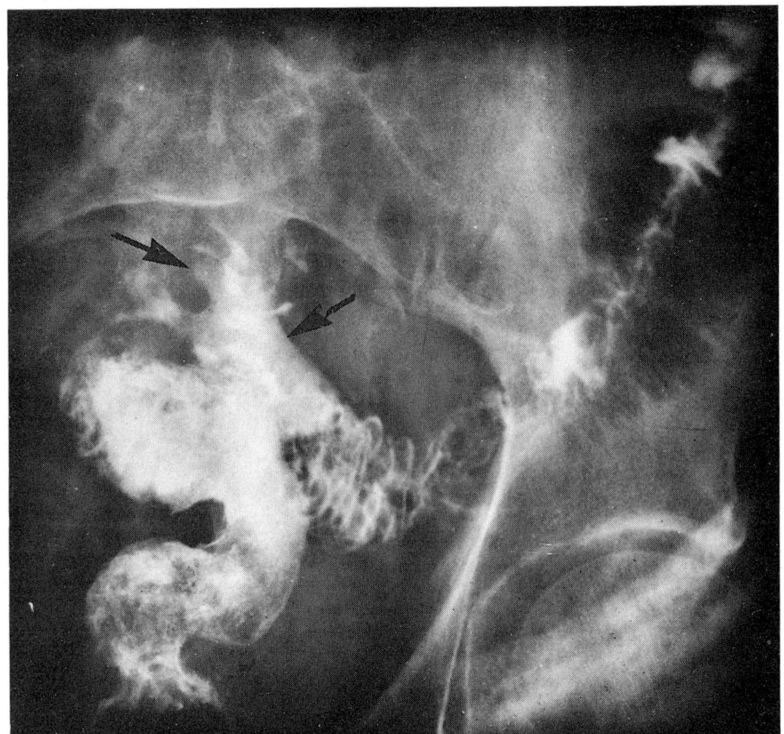

a

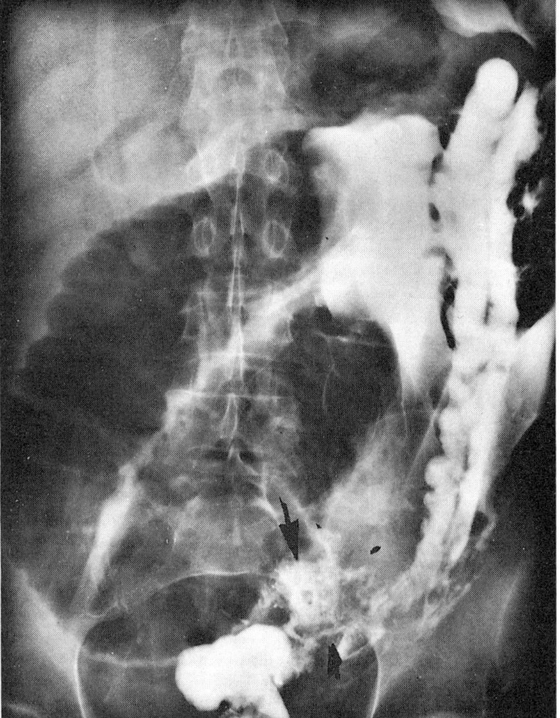

b

Fig. 1.7. Diverticulitis was suspected in this patient and because of a poor response to medical management he underwent a transverse colostomy. (a) A postevacuation radiograph after a barium enema revealed a localized extravasation (arrows). (b) Two years later the patient underwent sigmoid resection. Two months later, in contemplation of takedown of the colostomy, a barium enema was performed. There is intraperitoneal spill of barium through a leak at the sigmoid anastomosis (arrows).

The intraluminal pressure between two areas of spasm in the colon can exceed intraarterial pressure. Thus, the use of pharmacological agents to induce colon hypotonia and, hopefully, abolish excessive spasm, may help prevent some perforations due to increased pressure. Actually, perforations due to increased pressure are not limited to a barium enema but can occur with any other type of colon lavage, even with a tap water enema.

If a patient is having severe colon spasm, the fluoroscopist should lower the enema bag to the table level or below. The worst thing possible under such circumstances is to clamp off the enema tubing, since then one is dealing with a closed system and the resultant spasm can result in perforation or produce intramural extravasation.

The force necessary to burst the colon depends on Laplace's law: the total force is the product of intraluminal pressure times the radius of the colon (36). Thus, the cecum, having the greatest diameter, is where the greatest number of colon perforations occur due to increased intraluminal pressure in a normal colon.

e. Barium intravasation

Barium intravasation into blood vessels can occur not only during a barium enema examination, but also during an upper gastrointestinal examination (37). The mortality from barium intravasation is

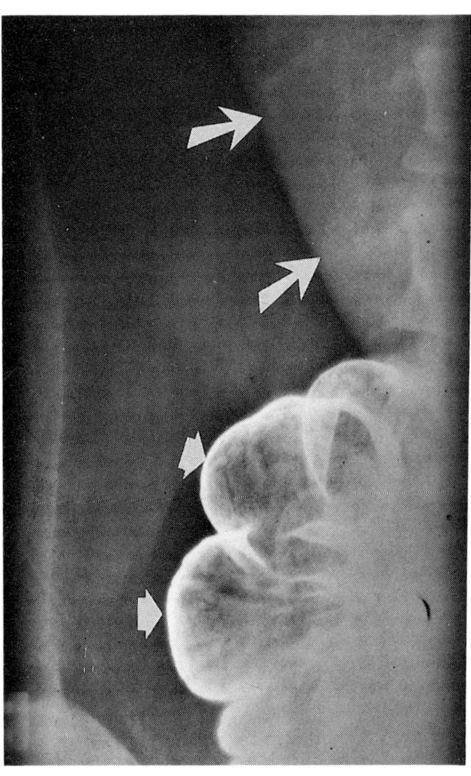

Fig. I.8. Massive pneumoperitoneum resulted during a double-contrast barium enema. The decubitus radiograph outlines barium in the right colon (arrowheads) and the liver edge surrounded by air (arrows). None of the radiographs revealed any barium spill into the peritoneal cavity and the patient recovered without any surgical intervention.

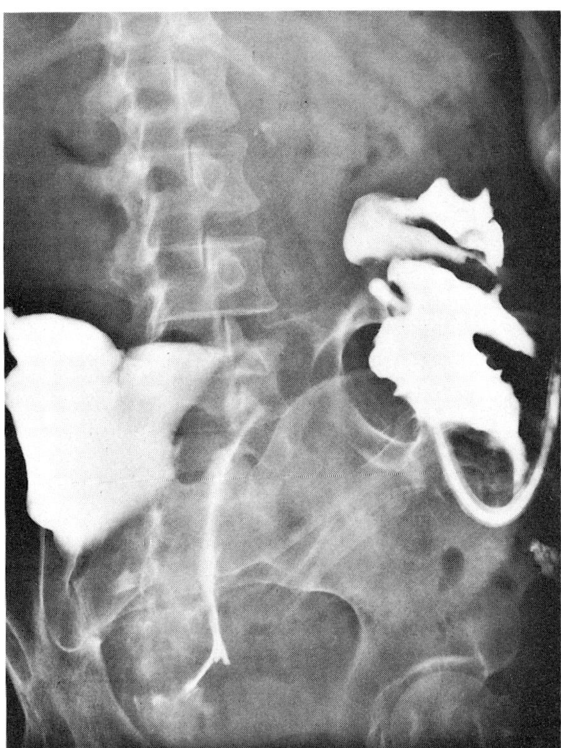

Fig. I.9. It was desired to ascertain the position of the tip of a feeding jejunostomy. Barium sulfate instead of one of the water soluble contrast media was injected through the feeding tube, resulting in spill of barium into the peritoneal cavity.

approximately 66% (38). Most patients expire within minutes of the accident; fortunately, this event is rare during a barium enema (39). Since most reports involve embolization to the lung, intravasation in the rectum into the drainage of the internal iliac veins must be postulated. Occasionally barium in the lung vessels may be a transient phenomenon (40). Portal intravasation (41) and a subsequent liver abscess is even less common (42).

Intravasation of gas may also occur (31, 34, 43), especially after a double-contrast examination (44). It may be argued that it is safer to intravasate gas (or air) rather than barium sulfate, with some of these patients reporting no significant sequelae.

f. Barium peritonitis

One survey reported an incidence of *intraperitoneal* perforation in 1 out of 17,000 barium enema examinations (4). The mortality from intraperitoneal colon perforation is probably close to 50%, with the outcome depending upon the amount of peritoneal soilage present. When barium sulfate and stool are mixed together in the peritoneal cavity the resultant toxicity is considerably greater than if each product is introduced separately (45), yet even relatively sterile barium sulfate can result in peritonitis (45) (Fig. I.9).

Barium peritonitis can be divided into an acute and chronic phase. Acutely, there is fluid sequestration into the peritoneal cavity and these patients may develop hypovolemic shock. If the patient survives the acute episode, chronic sequelae include extensive bowel adhesions and barium granuloma formation. Exuberant fibrosis surrounds the barium sulfate particles. The fibrosis quite often involves loops of bowel, resulting in numerous sites of obstruction (Figs. I.10 and I.11). Prior barium spillage should be readily identified radiographically.

The therapy of barium peritonitis should be individualized, with most of these patients being managed surgically. In addition to antibiotic coverage, these patients require large amounts of

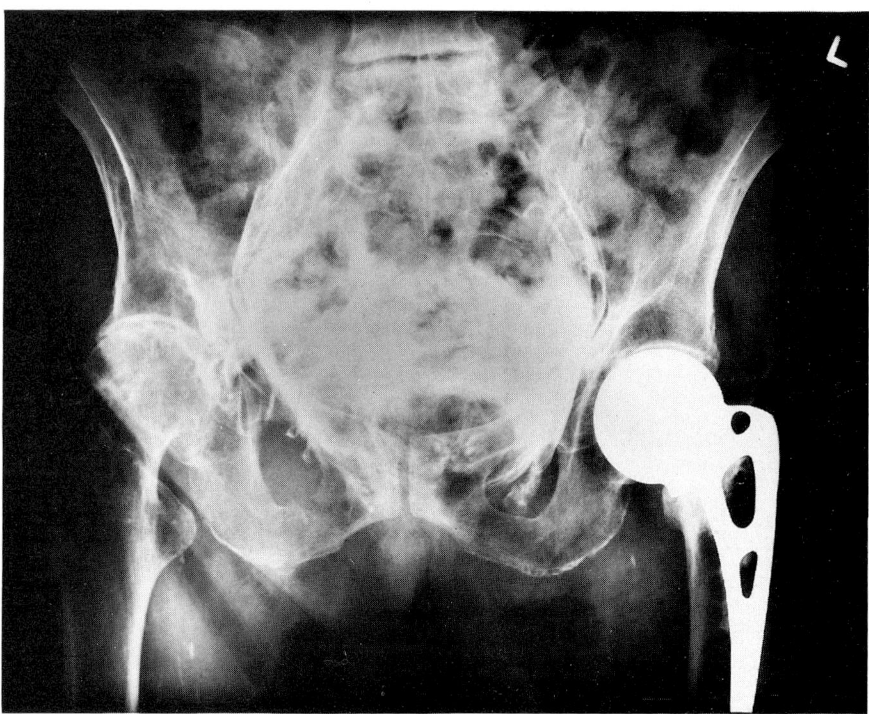

Fig. I.10. Prior colon perforation during barium enema. The perforation probably was in an area of diverticulitis. The residual barium sulfate is fixed in the pelvis and dense adhesions involve loops of bowel. (From R.E. Miller and J. Skucas (57), copyright 1977, University Park Press.)

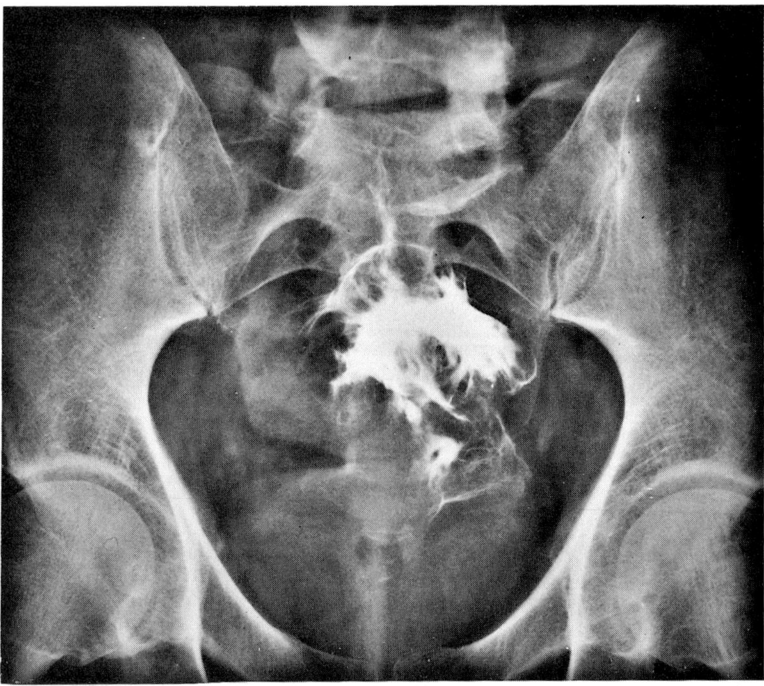

Fig. I.11. Prior colon perforation. Residual barium and loops of bowel are trapped in the pelvis.

intravenous fluid to compensate for the massive outpouring of fluid into the peritoneal cavity (46). One study of barium peritonitis in dogs found that most deaths occurred within 24 hours. Surgery was not a major factor in determining which dogs died and which did not, and the resultant mortality was lowest in those dogs where vigorous intravenous fluid therapy was used (47). At least in dogs, the commercial barium sulfate preparations resulted in more adverse reactions than USP barium sulfate (48).

g. Infection

Results are controversial as to whether bacteremia develops in some patients during a barium enema (49–51). It is thought that a diseased colon may predispose a patient to bacteremia. For instance, fatal septicemia following barium enema has been reported in a patient with leukemia (52). Those patients in whom bacteremia may be especially harmful, such as those with prosthetic valves or those who are immunosuppressed with chemotherapeutic agents, should be considered for antibiotic coverage.

Barium contamination by bacteria can occur (53), especially if liquid suspensions in opened containers are stored without refrigeration. Likewise, unsanitary mixing conditions can result in contamination but the disposable equipment can decrease this problem considerably.

h. Cardiac complications

ECG changes during an enema in elderly people are not uncommon. A study of patients over 60 years old found a 40% rate of significant arrhythmia and a 7% rate of ST-segment depression developing during the examination (54). Deaths due to myocardial infarction, during or immediately after a barium enema, have also been reported (55). In one study, premedication with B-receptor blocking agents helped reduce ECG changes (56). Glucagon apparently does not diminish the incidence of arrhythmias (54). It appears that a barium enema should be approached with caution in patients with cardiac disease. Little investigation is available to guide the practicing radiologist.

i. Autonomic dysreflexia

It is not unusual for a patient with a previous spinal cord injury, while undergoing a barium enema, to exhibit profuse sweating, nausea and abdominal pain. If the patient's blood pressure is measured, considerable elevation above normal may be present in the face of bradycardia.

Such a reaction starts with impulses originating from the colon afferent sensory nerve endings, ascending the spinal cord to the point of injury, and resulting in a marked release of sympathetic motor impulses in the efferent tracts. These efferent impulses result in arteriolar spasm and hypertension. The resultant hypertension triggers carotid and aortic baroreceptors, producing bradycardia and vasodilatation above the level of the cord injury. Below the level of injury, however, the sympathetic hyperreflexia results in spasm and vasoconstriction.

It should be realized that the treatment of autonomic dysreflexia is completely different from the treatment of typical contrast reactions. That is, the treatment is to remove the cause. Thus, when this condition is encountered, the barium enema should be stopped and the colon drained. The patient's pulse and blood pressure should be monitored and if significant hypertension is present, the hypertension should be treated to prevent hemorrhage or cardiac failure.

References

1. Gelfand DW: Complications of gastrointestinal radiologic procedures: I. Complications of routine fluoroscopic studies. Gastrointest Radiol 5:293–315, 1980.
2. Kahn SP, Lindenauer SM, Wojtalik RS: Perforation of the normal colon during barium contrast examination. Am Surg 42:789–792, 1976.
3. Gardiner H, Miller RE: Barium peritonitis. A new therapeutic approach. Am J Surg 125:350–352, 1973.
4. Masel H, Masel JP, Casey KV: A survey of colon examination techniques in Australia and New Zealand, with a review of complications. Austral Radiol 15:140–147, 1971.
5. Govindiah D, Bhaskar GR: An unusual case of barium poisoning. Antiseptic 69:675–677, 1972.
6. Gould DB, Sorrell MR, Lupariello HD: Barium sulfide poisoning. Arch Intern Med 132:891–894, 1973.
7. Lewi Z, Bar-Khayim Y: Food poisoning from barium carbonate. Lancet 2:342–343, 1964.
8. Jobba G, Renge B: Über die Neopol-Vergiftung. Arch Toxikol 27:106–110, 1971.
9. Ku D, Yen CK, Li CC: Acute poisoning by common salt containing barium chloride. Chin Med J 61:303–304, 1943.
10. Roza O, Berman LB: The pathophysiology of barium: hypokalemic and cardiovascular effects. J Pharmacol Exp Ther 117:433–439, 1971.
11. Miller RE: Laxative should not be routinely ordered after barium enema examination [Letter]. JAMA 239:970–971, 1978.

12. Miller RE, Lehman G: Localization of small bowel hemorrhage: complete reflux small bowel examination. Am J Dig Dis 17:1019–1023, 1972.
13. Miller RE: Reflux examination of the small bowel. Radiol Clin North Am 7:175–184, 1969.
14. Szunyogh B: Enema injuries. Am J Proctol 9:303–308, 1958.
15. Seaman WB, Wells J: Complications of the barium enema. Gastroenterology 48:728–737, 1965.
16. Lewis JW Jr, Kerstein MD, Koss N: Barium granuloma of the rectum: an uncommon complication of barium enema. Ann Surg 181:418–423, 1975.
17. Noveroske RJ: Perforation of a normal colon by too much pressure. J Indiana State Med Assoc 65:23–25, 1972.
18. McDonald CC, Rowe RJ: Retrorectal fistula secondary to barium-abscess granuloma: report of a case. Dis Colon Rectum 19:71–73, 1976.
19. Rockert H, Zettergren L: Tissue reaction to barium sulphate contrast medium. Acta Pathol Microbiol Scand 58:445–450, 1963.
20. Phelps JE, Sanowski RA, Kozarek RA: Intramural extravasation of barium simulating carcinoma of the rectum. Dis Colon Rectum 24:388–390, 1981.
21. Elliot JS, Rosenberg ML: Ureteral occlusion by barium granuloma. J Urol 71:692–694, 1954.
22. Herrington JL Jr: Barium granuloma within the peritoneal cavity: Ureteral obstruction 7 years after barium enema and colonic perforation. Ann Surg 164:162–166, 1966.
23. Broadfoot E, Martin G: Barium granuloma of the rectum. Austral Radiol 21:50–52, 1977.
24. Amberg JR: Complications of colon radiography. Gastrointest Endosc 26 (Suppl):15S–17S, 1980.
25. Nelson JA, Daniels AU, Dodds WJ: Rectal balloons: complications, causes, and recommendations. Invest Radiol 14:48–59, 1979.
26. Dodds WJ, Stewart ET, Nelson JA: Rectal balloon catheters and the barium enema examination. Gastrointest Radiol 5:277–284, 1980.
27. Wagget J, Bishop HC, Koop CE: Experience with gastrografin enema in the treatment of meconium ileus. J Pediatr Surg 5:649–654, 1970.
28. Beerman PJ, Gelfand DW, Ott DJ: Pneumomediastinum after double-contrast barium enema examination: a sign of colonic perforation. AJR 136:197–198, 1981.
29. Brunton FJ: Retroperitoneal emphysema as a complication of barium enema. Clin. Radiol 11:197–199, 1960.
30. Kozarek RA, Earnest DL, Silverstein ME, Smith RG: Air-pressure-induced colon injury during diagnostic colonoscopy. Gastroenterology 78:7–14, 1980.
31. Kees CJ, Hester CL Jr: Portal vein gas following barium enema examination. Radiology 102:525–526, 1972.
32. Desaulniers M: Intramural perforation of barium—transverse colon. J Can Assoc Radiol 29:194, 1978.
33. Seaman WB, Bragg DG: Colonic intramural barium: a complication of the barium-enema examination. Radiology 89:250–255, 1967.
34. Lazar HP: Survival following portal venous air embolization. Am J Dig Dis 10:259–264, 1965.
35. Gelfand DW, Ott DJ, Ramquist NA: Pneumoperitoneum occurring during double-contrast enema. Gastrointest Radiol 4:307–308, 1979.
36. Noveroske RJ; Intracolonic pressures during barium enema examination. AJR 91:852–863, 1964.
37. Mahboubi S, Gohel VK, Dalinka MK, Cho SY: Barium embolization following upper gastrointestinal examination. Radiology 111:301–302, 1974.
38. Juler GL, Dietrick WR, Eisenman JI: Intramesenteric perforation of sigmoid diverticulitis with non-fatal venous intravasation. Am J Surg 132:653–656, 1976.
39. Cove JKJ, Snyder RN: Fatal barium intravasation during barium enema. Radiology 112:9–10, 1974.
40. Zatzkin HR, Irwin GAL: Non-fatal intravasation of barium. AJR 92:1169–1172, 1974.
41. Schumacher F: $BaSO_4$ — Übertritt in die Vena mesenterica inferior bei Kolonkontrastuntersuchung — eine seltene Komplikation. ROEFO 133:99–100, 1980.
42. Isaacs I, Nissen R, Epstein BS: Liver abscess resulting from barium enema in a case of chronic ulcerative colitis. NY State J Med 50:332–334, 1950.
43. Weinstein GE, Weiner M, Schwartz M: Portal vein gas. Am J Gastroenterol 49:425–429, 1968.
44. Sadhu VK, Brennan RE, Madan V: Portal vein gas following air-contrast barium enema in granulomatous colitis: report of a case. Gastrointest Radiol 4:163–164, 1979.
45. Sisel RJ, Donovan AJ, Yellin AE: Experimental fecal peritonitis. Influence of barium sulfate or water-soluble radiographic contrast material on survival. Arch Surg 104:765–768, 1972.
46. Gardiner H, Miller RE: Barium peritonitis. Am J Surg 125:350–352, 1973.
47. Nahrwold DL, Isch JH, Benner DA, Miller RE: Effect of fluid administration and operation on the mortality rate in barium peritonitis. Surgery 70:778–781, 1971.
48. Cochran DQ, Almond CH, Shucart WA: An experimental study of the effects of barium and intestinal contents on the peritoneal cavity. AJR 89:883–887, 1963.
49. Butt J, Hentges O, Pelican G, Henstorf H, Haag T, Rolfe R, Hutcheson D: Bacteremia during barium enema study. AJR 130:715–718, 1978.
50. Le Frock J, Ellis CA, Klainer AS, Weinstein L: Transient bacteremia associated with barium enema. Arch Intern Med 135:835–837, 1975.
51. Schimmel DH, Hanelin LG, Cohen S, Goldberg HI: Bacteremia and the barium enema. AJR 128:207–208, 1977.
52. Richman LS, Short WI, Cooper WM: Barium enema septicemia. Occurrence in a patient with leukemia. JAMA 226:62–63, 1973.
53. Amberg JR, Unger JD: Contamination of barium sulfate suspension. Radiology 97:182–183, 1970.
54. Higgins CB, Roeske WR, Karliner JS, O'Rourke R, Berk RN: Predictive factors and mechanism of arrhythmias and myocardial ischaemic changes in elderly patients during barium enema. Br J Radiol 49:1023–1027, 1976.
55. Kiser JL, Spratt JS Jr, Johnson CA: Colon perforations occurring during sigmoidoscopic examinations and barium enemas. Mo Med 65:969–974, 1968.
56. Yigitbasi O, Sari S, Kiliccioglu, Nalbantgil I: Recherche par l'ECG dynamique des modifications cardiaques pouvant survenir pendant l'administration de lavements opaques. J Radiol Electrol 59:125–128, 1978.
57. Miller RE, Skucas J: Barium sulfate: clinical properties. In: Miller RE, Skucas J (ed) Radiographic Contrast Agents, p 137. University Park Press, Baltimore, 1977.

PART II

THE NORMAL COLON

II.A. Introduction

Embryologically, the colon can be divided into two parts. The right side of the colon and portions of the transverse colon originate from the mid-gut and receive their blood supply from the superior mesenteric artery. The bowel from the distal transverse colon through the rectum originates from the hindgut and receives much of its blood supply from the inferior mesenteric artery, with some supply to the rectum coming from the internal iliac arteries. The arterial branches pierce the colon at select sites of defects in the muscle layer and end eventually in a capillary plexus.

From a simplistic viewpoint, the distal half of the colon is primarily involved in evacuation and storage while the proximal half functions primarily as a water and electrolyte transport system. In general, sodium and chloride are absorbed while potassium and bicarbonate are secreted. The transverse colon acts simply as a connection between the two sides.

II.B. Bowel wall

The outer layer of the colon is the serosa, also called the tunica serosa, consisting of the partially overlying peritoneum and surrounding fat tissue. The fat is concentrated in discrete pockets or 'appendages' called the epiploic appendages and is arranged along several rows, which gives the outside of the colon an irregular appearance. These appendages are absent in the rectum. Because of these discrete collections of fat and the relatively thick underlying colon wall, it can be difficult for a surgeon to palpate a small intraluminal polyp. This problem does not exist in the small bowel since there the thin wall of the bowel allows ready palpation of even small polyps. Occasionally the colon epiploic appendages calcify and amputate, resulting in a mobile calcified intraperitoneal mass (1).

The next layer inward consists primarily of nonstriated muscle and is known as either the muscular coat, tunica muscularis, muscularis propria or muscularis externa. This layer consists of an outer longitudinal muscle layer arranged in discrete bands and an inner circular muscle layer. The myenteric or Auerbach's neural plexus is located in between these two muscle layers. The next layer inward in the submucosa, consisting of connective tissue, fat, and vascular and lymphatic ramifications.

The next inward layer is the mucosa, whose outermost portion is the muscularis mucosa and consists of an outer longitudinal and an inner circular layer of muscle. The muscularis mucosa effectively separates the mucosa from the submucosa and is useful to the pathologist in identifying invasion of the colon wall by tumors originating in the mucosa. The next inner layer of the mucosa is the lamina propria containing numerous lymph nodules and connective tissue. The overlying epithelium contains the crypts or glands of Lieberkühn. There is a lymphatic plexus around the muscularis mucosa, with no lymphatics located more superficially (2). Thus, lymphatic metastases from tumors located entirely in the mucosa superficial to the muscularis mucosae do not occur. There is, however, a rich capillary blood supply throughout the mucosa.

Quite often small spiculations or grooves are seen in the colon during a barium enema. Although initially believed to represent barium in the glands of Lieberkühn (3), subsequent investigation revealed closely spaced grooves or depressions in the colon mucosa (4, 5). These innominate grooves are usually spaced several millimeters apart, may be circumferential, and may form an interconnecting mesh network. Histological study reveals lymphatic follicles occurring in a linear distribution corresponding to these innominate grooves (6); the follicles are located in the mucosa with the muscularis mucosa interrupted at these sites. In addition, there are fewer glands in the mucosa overlying a lymph follicle, resulting in a thinner layer of mucosa. Radiographically visible lymphoid follicles are common in the colon and terminal ileum (7), although they may not be visible colonoscopically. The normal colon contains, on the average, 3 to 3.5 lymphoid follicles per square centimeter (8), there being a gradual increase in number from the ascending colon to the sigmoid. Children have more follicles than adults (9).

What is commonly called lymphoid hyperplasia actually represents a normal appearance of the lymph follicles (10). It is believed that in the vast majority of patients these lymph follicles have no malignant potential. Although these follicles are not neoplastic in origin, they may accompany both lymphoma and leukemia. In a rare patient lymphoid hyperplasia may precede the eventual development of either lymphoma or leukemia.

Why the lymphoid tissue is prominent in some patients is not known, although there appears to be a familial incidence. Some patients with an immunoglobulin deficiency condition may exhibit very prominent lymph follicles (11). There are occasional reports of familial adenomatous polyposis being associated with lymphoid hyperplasia (12), although the relationship is not clear. Likewise, true hyperplasia is present in regional enteritis, especially early in the disease process.

Radiographically these lymphoid follicles are under 5 mm in diameter, tend to be uniform in size in any one patient, are smooth and oval in outline, and may have a central umbilication which tends to trap barium (7, 13, 14). The overall appearance is that of a small 'doughnut' lesion (Fig. B.1). Diag-

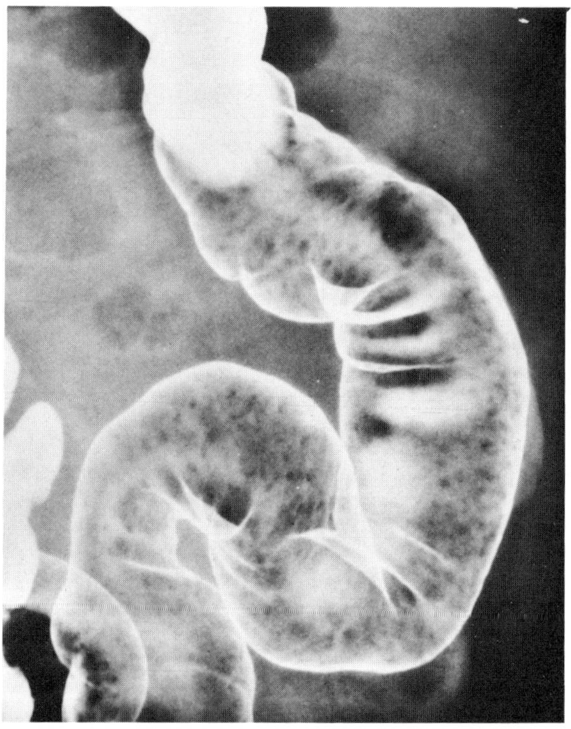

a

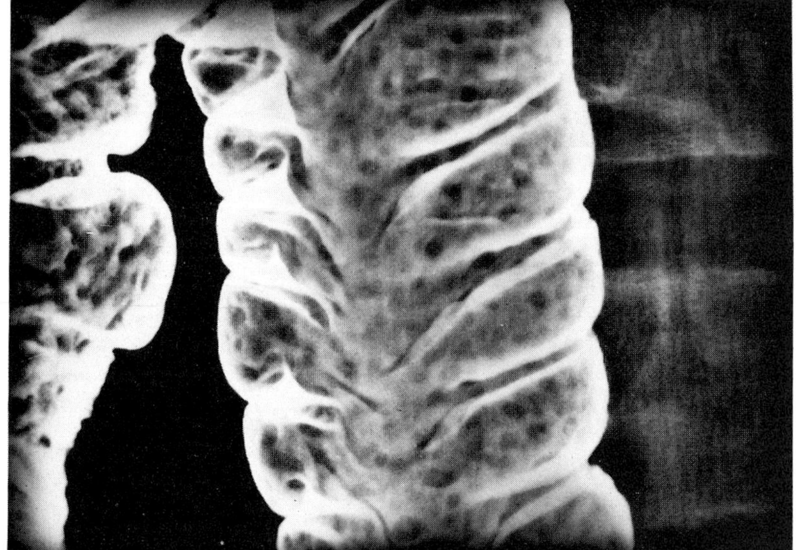

b

Fig. B.1. (a) Subtle lymph follicle prominence in a 20-year-old male. (b) More prominent lymph follicles in a 15-year-old male. Both appearances are considered as variations of normal.

nosis is generally easy due to the central umbilication, because few other polyps, with the exception of aphthoid ulcers as seen in regional enteritis or an unusual presentation of lymphoma, have such a configuration.

II.C. Vascular anatomy

The lymphatic drainage of the colon essentially parallels the vessels. The main colic lymphatics and nodes are adjacent to the ileocolic, right colic, middle colic and left colic vessels. The descending and sigmoid colic nodes eventually drain into the periaortic lymph nodes close to the origin of the inferior mesenteric artery. The rest of the colic nodes drain into the superior mesenteric nodes and eventually into the periaortic nodes and ultimately into the cisterna chyli. There is no lymphatic communication between the ileal and cecal sides of the ileocecal valve (15). Thus, cecal cancers tend not to spread to the terminal ileum except by direct invasion.

The blood supply to the bowel exhibits considerable variation, with over 50 collateral pathways having been described (16). Branches from the superior mesenteric artery (SMA) supply the colon approximately to the splenic flexure through the ileocolic, right colic and middle colic arteries (Fig. C.1). The descending and sigmoid colon are supplied by branches of the inferior mesenteric artery (IMA) (17). Both the SMA and the IMA arise directly from the aorta. The ileocolic artery, the termination of the superior mesenteric artery, is the most constant in location. It supplies the terminal ileum and portions of the right colon. The right colic artery usually originates from the superior mesentery artery; however, it can be part of the middle colic or even the ileocolic artery. Occasionally the right colic artery is absent and the ascending colon is supplied by branches from the middle colic artery. The middle colic artery usually originates from the proximal portion of the superior mesenteric artery just distal to the inferior pancreaticoduodenal artery. There may be two middle colic arteries present or, occasionally, the middle colic artery is absent (18). It may arise from a celiac axis branch.

The descending branch of the IMA terminates as the superior hemorrhoidal artery. The left colic artery originates from the IMA and supplies the colon roughly from the splenic flexure through the sigmoid. It divides into an ascending and a descending branch, with the ascending branch anastomosing with a branch from the middle colic artery, although in some patients the anastomosis is absent (17). From this marginal anastomasing artery, described by Drummond (19), originate feeding vessels to the bowel wall itself. This marginal artery of Drummond can consist of portions of the middle colic, the left colic, and at times even branches of the sigmoid arteries (16). The anastomosis at the splenic flexure, emphasized by Griffiths (18), provides collateral circulation between the SMA and the IMA. Circulation to the colon at the splenic flexure area is dependent upon this critical Griffiths point which can be a potential weak point and lead to ischemia. Occasionally an artery arises from the middle colic and anastamoses directly with a branch of the IMA, forming the arc of Riolan and thus providing another collateral between the SMA

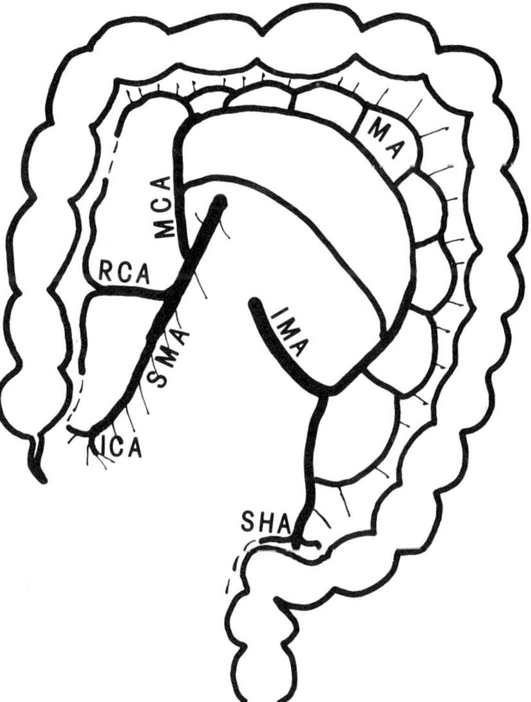

Fig. C.1. Schematic representation of arteries supplying the colon. There is considerable variation between individuals and at times even major vessels may have different origins. SMA – superior mesenteric artery, MCA – middle colic artery, RCA – right colic artery, ICA – ileo-colic artery, IMA – inferior mesenteric artery, MA – marginal artery of Drummond, SHA – superior hemorrhoidal artery.

and the IMA. These collateral pathways are potential sites for new flow patterns, especially with a gradual onset of obstruction in any one artery.

The rectum is supplied partly by the superior hemorrhoidal artery and partly by the bilateral inferior hemorrhoidal arteries originating from each of the internal iliac arteries. These inferior hemorrhoidal arteries provide additional systemic blood supply to the rectum and sometimes to the sigmoid, yet rectal ischemia is not rare (20). Underlying vascular disease, such as arteriosclerosis, trauma, surgery or tumor can modify the usual path of blood flow.

The venous drainage from the colon tends to parallel the major arteries. Most of the venous drainage eventually ends in the portal venous system. The inferior mesenteric vein drains into the splenic vein, while the superior mesenteric vein joins the splenic vein to form the portal vein. Drainage from the rectum is through the superior hemorrhoidal vein, which is the origin of the inferior mesenteric vein, and through the bilateral middle and inferior hemorrhoidal veins which drain into the internal iliac veins. A potential communicating pathway thus exists in the rectum between the portal and the systemic veins.

II.D. Gross appearance

In the neonate, the colon tends to be redundant and occupies a proportionately greater amount of space in the abdomen. The hepatic flexure tends to be depressed due to prominence of the liver. Haustra are not as distinct but are present.

In adults, the ascending and descending portions of the colon do not usually have a mesentery and are posterior in location. Thus, these segments are surrounded by peritoneum on three sides and are in contact with the extraperitoneum posteriorly. On the other hand, the transverse and sigmoid portions of the colon usually do have a mesentery of varying length and are anteriorly located. The cecum likewise can be completely surrounded by peritoneum.

There is considerable variation in colon length and redundancy even in asymptomatic patients. Redundant loops should be considered as a normal variant unless there is extreme elongation (Fig. D.1). A foreshortened colon, on the other hand, usually implies prior resection or disease.

The diameter of a normal colon can also vary considerably. A routine barium enema in normal volunteers revealed the average diameter of the cecum to be 7.8 cm, ascending colon 6.5 cm, transverse colon 5.4 cm, descending colon 2.7 cm, and sigmoid 3 cm (21). In general, the cecum should be the widest part of the colon with the distal descending or sigmoid colon the narrowest.

Occasionally encountered during a barium enema are inconstant transient segments of narrowing at discrete points in the colon. The fluoroscopist generally attributes these segments to spasm, although occasionally the narrowing can persist and mimic a neoplasm (22). With sufficient patience these narrowed segments can usually be distended. The most common such narrowing or 'sphincter' is known as Cannon's ring or Cannon's point and is located in the transverse colon (Fig. D.2). It is believed that Cannon's ring is the junction of the

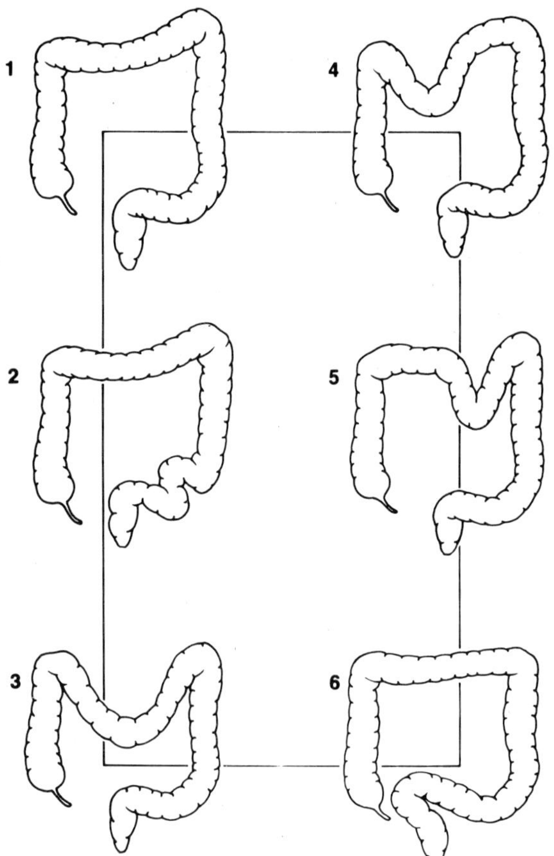

Fig. D.1. Variation in colon length and redundancy. All six patterns should be considered as variants of normal.

innervation between the mid-gut and hind-gut. The other narrow segments, many named after their original investigators, are usually curiosities of little significance. The Payr-Strauss ring, located at the splenic flexure, is a common site for the origin of a peristaltic wave involving the distal colon. These 'sphincters' are usually not as confusing during double contrast examinations as they are on a single contrast enema.

The colon differs considerably from the small bowel; it has a more fixed position and a saccular contour. Unlike the small bowel where the longitudinal muscles form a continuous layer around the bowel circumference, in the colon these longitudinal muscles are arranged in three discrete longitudinal bands, have fixed anatomic positions, and are known as the taeniae coli. In adults the taeniae are approximately one-sixth shorter than the overall length of the colon. The colon wall in between the taeniae is thus redundant, forming saccular outpouchings known as haustra. The circular muscles in the haustra are attached to the longitudinal taeniae. Since there are three taeniae in the circumference of the colon, in a cross-sectional view there are also three haustra. The circular muscles can contract independently of each other, resulting in segmental and asymmetrical contractions (23). There is considerable variation in the appearance of haustra not only between the right and the left side of the colon, but also in different individuals. The circular muscle layers in the cecum are thinner than in the remainder of the colon. The haustra are more apparent when the colon is partially collapsed than when fully distended. With distension it is possible to obliterate completely the haustra in portions of the descending and sigmoid colon even in normal individuals (Fig. D.3).

It should be emphasized that the haustra are the

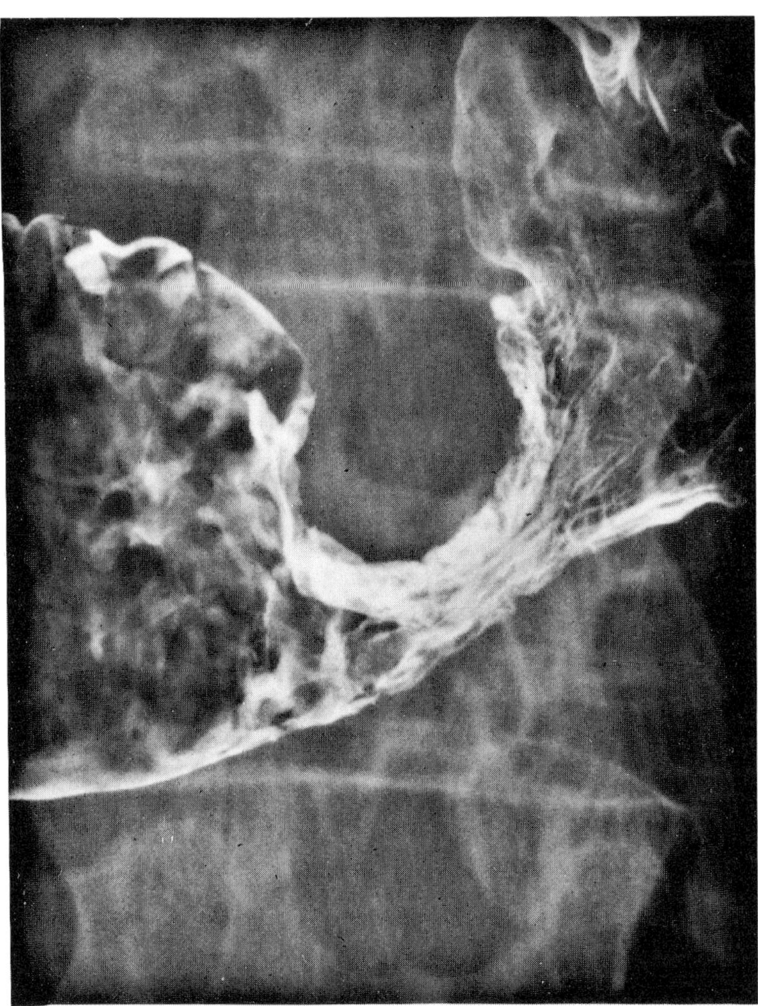

Fig. D.2. An asymmetrical narrowed segment was present in the mid-transverse colon. With further distension and change in patient position this area distended fully. This spastic segment corresponds to Cannon's point.

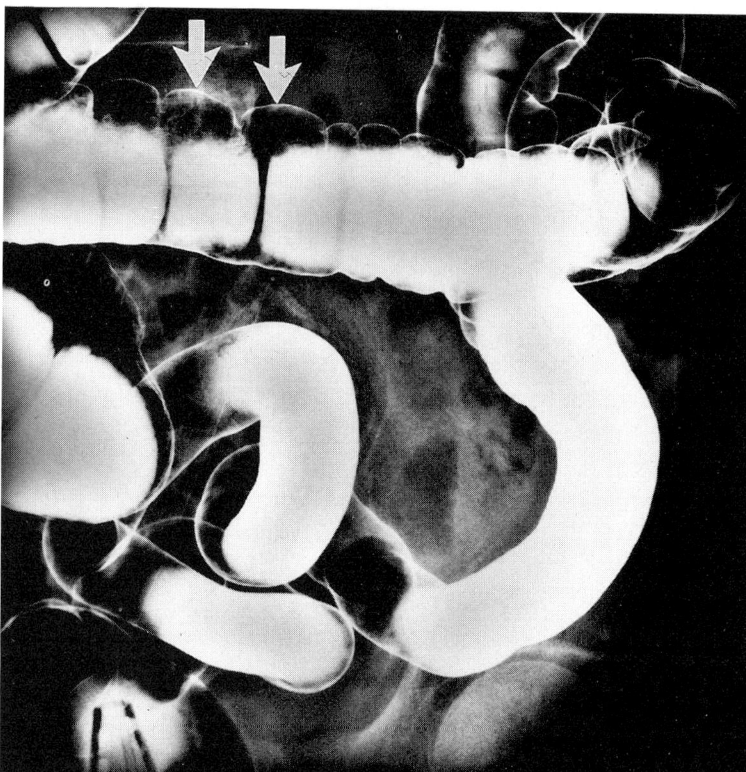

Fig. D.3. With adequate distension the haustra are still visible in the transverse colon (arrows) but are completely obliterated in the distal descending and sigmoid portions of the colon.

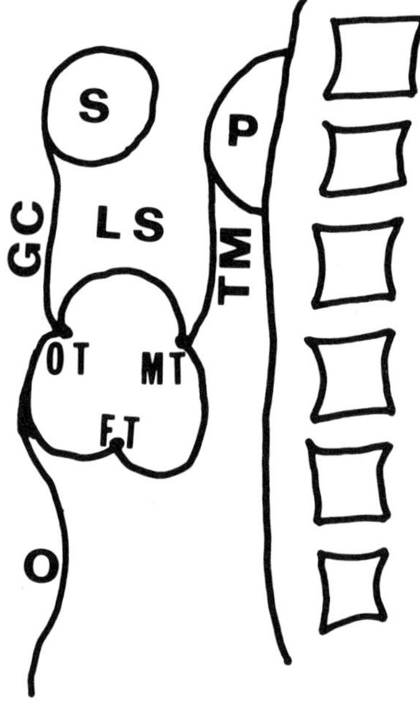

Fig. D.5. Cross-section of the transverse colon showing the relationship of the taeniae to surrounding structures. S – stomach, P – pancreas, LS – lesser sac, GC – gastro-colic ligament, O – greater omentum, TM – transverse mesocolon, OT – omental taenia, MT – mesocolic taenia, FT – free taenia.

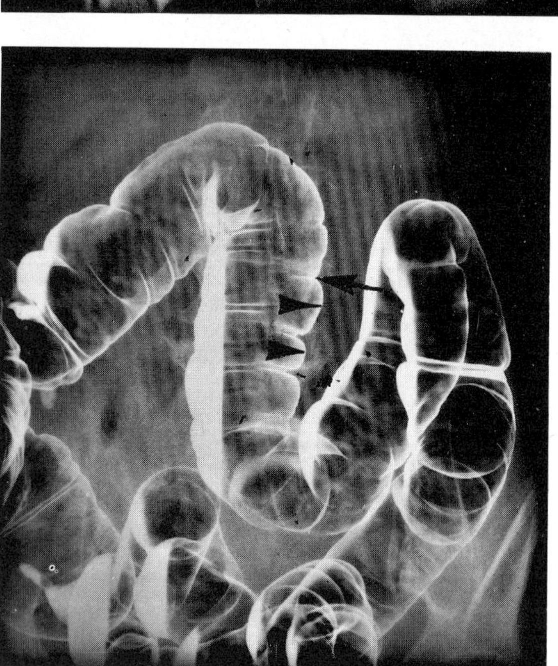

Fig. D.4. The haustra (arrowheads) are outpouchings between the plicae semilunares (arrows).

sac-like out-pouchings and *not* the indentations (Fig. D.4). These latter crescent-shaped folds are known as the plicae semilunares and run between the taeniae. Unlike the small bowel, where the folds do not contain muscle, the plicae contain a portion of the circular muscle layer.

The radiological anatomy of the taeniae and haustra has been elegantly studied by Meyers et al. (24). The taenia are most prominent in the right colon and gradually become inconspicuous in the distal sigmoid. The three taeniae are: omental taenia (taenia omentalis), mesocolic taenia (taenia mesocolica), and free taenia (taenia libera). The location of these three taenia is best visualized if one considers the transverse colon (Fig. D.5). Here the greater omentum extends inferiorly and the gastrocolic ligament superiorly from the omental taenia. The transverse mesocolon attaches superiorly and posteriorly to the mesocolic taenia. The free taenia,

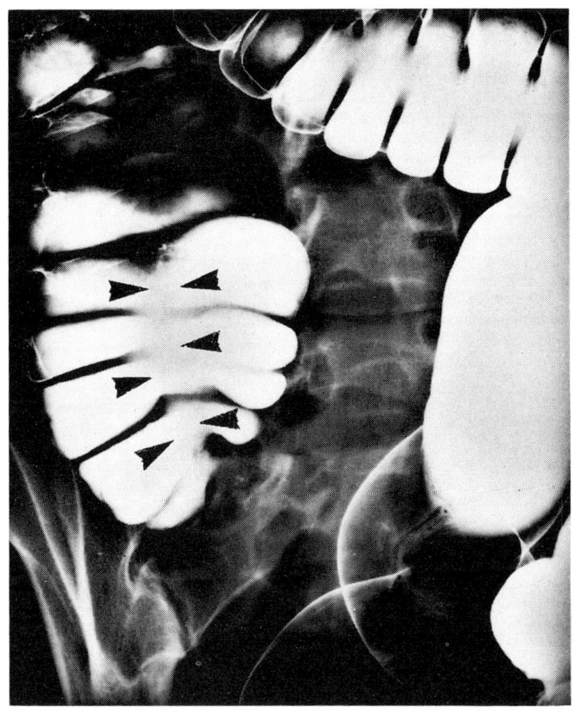

Fig. D.6. With the patient prone, barium outlines the longitudinal anteriorly located taenia libera (arrowheads).

as its name implies, has no mesenteric attachment and is inferior and posterior to the omental taenia. In the ascending and descending parts of the colon there is 90° rotation along the longitudinal axis and the free taenia faces anteriorly, the mesocolic taenia medially and the omental taenia laterally (Fig. D.6).

The colon haustra, oriented between the taenia, have a similar relationship (24). In the transverse colon the haustra located between the omental and mesocolic taeniae face superiorly and represent the inferior boundary of the lesser sac. Diseases involving the lesser sac thus involve the superior haustral row in the transverse colon. In both the ascending and descending portions of the colon, this superior row of haustra faces posteriorly, i.e., towards the extraperitoneal structures. With a patient supine, on a double-contrast examination barium pools in these haustra; this is more obvious in the ascending colon where the haustra are more prominent (Fig. D.7).

In the ascending and descending portions of the colon, the haustra between the omental and free taenia are adjacent to the lateral paracolic gutter and face the peritoneal surface. The haustra be-

Fig. D.7. With the patient supine, barium pools in the posteriorly located haustra running between the omental and mesocolic taeniae (arrowheads).

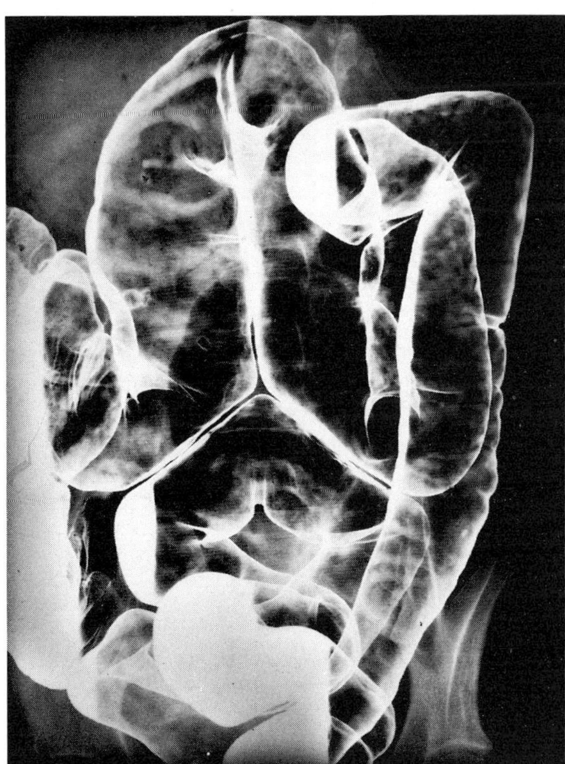

Fig. D.8. Redundant colon with the sigmoid and transverse portions of the colon indenting each other.

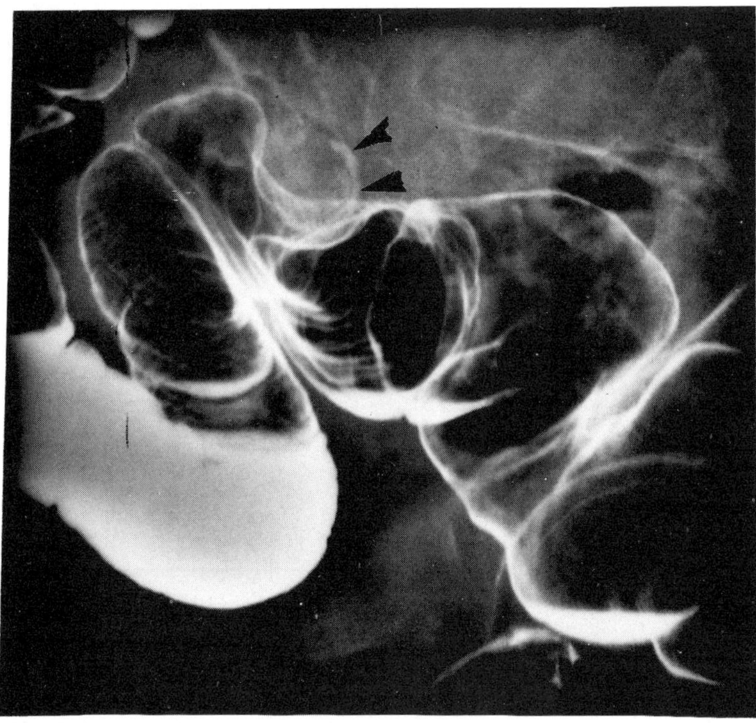

Fig. D.9. A dilated artery indents the sigmoid colon. Extensive calcifications are present in the arterial wall (arrowheads).

tween the mesocolic and free taenia are adjacent to the medial paracolic gutter and also face the peritoneal surface.

Some of the colitides are associated with a loss of haustration. This loss may be segmental or generalized, depending upon the extent of disease. It may be only a transient phenomenon, with haustra reappearing once the disease has cleared.

Adjacent structures may indent the colon. Unless adhesions are present, the indentation generally changes as the patient is rotated or stood up. The normal liver, spleen, gall bladder, and loops of bowel may all indent the colon (Fig. D.8). Similarly, enlarged organs, inflammatory masses and neoplasms may have a prominent impression on the colon (Fig. D.9).

II.E. Appendix

The appendix is developed by the twelfth week of intrauterine life into a funnel-shaped outpouching of the cecum (25). In children, the appendix is relatively short and has a wide diameter and only later on in life does it elongate and assume its usual adult vermiform appearance.

The appendix is thought to be a structure with little function. The rich lymphatic tissue in the appendix points towards an immunological function and the appendix may be involved in antibody formation.

In any group of patients the length of the appendix varies tremendously and the published figures of an average length only tend to mislead. Of more interest to the radiologist is that the tip of the appendix often has a bulbous dilatation, while the neck, close to its insertion into the cecum, can be narrowed.

The intraabdominal location of the appendix can vary considerably. It has been found in various internal fossae and in external hernial sacs (26, 27). The major factor determining the subsequent location of the appendix is prenatal rotation of the mid-gut. In most patients the appendix is in the right lower quadrant. It can be behind the cecum, point medially, extend over the pelvic brim, or point laterally (28). In the most common position, which is retrocecal, the appendix may be either intraperitoneal or extraperitoneal in location. With partial rotation or lack of rotation, however, the appendix can be located in any quadrant of the abdomen.

The appendix arises at the tip of the cecum and at the origin of the three taenia coli. It may have a short mesentery at its base, called the mesoap-

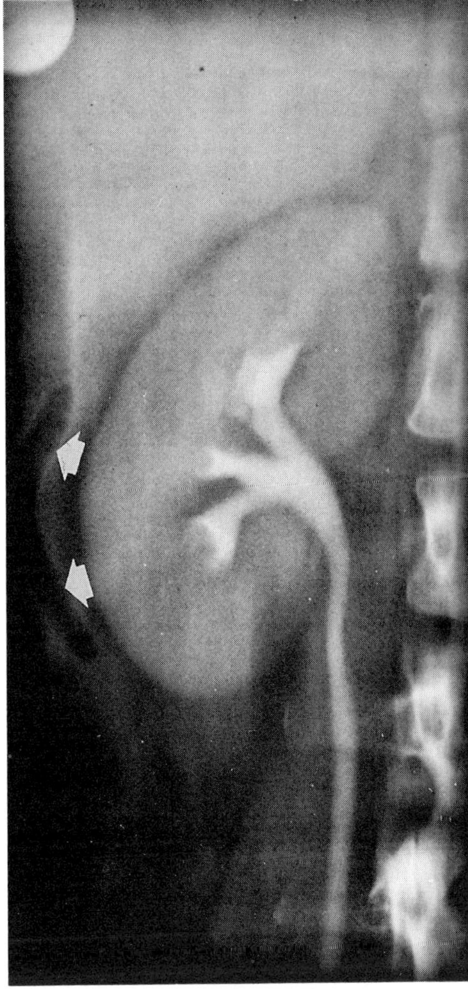

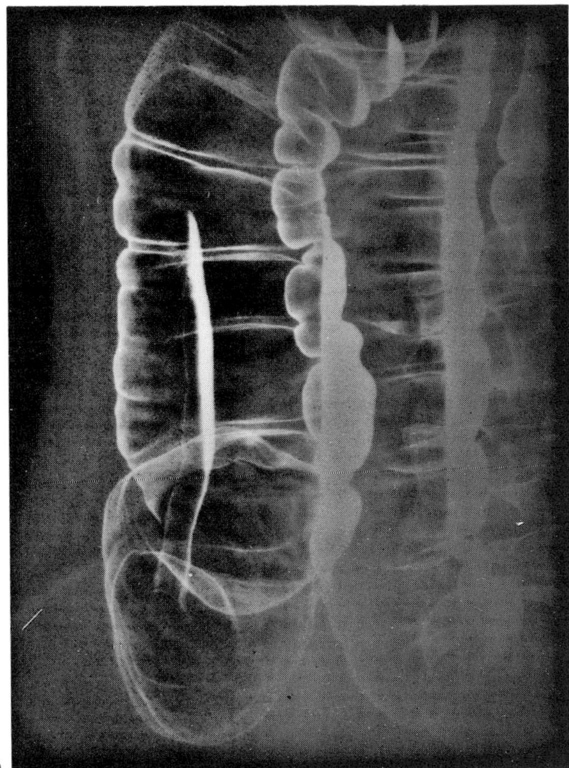

Fig. E.1. (a) Tomography during intravenous pyelography revealed a linear, gas-filled structure adjacent to the right kidney (arrowheads). (b) Subsequent barium enema shows that this structure is a relatively long retrocecal appendix. The patient had no symptoms referrable to the appendix.

pendix. The tip is usually free. The appendix can be relatively mobile and can change its position between two examination.

There may be occasional peristaltic waves present in the appendix, although in general, little contraction is present on any one examination. Contrast retained in the appendix for weeks or even occasionally months is not unusual.

Following appendectomy, a mass may be present in the cecum at the site of insertion of the appendix (29). This mass represents the intraluminal extension of an inverted edematous appendiceal stump and may be especially prominent shortly after surgery. Usually the history of a prior appendectomy and the characteristic location provide ready differentiation. Although the inverted stump can act as a lead point for an intussusception, associated adhesions from the patient's surgery generally prevent such a complication.

Occasionally, even with adequate cecal distension, the appendix does not fill during a barium enema. If a prior appendectomy has been excluded, then one must postulate either appendiceal obstruction or a prior 'autoamputation'. Sometimes a gas-filled appendix is seen on noncontrast radiographs of the abdomen. This is a normal finding (30) (Fig. E.1).

II.F. Right colon

The cecum is a wide pouch situated inferiorly to the ileocecal valve. In some patients, the peritoneal reflection posterior to the cecum is low and the cecum, and at times even the terminal ileum, are firmly attached to the posterior abdominal wall. At other times, the peritoneal reflection occurs so high that even a portion of the ascending colon is surrounded by peritoneum.

The cecum can be quite mobile and may extend to the left side of the abdomen or into the pelvis (Fig. F.1). When distended, the cecum may displace surrounding structures and abut on the anterior abdominal wall.

Cecal duplication is rare; when present, it is not uncommon to also have appendiceal duplication since the appendix originates from the cecum. The cecum tends to be absent or hypoplastic when there is agenesis of the appendix.

An excellent review of the radiography of the ileocecal valve has been published by Short et al. (31). In the average patient, this valve, also known in Europe as Bauhin's valve, points medially and posteriorly. The valve is usually located one major haustrum distal to the appendix and is on the same side as the appendix. The reason is that the medial cecal haustrum does not grow as rapidly as the more laterally placed haustrum, resulting in asymmetry. With partial malrotation both the ileocecal valve and the appendix can be laterally placed.

The valve is bilobed and consists of a larger superior and smaller inferior lips, both being semilunar in shape. When viewed *en face*, the valve has an oval appearance with radiating folds towards a central collection of barium mimicking an ulcer (Fig. F.2). Because of the valve's known location there should be little chance of confusing it with a tumor. Although it is commonly assumed that the function of the valve is simply to prevent reflux of colon content into the terminal ileum, it may also act as a sphincter preventing ileal contents from spilling into the colon too quickly.

There is considerable variation in the size of the valve. The apparent size of the valve may also change with the degree of distension (31). With compression the valve may become larger and more prominent in outline.

The most common cause of a large ileocecal valve is excess fat, a condition more common in women than men. Such fatty infiltration, or lipomatosis, is of little significance; radiographically, the problem is differentiating lipomatosis from a neoplasm. A valve infiltrated with fat generally is quite soft and

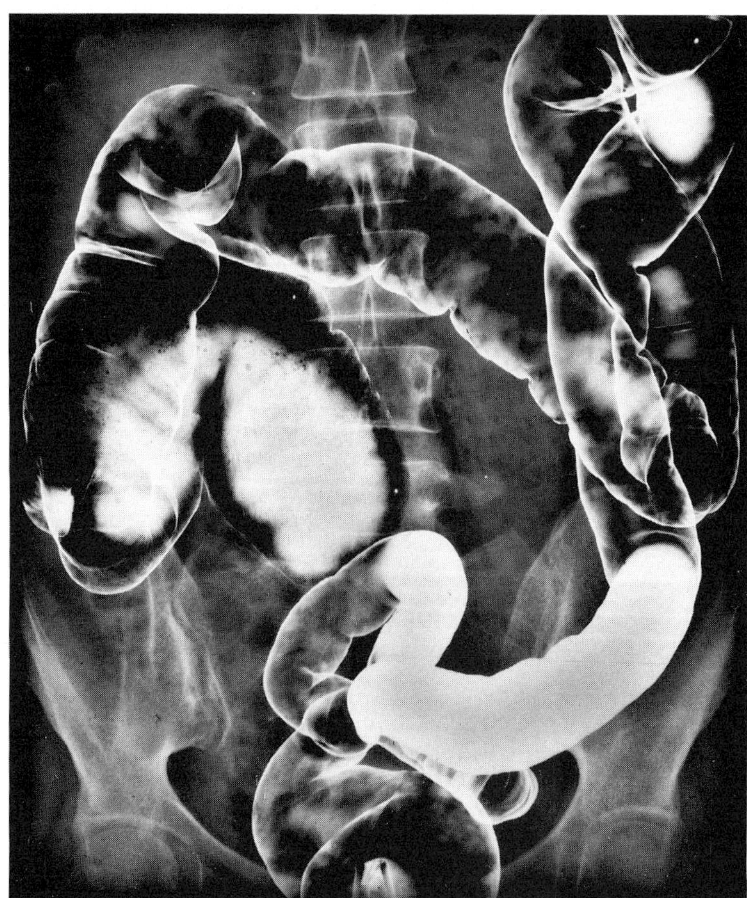

Fig. F.1. A mobile cecum and redundant ascending colon. A portion of the ascending colon is intraperitoneal in location.

changes shape with compression, while most tumors are quite firm in consistency. Also, fatty infiltration generally results in both lips of the valve being symmetrically involved, while malignant tumors tend initially to infiltrate either one or the other lip, resulting in considerable asymmetry. In children, lymphoid hyperplasia is a rare cause of a large valve (32).

Transient prolapse of the ileocecal valve is not abnormal. A postevacuation radiograph may reveal prolapse as a prominent mass at the valve; with distension the prolapse is reduced and the mass can no longer be identified. Retrograde prolapse of the ileocecal valve also occurs and should be considered a normal variant (33).

The terminal ileum usually lies parallel to the cecum and makes a sharp 90° turn to the right to insert at the ileocecal valve (Fig. F.3). The terminal ileum may be either partly fused to the cecum or, more commonly, it may be attached to the medial wall of the cecum by a fold originating on the antimesenteric (lateral) border of the terminal ileum. Occasionally, this fold is lax or completely absent and the terminal ileum then extends horizontally across the abdomen before inserting into the ileocecal valve.

Reflux during a barium enema is normal. Only occasionally will a patient not reflux, with the incidence of reflux reflecting the persistence and experience of the examiner.

The ascending colon originates from a horizontal line drawn through the ileocecal valve and becomes the transverse colon at the hepatic flexure, with the flexure acting as a transition zone. At the hepatic flexure, the colon turns anteriorly and is initially in close proximity to the right kidney and then in contact with the descending portion of the duodenum. Usually just distal to this point the colon becomes intraperitoneal in location, acquires a mesentery, and continues to swing anteriorly. In approximately 80% of patients, the superior and medial aspect of the hepatic flexure is adjacent to the gall bladder (34). Thus, gall bladder disease may affect the colon.

Occasionally the hepatic flexure extends far superiorly and lies just beneath the right hemi-

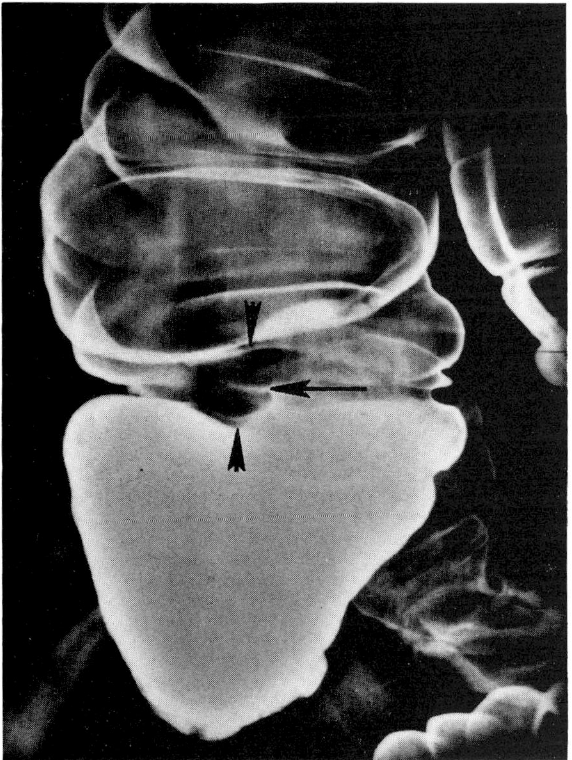

Fig. F.2. *En face* appearance of the ileocecal valve (arrowheads). The linear collection of barium (arrow) represents contrast between the two valve lips.

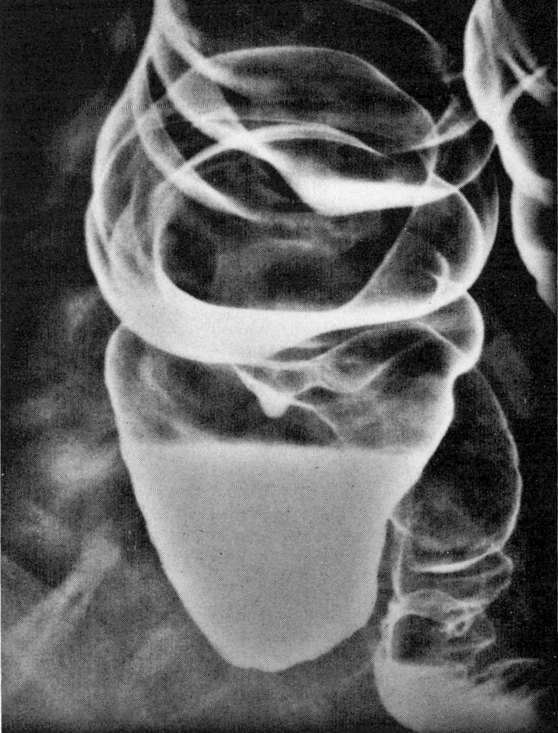

Fig. F.3. Usual relationship between terminal ileum and cecum. Such close approximation is due to a short fold connecting the terminal ileum to the cecum.

diaphragm. Such colon interposition between the liver and diaphragm, known as Chilaiditi's syndrome (35), implies a failure of fusion of the posterior abdominal wall in association with lax mesenteric attachments. The vast majority of these patients are asymptomatic and the condition is simply a curiosity.

II.G. Transverse colon

The most mobile portion of the colon is the transverse colon; it is surrounded by peritoneum and is usually far anterior in location. In women the mesocolon tends to be elongated, with the transverse colon extending far inferiorly into the abdomen, while in men the transverse colon has a straighter course.

In the left upper quadrant the transverse colon is attached to the diaphragm at the anatomic splenic flexure by the phrenicocolic ligament. The 'radiologic' splenic flexure, which differs from the anatomic flexure, is usually the most superior aspect of the colon (Fig. G.1). The radiologic flexure simply represents a sharp angulation in the distal transverse colon, with the anatomic splenic flexure being located more distally (36).

II.H. Left colon

The descending or left colon starts at the anatomic splenic flexure. In its proximal portion, it is adjacent to the medially and posteriorly placed left kidney. This part of the colon is enveloped by the peritoneum on three sides, with its posterior portion facing the extraperitoneal structures. It is not unusual to see some redundancy in this portion of the colon.

II.I. Sigmoid colon

The junction of the descending and sigmoid colon is ill-defined and controversial in location. Although anatomically the sigmoid colon can be outlined by its attached mesentery, radiographically the point where the descending colon acquires a mesentery is difficult to define. A rough landmark for the proximal end of the sigmoid is the point where the colon crosses the iliac crest. Sometimes, however, the level of the external iliac artery or the psoas muscle border is used to define the proximal end of the sigmoid. In general, if there is a short descending colon, the sigmoid tends to be long and vice versa.

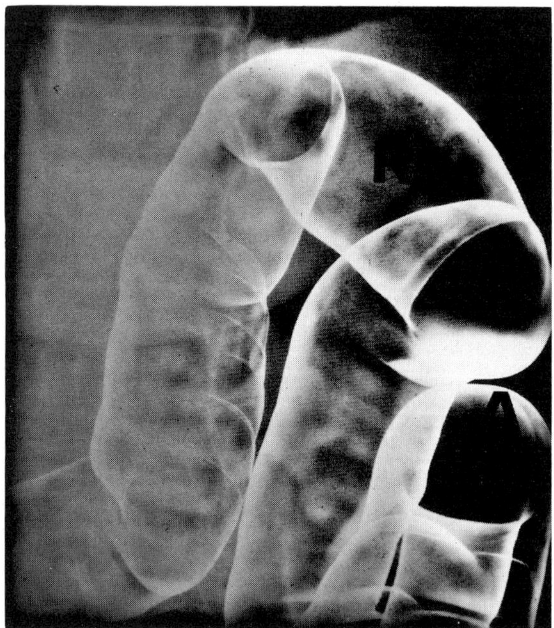

Fig. G.1. The 'radiologic' splenic flexure (R) is still part of the transverse colon. The anatomic splenic flexure (A) is more distal and inferior.

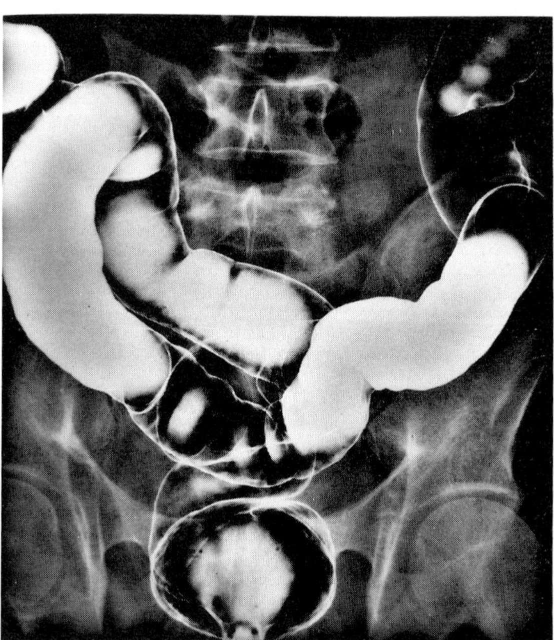

Fig. I.1. A redundant sigmoid, located intraperitoneally, predisposes to sigmoid volvulus.

The sigmoid colon is surrounded by peritoneum and thus is intraperitoneal in location. The peritoneum forms a mesentery called the sigmoid mesocolon. Because of variation in length of the sigmoid there is considerable mobility and redundancy (Fig. I.1). When collapsed the sigmoid usually lies in the pelvis, however, with distention it rises into the abdomen. Because of a commonly associated long mesentery, the most common site of colon volvulus is in the sigmoid colon.

II.J. Rectum

The intraperitoneally located sigmoid passes posteriorly and inferiorly and becomes the extraperitoneal rectum. The peritoneal reflection does not stop abruptly; rather, it extends slightly more inferiorly along the anterior and lateral margins of the rectum. The actual point where the colon becomes extraperitoneal is difficult to judge radiographically because there is considerable individual variation to the inferior peritoneal reflections. Radiographically the rectosigmoid junction is often assumed to be opposite the sacral promontory.

The peritoneal reflection anterior to the rectum results in a space known as the pouch of Douglas. In the female, this space is the rectovaginal pouch, while in the male it represents the rectovesical pouch. The pouch of Douglas can vary in its inferior extent not only upon the course of the peritonal reflection but also upon the degree of bladder filling. Laterally, the pouch extends into the lateral paravesical recesses. The inferior surface of the pouch of Douglas is formed by fusion of the peritoneum to the rectovesical septum (rectovaginal septum in the female). This septum, also known as Denonvillier's fascia, is a pathway for inflam-

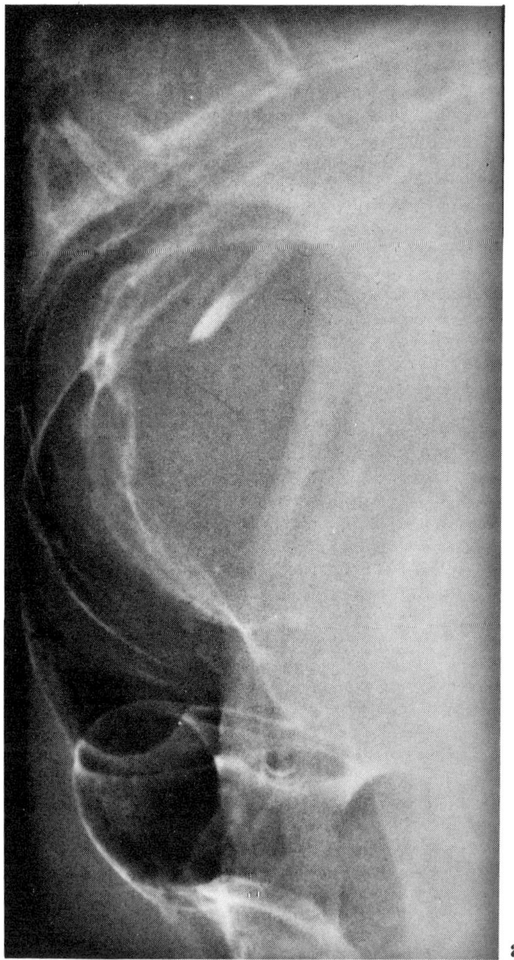

a

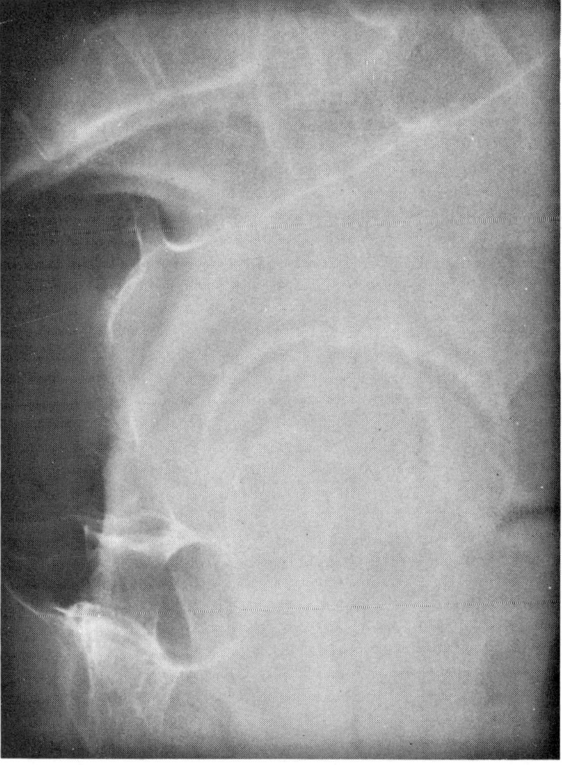

b

Fig. J.1. Ascites mimicking a tumor in the pouch of Douglas. (a) The mass is prominent with the patient upright. (b) Mass disappears when the patient is recumbent. (Courtesy of Drs. A. Schulman and S. Fataar (38), copyright 1979, Royal College of Radiologists.)

matory and tumor spread from the pelvic organs to the rectum (37). Likewise, intraperitoneal fluid and tumor tend to gravitate to the pouch of Douglas, resulting in extrinsic narrowing of the rectosigmoid junction and proximal portions of the rectum (38). With the patient upright, ascites may mimic a tumor at this location; a change in size of the mass with the patient recumbent should suggest the correct diagnosis (Fig. J.1).

The rectum does not have sacculations as seen in the rest of the colon. There are, however, several transverse semilunar folds, known as the valves of Houston, produced by thickening of the muscles. In most patients there are three such valves, with the superior and inferior valves on the left side and the middle valve usually extending to the right (Fig. J.2). These valves serve as convenient radiographic landmarks. Occasionally, a tumor may be hidden along the superior aspect of one of the valves and be missed on sigmoidoscopy or colonoscopy.

The distal end of the rectum turns inferiorly and posteriorly and becomes the anal canal. Vertical folds, called the columns of Morgagni, run through the anal canal. The internal hemorrhoidal veins are located in the submucosa at the level of the columns of Morgagni. When enlarged, these veins are readily visible radiologically, especially on collapsed views of the rectum (Fig. J.3). A prolapsing hemorrhoidal tag may mimic a neoplasm (Fig. J.4).

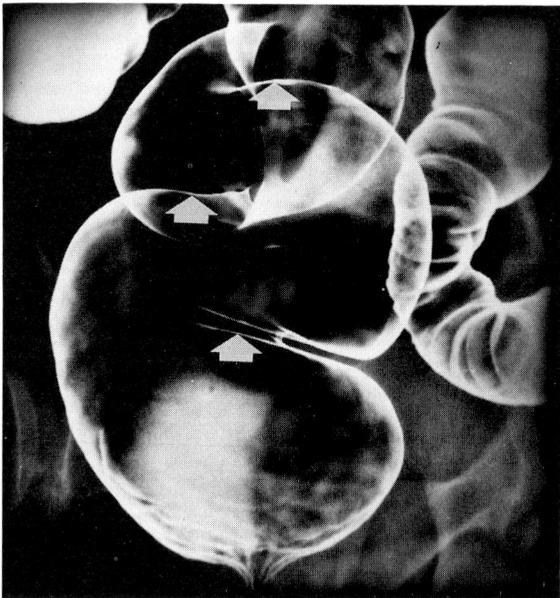

Fig. J.2. Frontal view of the rectum shows the three valves of Houston (arrowheads). A tumor located just proximal to one of the valves can be missed on sigmoidoscopy.

The mucocutaneous junction between the colon and skin is within the anal canal; this junction is variable, not well defined, and is difficult to outline radiographically.

The presacral space is bound superiorly by the peritoneal reflection and inferiorly by the pelvic floor muscles. Fascial layers over the rectum and sacrum define the anterior and posterior borders. This space contains fat, lymphatics, blood vessels, nerves, and fibrous tissue, with a lesion in any of these structures or any of the adjacent structures potentially resulting in widening of the presacral space (Table J.1) (Fig. J.5). This space is generally the same width throughout its length. There may be apparent widening if the rectum is displaced from midline or if a radiograph is obtained with the patient in an oblique position. It is difficult to assign a normal range to the width of this space,

Table J.1. Conditions associated with widening of the presacral space

1. Diffuse widening
   a. Colitides
      1. Ulcerative colitis
      2. Regional enteritis
      3. Ischemic colitis
      4. Infectious colitis
      5. Radiation colitis
   b. Other
      1. Normal variation
      2. Inferior vena cava occlusion
      3. Periaortic lymphatic occlusion
      4. Steroid therapy or related conditions
      5. Obesity or pelvic lipomatosis
      6. Prior pelvic surgery
      7. Diffuse tumor infiltration
      8. Diffuse infiltration such as amyloidosis
2. Localized widening
   a. Tumors
      1. Bone tumors
      2. Soft tissue tumors
      3. Tumors in adjacent pelvic organs
      4. Colon tumors
      5. Neurogenic tumors
      6. Lymphoma
      7. Metastatic tumors
   b. Other
      1. Normal variation
      2. Trauma or prior surgery
      3. Infection
      4. Developmental cysts

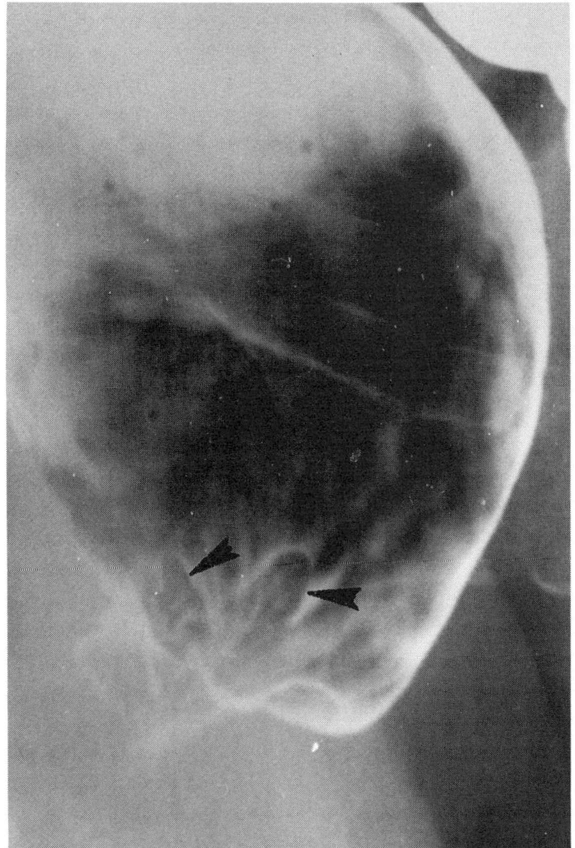

a

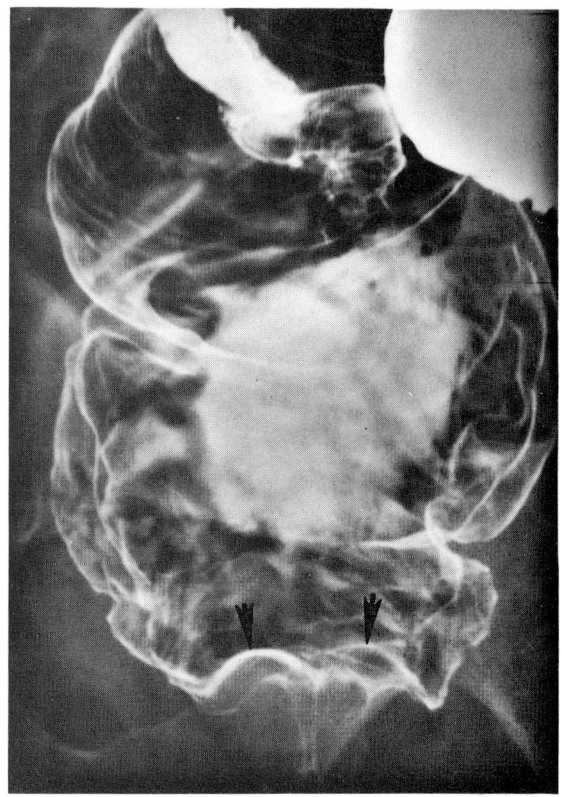

b

Fig. J.3. Two examples of internal hemorrhoids (arrowheads). These are best seen with the enema tip removed.

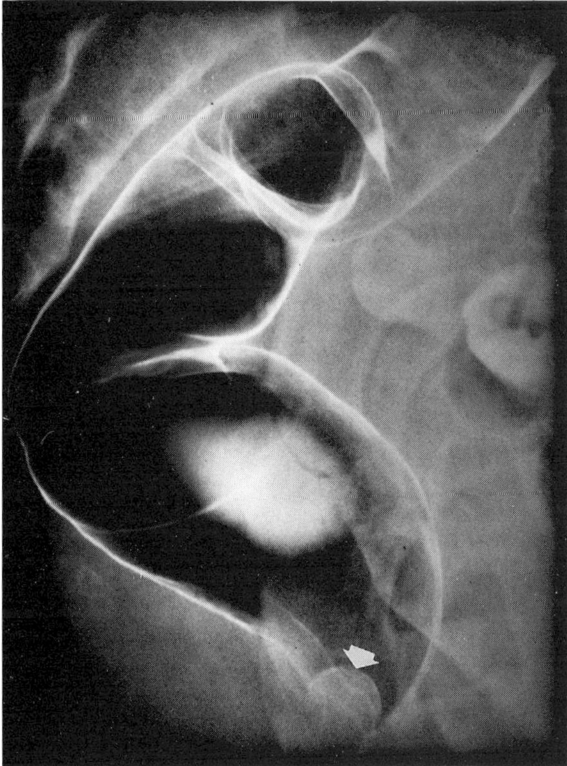

a

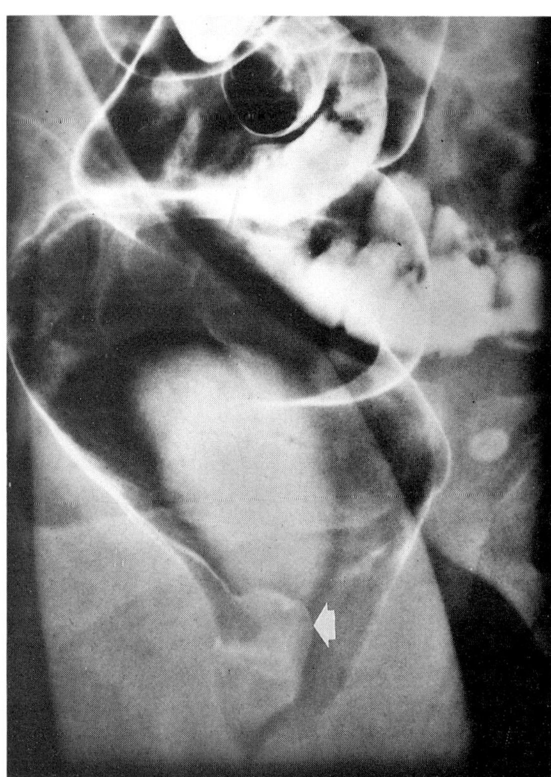

b

Fig. J.4. (a) Lateral and (b) oblique views of the rectum show a smooth polyp in the rectum (arrowheads). The polyp was a hemorrhoidal tag. (Courtesy of D. Maglinte, M.D., Indianapolis, Indiana.)

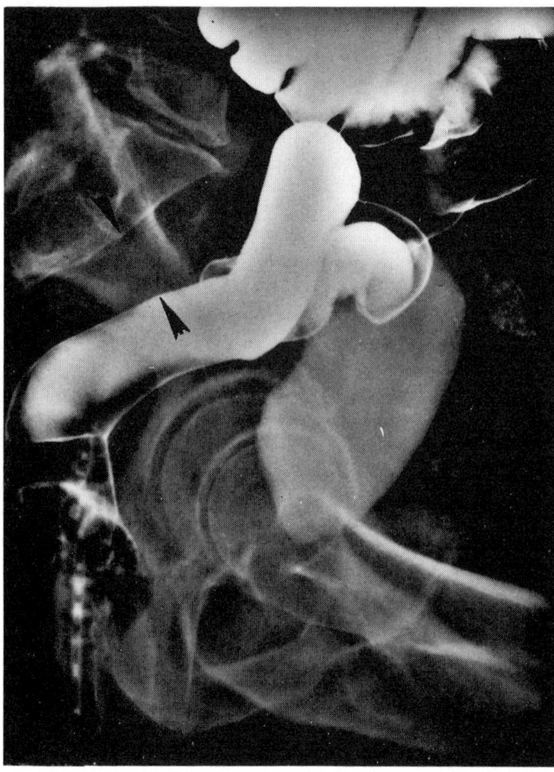

Fig. J.5. An example of diffuse widening of the presacral space (arrowheads). Contrast is present in the colon, bladder, and several lymph nodes. In this patient the etiology of the widened presacral space was inferior vena caval obstruction.

although various numbers have appeared in the literature (39). There is considerable variation between individuals. Obesity is a major factor in determining the width of the presacral space. Likewise, different degrees of colon distension will influence the apparent width. An apparent widening by itself does not mean that an abnormality is present (40). Generally, further substantiation is necessary.

References

1. Borg SA, Whitehouse GH, Griffiths GJ: A mobile calcified amputated appendix epiploica. AJR 127:349–350, 1976.
2. Fenoglio CM, Kaye GI, Lane N: Distribution of human colonic lymphatics in normal, hyperplastic, and adenomatous tissue. Its relationship to metastasis from small carcinomas in pedunculated adenomas, with two case reports. Gastroenterology 64:51–66, 1973.
3. Dassel PM: Innocuous filling of the intestinal glands of the colon during barium enema (spiculation) simulating organic disease. Radiology 78:799–801, 1962.
4. Williams I: Innominate grooves in the surface of mucosa. Radiology 84:877–880, 1965.
5. Matsuura K, Nakata H, Takeda N, Nakata S, Shimoda Y: Innominate lines of the colon. Radiological–histological correlation. Radiology 123:581–584, 1977.
6. Cole FM: Innominate grooves of the colon: morphological characteristics and etiologic mechanisms. Radiology 128:41–43, 1978.
7. Kelvin FM, Max RJ, Norton GA, Oddson TA, Rice RP, Thompson WM, Garbutt JT: Lymphoid follicular pattern of the colon in adults. AJR 133:821–825, 1979.
8. Dukes C, Bussey HJR: The number of lymphoid follicles of the human large intestine. J Pathol Bacteriol 29:111–116, 1926.
9. Riddlesberger MM Jr, Lebenthal E: Nodular colonic mucosa of childhood: normal or pathologic. Gastroenterology 79:265–270, 1980.
10. Franken EA: Lymphoid hyperplasia of the colon. Radiology 94:329–334, 1970.
11. Crooks DJM, Brown WR: The distribution of intestinal nodular lymphoid hyperplasia in immunoglobulin deficiency. Clin Radiol 31:701–706, 1980.
12. Shaw EB, Hennigar GR: Intestinal lymphoid polyposis. Am J Clin Path 61:417–422, 1974.
13. Capitano MA, Kirkpatrick JA: Lymphoid hyperplasia of the colon in children. Radiology 94:323–327, 1970.
14. Theander G, Trägardh B: Lymphoid hyperplasia of the colon in childhood. Acta Radiol (Diagn) 17:631–640, 1976.
15. Bargen JA, Wesson HR, Jackman RJ: Studies on the ileocecal junction (ileocecus). Surg Gynecol Obstet 71:33–38, 1940.
16. Michels NA, Siddharth P, Kornblith PL, Parke WW: The variant blood supply to the small and large intestines: its import in regional resections. J Int Coll Surg 39:127–170, 1963.
17. Meyers MA: Griffiths' point: critical anastomosis at the splenic flexure. AJR 126:77–94, 1976.
18. Griffiths JD: Surgical anatomy of the blood supply of the distal colon. Ann R Coll Surg 19:241–256, 1956.
19. Drummond H: Some points relating to the surgical anatomy of the arterial supply of the large intestine. Proc R Soc Med 7:185–193, 1913.
20. Kilpatrick ZM, Farman J, Yesner R, Spiro HM: Ischemic proctitis. JAMA 205:74–80, 1968.
21. Miller RE, Chernish SM, Skucas J, Rosenak BD, Rodda BE: Hypotonic colon examination with glucagon. Radiology 113: 555–562, 1974.
22. Templeton AW: Colon sphincters simulating organic disease. Radiology 75:237–241, 1960.
23. Ritchie JA: Movement of segmental constrictions in the human colon. Gut 12:350–355, 1971.
24. Meyers MA, Volberg F, Katzen B, Abbott G: Haustral anatomy and pathology: a new look — I. Roentgen identification of normal patterns and relationships. Radiology 108:497–504, 1973.
25. Balthazar EJ, Gade M: The normal and abnormal development of the appendix. Radiology 121:599–604, 1976.
26. Collins DC: 71,000 human appendix specimens: a final report, summarizing forty years' study. Am J Proctol 14:365–381, 1963.
27. Joffe N: Radiology of acute appendicitis and its complications. Crit Rev Clin Radiol 7:97–160, 1975.
28. Wakely CPG: The position of the vermiform appendix as ascertained by an analysis of 10,000 cases. J Anat 67:277–283, 1933.

29. Ekberg O: Cecal changes following appendectomy. Gastrointest Radiol 2:57–60, 1977.
30. Lim MS: Gas-filled appendix: lack of diagnostic specificity. AJR 128:209–210, 1977.
31. Short WF, Smith BD, Hoy RJ: Roentgenologic evaluation of the prominent or the unusual ileocecal valve. Med Radiogr Photogr 52:2–26, 1976.
32. Selke AC, Jr., Jona JZ, Belin RP: Massive enlargement of the ileocecal valve due to lymphoid hyperplasia. AJR 127:518–520, 1976.
33. Hatten HP Jr, Mostowycz L, Hagihara PF: Retrograde prolapse of the ileocecal valve. AJR 128:755–757, 1977.
34. Ghahremani GG, Meyers MA: The cholecysto-colic relationships. A Roentgen-anatomic study of the colonic manifestations of gall bladder disorders. AJR 125:21–34, 1975.
35. Chilaiditi D: Zur Frage der Hepatoptose und Ptose im Allgemeinen im Anschluss und drei Fälle von temporärer, partieller Leberverlagerung. Fortschr Geb Roentgenstr 16:173–208, 1910–11.
36. Whalen JP: Anatomy of the colon. Guide to intra-abdominal pathology. AJR 125:3–20, 1975.
37. Hultborn KA, Morales O, Romanus R: The so-called shelf tumour of the rectum. Acta Radiol Suppl 124:1–46, 1955.
38. Schulman A, Fataar S: Extrinsic stretching, narrowing and anterior indentation of the rectosigmoid junction. Clin Radiol 30:463–469, 1979.
39. Gardiner GA: Routine lateral view of the barium filled rectum: is it worthwhile? A review of 2500 consecutive examinations. AJR 104:571–579, 1968.
40. Teplick SK, Stark P, Clark RE, Metz JR, Shapiro JH: The retrorectal space. Clin Radiol 29:177–184, 1978.

PART III

LESIONS

III.1. THE COLITIDES

III.1.A. Introduction

The various colitides are arbitrarily included in this section. The exception is diverticulitis, which is discussed in its associated setting of diverticulosis. The colitides are arbitrarily divided into several broad categories, based either on etiology or on the clinical presentation. They have different rates of incidence throughout the world; some are associated with poverty and low living standards, while others have a high incidence in the well-developed industrial countries.

Some colitides, such as the infectious, are considerably more prevalent in the tropical regions. Other colitides, such as ulcerative colitis and regional enteritis, are encountered considerably less frequently in those areas where infectious colitis is prevalent. Likewise, diverticular disease and colon cancers are less frequently encountered in the tropical regions where infectious colitis is more rampant. Whether repeated infection of the colon, diet, or other associated environmental influences have a significant role in determining the incidence of a particular type of colitis is still poorly understood.

The radiographic appearance of some colitides may be almost pathognomonic. However, microscopic examination, culture, and at times serological testing are generally necessary not only to confirm the diagnosis, but also to exclude other similar appearing diseases. In particular, the radiographic appearance of both regional enteritis and ulcerative colitis may be closely mimicked by some of the infectious colitides and cultures should be obtained even in those patients where the radiographic appearance is 'classic'.

Occasionally encountered are unusual colitides. These range from a 'herbal-enema' colitis encountered in Africa (1), a soapsuds enema colitis due to possible hypersensitivity (2), hydrogen peroxide enema colitis (3), thermal colitis following irrigation with hot water (4), chrysotherapy-induced enterocolitis when gold therapy is used in rheumatoid arthritis (5–7), to an unclassifiable colitis associated with an immunodeficiency state (8). New colitides continue to be discovered. As an example, colitis developing in the excluded segment following a colostomy has recently been described (9).

Although regional enteritis and ulcerative colitis are discussed separately, at present there is little evidence to prove that they are indeed different entities. It is likewise not known whether one or the other actually represents the manifestation of several 'diseases'. In an occasional patient, neither the clinical presentation, radiographic appearance nor pathological examination allows ready classification. Some investigators label these patients as having 'colitis indeterminate' (10) or having 'inflammatory bowel disease' (IBD). The medical therapy for both ulcerative colitis and regional enteritis is essentially the same. The major difference is in prognosis. Occasionally ulcerative colitis will regress and follow-up colon examinations will be normal, while it is unusual for regional enteritis to regress. The latter entity either progresses or smoulders for the patient's remaining lifetime. The incidence of malignancy in regional enteritis is small, while in ulcerative colitis involving the entire colon the threat of malignancy is so high that an eventual colectomy is considered in these patients. A total proctocolectomy 'cures' ulcerative colitis, while regional enteritis may recur after surgery. It is because of this difference in prognosis that most investigators do not simply label all of these patients as having IBD, but still attempt to differentiate into the two entities.

The pathogenesis of diarrhea in patients with inflammatory bowel disease is poorly understood. Presumably, the electrolyte transport mechanism across the mucosa is deranged. Diseased mucosa has an abnormal electric potential difference and a lower electric resistance across the mucosa (11).

It is difficult to assess the relative accuracy of diagnosis of colonoscopy, single-contrast and double-contrast barium enema. Resected specimens cannot be used as a valid standard because they generally represent examples of severe and long-standing disease. Most studies have relied considerably on colonoscopic or sigmoidoscopic biopsies to establish the presence of a 'colitis'.

Some radiologists still claim that the single contrast barium enema is sufficient in the study of colitis. Yet studies have clearly shown the superiority of the double-contrast examination in detecting disease. Colitis was missed in 20 to 81% of patients when a single contrast examination was performed (12–14). Obviously, the false negative rate will vary depending upon the relative severity of the findings.

When comparing the results of a double-contrast examination against the endoscopic findings, the overall agreement has ranged from 82 to 96.8% (15–18). Early changes can be detected with a double-contrast examination (19). The false-negative examinations are generally associated with mild findings during endoscopy.

The relative sensitivity of the double-contrast barium enema depends upon the severity of disease and the type of colitis. One study accurately correlated with the final diagnosis in 98% of patients with regional enteritis but only 83% in ulcerative colitis (20); others have found the correlation to be 94% and 98% respectively (18). The barium enema was more specific in differentiating ulcerative colitis from other colitides, with endoscopy incorrectly classifying 11% of these patients as regional enteritis (18).

Endoscopic visualization of the mucosa is not foolproof. Especially with regional enteritis, biopsy of endoscopically normal appearing mucosa can reveal IBD in a number of patients (21). Ideally, the colon must be studied with multiple biopsies even of those areas which appear endoscopically normal.

References

1. Young WS: Herbal-enema colitis and stricture. Br J Radiol 53:248–249, 1980.
2. Barker CS: Acute colitis resulting from soapsuds enema. Can Med Assoc J 52:285, 1945.
3. Meyer CT, Brand M, DeLuca VA, Spiro HM: Hydrogen peroxide colitis: a report of three patients. J Clin Gastroenterol 3:31–35, 1981.
4. Jackson FR, Ott DJ, Gelfand DW: Thermal injury of the colon due to colostomy irrigation. Gastrointest Radiol 6:231–233, 1981.
5. Kaplinsky N, Pras M, Frankl O: Severe enterocolitis complicating chrysotherapy. Ann Rheum Dis 32:574–577, 1973.
6. Stein HB, Urowitz MB: Gold-induced enterocolitis. Case report and literature review. J. Rheumatol 3:21–26, 1976.
7. Martin DM, Goldman JA, Gilliam J, Nasrallah SM: Gold-induced eosinophilic enterocolitis: response to oral cromolyn sodium. Gastroenterology 80:1567–1570, 1981.
8. Strauss RG, Ghishan F, Mitros F, Ebensberger JR, Kisker CT, Tannous R, Younoszai MK: Rectosigmoidal colitis in common variable immunodeficiency disease. Dig Dis Sci 25:798–801, 1980.
9. Glotzer DJ, Glick ME, Goldman H: Proctitis and colitis following diversion of the fecal stream. Gastroenterology 80:438–441, 1981.
10. Price AB: Overlap in the spectrum of non-specific inflammatory bowel disease — 'colitis indeterminate.' J Clin Pathol 31:567–577, 1978.
11. Hawker PC, McKay JS, Turnberg LA: Electrolyte transport across colonic mucosa from patients with inflammatory bowel disease. Gastroenterology 79:508–511, 1980.
12. Fennessy JJ, Sparberg M, Kirsner JB: Early roentgen manifestations of mild ulcerative colitis and proctitis. Radiology 87:848–858, 1966.
13. Nugent FW, Voidenheimer MC, Zuberi S, Garabedian MM, Parikh NK: Clinical course of ulcerative proctosigmoiditis. Am J Dig Dis 15:321–326, 1970.
14. Myren J, Eie H, Serck-Hanssen A: The diagnosis of colitis by colonoscopy with biopsy and x-ray examination. A blind comparative study. Scand J Gastroenterol 11:141–144, 1976.
15. Simpkins KC, Stevenson GW: The modified Malmö double-contrast barium enema in colitis: an assessment of its accuracy in reflecting sigmoidoscopic findings. Br J Radiol 45:486–492, 1972.
16. Kinsey I, Horness N, Anthonisen P, Riis P: The radiological diagnosis of nonspecific hemorrhagic proctocolitis (hemorrhagic proctitis and ulcerative colitis). Acta Med Scand 176:181–186, 1964.
17. Laufer I, Mullens JE, Hamilton J: Correlation of endoscopy and double-contrast radiography in the early stages of ulcerative and granulomatous colitis. Radiology 118:1–5, 1976.
18. Williams HJ, Stephens DH, Carlson HC: Double-contrast radiography: colonic inflammatory disease. AJR 137:315–322, 1981.
19. Fraser GM, Findlay JM: The double contrast enema in ulcerative and Crohn's colitis. Clin Radiol 27:103–112, 1976.
20. Kelvin FM, Oddson TA, Rice RP, Garbutt JT, Bradenham BP: Double contrast barium enema in Crohn's disease and ulcerative colitis. AJR 131:207–213, 1978.
21. Geboes K, Vantrappen G: The value of colonoscopy in the diagnosis of Crohn's disease. Gastrointest Endosc 22:18–23, 1975.

III.1.B. Ischemic colitis and related vascular disorders

a. Introduction

There is a rich blood supply to the colon and, as expected, a wide variety of vascular disorders can be encountered. Some of these disorders are now understood; others still defy understanding and can only be described. Discussed in this section are those disorders manifesting themselves primarily through their vasculature. Although various classifications have been proposed for vascular lesions of the bowel, none are satisfactory because of overlap and diverse conditions encountered. Some of the entitics covered in this section are considered to be tumors rather than colitides. They are included here simply as a matter of convenience.

Ischemic colitis results from an impaired blood supply to the colon. The initial changes are first seen in the mucosa, because it is more sensitive than the muscle layers (1); acute ischemia results in epithelial desquamation at the tips of the villi together with vascular congestion in the capillaries (2). Initially there is a marked loss of water and electrolytes into the lumen. With extended damage the insult is potentiated by bacterial invasion (3). Mucosal damage can lead to submucosal edema and hemorrhage into the lumen, with sloughing and ulceration the next step. With a more severe injury the muscle layers become involved and can lead to bowel wall necrosis.

Experimental studies in animals have shown that edema can be seen as early as four hours after the insult (4). In dogs, this initial edema appears as a fine 'saw-tooth' irregularity. Thumbprinting is generally present 12 to 24 hours later, with regression of these findings occurring in several weeks. Bowel infarction may take place as soon as six hours after the onset of the attack (5).

Ischemic colitis may be due to arterial occlusion, venous occlusion, or a 'nonocclusive' condition. Drugs such as oral contraceptives (6–9) ergot (10, 11) and digitalis have been associated with bowel ischemia. Although patients taking digitalis also generally have poor cardiac perfusion, digitalis increases vasoconstriction of the mesenteric arteries (12, 13).

b. Mesenteric thrombosis, embolus, and low flow states

Considerable interest has developed in this entity since the initial description by Boley et al. in 1963 (14). Ischemia is not a single disease but consists of a complex set of conditions resulting in bowel ischemia. The clinical manifestations of mesenteric thrombosis or embolus will vary depending upon the chronicity and intensity of the insult. There can be a sudden, severe life-threatening episode leaving the patient in shock. On the other hand, with mild, chronic disease the patient will simply complain of nonspecific abdominal pain, diarrhea, or nausea. The pain can be severe and often of sudden onset. Ischemia limited to the colon generally results in fewer clinical signs than generalized mesenteric ischemia. It is not unusual during the acute attack to have rectal bleeding, with the bleeding often being maroon or burgundy in color. Obviously the clinical picture will be influenced by the particular vessels involved, the extent of the vascular obstruction, and whether adequate collateral channels have developed (15). A combination of factors may be present; as an example, decreased mesenteric blood flow in a setting of atherosclerosis is not as well tolerated as it is with normal vessels (16).

The sequelae of ischemic bowel disease can take several alternative pathways: the patient can develop gangrene with perforation and peritonitis, there can be bowel fibrosis with stricture and a 'tube-like' appearance, or the ischemia can clear with no residual recognizable radiographic changes. Unfortunately, it is not always possible to predict the eventual outcome from the initial presentation.

There is controversy about the most common sites of involvement. Some report the splenic flexure as being commonly involved (17–19), while others have found the splenic flexure an unusual site of involvement (15). Occasionally there may be several sites (17) with skip areas mimicking regional enteritis. Rectal ischemia is not uncommon (19).

The extensive collateral blood supply to the colon can adjust to gradual occlusion and result in strange and complex pathways. As an example, with gradual onset of occlusion, even with only the inferior mesenteric artery being patent, there may be a viable blood supply not only to the entire intestine, but also to the liver and pancreas as well. Obviously, rapid occlusion of one of the major vessels can lead to gangrene. Because many adults do have some degree of atherosclerotic disease involving the mesenteric vessels, changes identified on an angiogram may not necessarily be the cause of a patient's immediate symptomatology. Thus, the angiographic findings should be interpreted with caution.

The cause of major arterial thrombosis usually is underlying arteriosclerosis, generally involving the proximal portion of the artery. Embolization is a rapid event, with many of the emboli originating from the heart. The emboli tend to lodge at the arterial bifurcations. Occasionally abdominal vascular surgery, such as aortic reconstruction, may result in ischemia (20, 21). Acute ischemia may also result from a low flow state, vasoconstriction of the smaller vessels, or a combination of factors. Likewise, a dissecting abdominal aortic aneurysm may occlude the mesenteric arteries.

Approximately 25 or more percent of patients with acute ischemia have occlusion of a major arterial supply, 25% have occlusion of venous drainage, and approximately 50% have 'nonocclusion' or occlusion at the 'capillary level'. In the latter group of patients, labelled as having 'nonocclusive' mesenteric ischemia (22), even selective angiography does not demonstrate any obvious obstruction. The angiographic signs for such nonocclusive ischemia are (23):

1. Narrowing at the origin of major arterial branches.
2. Irregular vessel outline with narrowing and beading.
3. Spasm at the arcade level.
4. Poor filling of the intramural vessels with a decreased flow rate.

Although these signs may also be present in a patient in shock and other intraabdominal disease, correlation with the clinical findings generally allows ready differentiation. One presumably is dealing with increased resistance at the small vessel level when a clinical course strongly suggests an ischemic etiology in spite of no angiographically demonstrated obstruction. Reflux peripheral vasoconstriction due to a systemic or local low flow state may be the etiology in some patients (19) with either cardiac failure or increased colon intraluminal pressure producing such a low flow state (1).

Decreased mesenteric blood flow is difficult to detect clinically. In dogs, sufficient hypovolemia to produce a reduction of 50–75% in mesenteric blood flow does not result in any significant systemic blood pressure changes (16), nor does a reduction in mesenteric arterial blood flow to 75% of normal for 12 hours result in any identifiable ischemic changes (19).

In all patients with suspected ischemic bowel disease an acute abdominal examination should be initially obtained. Unfortunately, abnormal findings are seen only late in the course; noncontrast radiographs reveal changes only 10–12 hours after the insult (24). Linear or cystic collections of gas within the bowel wall are a late finding and suggest gangrene (Fig. B.1), yet gas within the bowel wall may be present as an unrelated innocuous finding (25). Gas in the portal venous system is an ominous sign (Fig. B.2). 'Thumbprinting' generally implies significant bowel wall edema (Fig. B.3). Quite often initially there is considerable spasm with narrowing of the small bowel and colon, resulting in a radiographic appearance of an 'empty abdomen'. Delayed evaluation may result in

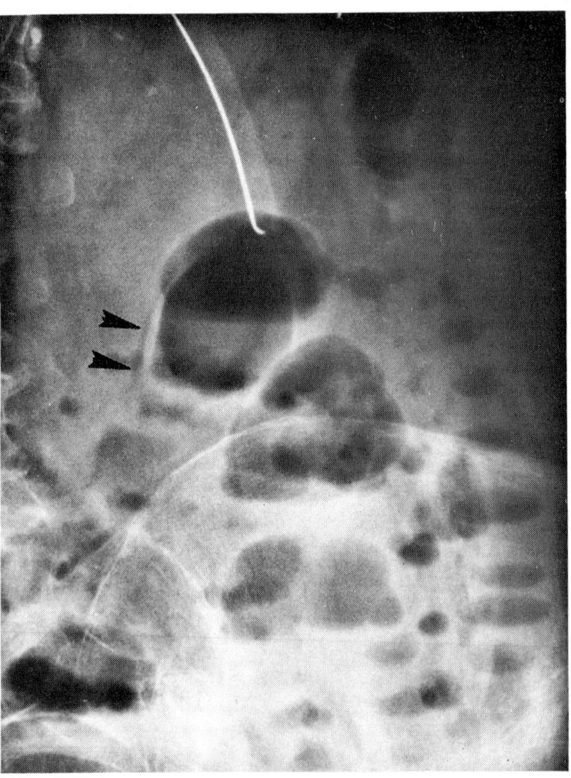

Fig. B.1. Linear collections of gas are present in the bowel wall (arrowheads). Surgery revealed infarcted bowel from the ileum to the sigmoid.

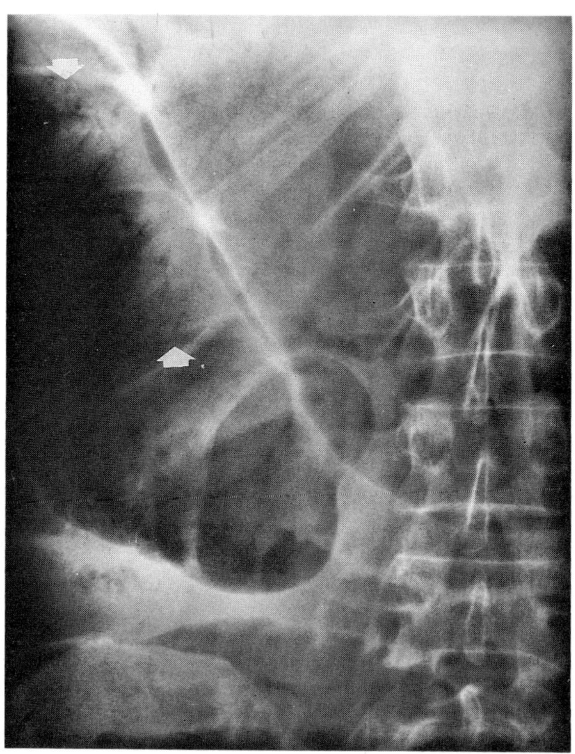

Fig. B.2. This 48-year-old male had gangrene of the distal small bowel and proximal part of the colon. Gas is present in the intrahepatic radicles of the portal venous system (arrowheads). A barium enema is contraindicated in such a situation.

an appearance similar to toxic megacolon as seen in ulcerative colitis (26). Dilated bowel can be present proximal to the ischemic segment. The primary purpose of the acute abdominal examination is to exclude other intraabdominal catastrophes.

When there is strong clinical suspicion of ischemia, the acute abdominal, examination should lead to angiography. In addition to showing vascular ischemia, the angiogram may also demonstrate a tumor, aneurysm, or possibly even one of the arteritides.

It is difficult to judge at which point one should perform barium studies. If the acute abdominal examination suggests no overt ischemia, no colon obstruction, the patient is stable, and small bowel involvement is suspected, we generally perform a small bowel examination (enteroclysis) using the antegrade approach. If there is radiological evidence of gas in the bowel wall or if there is rebound tenderness, barium studies are contraindicated.

If colon involvement is suspected and there are no contraindications, a barium enema may provide definitive information (15, 17, 27). Because these patients cannot be cleansed normally, blood clots and retained stool may result in extensive artifacts. The barium enema may reveal 'thumbprinting' due to bowel wall edema and intramural hemorrhage

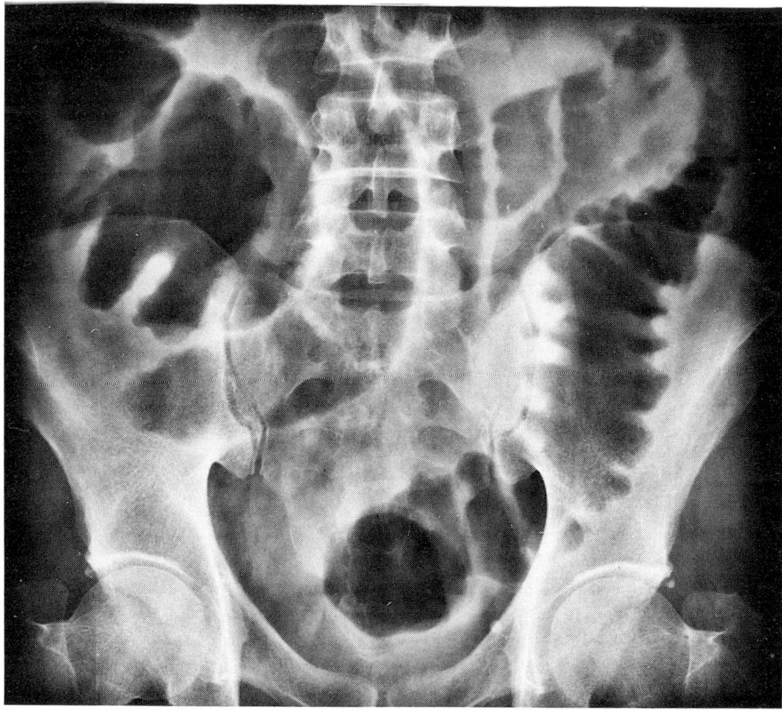

Fig. B.3. Left colon ischemia. Thickened folds and 'thumbprinting' are present in the descending and sigmoid portions of the colon.

(Fig. B.4). The degree of 'thumbprinting' can vary with the amount of intraluminal pressure; with increased pressure during a barium enema the 'thumbprinting' may be less apparent than on noncontrast radiographs (28).

With sufficient damage shallow ulcers and saccular outpouchings, or intramural barium disection can develop (29). Stenosis may be the end result (Fig. B.5). The overall radiographic appearance can be similar to regional enteritis or ulcerative colitis (30) except that the rectum is usually spared (Fig. B.6).

Generally, serial examinations allow one to differentiate between ischemic colitis and ulcerative colitis. A patient presenting with an acute episode of ischemia exhibits rapid changes on serial examinations; either the colon reverts back to a normal appearance, a stricture develops, or with a sufficiently large insult, gangrene and perforation intervene unless interrupted by surgery.

Even pathological examination of resected specimens may not reveal the etiology of the underlying disease (31). The colon can react only in a limited number of ways to an insult. Histologic examination may not differentiate between ischemic

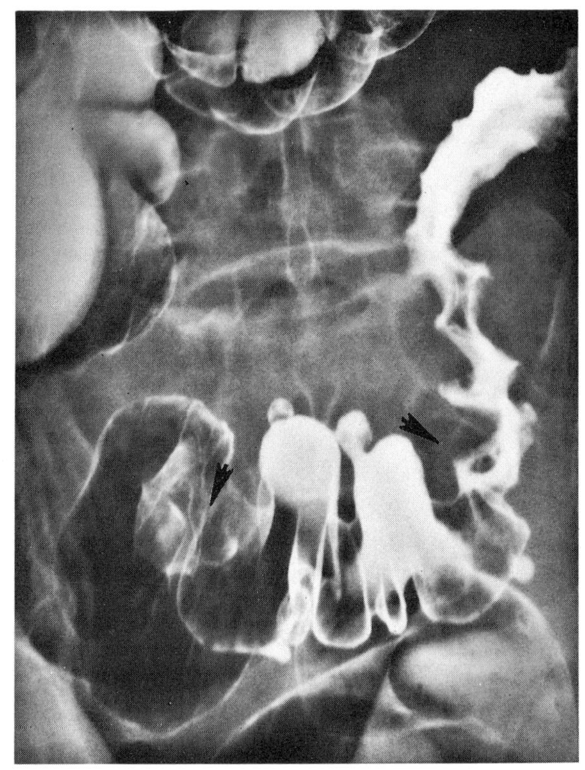

a

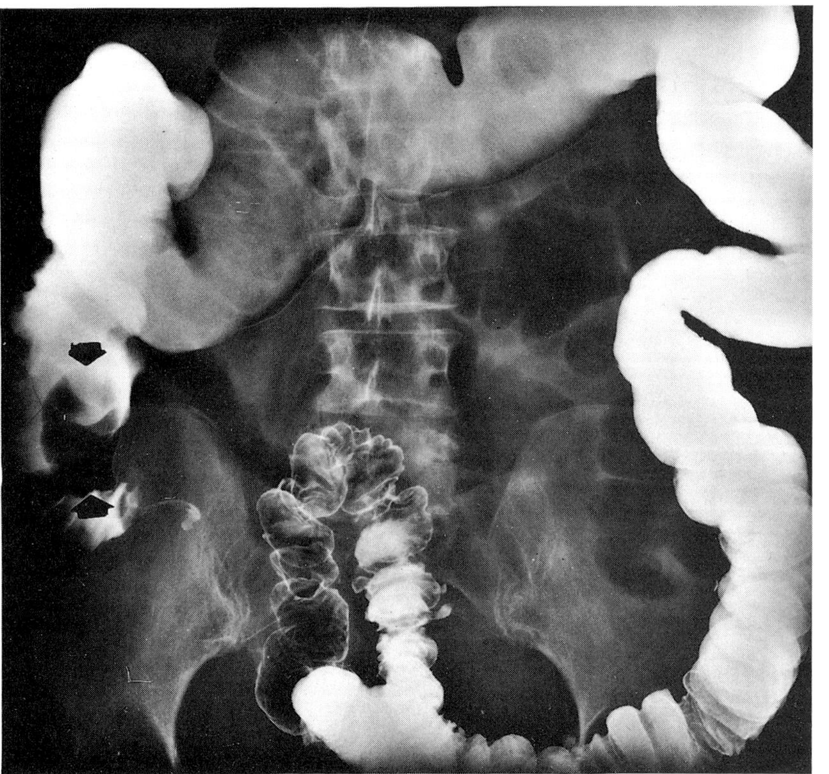

b

Fig. B.4. (a) 60-year-old female with severe cardiovascular disease developed rectal bleeding and diarrhea. The barium enema shows 'thumbprinting' (arrowheads) secondary to intramural hemorrhage and edema throughout the sigmoid. (b) Another patient with superior mesenteric artery thrombosis. The folds throughout the right colon are thickened and the ileocecal valve is enlarged; the edematous ileocecal valve (arrowheads) had resulted in small bowel obstruction.

colitis, regional enteritis, or ulcerative colitis. The clinical course of the patient, however, is a reliable differential between these entities (32).

Ischemia can develop proximal to a distal colon obstruction (17, 19, 33) or in a closed loop obstruction, such as a volvulus (34) (Fig. B.7). Present evidence suggests that the pathogenesis of such ischemia is the increased intraluminal pressure and resultant decreased blood flow, leading to a compromise in the blood supply initially to the mucosa and eventually to the deeper layers (16).

A curious form of transient or evanescent colitis is occasionally encountered in young adults. Women predominate, with many being on birth control medication (6–9). The patient usually has sudden onset of crampy abdominal pain followed by diarrhea and rectal bleeding. Vomiting, fever and abdominal tenderness can be present. The bleeding is burgundy or red in color. The acute abdominal examination can be normal or reveal intramural 'thumbprinting' or diffuse narrowing (Fig. B.8). A barium enema generally shows similar findings. Usually there is little problem in making the correct diagnosis because of the characteristic clinical presentation and radiographic appearance (Fig. B.9). With the appropriate history and age group we generally do not perform an immediate barium enema but wait until the patient's symptoms have cleared. An examination performed then should reveal a normal colon. The follow-up examination is designed to exclude some other cause for the patient's bleeding. Occasionally the condition leads to bowel necrosis, although colon involvement is generally more often reversible than small bowel involvement. Angiography appears to be of little use in making a diagnosis in these patients.

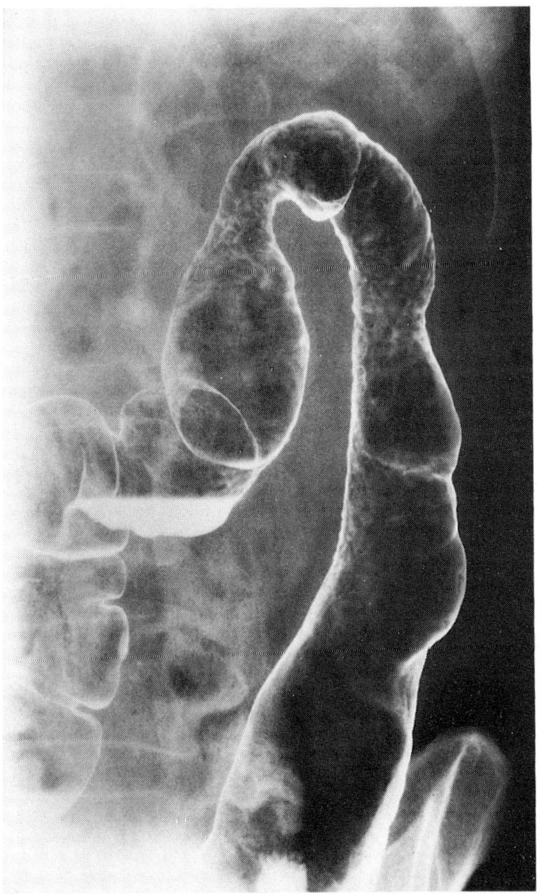

Fig. B.5. This patient with abdominal pain had a thrombus in the abdominal aorta. A stricture and numerous shallow ulcers are present at the splenic flexure.

An 'evanescent colitis' has been described in a child (35). Whether this is the same entity as seen in adults remains to be determined.

c. Vasculitis

A vasculitis, such as associated with polyarteritis nodosa, systemic lupus erythematosus (36), scleroderma (37), or renal transplant (38) may result in ischemic changes in the bowel. Usually, the changes are more prominent within the small bowel, although the colon can be extensively involved (39). Polyarteritis nodosa can lead to colon ulcers, strictures, aneurysms, or perforation (40) (Fig. B.10). Some of the vasculitides may be associated with an asymptomatic pneumatosis.

An unusual cause of rectal bleeding is due to an aneurysm, such as an aneurysm of the superior hemorrhoidal artery (41).

Although Henoch-Schönlein purpura tends to be self limiting, the symptoms can be indistinguishable from those of polyarteritis nodosa. The characteristic clinical findings are pain and tenderness. Radiographic changes are similar to ischemic colitis and consist of bowel wall thickening and 'thumbprinting' because of edema and intramural hemorrhage (42). If the damage is localized, the resultant radiographic appearance may resemble an infiltrating tumor (Fig. B.11).

A patient with the hemolytic-uremic syndrome may present with hemolytic anemia, renal failure, or an ileocolitis (43). The colitis can be the initial finding of this entity, with the bowel changes being

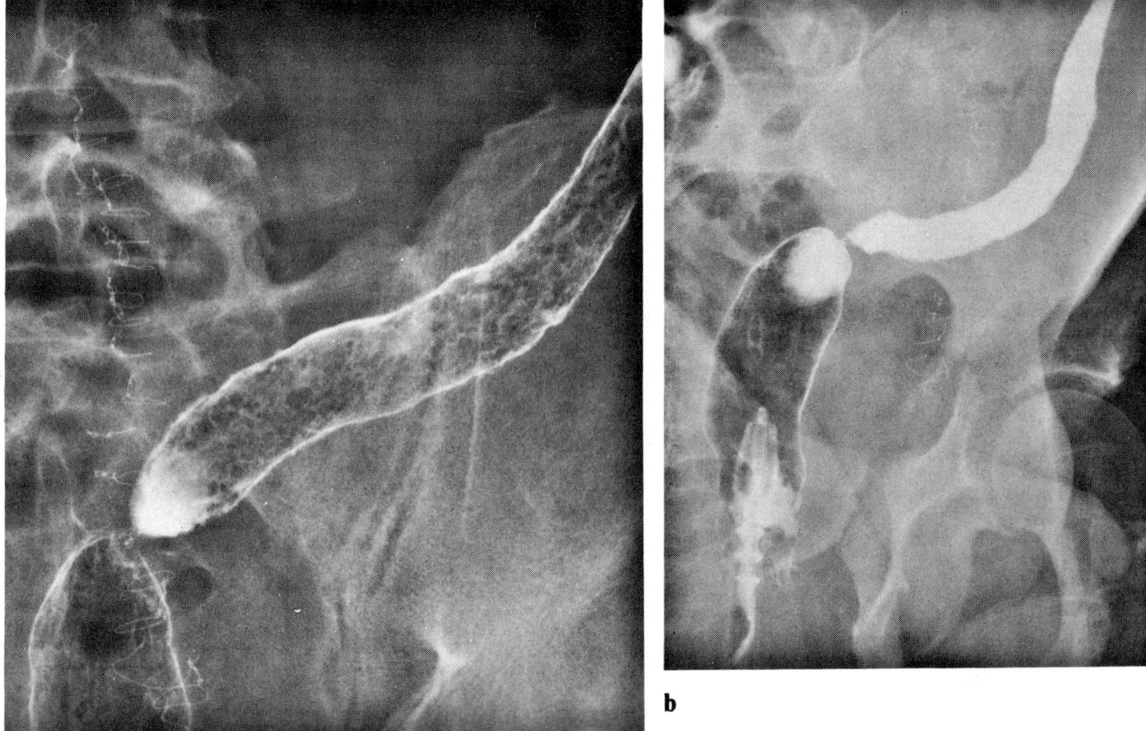

Fig. B.6. A 44-year-old patient underwent sigmoid resection for sigmoid carcinoma. A transverse colostomy was also performed at which time the middle colic artery was ligated. Several months later the colostomy was taken down and the patient developed abdominal pain and intractable diarrhea. (a) A stricture is present at the anastomosis. Proximal to the anastomosis the colon is diffusely narrowed, the haustra are obliterated and multiple shallow ulcers are present. (b) Although the rectum was also involved, the sigmoid colon revealed the most severe changes. Ischemia probably developed in this patient because both the middle colic artery and the inferior mesenteric artery were sacrificed at surgery and the patient did not have sufficient collateral circulation.

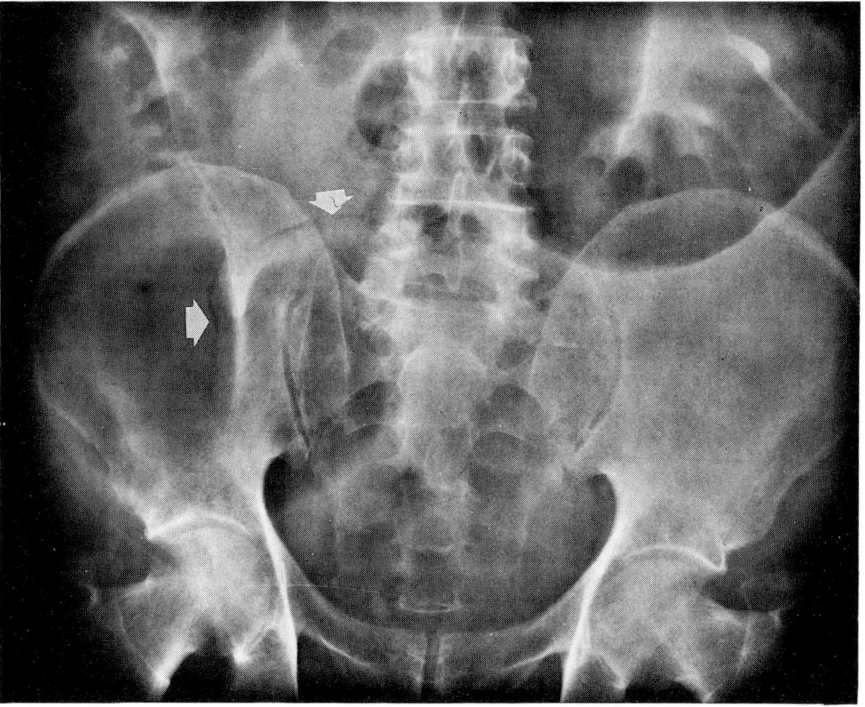

Fig. B.7. Right colon ischemia developing in a setting of distal colon obstruction. The obstruction was caused by a carcinoma. Ischemia manifests as gas in the bowel wall (pneumatosis coli) (arrowheads). Emergency surgery revealed an already gangrenous right colon. A barium enema is contraindicated in such a setting because of the danger of perforation.

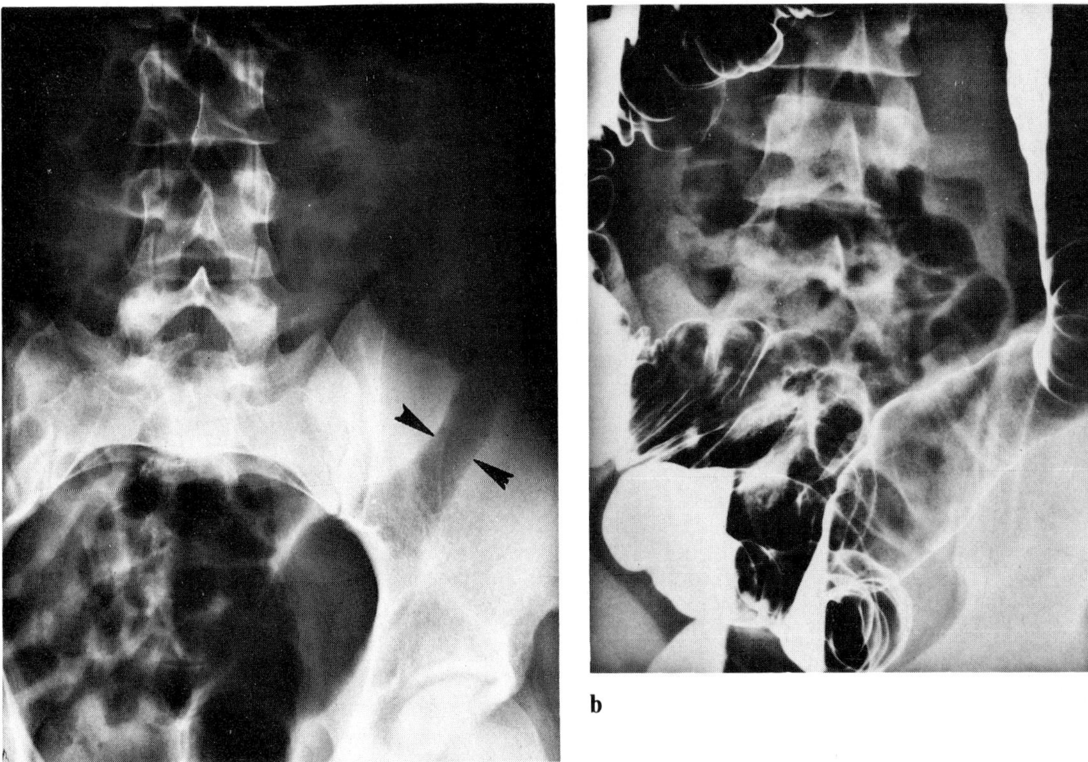

Fig. B.8. Evanescent colitis in a 19-year-old male with sudden rectal bleeding and left lower quadrant pain. (a) The acute abdominal examination shows a hypotonic and narrowed distal descending colon (arrowheads). (b) Three days later the symptoms had cleared and a barium enema is normal.

ischemic in origin and due to the intravascular obstruction by fibrin. Examination during an acute attack reveals bowel wall thickening, ulceration, edema, and hemorrhage manifesting as 'thumbprinting' (44). The presentation may mimic ulcerative colitis (45). Long-term sequellae can be colon strictures (46).

d. Benign colon ulcers

Colon ulcers were first described by Cruveilhier in the previous century (47) and although these benign ulcers can be found anywhere in the colon most are in the cecum. Their incidence is low and they can be readily misdiagnosed as appendicitis (48).

Most patients have no underlying disease, although occasionally patients with lupus erythematosus (36), Behçet's disease (3), renal transplantation (49), or patients on oral contraceptives (6) will develop colon ulcers. Most patients who develop colon ulcers after renal transplantation die (49).

The etiology of these ulcers is not understood. Ischemia probably is a major factor, with throm-

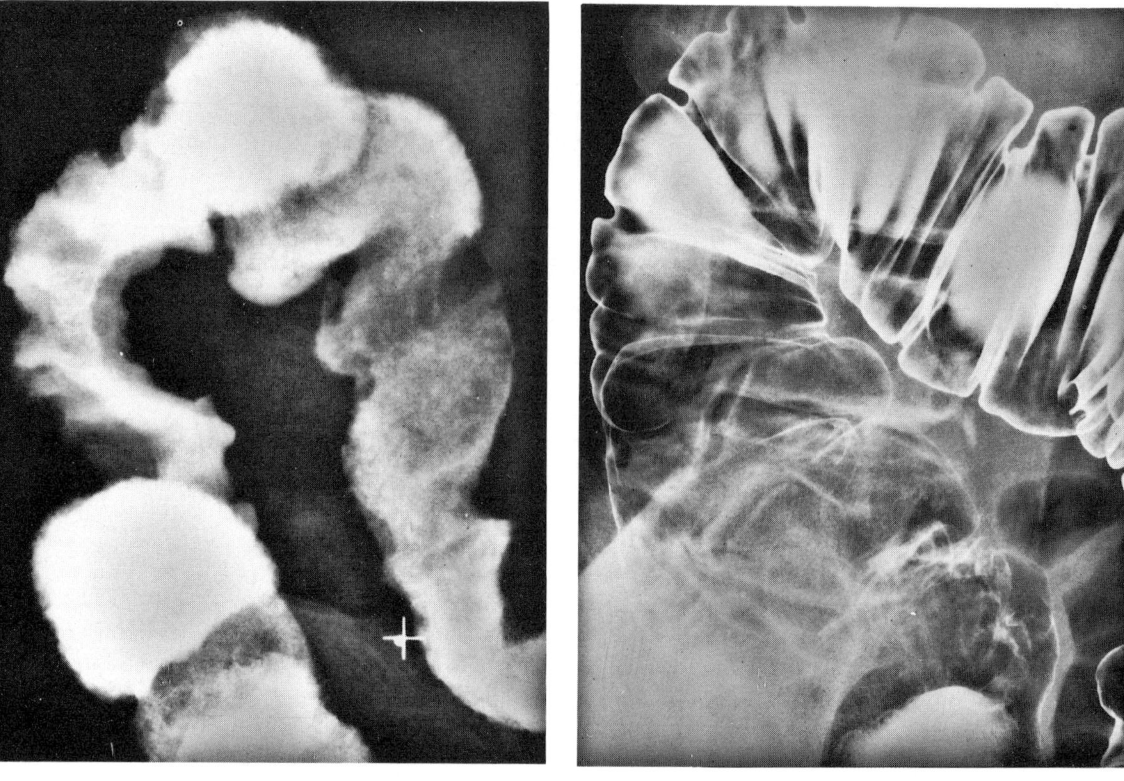

Fig. B.9. Evanescent colitis. (a) An emergency barium enema was performed shortly after admission because of sudden onset of abdominal pain and burgundy-colored bleeding. Extensive 'thumbprinting', presumably secondary to intramural bleeding, is centered around the hepatic flexure. (b) Barium enema 5 weeks later is normal.

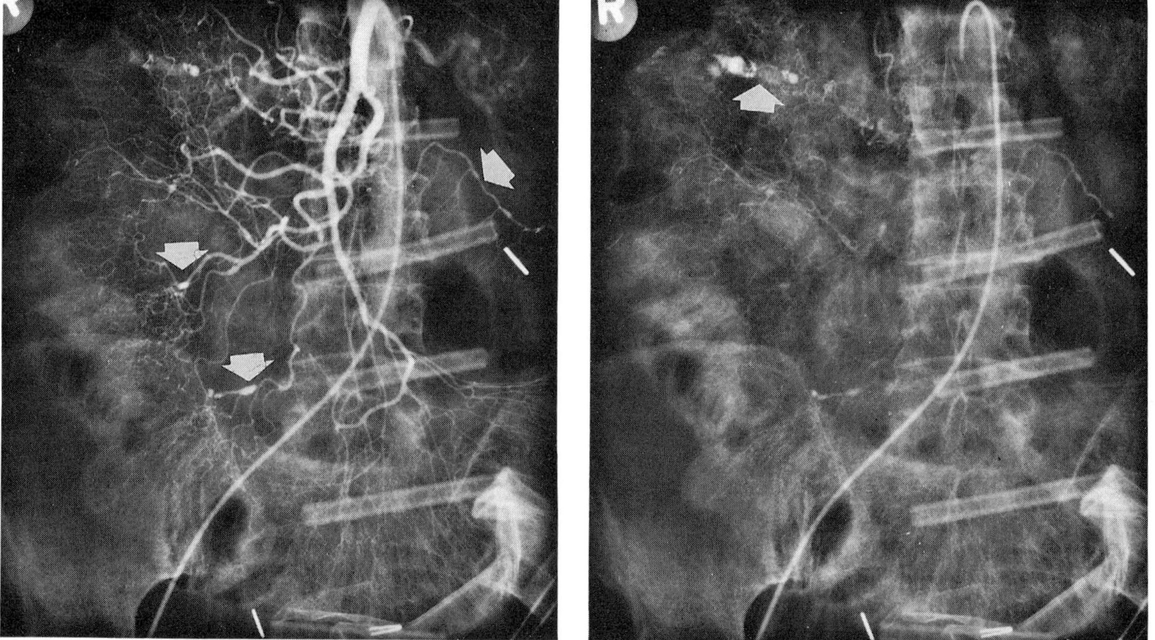

Fig. B.10. This patient with polyarteritis nodosa developed gastrointestinal bleeding. (a) Numerous sites of aneurysmal dilation, seen as beaded areas (arrowheads), are scattered throughout the superior mesenteric artery distribution. (b) The extravasation (arrowhead) is apparent during the venous phase. (Courtesy of Dr. O. Gutierrez, Rochester, NY.)

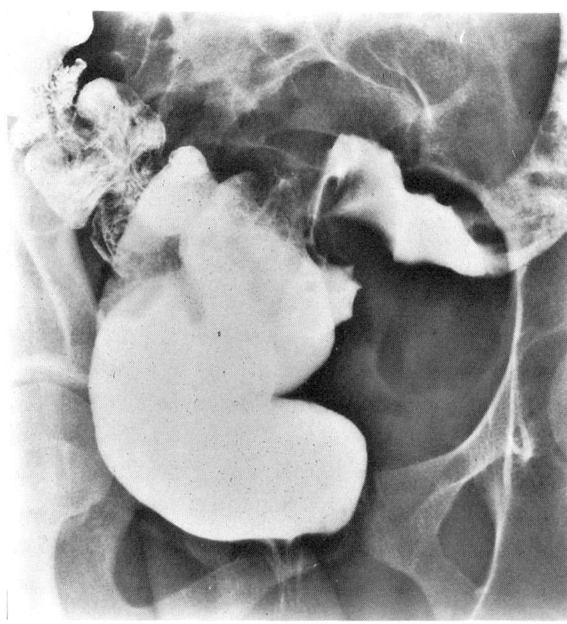

Fig. B.11. A 22-year-old woman with Henoch-Schoenlein purpura involving the colon. Intramural masses in the sigmoid mimic a carcinoma. Ischemic changes were present in the colon proximal to this lesion. (Courtesy of Drs. Van den Bosch and Blomme (42); copyright, Georg Thieme Verlag, 1980.)

bosis of the small vessels playing a major role (48). These ulcers may also be due to localized diverticulitis, especially if the ulcer is seen in the cecum. Clinically, the patients exhibit a wide variety of symptoms ranging from those typical for inflammatory disease and appendicitis to those who present with bleeding. Similar to gastric ulcers, there can be perforation with subsequent peritonitis. The ulcers may be single or multiple.

The pathological changes include thickening of bowel wall, mucosal ulceration, infarction of a portion of the mucosa, and adjacent microcirculatory thrombosis (48). The ulcer is typically on the antimesenteric wall of the cecum close to the ileocecal valve.

A barium enema in these patients reveals a mass indenting the colon or 'thumbprinting'. Reports of full-column barium enemas mention the difficulty in differentiating benign ulcer from malignancy (50, 51). In some patients the examination is normal. Some of the more superficial ulcers may be missed. Considerable difficulty can be encountered in adequately visualizing the area because of irritability and spasm.

Colonoscopy can visualize the ulcer (52), although a specific diagnosis may be difficult. Angiography can localize the bleeding site in patients with brisk bleeding (49, 53). No specific angiographic appearance has been described for these lesions.

e. Bleeding diathesis

In adults the most common cause for intramural bleeding is an underlying coagulation defect, sometimes induced by anticoagulation medication. Patients with leukemia, lymphoma, myeloma, or metastatic carcinoma are prone to develop a coagulation disorder. Usually the small bowel is involved but there may be changes only in the colon. Noncontrast radiographs are usually not helpful but contrast studies can usually localize the involved segment. Colon involvement tends to be in the respective distribution of the two major vascular systems; thus, one sees either right-sided or transverse colon changes with superior mesenteric artery involvement, or, if the inferior mesenteric distribution is involved, left colon or sigmoid changes are seen.

Blunt abdominal trauma can lacerate major vessels, with subsequent extraperitoneal, intraperitoneal, intramural or intraluminal bleeding (54). If the patient survives the acute episode, subsequent bowel ischemia because of compromised vasculature can result in an eventual stricture.

Bleeding can also result from diverticula, fissures, ulcers, tumors, and the various colitides. These entities are discussed in their respective sections.

f. Vascular malformations

Vascular malformations in the colon can be classified histologically into either benign or malignant lesions (Table B.1). Although some investigators consider these lesions as neoplasms, they are discussed in this section because of their primary vascular appearance.

Clinically, these lesions have been classified according to angiographic appearance, location and age (55). The nomenclature is confusing, with some calling similar lesions arteriovenous malformations (55, 56), angioma (57), hemangioma (58), vascular ectasia (59, 60) and simply as vascular malformations (61). The terms vascular dysplasia (62) and angiodysplasia are used for some of these lesions

(63). The histological appearance of angiodysplasia is that of numerous thin-walled dilated blood vessels. The pathologist can generally distinguish between angiodysplasia and arteriovenous malformation. Angiographically, it is difficult to differentiate between a hemangioma, a hamartoma, or a telangiectasia. Some arteriovenous communications simply show a shunting of blood with prominent drainage (Fig. B.12).

Patients with a diffuse cavernous hemangioma of the rectum can have obstruction, bleeding, or prolapse. Resection can be difficult if not impossible because of the tumor's infiltration. Many of these patients also have cutaneous hemangiomata. An acute abdominal examination may reveal numerous phleboliths at the site of a hemangioma. A barium enema is normal with most small hemangiomata; an occasional large submucosal hemangioma will show pliable, well-defined masses, similar to localized varices, in the involved colon segment (Fig. B.13). An angiogram defines the extent of these lesions (Fig. B.14).

Patients with the Klippel-Trenaunay syndrome appear to have a higher incidence of diffuse cavernous hemangioma of the colon than the normal population (64). Bowel angiomata can be present in patients with Rendu-Osler-Weber syndrome. These lesions are probably different pathogenetically from the more common lesions known as angiodysplasia (65), although radiographically, these lesions may appear to be similar (66). Some consider vascular ectasias as representing a spectrum, with the inherited Rendu-Osler-Weber syndrome at one end of the spectrum and the acquired lesions at the other end (67).

The vascular malformations known as angiodysplasias can be a source of chronic bleeding. These

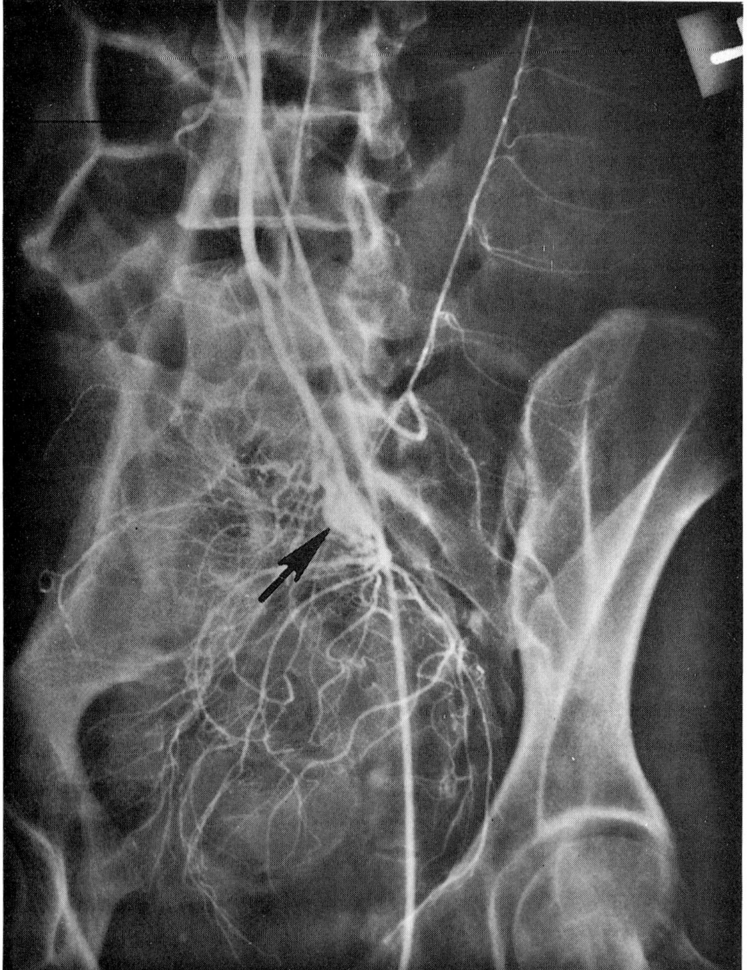

a

Fig. B.12. Arteriovenous communication. (a) Inferior mesenteric artery injection reveals sacular dilation of the artery (arrow). (b) Prominent veins are already apparent in the capillary phase. (c) The venous phase shows extensive and prominent tortuous veins (arrowheads), indicative of the extra blood flow through these vessels. (Courtesy of Dr. O. Gutierrez, Rochester, NY.)

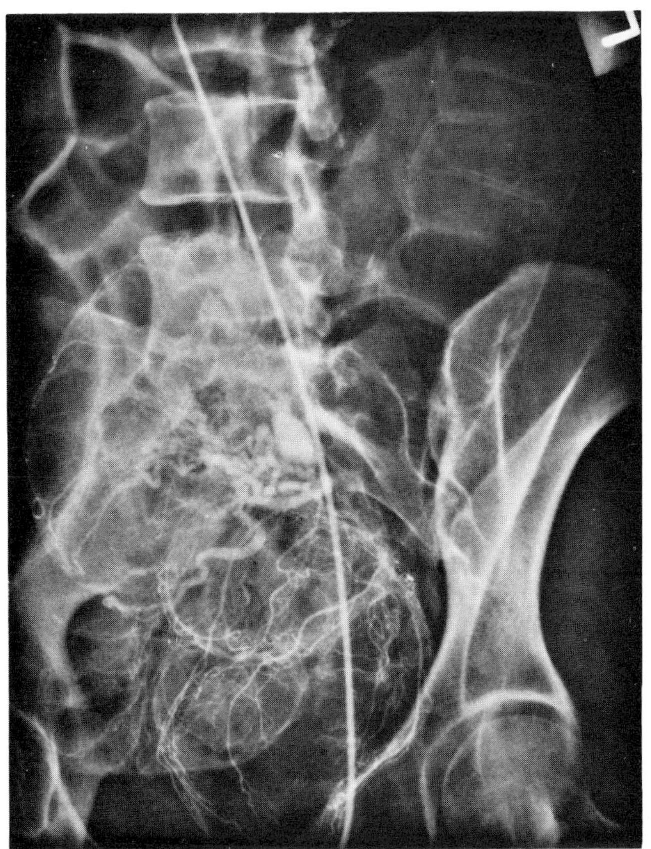

b

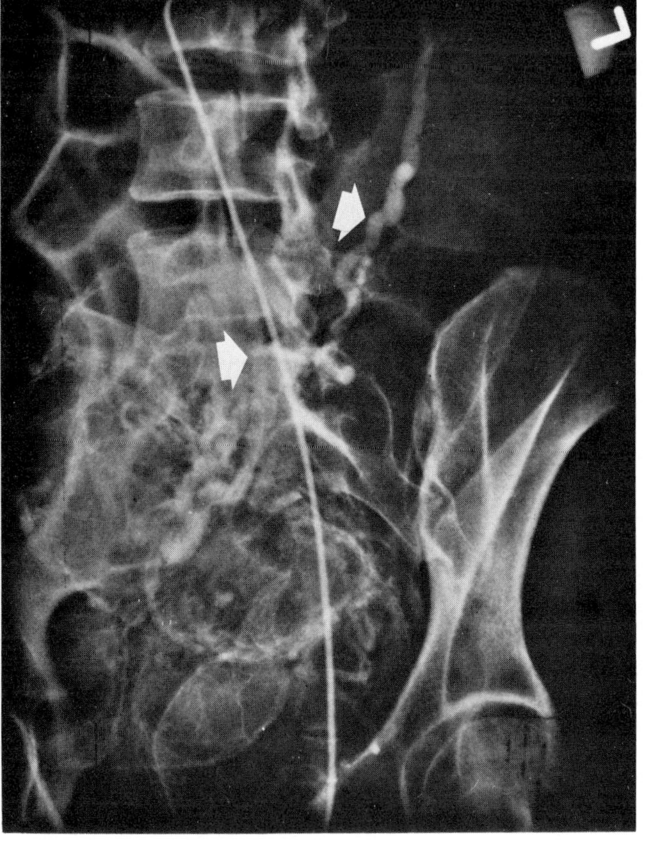

c

a

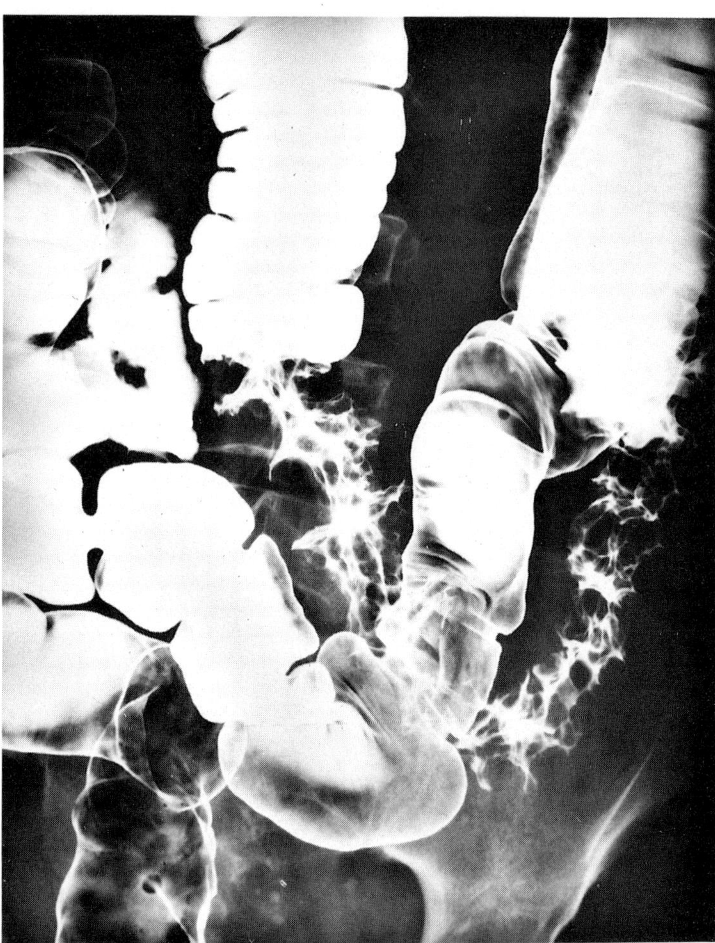

Fig. B.13. Transverse colon hemangioma in a 33-year-old male. (a) The involved colon shows well-defined intramural masses with considerable narrowing of the colon lumen. (b) With further distension the intramural location of the hemangioma is better appreciated. Intramural hemorrhage or edema are usually not as sharply marginated as this lesion. Benign neoplasms are not as extensive, while a carcinoma should result in significant destruction.

b

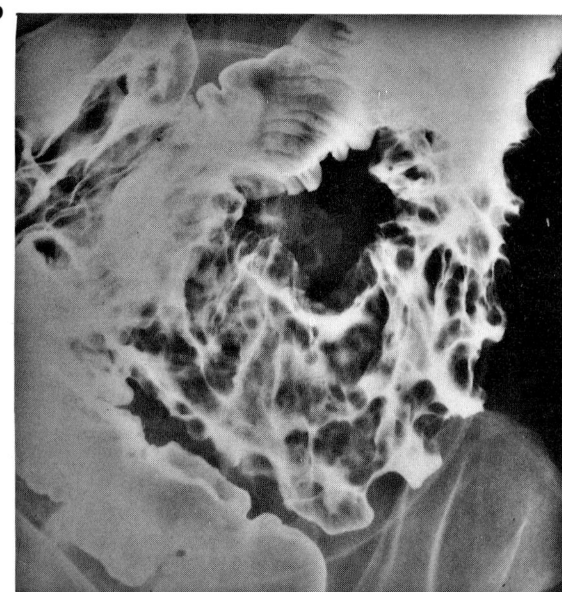

Table B.1. Vascular malformations of the colon: a histological classification.

BENIGN
Telangiectasia
Hemangioma
  Capillary hemangioma
  Mixed capillary and cavernous hemangioma
  Cavernous hemangioma

MALIGNANT
Hemangioendothelioma
'Benign metastasizing hemangioma'
Kaposi's sarcoma
Angiosarcoma

lesions are usually located in the right side of the colon and, because they are seen in an older age group (68), an acquired etiology is postulated. Most of these patients are investigated because of unexplained lower gastrointestinal bleeding. The bleeding episodes tend to recur, the patients require blood transfusions, and they often undergo exploratory laparotomy. The angiographic discovery of vascular lesions is then associated with the prior blood bloss. Shallow ulcers can occur (65). A rare dysplasia may result in hemoperitoneum(69).

The pathogenesis of these lesions is not known. They tend to occur on the antimesenteric border of the colon. It is thought that chronic bowel ischemia may play a part (70). Some evidence suggests that increased intraluminal pressure results in opening of arteriovenoús shunts which then progress to angiodysplasia (60). On the other hand, angiodysplasia may simply be a degenerative process of aging (60); intermittent venous obstruction may contribute to this condition.

Angiodysplasia has been associated with aortic valve disease, although the reason for this association is still not clear (61, 71, 72). The incidence of gastrointestinal bleeding in patients with aortic valve disease certainly is higher than that expected in the general population (60, 71, 73). There appears to be an association between angiodysplasia and von Willebrand's disease (31, 74).

The true incidence of angiodysplasia is not known. It is generally assumed that the incidence increases with age. An incidence of 53% was found in the colons of patients who had resection for carcinoma (60).

Mesenteric angiography can readily diagnose angiodysplasia in patients with lower gastrointestinal bleeding (70, 75–78) (Figs. B.15 and B.16). Angiography should be employed only after conventional studies have failed to reveal any other source of bleeding. Careful attention to technique, including magnification angiography, gives the highest yield. Multiple lesions may be present (79). Often the lesions are on the antimesenteric border (80).

In patients with colon angiodysplasia the following angiographic findings are seen (66, 70, 80, 81):

1. Prominent small arterial clusters.
2. Intense opacification of a portion of the bowel wall.
3. Early opacification of a draining vein which may be enlarged.
4. Delayed emptying of a dilated and tortuous draining vein.

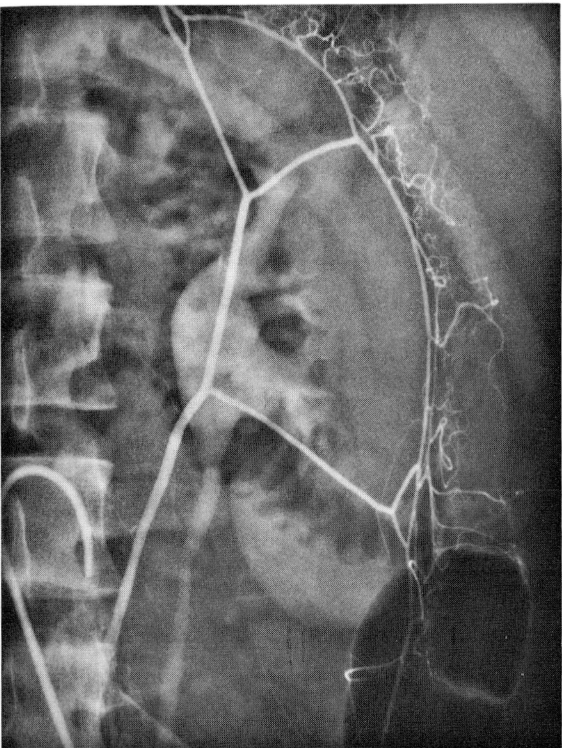

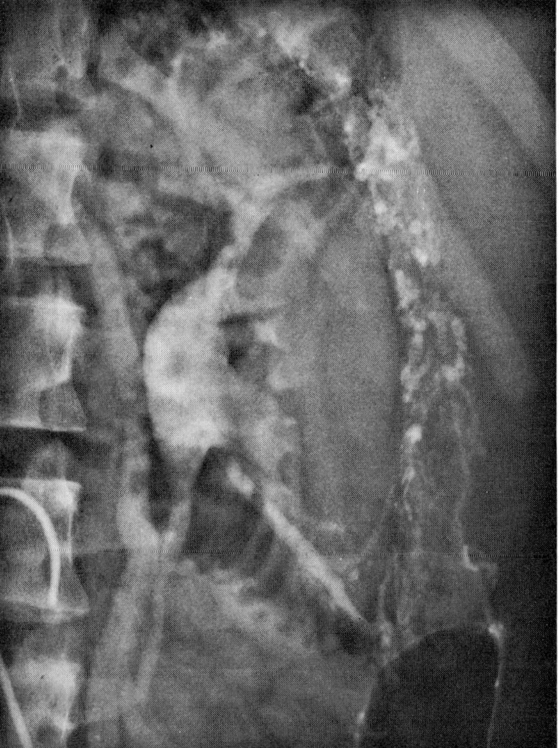

Fig. B.14. Cavernous hemangioma in a 21-year-old male. (a) The arterial phase shows slightly prominent vessels. (b) The venous phase reveals striking vascular dilatation throughout the descending colon. (Courtesy of Dr. O. Gutierrez, Rochester, NY.)

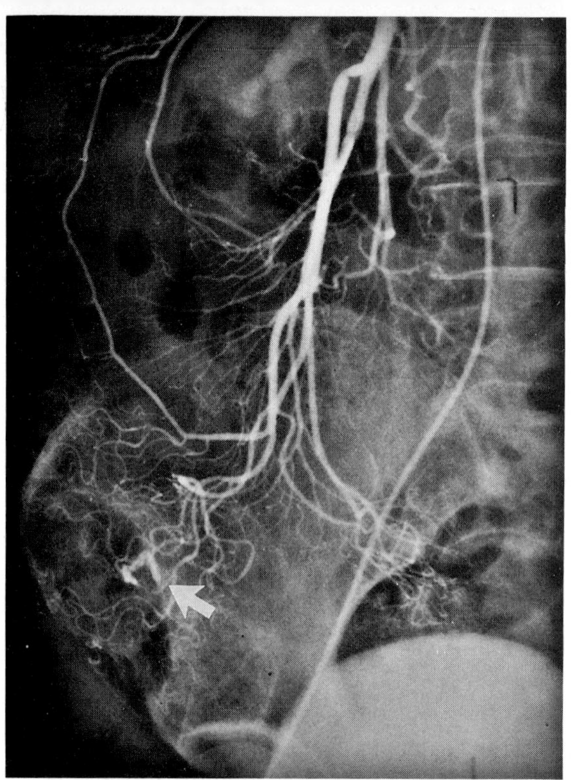

5. Although rarely seen, during active bleeding there can be extravasation of contrast into the lumen.

Barium studies cannot diagnose these lesions because they are submucosal in location, the lesions are small, and no intraluminal mass is present. Even if there is mucosal erosion and ulceration with resultant bleeding, the changes are too minute to be picked up on a barium enema study. The role of barium enema is simply to exclude any other underlying cause for gastrointestinal bleeding; angiography may reveal only abnormal vessels but not identify the specific etiology. For example, colon carcinoma can be misdiagnosed as angiodysplasia on an arteriogram (70) (Fig. B.17). The

Fig. B.15. Cecal angiodysplasia. There is a cluster of small vessels in the cecum (arrow). A dilated draining vein with early opacification was seen later in the study.

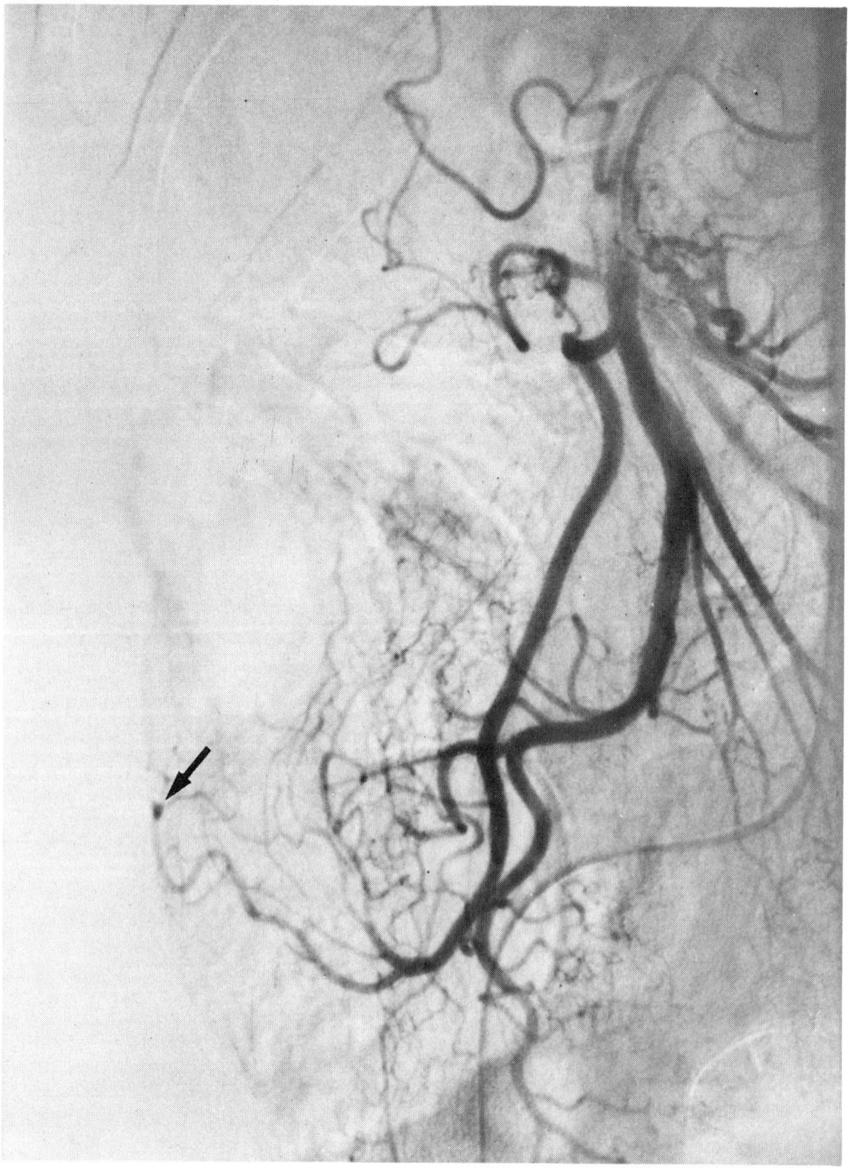

a

Fig. B.16. Cecal angiodysplasia in a 61-year-old man with chronic gastrointestinal bleeding over a 3-year period. (a) The arterial phase of an ileocolic arteriogram reveals an abnormal vascular lake on the antimesenteric border of the cecum (arrow). (b) An early draining vein (arrows) is later present (Courtesy of Drs. D.J. Allison and A.P. Hemingway (88); copyright, Br J Hosp Med, 1980.)

subsequent intraoperative surprise is not appreciated by a surgeon. Inflammatory diseases, such as regional enteritis, may also present with early opacification of draining veins (82).

Although colonoscopy can be diagnostic (83–85), the role of colonoscopy in the evaluation of angiodysplasia is not yet settled. In one study of 20 patients with angiographically shown angiodysplasia, colonoscopy could identify a lesion in areas corresponding to the arteriographic site only in seven patients (80). However, colonoscopy can be used for electrocoagulation of these lesions (72).

Because the lesions of angiodysplasia are small and after resection the blood vessels tend to collapse, identification of a lesion can be difficult. An injection technique aids the pathologist in identifying the extent of the underlying disease (76). Some advocate injection of silicone rubber (63), while others prefer a barium sulfate–gelatin suspension (65, 86). If barium is used, radiographic study is possible as an aid in an analysis of the lesions (Fig. B.18).

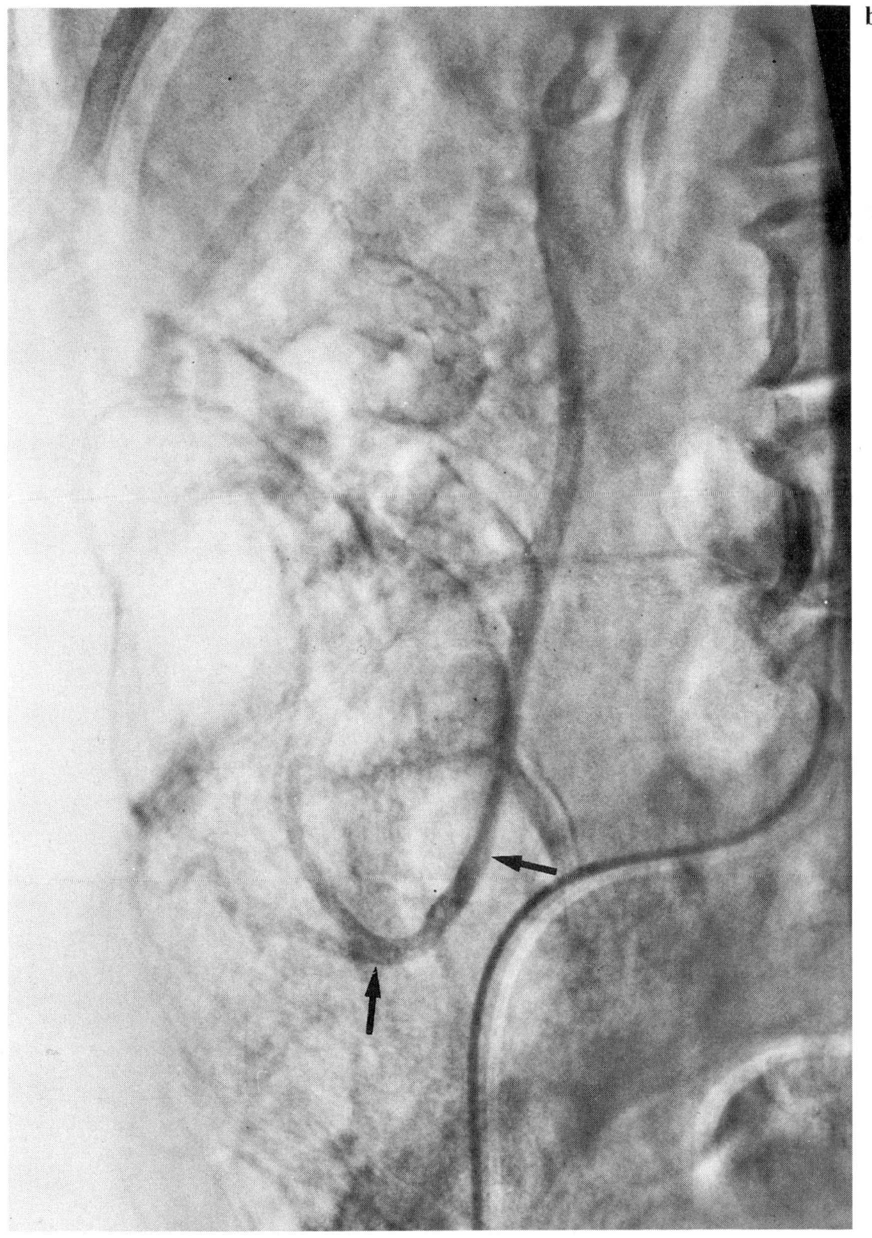

b

The current management of patients with gastrointestinal bleeding from angiodysplasia is generally segmental resection, although successful transcatheter gelfoam embolization has been reported (87). A more complex issue involves that patient where angiodysplasia is diagnosed as an incidental finding in a patient with little or no colon bleeding. Currently most investigators are recommending surgery only in those patients where gastrointestinal bleeding is present.

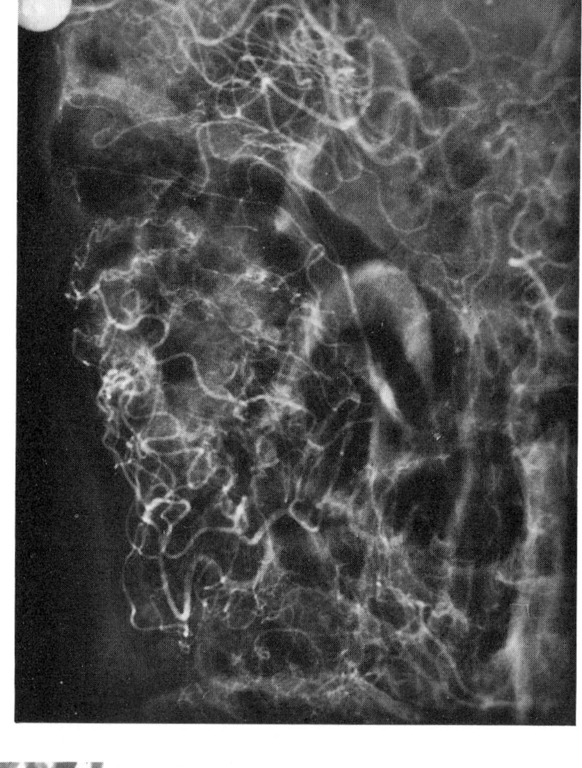

Fig. B.17. An angiogram revealed prominent arterial clusters with prompt opacification of the venous drainage. An angiodysplasia was suspected in this patient with chronic gastrointestinal bleeding. Surgery revealed a right colic adenocarcinoma.

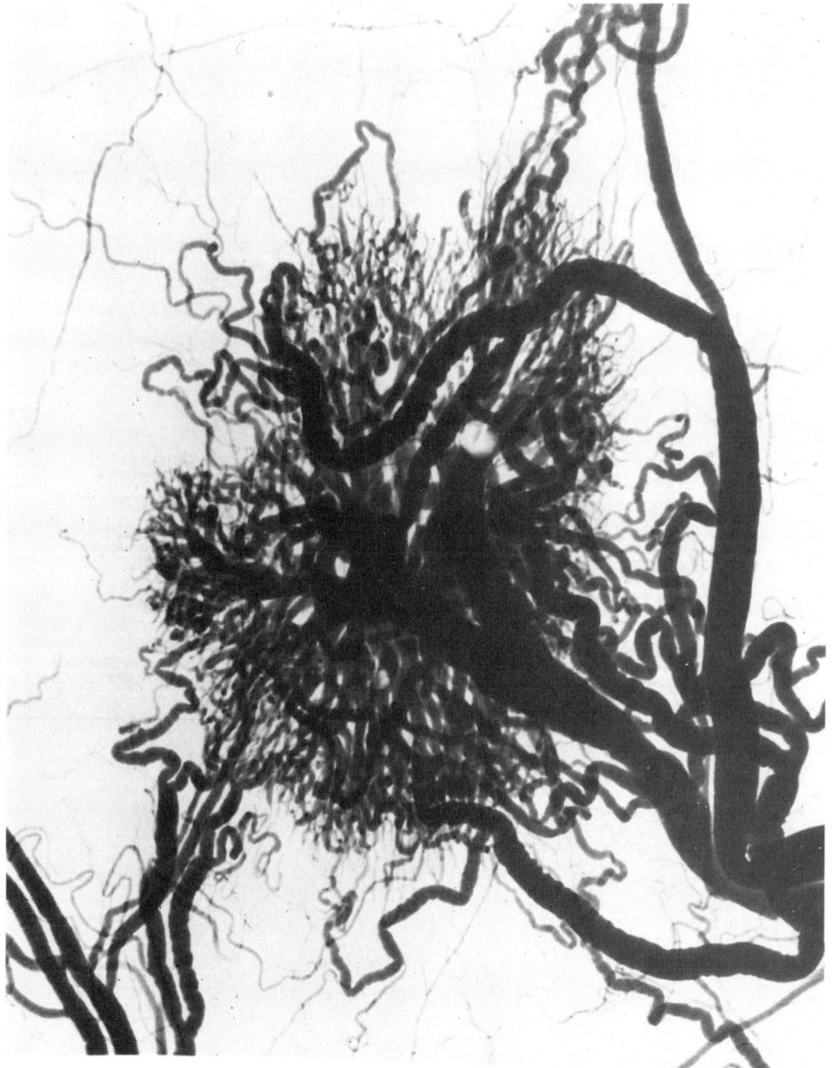

Fig. B.18. Microangiogram of an area of angiodysplasia in a resected specimen. A barium–gelatin mixture was used for injection. The numerous abnormally dilated vessels are clearly seen. (Courtesy of Drs. D.J. Allison and A.P. Hemingway (86); copyright, World Medicine 1981.).

References

1. Bookstein JJ: Non-occlusive ischemic colitis: angiographic aspects in a canine model. Invest Radiol 13:506–513, 1978.
2. Robinson JWL, Winistörfer B, Mirkovitch V: Source of net water and electrolyte loss following intestinal ischemia. Res Exp Med (Berl), 176:263–275, 1980.
3. Stanley RJ, Tedesco FJ, Melson GL, Geisse G, Herold SL: The colitis of Behçet's disease: a clinical–radiographic correlation. Radiology 114:603–604, 1975.
4. Matthews JGW, Parks TG: Ischemic colitis in the experimental animal. I. Comparison of the effects of acute and subacute vascular occlusion. Gut 17:671–676, 1976.
5. Mavor GE: Acute occlusion of the superior mesenteric artery. Clin Gastroenterol 1:639–653, 1972.
6. Bernardino ME, Lawson TL: Discrete colonic ulcers associated with oral contraceptives. Am J Dig Dis 21:503–506, 1976.
7. Barcewicz PA, Welch JP: Ischemic colitis in young adult patients. Dis Colon Rectum 23:109–114, 1980.
8. Nesbit RR Jr, DeWeese JA: Mesenteric venous thrombosis and oral contraceptives. South Med J 70:360–362, 1977.
9. Ghahremani GG, Meyers MA, Farman J, Port RB: Ischemic disease of the small bowel and colon associated with oral contraceptives. Gastrointest Radiol 2:221–228, 1977.
10. Stillman AE, Weinberg M, Mast WC, Palpant S: Ischemic bowel disease attributable to ergot. Gastroenterology 72:1336–1337, 1977.
11. Lévy E, Cosnes J, Bognel J-C, Liégeois A, Milliez J, Loygue J: Le syndrome de colite aiguë grave et ses éléments de pronostic (100 cas). Gastroenterol Clin Biol 3:637–646, 1979.
12. Shanbour LL, Jacobson ED: Digitalis and the mesenteric circulation. Am J Dig Dis 17:826–828, 1972.
13. Hess T, Stucki P: Mesenterialinfarkt bei Digitalis Intoxikation. Schweiz Med Wochenschr 105:1237–1240, 1975.
14. Boley SJ, Schwartz S, Lash J, Sternhill V: Reversible vascular occlusion of the colon. Surg Gynecol Obstet 116:53–60, 1963.
15. Wittenberg J, Athanasoulis CA, Williams LF Jr, Paredes S, O'Sullivan P, Brown B: Ischemic colitis. AJR 123:287–300, 1975.
16. Matthews JGW, Parks TG: Ischemic colitis in the experimental animal. II. Role of hypovolemia in the production of the disease. Gut 17:677–684, 1976.
17. O'Connell TX, Kadell B, Tompkins RK: Ischemia of the colon. Surg Gynecol Obstet 142:337–342, 1976.
18. Meyers MA: Griffiths' point: critical anastomosis at the splenic flexure. AJR 126:77–94, 1976.
19. Boley SJ, Brandt LJ, Veith FJ: Ischemic disorders of the intestines. Curr Probl Surg 15:1–85, 1978.
20. Ernst CB, Hagihara PF, Dougherty ME, Sachatello CR, Griffen WO Jr: Ischemic colitis incidence following abdominal aortic reconstruction: a prospective study. Surgery 80:417–421, 1976.
21. Ottinger LW, Darling RC, Nathan MJ, Linton RR: Left colon ischemia complicating aorto-iliac reconstruction. Arch Surg 105:841–846, 1972.
22. Williams LF Jr, Kim J-P: Nonocclusive mesenteric ischemia. In Boley JS (ed) Vascular Disorders of the Intestine, p 519. Appleton-Century-Crofts, New York, 1971.
23. Siegelman SS, Sprayregen S, Boley SJ: Angiographic diagnosis of mesenteric arterial vasoconstriction. Radiology 112:533–542, 1974.
24. Probst P, Hirschmann DM, Haertel M, Fuchs WA: Die Röntgendiagnostik der akuten intestinalen Ischämie. ROEFO 132:527–534, 1980.
25. Meyers MA, Ghahremani GG, Clements JL Jr, Goodman K: Pneumatosis intestinalis. Gastrointest Radiol 2:91–105, 1977.
26. Miller WT, Scott J, Rosato EF, Rosato FE, Crow H: Ischemic colitis with gangrene. Radiology 94:291–297, 1970.
27. Schmutz G, Schutz J-F, Kempf F, Baumann R, Weill J-P: Aspects radiologiques de l'ischémie colique non gangreneuse. J Radiol 61:603–609, 1980.
28. Bartram CI: Obliteration of thumbprinting with double-contrast enemas in acute ischemic colitis. Gastrointest Radiol 4:85–88, 1979.
29. Greves JH III, Bohlman TW, Frische LH, Katon RM: Intramural barium in ischemic colitis. A new radiographic finding. Am J Dig Dis 21:257–262, 1976.
30. Gore RM, Calenoff L, Rogers LF: Roentgenographic manifestations of ischemic colitis. JAMA 241:1171–1173, 1979.
31. Cass AJ, Bliss BP, Bolton RP, Cooper BT: Gastrointestinal bleeding, angiodysplasia of the colon and acquired von Willebrand's disease. Br J Surg 67:639–641, 1980.
32. Eisenberg RL, Montgomery CK, Margulis AR: Colitis in the elderly: ischemic colitis mimicking ulcerative and granulomatous colitis. AJR 133:1113–1118, 1979.
33. Whitehouse GH, Watt J: Ischemic colitis associated with carcinoma of the colon. Gastrointest Radiol 2:31–35, 1977.
34. Meyers MA, Ghahremani GG, Govoni AF: Ischemic colitis associated with sigmoid volvulus: new observations. AJR 128:591–595, 1977.
35. Friedland GW, Filly R: Evanescent colitis in a child. Pediatr Radiol 2:73–74, 1974.
36. Tsuchiya M, Okazaki I, Asakura H, Ohkubo T: Radiographic and endoscopic features of colonic ulcers in systemic lupus erythematosus. Am J Gastroenterol 64:277–285, 1975.
37. Levesque M, Fauck C, Mornet P, Barsamian L, Lecronier M, Vital C: Manifestations digestives de la dermatomyosite. J Radiol 62:13–18, 1981.
38. Perloff LJ, Chon H, Petrella E, Grossman RA, Barker CF: Acute colitis in the renal allograft recipient. Ann Surg 183:77–83, 1976.
39. Wood MK, Read DR, Kraft AR, Barreta TM: A rare cause of ischemic colitis: polyarteritis nodosa. Dis Colon Rectum 22:428–433, 1979.
40. Scully RE, McNeely BU: Case Records of the Massachusetts General Hospital: case 45-1974. N Engl J Med 291:1073–1080, 1974.
41. Pond GD, Ovitt TW, Witte CL, Farrell K: Aneurysm of the superior hemorrhoidal artery: an unusual cause of massive rectal bleeding. J Can Assoc Radiol 28:146–147, 1977.
42. Van den Bosch A, Blomme G: Henoch-Schoenlein purpura with colonic involvement. A case report. ROEFO 132:457–459, 1980.
43. Peterson RB, Meseroll WP, Shrago GG, Gooding CA: Radiographic features of colitis associated with the hemolytic-uremic syndrome. Radiology 118:667–671, 1976.
44. Bar-Ziv J, Ayoub JIG, Fletcher BD: Hemolytic uremic syndrome: a case presenting with acute colitis. Pediatr Radiol 2:203–205, 1974.
45. Yates RS, Osterholm RK: Hemolytic-uremic syndrome colitis. J Clin Gastroenterol 2:359–363, 1980.
46. Sawaf H, Sharp MJ, Youn KJ, Jewell PA, Rabbani A: Ischemic colitis and stricture after hemolytic-uremic syndrome. Pediatrics 61:315–316, 1978.

47. Cruveilhier J: Un beau cas de cicatrisation d'un ulcère de l'intestin grêle, datant d'une douzaine d'années. Bull Soc Anat 7:1–2, 1832.
48. Hardie IR, Nicoll P: Localized ulceration of the caecum due to microcirculatory thrombosis. Aust NZ J Surg 43:149–157, 1973.
49. Sutherland DER, Chan FY, Foucar E, Simmons RL, Howard RJ, Najarian JS: The bleeding cecal ulcer in transplant patients. Surgery 86:386–398, 1979.
50. Gardiner GA, Bird CR: Nonspecific ulcers of the colon resembling annular carcinoma. Radiology 137:331–334, 1980.
51. Brodey PA, Hill RP, Baron S: Benign ulceration of the cecum. Radiology 122:323–327, 1977.
52. Blundell CR, Earnest DL: Idiopathic cecal ulcer. Diagnosis by colonoscopy followed by nonoperative management. Dig Dis Sci 25:494–503, 1980.
53. Sutherland D, Frech RS, Weil R, Najarian JS, Simmons RL: The bleeding cecal ulcer: pathogenesis, angiographic diagnosis, and non-operative control. Surgery 71:290–294, 1972.
54. Westcott JL, Smith JRV: Mesentery and colon injuries secondary to blunt trauma. Radiology 114:597–600, 1975.
55. Moore JD, Thompson NW, Appelman HD, Foley D: Arteriovenous malformation of the gastrointestinal tract. Arch Surg 111:381–388, 1976.
56. Cooperman AM, Kelly KA, Bernatz PE, Huizenga KA: Arteriovenous malformations of the intestine. Arch Surg 104:284–287, 1972.
57. Bentley PG: The bleeding caecal angioma: a diagnostic problem. Br J Surg 63:455–457, 1976.
58. Hollingsworth G: Haemangiomatous lesions of the colon. Br J Radiol 24:220–222, 1951.
59. Baum S, Athanasoulis CA, Waltman AC, Ring EJ: Gastrointestinal hemorrhage. II. Angiographic diagnosis and control. Adv Surg 7:149–198, 1973.
60. Boley SJ, Sammartano R, Adams A, DiBiase A, Kleinhaus S, Sprayregen S: On the nature and etiology of vascular ectasias of the colon: degenerative lesions of aging. Gastroenterology 72:650–660, 1977.
61. Galloway SJ, Casarella WJ, Shimkin PM: Vascular malformations of the right colon as a cause of bleeding in patients with aortic stenosis. Radiology 113:11–15, 1974.
62. Genant HK, Ranniger K: Vascular dysplasias of the ascending colon: report of two cases and review of the literature. AJR 115:349–354, 1972.
63. Athanasoulis CA, Galdabini JJ, Waltman AC, Novelline RA, Greenfield AJ, Ezpeleta ML: Angiodysplasia of the colon: a cause of rectal bleeding. Cardiovasc Radiol 1:3–13, 1978.
64. Ghahremani GG, Kangarloo H, Volberg F, Meyers MA: Diffuse cavernous hemangioma of the colon in the Klippel-Trenaunay syndrome. Radiology 118:673–678, 1976.
65. Baer JW, Ryan S: Analysis of cecal vasculature in the search for vascular malformations. AJR 126:394–405, 1976.
66. Sing AK, Agenant DMA, Hausman R, Tijtgat GN: Vascular ectasias (angiodysplasias) of the cecum and the ascending colon. ROEFO 132:534–541, 1980.
67. Weaver GA, Alpern HD, Davis JS, Ramsey WH, Reichelderfer M: Gastrointestinal angiodysplasia associated with aortic valve disease: part of spectrum of angiodysplasia of the gut. Gastroenterology 77:1–11, 1979.
68. Sprayregen S, Boley SJ: Vascular ectasias of the right colon. JAMA 239:962–964, 1978.
69. Sarles J-C, Horta ME, Castelo HB, Delecourt P: Arterial dysplasia of the colonic arteries: a rare cause of hemoperitoneum. Dis Colon Rectum 23:411–417, 1980.
70. Baum S, Athanasoulis CA, Waltman AC, Galdabini J, Schapiro RH, Warshaw AL, Ottinger LW: Angiodysplasia of the right colon: a cause of gastrointestinal bleeding. AJR 129:789–794, 1977.
71. Galloway SJ, Casarella WJ, Shimkin PM: Vascular malformations of the right colon as a cause of bleeding in patients with aortic stenosis. Radiology 113:11–15, 1974.
72. Rogers BHG, Adler F: Hemangiomas of the cecum. Gastroenterology 71:1079–1082, 1976.
73. Cody MC, O'Donovan PB, Hughes RW Jr: Idiopathic gastrointestinal bleeding and aortic stenosis. Am J Dig Dis 19:393–398, 1974.
74. Rosborough TK, Swaim WR: Acquired von Willebrand's disease, platelet-release defect, and angiodysplasia. Am J Med 65:96–100, 1978.
75. Athanasoulis CA, Waltman AC, Novelline RA, Krudy AG, Sniderman KW: Angiography: its contribution to emergency management of gastrointestinal hemorrhage. Radiol Clin North Am 14:265–280, 1976.
76. Baum S, Athanasoulis CA: Diagnostic studies in colonic affections. In: Bockus HL (ed). Gastroenterology, 3rd edn, Part V: Angiography, Vol II, pp 866–886. Saunders, Philadelphia, 1976.
77. Boley SJ, Sprayregen S, Sammartano RJ, Adams A, Kleinhaus S: The pathophysiologic basis for the angiographic signs of vascular ectasias of the colon. Radiology 125:615–621, 1977.
78. Nyman U, Boijsen E, Lindström C, Rosengren J-E: Angiography in angiomatous lesions of the gastrointestinal tract. Acta Radiol Diagn 21:21–31, 1980.
79. Tedesco FJ, Griffin JW Jr, Khan AQ: Vascular ectasia of the colon: clinical, colonoscopic, and radiographic features. J Clin Gastroenterol 2:233–238, 1980.
80. Miller KD, Tutton RH, Bell KA, Simon BK: Angiodysplasia of the colon. Radiology 132:309–313, 1979.
81. Menanteau B, Amselle M, Bonnet F, Ducreux A, Sénécail B: Angiodysplasie du côlon droit. J Radiol 61:717–721, 1980.
82. Brahme F, Hildell J: Angiography in Crohn's disease revisited. AJR 126:941–951, 1976.
83. Max MH, Richardson JD, Flint LM Jr, Kautson CO, Schwesinger W: Colonoscopic diagnosis of angiodysplasias of the gastrointestinal tract. Surg Gynecol Obstet 152:195–199, 1981.
84. Thanik KD, Chey WY, Abbott J: Vascular dysplasia of the cecum as a repeated source of hemorrhage. Role of colonoscopy in diagnosis. Gastrointest Endosc 23:167–169, 1977.
85. Wolff WI, Grossman MB, Shinya H: Angiodysplasia of the colon: diagnosis and treatment. Gastroenterology 72:329–333, 1977.
86. Allison DJ: Who's aware of angiodysplasia? World Med 16:59–60, 1981.
87. Sniderman KW, Franklin J Jr, Sos TA: Successful transcatheter gelfoam embolization of a bleeding vascular ectasia. AJR 131:157–159, 1978.
88. Allison DJ: Gastrointestinal bleeding: radiological diagnosis. Br J Hosp Med 23:358–365, 1980.

III.1.C. Regional enteritis

a. Introduction

During the last century and early part of this century there were case reports describing isolated thickening of the bowel wall and long benign bowel strictures. Many of the changes described were primarily in the ileum and consisted of 'diffuse ileitis'. Descriptions of the microscopic appearance mention inflammatory granulomata as being scattered throughout the involved segment. Many of these were believed to represent tuberculosis. Undoubtedly, several disease entities were being lumped together by these early investigators into a nonspecific granulomatous bowel disease.

In 1932, Crohn, Ginzburg and Oppenheimer first described 14 patients with a necrotizing inflammation involving the terminal ileum (1). Although initially similar findings in the colon were thought to represent ulcerative colitis, Lockhart-Mummery and Morson clearly showed in 1959–1960 that this nonspecific granulomatous inflammatory disease of the colon was also the same entity (2, 3). It became apparent that such a granulomatous disease could be found in the small bowel alone, the colon alone, or that it could involve both the small bowel and the colon. As a result, this disease became known as ileocolitis. Pathologic features tend to distinguish this entity from nonspecific ulcerative colitis.

When limited to the colon, generally the terms Crohn's colitis or granulomatous colitis are commonly used (4), although currently there is no consensus for a single term. Some investigators use the term regional enteritis even when the disease is limited to the colon, while others use a descriptive term depending upon the site of involvement, such as jejunoileitis, or enterocolitis. These terms are descriptive only; ileitis can mean Crohn's disease, infection with *Yersinia* or even tuberculosis. When only the colon is involved it may be best to use either 'Crohn's colitis', 'granulomatous colitis' or 'regional enteritis limited to the colon' to describe this condition. When both the small bowel and colon are involved, the terms 'Crohn's disease' or 'regional enteritis' appear reasonable. Just for consistency, we will use the latter term to describe this entity, regardless of site of involvement. The many names for this disease attest to the confusion existing in defining its pathogenesis. The etiology of this disease is not known.

Why regional enteritis was discovered only several decades ago is puzzling. Some evidence suggests that this disease was rare previous to its discovery (5). As late as the 1964 edition of Bockus' *Gastroenterology*, it is stated that 'unquestionably there are many general practitioners in the United States who have never encountered a patient with regional enteritis' (6).

There are certain distinct and unusual geographic distributions for this entity. For example, it is uncommon in Japan and most of the other Asian countries where infectious colitis is more common. In Japan, the number of patients with colon tuberculosis exceeds the number with regional enteritis. Regional enteritis is seen most often in North America and Europe. Whether the incidence in Asia is truly less than in North America or whether the number of reported cases is less simply due to a lower index of suspicion is conjecture. This disease appears to be more prevalent among American Jews (7) and relatively unusual among American Blacks (8, 9). It is a disease primarily of young adults. In adults the colon is frequently involved while in children the majority have disease limited to the small bowel (10).

There is a familial occurrence of regional enteritis, with the disease being more frequently encountered in some families (11–13). It has been found in some sets of identical twins (14).

In 1937, Hulusi Behçet, a Turkish dermatologist, described an association or oral ulcers, genital lesions and ocular inflammation (15). A further association of arthritis, colitis, inflammation, and other manifestations has been subsequently added to this syndrome. Noncaseating granuloma can be found in a biopsy specimen (16). Radiographically the colitis tends to mimic regional enteritis both in distribution and appearance (17–19). The rectum is usually involved (16) and there may also be small bowel disease. The presacral space can be widened (16), generally in association with rectal disease. Aphthous ulcers may be present (16, 20) or there can be numerous discrete ulcers with normal intervening colon. The ulcers tend to be deep and may result in perforation (20). Toxic megacolon has been reported (19, 21). Because of the unrelenting course of the disease, in most patients with an established diagnosis of Behçet's disease and intestinal involvement the prognosis is grim. The terminal episode can be bowel perforation and peritonitis. Because of extensive involvement, surgery may offer little hope. The incidence of postoperative complication and recurrence of ulcers is high (22). In an occasional patient the symptoms clear and the radiographic findings revert to normal (19).

It is not known if Behçet's syndrome is a separate entity or whether it is part of a spectrum that also includes regional enteritis.

b. Clinical considerations

Patients with regional enteritis involving the colon tend to present with fever, abdominal pain, and diarrhea. Bleeding is not usually a prominent feature in most patients. Melena may occur in regional enteritis, although bloody diarrhea to the extent seen in ulcerative colitis is unusual. An occasional patient may first present with massive lower gastrointestinal hemorrhage (23, 24). The first indication of regional enteritis can be a perirectal fistula that appears even before there is any other evidence of disease. Even with extensive fistulae, the rectum may appear to be normal sigmoidoscopically.

Patients with regional enteritis have an increased incidence of various arthritides (Fig. C.1) and diseases involving the bile ducts (25). The incidence, however, is lower than seen with ulcerative colitis. There is a higher incidence of cholelithiasis, sclerosing cholangitis and bile duct carcinoma than in the normal population. Arthralgia tends to parallel activity of the bowel disease. Regional enteritis is also associated with erythema nodosum, pyoderma gangrenosum, and with sarcoid granuloma-containing skin ulcerations. The latter are found primarily in the perineum. There appears to be an increased association with ankylosing spondylitis. Ocular inflammation is an unusual asssociation. One patient with regional enteritis developed a vasculitis in striated muscles, a distinctly unusual association (26).

Regional enteritis is a chronic, and often a relentless disease. These patients have a twofold increased risk of dying compared to the general population (27). Remissions may last for years and most patients can be managed with medical therapy, consisting primarily of treatment of the patient's symptoms with steroids and azulfidine. Sometimes a change in diet gives symptomatic

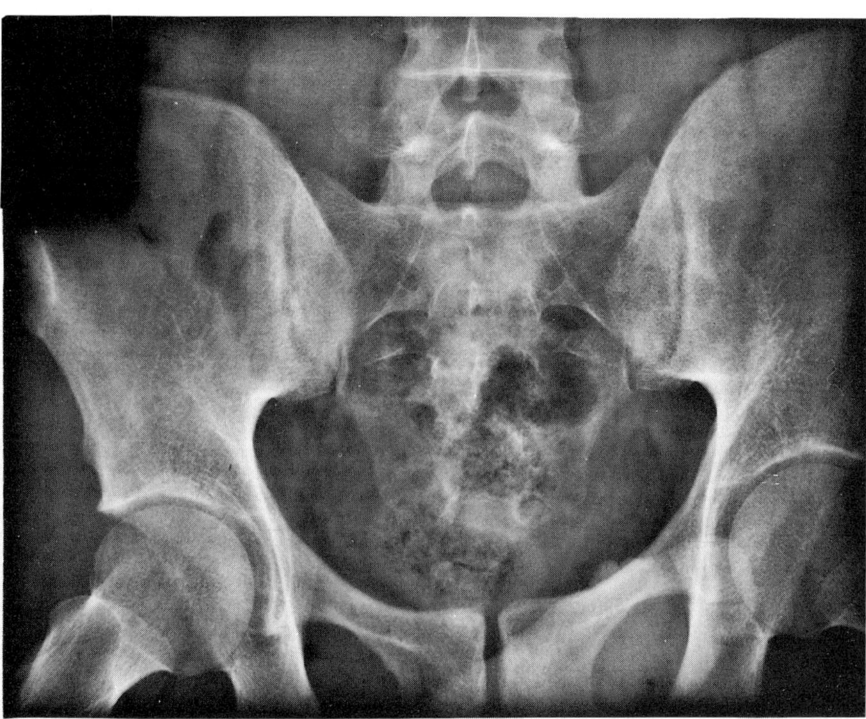

Fig. C.1. 25-year-old male with regional enteritis and sacroileitis. The sacroiliac joints are poorly defined.

relief. A restriction of the intake of fat or milk can be helpful and some patients develop an iron deficiency anemia. Pain medication is used empirically. Antibiotic therapy should be considered on a trial basis and may lead to clinical and radiographic evidence of improvement (28). One reason for improvement with antibiotics may be the eradication of overgrowth with such organisms as *Clostridium difficile* (29), although this organism appears to be an unlikely factor in the etiology and pathogenesis of the underlying disease (30). Hyperalimentation may also relieve symptoms temporarily. The role of immunosuppressive drugs has still not been established. Although rarely encountered today, radiation therapy has been used in the past with some improvement in symptoms (8, 31).

Surgery is generally considered only after failure of medical therapy or if complications are encountered. Currently, surgery is considered if there are signs of obstruction, abscess, sepsis, extensive fistulae including severe perirectal fistulae, or toxic megacolon. If inflammation due to regional enteritis results in ureteral obstruction, the obstructed kidney may eventually be destroyed. Surgery consists of resection of the involved bowel segment and any associated inflammatory masses. A colectomy is performed if the entire colon is diseased. Fecal diversion around a diseased colon segment has invariably failed.

There appears to be an increased incidence of small bowel obstruction after excisional surgery for inflammatory bowel disease. In some series the majority of obstructions were due to adhesions and stomal malfunction, with recurrent disease being a rare cause (32), while others have found the reverse to be true (33). Unfortunately, many of the patients who have disease involving the colon and undergo surgery have a recurrence of their disease (34, 35).

After resection, recurrence usually occurs proximal to the anastomosis (Fig. C.2), although recurrence may be in the distal segment but this is rare (36) (Fig. C.3). The recurrence rate varies but most investigators agree that the incidence of recurrence increases with time (37, 38). Recurrence appears to be inversely proportional to the age of the patient (38).

It is not unusual to see histologic evidence of disease at the resection margins even when gross disease is not present. Some investigators believe that the presence of *microscopic* disease at the anastomosis does not predispose to future recurrence of the disease (35), although others differ (39–41). Grossly diseased bowel left behind is associated with postoperative colitis (36).

c. Pathology

Regional enteritis is an inflammatory disease which can involve any part of the alimentary tract. When well established, there are several characteristic features. In extensive involvement with regional enteritis the entire bowel wall is thick, all layers are involved, and there is narrowing of the lumen. Single or multiple strictures are present. Extensive ulcers are common and the surface can have an irregular cobblestone appearance. The terminal ileum, if involved, likewise shows thickening of the wall and a stenotic lumen. Generally, the valvulae conniventes are destroyed and there is an irregular cobblestone appearance. Deep ulcers and fistulae may be present (Fig. C.4).

When the distal ileum is involved the associated mesentery is thickened and edematous. Numerous loops of bowel tend to be matted together in an inflammatory mass. With stenosis and partial obstruction there is dilation of the bowel proximal to the area of involvement. At times even the dilated segment can be diseased although usually the dilation is either due to the distal obstruction or to a localized adynamic ileus from the surrounding inflammation. Skip areas, with normal bowel in between the diseased segments, are not uncommon.

The disease often starts in the ileocecal region. Whether it then spreads distally, or whether the eventually involved colon segment may have been previously diseased is still debatable. Some observers believe that the disease does not spread either proximally or distally in the absence of surgical manipulation (42, 43); others do describe extension of the disease (44–47).

With terminal ileal disease the appendix may also be involved even when the adjacent cecum is not diseased. These changes are generally better seen by the pathologist than the radiologist.

With early disease the lesions are primarily in the submucosa and mucosa. Initially there are nonulcerated granulomatous lesions with giant cell formation (48). Hyperplastic lymphoid follicles ap-

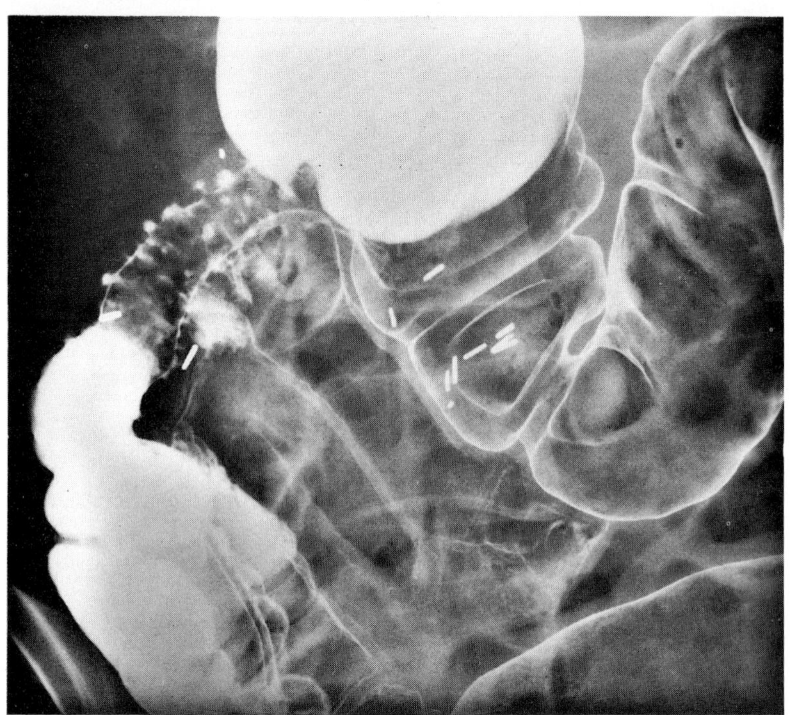

Fig. C.2. 32-year-old female with ileotransverse colostomy and recurrence proximal to the anastomosis. Deep ulcers are scattered throughout the involved segment. Such recurrence *proximal* to an anastomosis is more common than distal recurrence.

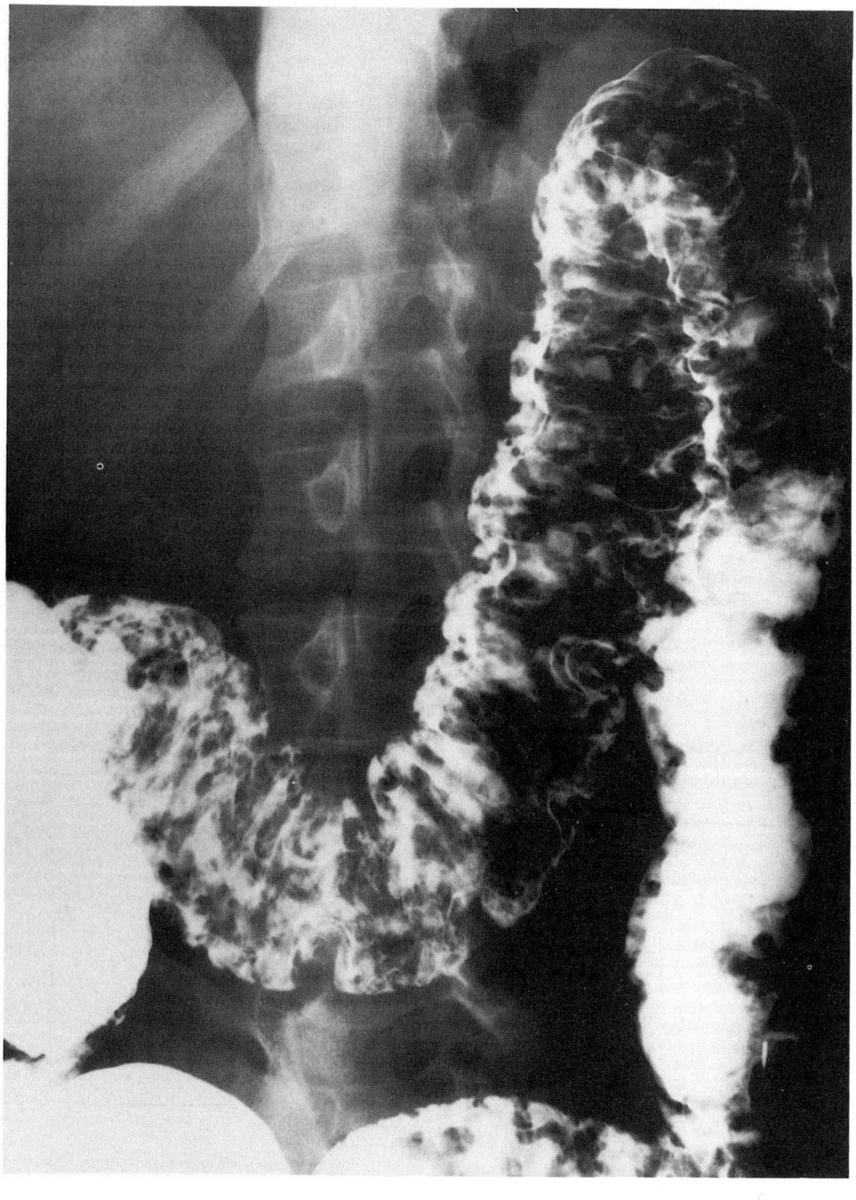

Fig. C.3. One year previously this 34-year-old male had a normal barium enema. Because of known distal ileal regional enteritis and resultant small bowel obstruction patient underwent an ileocolostomy. One year later there is striking involvement of the entire colon. There are deep ulcers and inflammatory polyps throughout the colon, changes developing suddenly after surgery.

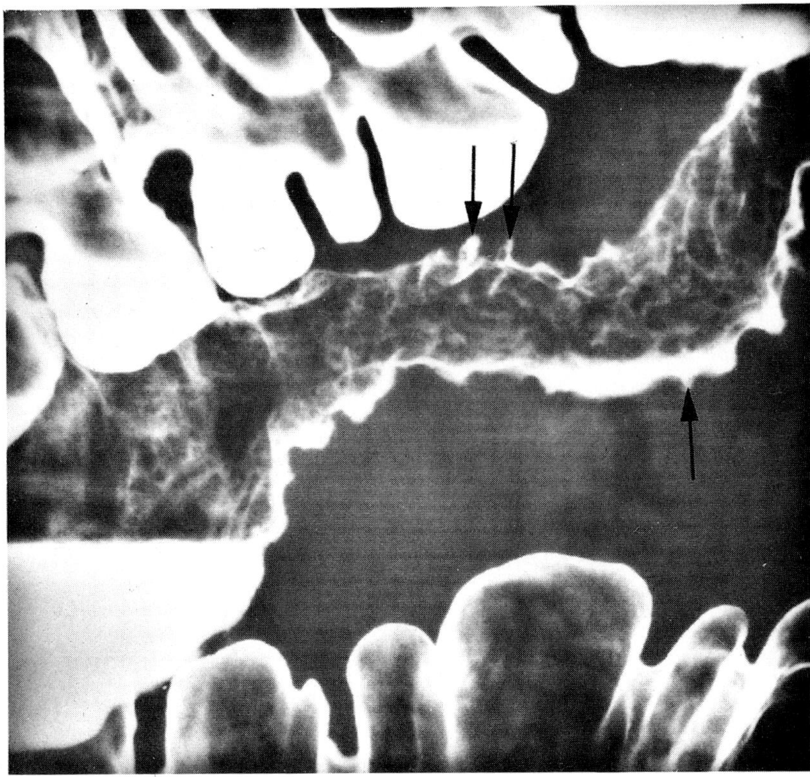

a

Fig. C.4. (a) Regional enteritis involving the distal ileum. The valvulae conniventes are destroyed, the lumen narrowed, and numerous deep ulcers (arrows) are present. (b) Another patient with extensive terminal ileal involvement. Numerous inflammatory polyps are scattered throughout the involved segment.

b

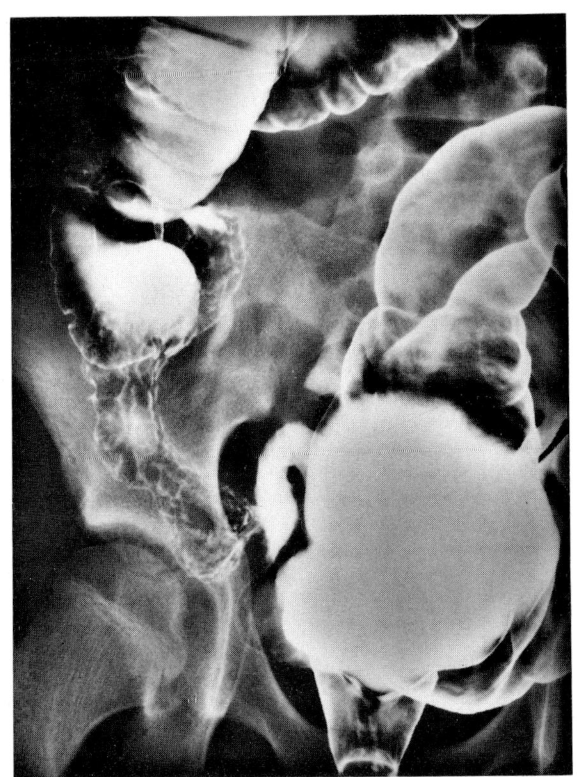

pear as small polyps with a centrally located ulcer, usually less than 3 mm in diameter (49). The ulcers, commonly called aphthous ulcers, are believed to be due to pressure necrosis over the lymph follicle.

Overall, the diseased segment if inflammed and ulcerated with considerable variation in histology seen with progression of the disease, there is commonly lymphocytic infiltration and transmural inflammation. The muscularis mucosa tends to be thickened considerably and there can be submucosal edema. Ulcers varying in size can be scattered throughout the colon. These ulcers may be small and located between normal appearing mucosa or they may be so extensive and confluent that there are large areas of denuded mucosa. Crypt abscesses, commonly seen with ulcerative colitis, can also be present in regional enteritis. Deep fissures are common in regional enteritis, a finding not seen in ulcerative colitis. There is an exuberant fibrotic reaction, with the fibrosis being disproportionate to the amount of inflammation involved. Bowel wall edema and significant lymphangiectasia due to lymphatic obstruction is a feature consistently seen in regional enteritis (50).

The hallmark of regional enteritis is the presence of noncaseating granulomata. Unfortunately, granulomata are not always present even in surgical specimens. When present, granulomata in regional enteritis are both in the colon wall or in the regional lymph nodes. The granulomata consist of epithelioid cells and may contain giant cells, called Langhans' cells, which are multinucleated giant cells with nuclei arranged at the periphery of the cell. These cells are not specific for regional enteritis but are also seen in other granulomatous diseases. If caseation is present another disease, such as tuberculosis, should be suspected. The presence of granulomata, likewise, is not pathognomonic for this disease. As an example, infectious colitis due to *Entamoeba histolytica* may result in granulomata. Granulomata, however, are not seen in ulcerative colitis and, if present, should exclude this disease from the differential diagnosis. Tuberculosis is also associated with granulomata, although caseation is generally present. Other rare causes of colon granulomata include schistosomiasis, infection by some fungi, sarcoidosis, and Whipple's disease. Granulomata are also found in such entities as primary biliary cirrhosis (51).

Occasionally when disease is limited to the terminal ileum, a biopsy of the rectum reveals granulomata even in the absence of clinical disease of the rectum. Although helpful in establishing the diagnosis in some patients, such a finding is not always seen (52).

The etiology and pathogenesis of regional enteritis are unknown. There may be some genetic influence (53). Although there are reports of possible transmissible agents (54, 55), including cell-wall-defective variants of microorganisms (56), the overall evidence at present is against an infectious etiology (57, 58). The final diagnosis currently rests on the clinical picture, radiographic appearance, and pathology. No pathognomonic features are seen exclusively in regional enteritis. There also is poor correlation between the microscopic appearance and future clinical course of the disease (59).

Some patients in Japan with acute regional ileitis have infestation with *Anisakis* larvae (60). A high incidence of acute regional ileitis occurs on the west coast of Hokkaido in the winter. One case of *Anisakis* ileocolitis has been reported in the United States (61). It is believed that reinfection with *Anisakis* larvae produces an Arthus-type allergic reaction resulting in the acute regional ileitis (60). Whether some other allergic reaction is responsible for the typical findings in regional enteritis as seen in the Western world in pure speculation.

d. Radiology

The colon can be involved with or without small bowel involvement. Isolated left-sided colitis is rare; involvement of the left side usually occurs together with colitis of the right side of the colon (43). Segmental disease can occur with normal-appearing colon in between (Fig. C.5), the entire colon can be involved, or, occasionally regional enteritis is limited primarily to the small bowel but the colon is involved only secondarily due to the formation of a fistula or an adjacent inflammatory mass (Fig. C.6). Segmental disease is more common than pancolitis. With secondary colon involvement, once the primary diseased bowel is resected the colon lesion heals. It is common to see asymmetric and eccentric bowel wall involvement. The transition between normal and abnormal bowel is abrupt (Fig. C.7), although the transition may be difficult to identify when only early changes are present. Such an abrupt transition usually is not seen with ulcerative colitis.

It has been claimed that the earliest changes, consisting of submucosal and mucosal edema, are seen radiographically as fine transverse streaks of barium (62). Others believe that these streaks represent innominate lines and are normal (63). Some consider a very fine granular pattern and the nodular pattern as seen in lymphoid hyperplasia as signs of early regional enteritis (64). Unfortunately, prominent lymph follicles are often found in normal patients, especially children and young adults, and thus this sign is nonspecific but can be seen early in regional enteritis (Fig. C.8). Most investigators agree that the earliest definitive changes in regional enteritis are 'doughnut' shaped aphthous ulcers scattered throughout the involved segment (65–69) (Fig. C.9). (The definition of *aphtha* is a 'small ulcer' and the term *aphthous ulcer* is thus redundant. Yet the pathologic, radiologic and medical literature uses *aphthous ulcer* to represent the small ulcers with surrounding edema as seen in

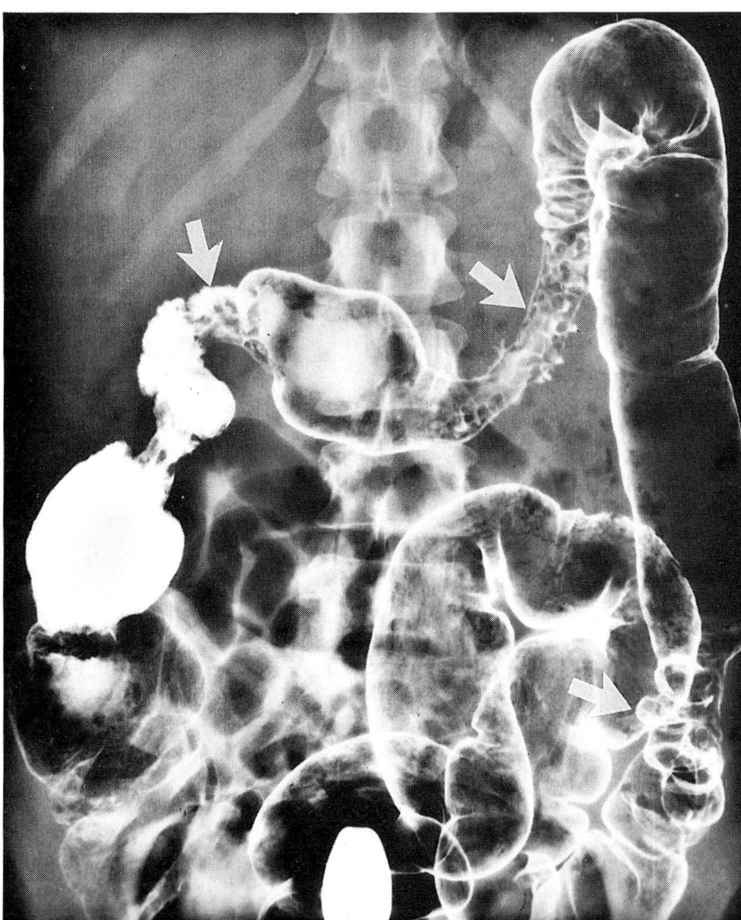

Fig. C.5. Segmental regional enteritis at the hepatic flexure, transverse colon and descending colon (arrows). The intervening colon appears normal.

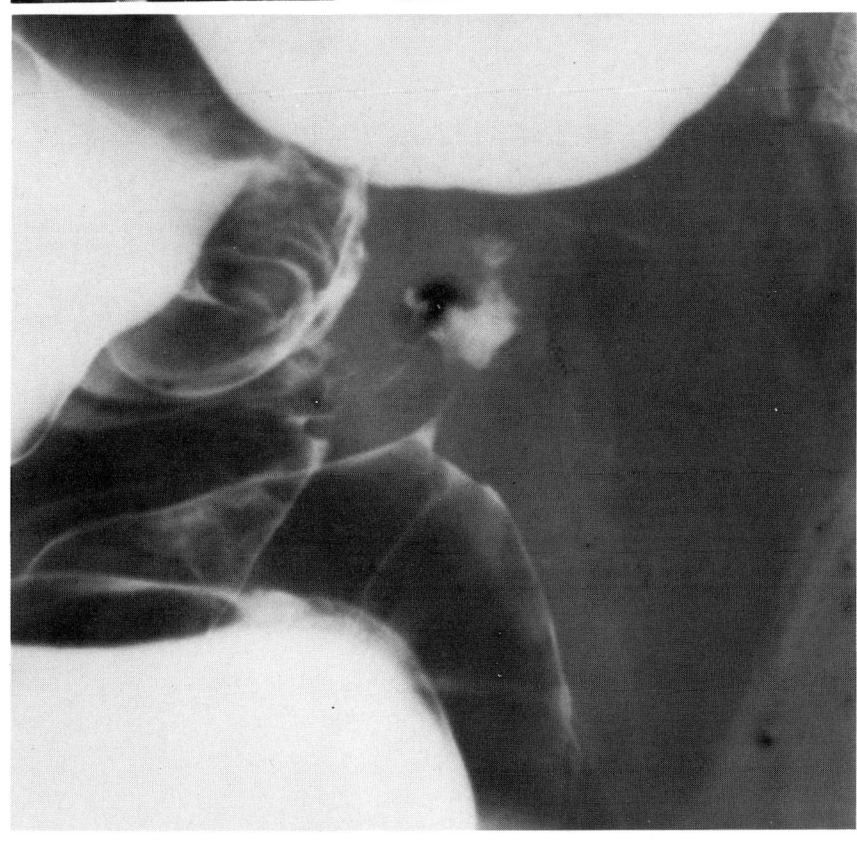

Fig. C.6. The sigmoid is secondarily involved by the inflammatory changes, although regional enteritis is primarily limited to the ileum and right colon.

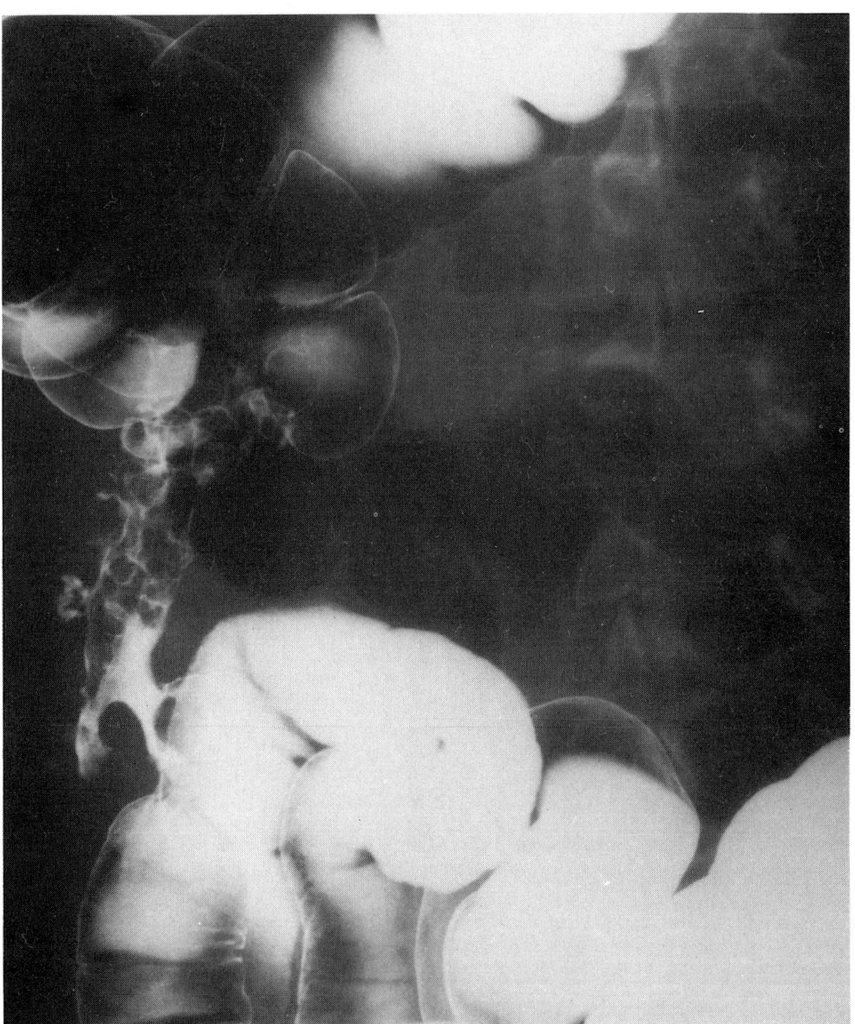

Fig. C.7. The junction between abnormal right colon and normal hepatic flexure is sharply defined, characteristic of regional enteritis. The involved segment is stenotic and numerous deep ulcers are present. The cecal lumen has been almost completely obliterated.

regional enteritis.) Still others have questioned whether the aphthous ulcers are really the *earliest* changes and believe that these ulcers simply represent one radiographic sign seen in regional enteritis (70, 71). From our experience, we agree with the latter investigators. In either case, aphthous ulcers are not pathognomonic of regional enteritis and have occasionally been seen in other diseases (72).

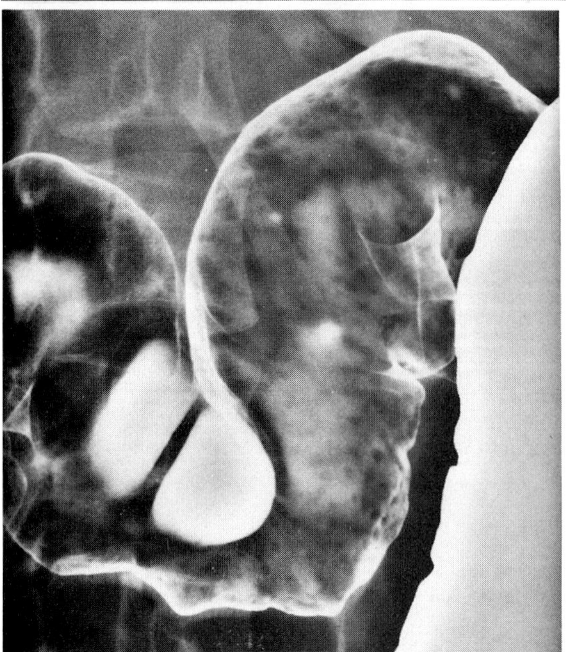

Fig. C.8. Multiple small polyps are scattered throughout the transverse colon in this 35-year-old patient. Almost no central ulceration can be identified and the pattern appears similar to that seen with prominent lymph nodes. The patient had regional enteritis.

These lesions appear as small nodules with central ulcerations and a double-contrast examination is essential to recognize them (Fig. C.10). The lesions are surrounded by normal-appearing mucosa (73).

With progression of disease, these small ulcers become confluent and result in deep linear ulcers (Fig. C.11); when extensive, linear ulcers intercept retained areas of mucosa and result in a 'cobblestone' appearance (64). If the ulcers penetrate deeply, eventually the appearance mimics wide-neck diverticula (74).

Progression between serial examinations is common (44). The lesions can become arrested at any stage except for the minute ulcers; these ulcers

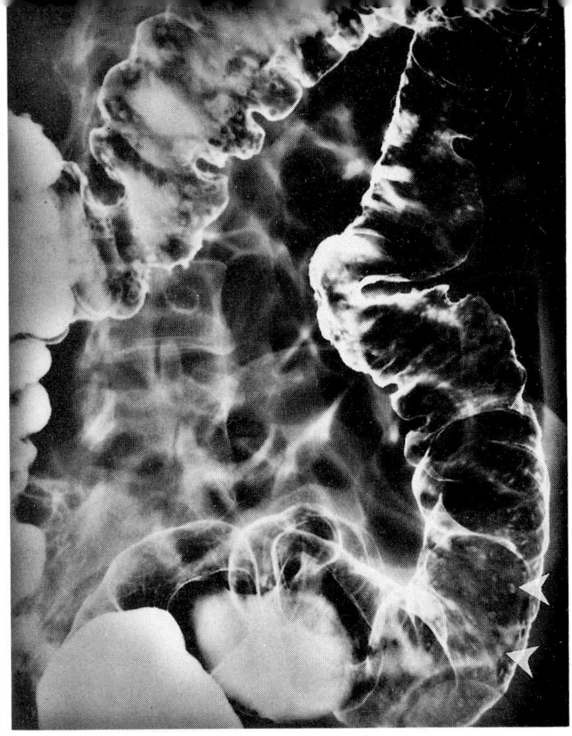

a

b

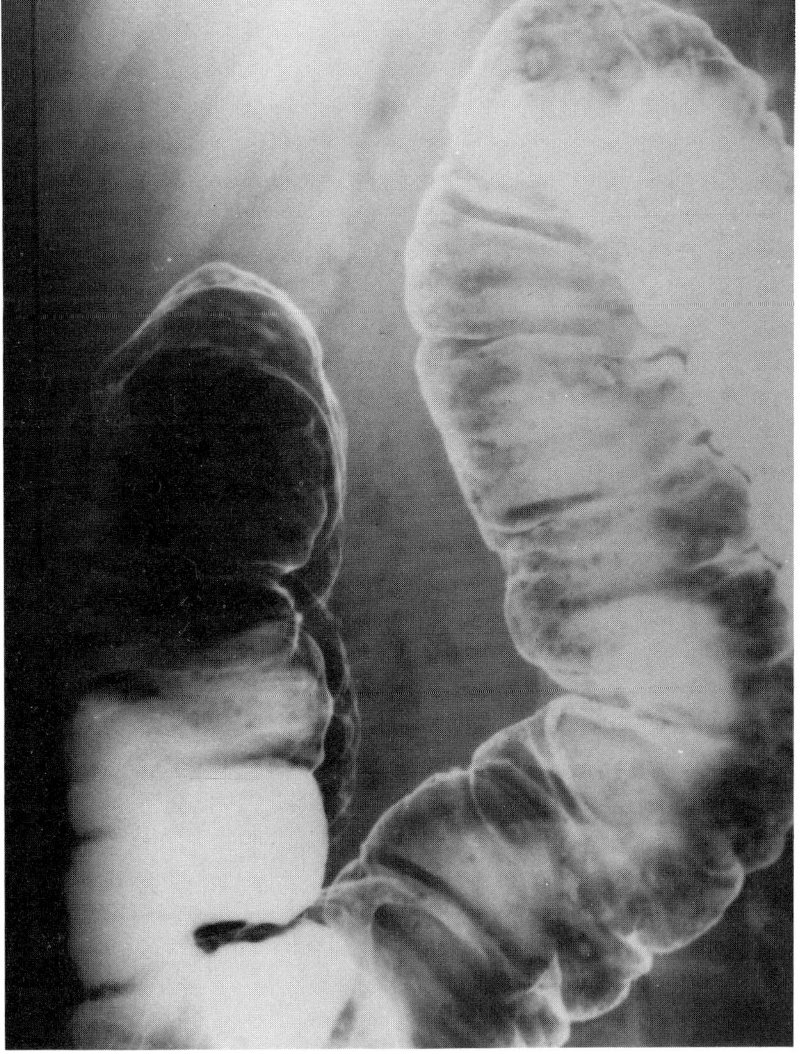

Fig. C.9. (a) Numerous 'doughnut' shaped ulcers (arrowheads) are scattered in the descending colon in this patient with regional enteritis. (b) Another patient with numerous ulcers throughout the transverse colon.

either disappear or, more commonly, progress. Progression of radiographic findings tends to occur in a steplike manner rather than as a continuous spectrum (44).

Occasionally extensive disease in the right colon with mild involvement of the left colon will change with time and result in regression of the right colic disease with progression on the left (43). Such migration may occur almost to the point of the right colon appearing 'normal', but histologically the involved segment is still diseased. Rarely, left colic involvement can clear radiographically (Fig. C.10). At times there are present elongated or oval inflammatory masses (75), called filiform polyps (76) (Fig. C.12). These polyps are sometimes so large that the lumen is narrowed considerably (77, 78) (Fig. C.13). If irregular, they can mimic a cancer (79). Such polyps are not specific and have been described both in regional enteritis (80, 81) and in ulcerative colitis (75, 82).

With further progression, the lumen narrows, the colon becomes foreshortened, and the colon and adjacent small bowel become surrounded by inflammatory masses. Adjacent normal bowel can be either simply displaced or fixed and distorted by the inflammatory mass. Internal fistulae are more commonly seen with involvement of the terminal ileum (Fig. C.14). A fistula may develop into an abscess. Eventually, either long or short stenotic segments appear and multiple stenoses can be present.

The presacral space can be widened either due to the disease itself or to subsequent steroid therapy or both (Fig. C.15). Widening may also result from sinus tracts extending posteriorly from the rectum and from abscesses within this space.

Although unusual, pneumatosis intestinalis can develop in a setting of regional enteritis (70). The most likely explanation is mucosal destruction leading to intramural gas dissection.

Bowel wall thickness can sometimes be measured

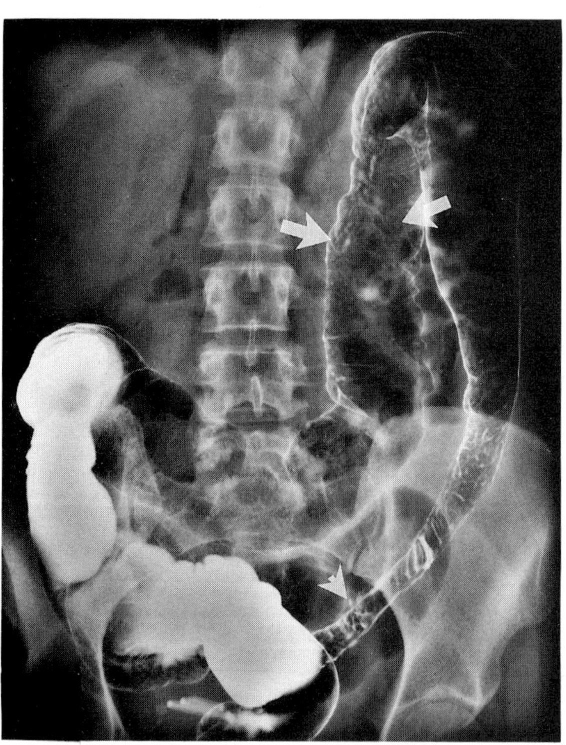
a

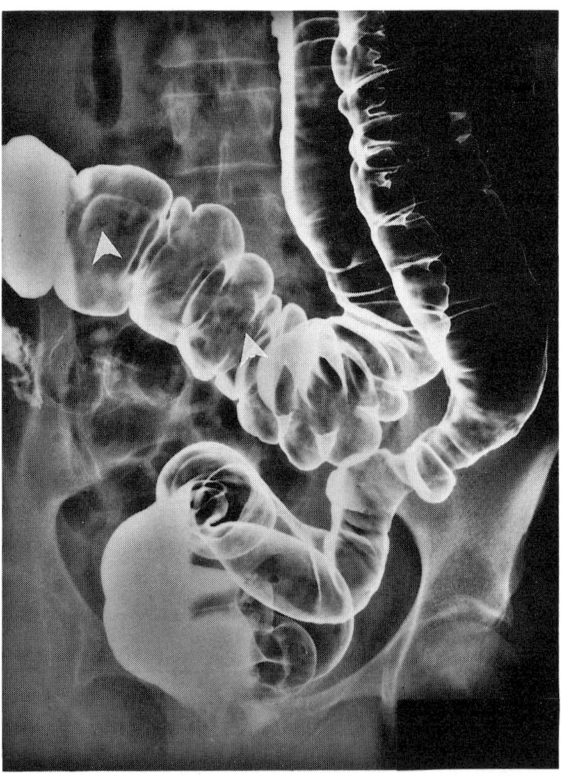
b

Fig. C.10. (a) Pan colitis is present in this 46-year-old female with long-standing regional enteritis. The distal ileum was also severely involved. The descending colon is involved the most with loss of haustra, a long stricture, and deep ulcers (arrowhead). Aphthous ulcers are present in the transverse colon (arrows). Because of the severe ileal disease the patient underwent a distal ileohemicolectomy with ileocolostomy. (b) Two years later the left colic disease has cleared radiographically. Aphthous ulcers are present in the transverse colon (arrowheads). Seventeen months later the patient underwent resection of the anastomosis because of stenosis. Both resection margins were involved by the disease. The left colon was not explored.

on a double contrast barium enema if the serosal surface can be outlined by fat. If an examination is inconclusive in differentiating between regional enteritis and ulcerative colitis, a bowel wall thickness in excess of 5 mm is suggestive of regional enteritis (83). A thickness less than 5 mm, however, may be seen with both entities.

The angiographic signs of regional enteritis include thickening of the bowel wall (as judged by colon wall vascularity), an intensely vascular inner core (probably representing the submucosa and mucosa) and a hypovascular outer core (probably the muscularis propria) (84, 85). Angiography is currently of limited value in the evaluation of regional enteritis, except in patients presenting with massive hemorrhage (23).

After good response to medical management the radiographic changes of regional enteritis can become less apparent. Yet, pathologically the disease is generally still present. Although in ulcerative colitis the colon may occasionally become normal again, both radiologically and pathologically, this is unusual in regional enteritis once the disease has become fully established. Generally, the disease recurs in that rare patient who does revert to a normal appearance (44). Occasionally, one encounters 'burned out' regional enteritis with an appearance similar to that seen in other end-stage colitides.

e. Complications

Although an internal fistula is relatively common, free peritoneal perforation is rare in this disease (86, 87). When perforation does occur, the patient will present with an acute abdomen. The patient can have varying degrees of bowel obstruction, but obstruction is more common with small bowel rather than with colon involvement.

Growth retardation and osteopenia are common in adolescents with chronic disease (88). The osteoporosis can develop because of the poor nutritional status of these patients or from therapy with steroids.

Inflammatory involvement of adjacent structures such as the genitourinary tract is not unusual. Regional enteritis of the terminal ileum and right colon can result in an inflammatory mass involving and obstructing the right ureter (89) (Fig. C.16). Thus, in these patients it is imperative to perform an intravenous pyelogram to exclude ureteral obstruc-

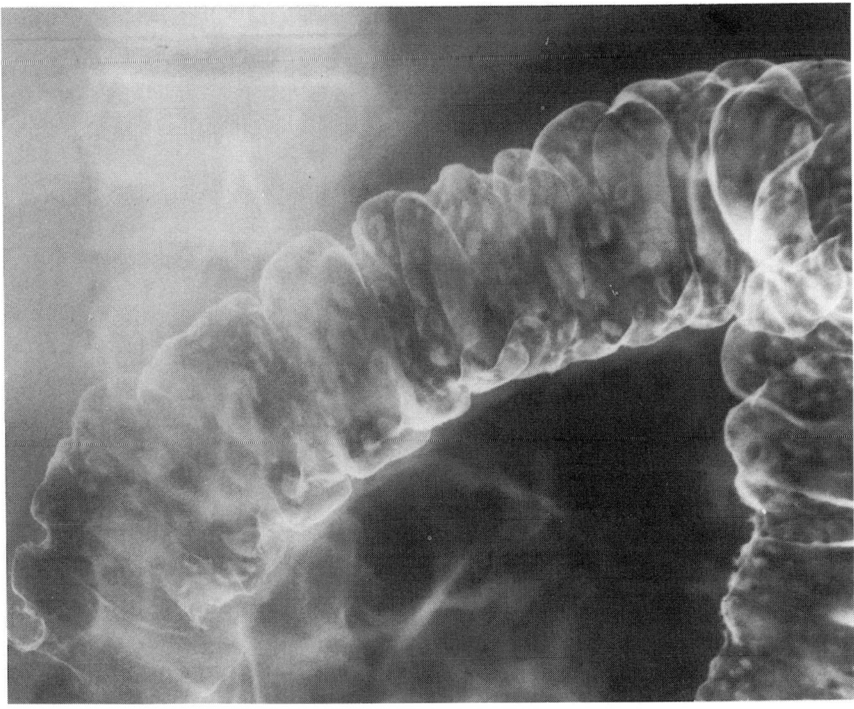

Fig. C.11. Intramural ulcers are in profile in the descending colon. Similar ulcers are seen en face in the distal transverse colon.

tion and subsequent renal damage.

Internal fistulae can connect loops of bowel, can run between the colon and an inflammatory mass, or can be primarily in the mesentery of the involved segment. Osteomyelitis of the sacrum, although rare, can result from a rectal fistula extending posteriorly. A fistula may burrow for long distances and eventually appear cutaneously. Fistula to unusual sites can occur (90).

Toxic megacolon can develop in regional enteritis (42, 91) although the incidence is considerably less than with ulcerative colitis. Toxic dilatation sometimes, though rarely, occurs in the ileum (92). The distinguishing features of toxic megacolon in a setting of granulomatous colitis are prominent edema and thickening of the bowel wall (Fig. C.17); these changes are not usually seen with ulcerative colitis, where the wall tends to be thin.

An unusual complication of chronic regional enteritis is retroperitoneal fibrosis (93).

Unlike ulcerative colitis, the subsequent development of carcinoma is not common, although the incidence is still higher than that in a comparable

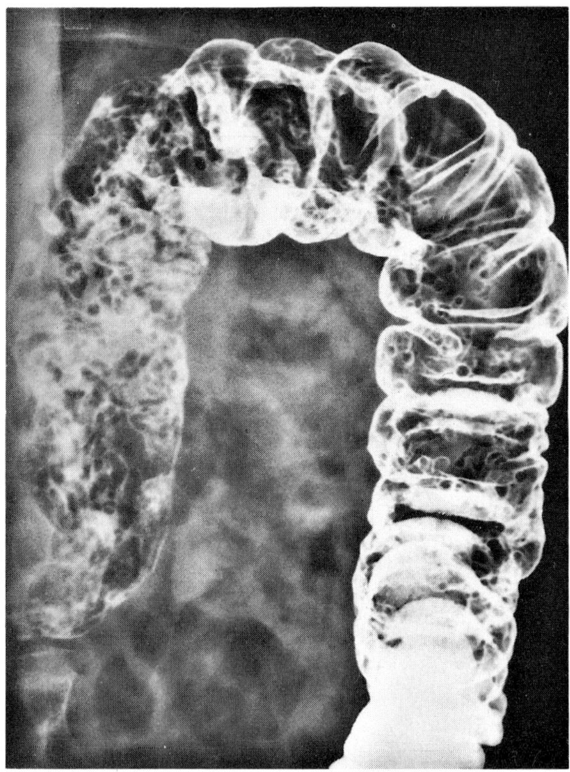

a

b

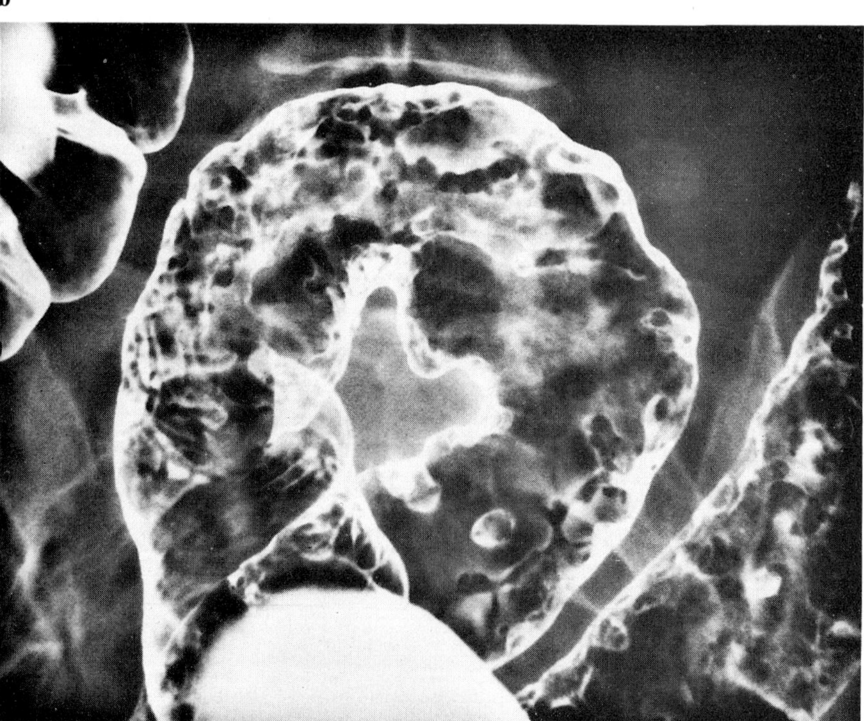

Fig. C.12. (a) Numerous elongated inflammatory masses are centered around the splenic flexure, typical of 'filiform polyposis'. (Courtesy of Dr. H.F. Gramm, New England Deaconess Hospital, Boston, MA.) (b) Another patient with filiform polyposis of the sigmoid.

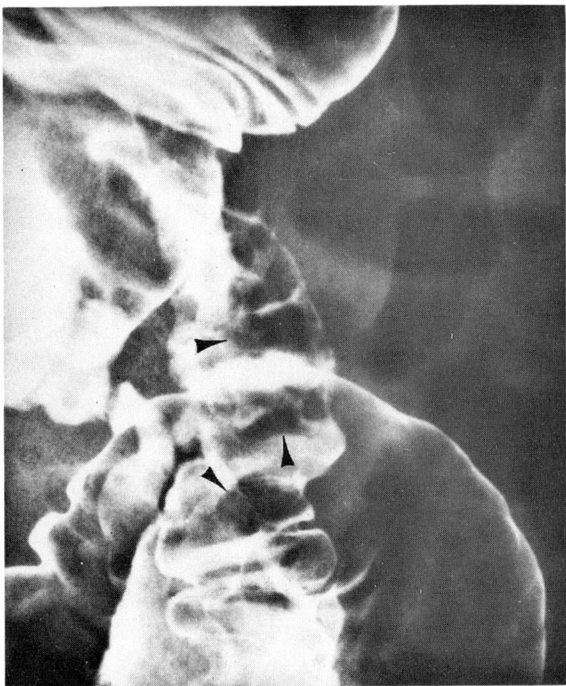

Fig. C.13. Inflammatory polyps in the terminal ileum (arrows) with narrowing of the lumen.

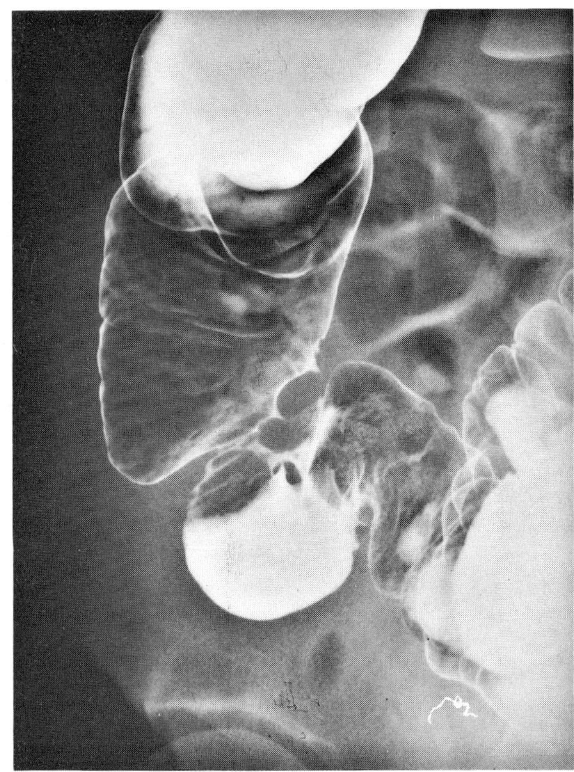

a

b

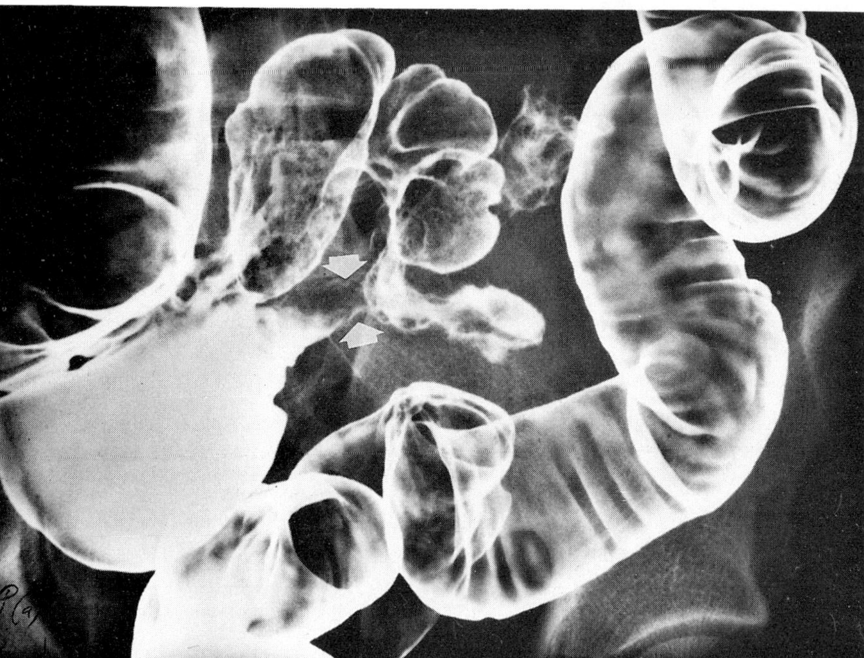

Fig. C.14. (a) An ileocecal fistula (arrowheads) is present in a 31-year-old male. (b) Another patient had an ileoascending colon fistula. (c) In general, these fistula are easier to demonstrate on a barium enema than an antegrade small bowel examination where the actual fistula may be poorly seen.

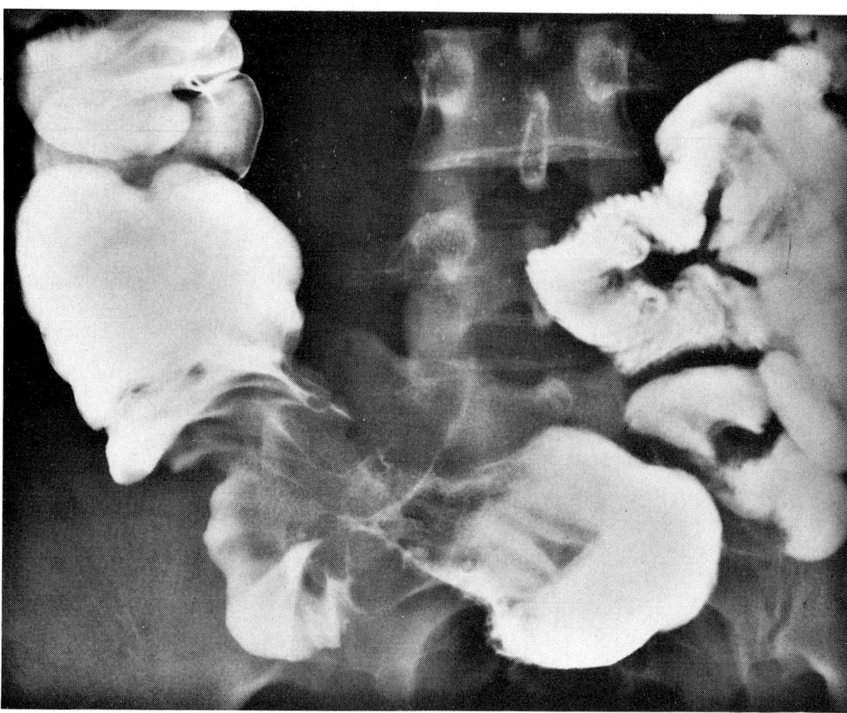

Fig. C.14.c

normal patient population group (94–96). The relative risk of alimentary tract cancer has been reported to be about three times higher than in the normal population (97). In addition, there appears to be an overall increased incidence of cancer of all sites (97). Regional enteritis may predispose neoplastic transformation of other tissues. Diversionary bypass surgery, leaving the diseased segment excluded, results in a higher incidence of cancer in the diverted segment than expected in the general population (98, 99).

The precancerous colon reveals epithelial dysplasia, an adenomatous growth pattern, or 'villiform mucosal proliferations' similar to those seen in ulcerative colitis (100). As a result, once the diagnosis of regional enteritis is established, follow-up for possible neoplastic transformation includes colonoscopy primarily with multiple biopsies for evaluation of epithelial dysplasia (101); currently there are no radiographic signs of dysplasia and radiology can detect only the more obvious findings.

Regional enteritis involving the small bowel is also associated with an increased incidence of small bowel carcinomata (102, 103); these cancers occur in a younger population than usually encountered, the tumors are less differentiated, and the survival rate is considerably less than with de novo cancers (104).

f. Differential diagnosis

The radiologist should use *all* available clinical data together with the radiographic findings in suggesting a diagnosis of regional enteritis. This diagnosis should be questioned if the clinical presentation is atypical or if there is a poor response to medical therapy, since other disease entities may mimic the radiographic picture (105).

In young people the main diagnostic problem is differentiating regional enteritis from ulcerative colitis (Table C.1). In the vast majority of patients the radiographic findings are specific (106). If there is significant small bowel involvement, if there are skip areas, or if the rectum appears normal then one is dealing with regional enteritis. If only the rectosigmoid is involved, either disease may be present. The ulcers seen initially in ulcerative colitis usually are small and have a 'grain of sand' appearance. The ulcers in regional enteritis tend to be larger and the appearance is that of scattered 'pebbles'. Deep fistula are unusual in ulcerative colitis but are relatively common in regional enteritis.

In an occasional patient it may not be possible to

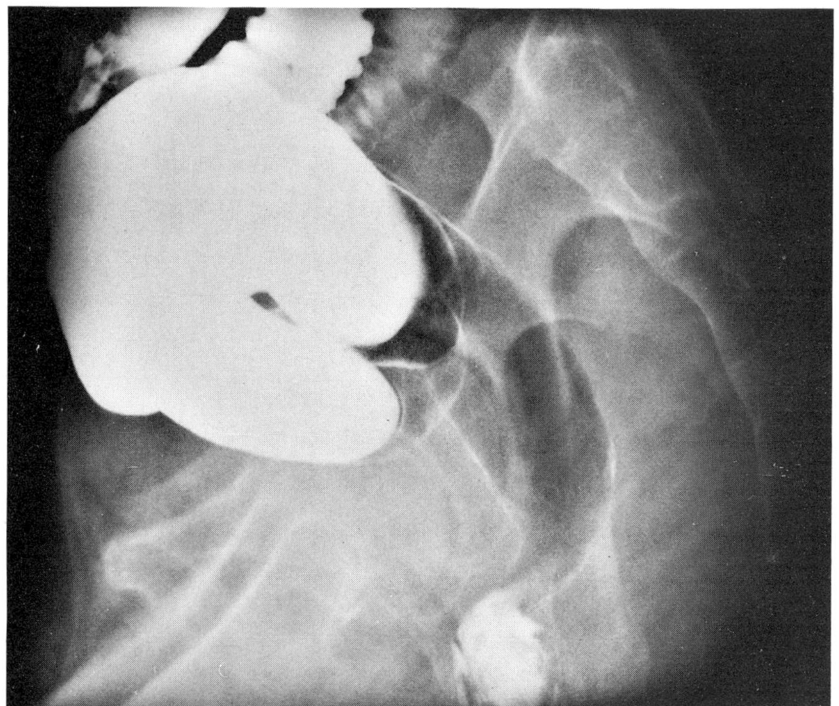

a

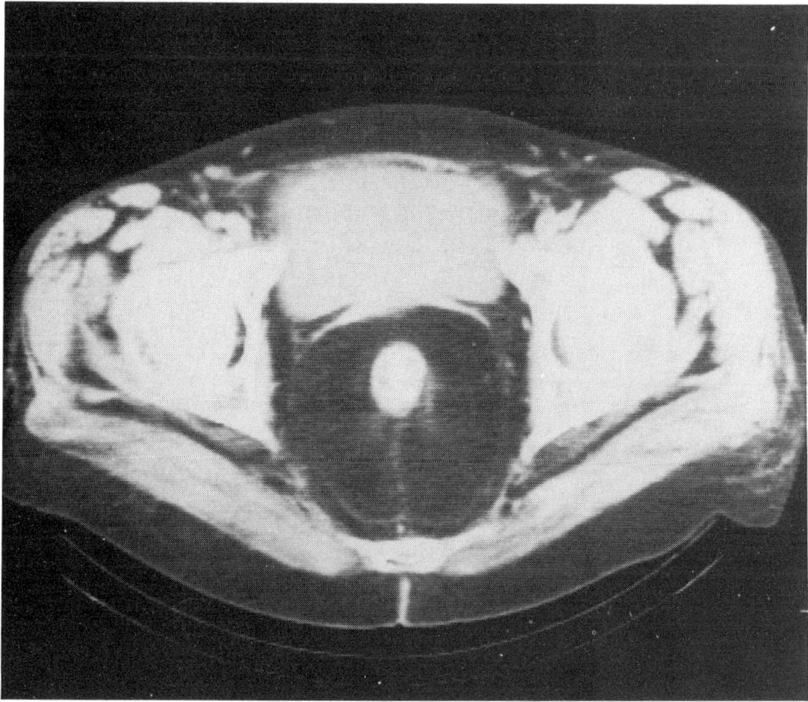

b

Fig. C.15. (a) Widened presacral space and narrowed tubelike rectum in a 31-year-old patient with long-standing regional enteritis. (b) A CT scan shows the extensive pelvic lipomatosis.

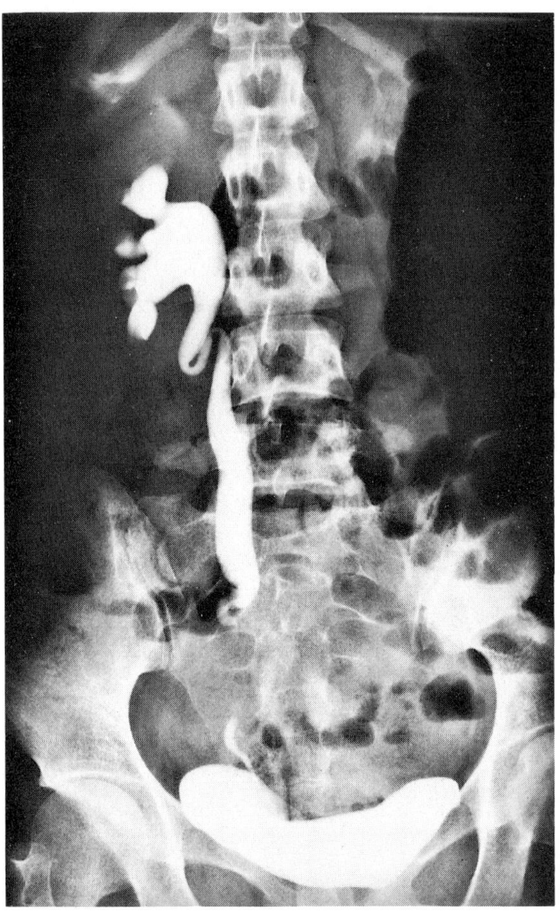

Fig. C.16. Right ureteric obstruction in a 25-year-old female. She has regional enteritis involving the terminal ileum. Although clinically her disease was under control, a phlegmon involving the terminal ileum has produced asymptomatic ureteric obstruction, a not unusual finding.

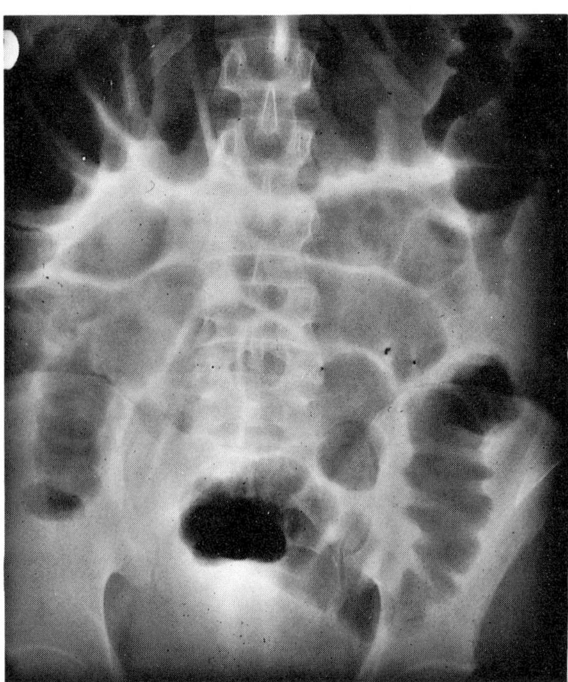

Fig. C.17. Toxic megacolon in a patient with regional enteritis. There is edema and considerable thickening of the bowel wall.

Table C.1. Differences between regional enteritis and ulcerative colitis.

	Regional enteritis	Ulcerative colitis
Significant small bowel involvement	Common	None (except for backwash ileitis)
Skip areas	May occur	None seen
Normal rectum	May occur	Rare, if ever
Size of ulcers	May be large	May appear flask-shaped
Fistulae	May occur (often perineal)	Unusual (occasionally to vagina)
Aphthous ulcers	Common early	Rare, if ever
Rectal bleeding	May occur	Almost always
Toxic megacolon	May occur	May occur
Reversion to normal radiographic appearance	Rare, if ever	May occur
End state 'burned out' colitis	May occur	May occur
Diverticulosis	May occur	Rare
Symmetrical involvement	May occur	Almost always
Separation of bowel loops	Common	Rare, if ever

differentiate between regional enteritis and the other colitides (107) (Fig. C.18). The term 'colitis indeterminate' (108) or inflammatory bowel disease (IBD) has been used by some investigators. Adequate tissue biopsy of multiple areas of the colon, obtained over a prolonged period of time, should generally point to a specific disease entity (109). Sometimes when the radiographic signs are nonspecific, the pathological findings will point towards one disease entity or the other. At other times, in the presence of nonspecific pathological findings, radiology will be diagnostic.

Amebiasis presenting with discrete ulcers can mimic regional enteritis (72). When amebiasis is limited to the cecum, differentiation between the two diseases may not be possible. Actually any chronic inflammation of the cecum can result in a narrowed small cecum and these changes are nonspecific.

Tuberculosis can mimic regional enteritis. Fortunately, tuberculosis involving only the colon is relatively rare in the United States although in some areas bowel tuberculosis is prevalent. Strictures may be present in both diseases.

Although the superficial radiographic appearance of ischemic colitis can mimic regional enteritis, the clinical and pathological picture usually allows one to differentiate these diseases in most patients. Differentiation may be impossible in an elderly patient with arteriosclerotic cardiovascular disease who develops diarrhea due to ischemic colitis, although acute ischemia generally results in a rapid change of the radiographic findings during serial examinations

Carcinoma can mimic regional enteritis. However, with cancer there usually is considerably more bowel destruction and the diseased segment is limited to one portion of the colon.

Confusion with diverticulitis can exist because similar long extraluminal sinus tracts can be seen in both diseases (110). Transmural inflammation may be present with both diseases. Diverticulitis and regional enteritis may likewise coexist (110, 111). Extensive internal fistulae, ileal disease, or the presence of aphthous ulcers should raise the suspicion of regional enteritis even if there is radiographic evidence of diverticulitis. The extent of diverticulosis seen radiographically may regress with a flare-up of regional enteritis, and vice versa (112).

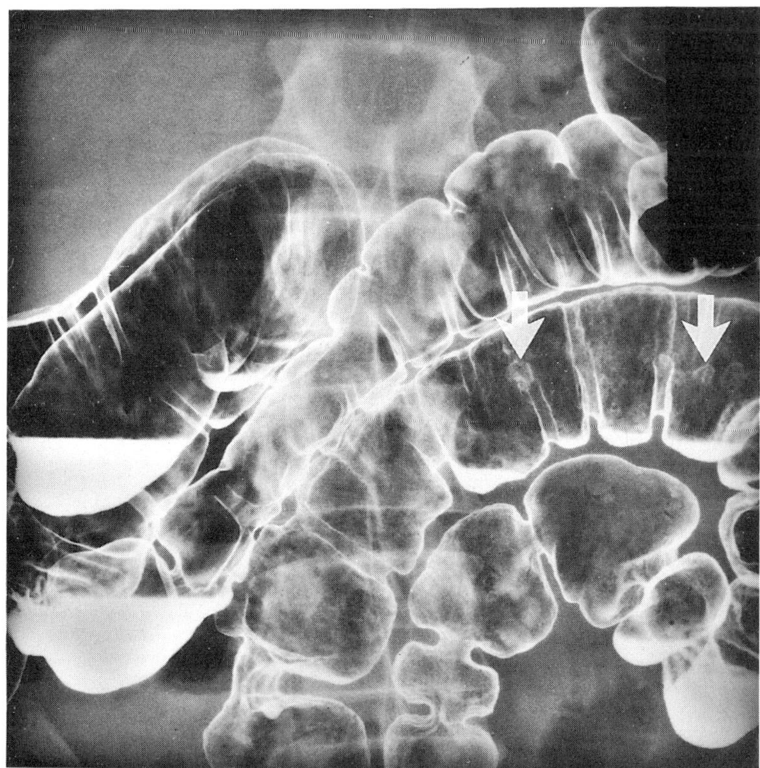

Fig. C.18. There are numerous polyps in the sigmoid colon (arrows). The transverse colon, located just superior to the sigmoid, appears normal. One biopsy revealed severe lymphoplasmacytic colitis with submucosal involvement most consistent with regional enteritis. A biopsy one week later showed changes consistent with ulcerative colitis. The patient was subsequently lost to follow-up.

References

1. Crohn BB, Ginzburg L, Oppenheimer GD: Regional ileitis. A pathologic and clinical entity. JAMA 99:1323–1329, 1932.
2. Lockhart-Mummery HE, Morson BC: Crohn's disease (regional enteritis) of the large intestine and its distinction from ulcerative colitis. Gut 1:87–105, 1960.
3. Morson BC, Lockhart-Mummery HE: Crohn's disease of the colon. Gastroenterologia 92:168–173, 1959.
4. Schachter H, Kirsner JB: Definitions of inflammatory bowel disease of unknown etiology. Gastroenterology 68:591–600, 1975.
5. Crohn BB, Janowitz HD: Reflections on regional enteritis twenty years later. JAMA 156:1221–1225, 1954.
6. Bockus HL: Gastroenterology, Vol II, p. 230. WB Saunders, Philadelphia, 1964.
7. Acheson ED: The distribution of ulcerative colitis and regional enteritis in United States veterans with particular reference to the Jewish religion. Gut 1:291–293, 1960.
8. Van Patter WN, Bargen JA, Dockerty MB, Feldman WH, Mayo CW, Waugh JM: Regional enteritis. Gastroenterology 26:347–450, 1954.
9. Marks JA, Fink SA: Regional enteritis in the Negro. Rev Gastroenterol 16:623–628, 1949.
10. Franken EA Jr, Smith JA, Fitzgerald JR: Regional enteritis in children: clinical and roentgen features. Crit Rev Diagn Imag 10:163–185, 1977.
11. Steigmann F, Shapiro S: Familial regional enteritis. Gastroenterology 40:215–218, 1961.
12. Sherlock P, Bell BM, Steinberg H, Almy TP: Familial occurrence of regional enteritis. Gastroenterology 42:770, 1962.
13. Hammer B, Ashurst P, Naish J: Disease associated with ulcerative colitis and Crohn's disease. Gut 9:17–21, 1968.
14. Hislop IG, Kerr Grant A: Genetic tendency in Crohn's disease. Gut 10:994–995, 1969.
15. Behçet H: Über rezidivierende aphthöse, durch ein Virus verursachte Geschwüre am Mund, am Auge und an den Genitalien. Dermatol Wochenschr 105:1152–1157, 1937.
16. O'Connell DJ, Courtney JV, Riddell RH: Colitis of Behçet's syndrome — radiologic and pathologic features. Gastrointest Radiol 5:173–179, 1980.
17. Goldstein SJ, Mackenzie Crooks DJ: Colitis in Behçet's syndrome. Radiology 128:321–323, 1978.
18. Stanley RJ, Tedesco FJ, Melson GL, Geisse G, Herold SL: The colitis of Behçet's disease: a clinical–radiographic correlation. Radiology 114:603–604, 1975.
19. Smith GE, Kime LR, Pitcher JL: The colitis of Behçet's disease: a separate entity. Am J Dig Dis 18:987–1000, 1973.
20. Baba S, Maruta M, Ando K, Teramoto T, Endo I: Intestinal Behçet's disease: report of five cases. Dis Colon Rectum 19:428–440, 1976.
21. Mir-Madjlessi SH, Farmer RG: Behçet's syndrome, Crohn's disease and toxic megacolon. Cleve Clin Q 39:49–55, 1972.
22. Kasahara Y, Tanaka S, Nishino M, Umemura H, Shiraha S, Kuyama T: Intestinal involvement in Behçet's disease: review of 136 surgical cases in the Japanese literature. Dis Colon Rectum 24:103–106, 1981.
23. Podolny GA: Crohn's disease presenting with massive lower gastrointestinal hemorrhage. AJR 130:368–370, 1978.
24. Rubin M, Herrington L, Schneider R: Regional enteritis with major gastrointestinal hemorrhage as the initial manifestation. Arch Intern Med 140:217–219, 1980.
25. Greenstein AJ, Janowitz HD, Sacher DB: The extra-intestinal complications of Crohn's disease and ulcerative colitis: a study of 700 patients. Medicine 55:401–412, 1976.
26. Gilliam JH III, Challa VR, Agudelo CA, Albertson DA, Huntley CC: Vasculitis involving muscle associated with Crohn's colitis. Gastroenterology 81:787–790, 1981.
27. Prior P, Gyde S, Cooke WT, Waterhouse JAH, Allan RN: Mortality in Crohn's disease. Gastroenterology 80:307–312, 1981.
28. Moss AA, Carbone JV, Kressel HY: Radiologic and clinical assessment of broad-spectrum antibiotic therapy in Crohn's disease. AJR 131:787–790, 1978.
29. Trnka Y, LaMont JT: Association of *Clostridium difficile* toxin with symptomatic relapse of chronic inflammatory bowel disease. Gastroenterology 80:693–696, 1981.
30. Meyers S, Mayer L, Bottone E, Desmond E, Janowitz HD: Occurrence of *Clostridium difficile* toxin during the course of inflammatory bowel disease. Gastroenterology 80:697–700, 1981.
31. Bargen JA: Nonsurgical management of regional enteritis. JAMA 165:2045–2047, 1957.
32. Hughes ESR, McDermott FT, Masterton JP: Intestinal obstruction following operation for inflammatory disease of the bowel. Dis Colon Rectum 22:469–471, 1979.
33. Greenstein AJ, Meyers S, Sher L, Heimann T, Aufses AH: Surgery and its sequelae in Crohn's colitis and ileocolitis. Arch Surg 116:285–288, 1981.
34. Greenstein AJ, Sachar DB, Pasternack BS, Janowitz HD: Reoperation and recurrence in Crohn's colitis and ileocolitis. N Engl J Med 293:685–690, 1975.
35. Pennington L, Hamilton SR, Bayless TM, Camerson JL: Surgical management of Crohn's disease. Influence of disease at margin of resection. Am Surg 192:311–317, 1980.
36. Hildell J, Lindström C, Wenckert A: Radiographic appearances in Crohn's disease. III. Colonic lesions following surgery. Acta Radiol (Diagn) 21:71–78, 1980.
37. Goligher JC: The outcome of excisional operations for primary and recurrent Crohn's disease of the large intestine. Surg Gynecol Obstet 148:1–8, 1979.
38. Block GE: Surgical management of Crohn's colitis. N Engl J Med 302:1068–1070, 1980.
39. Mühe E, Gall FP, Hager T, Angermann B, Söhnlein B, Schier F, Hermanek P: Die Chirurgie des Morbus Crohn. Dtsch Med Wochenschr 106:165–170, 1981.
40. Bergman L, Krause U: Crohn's disease: a long-term study of the clinical course in 186 patients. Scand J Gastroenterol 12:937–944, 1977.
41. Karesen R, Serch-Hanssen A, Thoresen BO, Hertzberg J: Crohn's disease: long-term results of surgical treatment. Scand J Gastroenterol 16:57–64, 1981.
42. Marshak RH: Granulomatous disease of the intestinal tract (Crohn's disease). Radiology 114:3–22, 1975.
43. Hildell J, Lindström C, Wenckert A: Radiographic appearances in Crohn's disease. II. The course as reflected at repeat radiography. Acta Radiol (Diagn) 20:933–944, 1979.
44. Brahme F, Fork FT: Dynamic aspects of Crohn's disease. Radiologe 15:463–468, 1975.
45. Goldberg HI, Caruthers SB Jr, Nelson JA, Singleton JW: Radiographic findings of the National Cooperative Crohn's Disease Study. Gastroenterology 77:925–937, 1979.
46. Truelove SC, Pena AS: Course and prognosis of Crohn's disease. Gut 17:192–201, 1976.

47. Julien M, Vignal J: La maladie de Crohn recto-colique. J Chir (Paris) 112:51–68, 1976.
48. Watier A, Devroede G, Perey B, Haddad H, Madarnas P, Grand-Maison P: Small erythematous mucosal plaques: an endoscopic sign of Crohn's disease. Gut 21:835–839, 1980.
49. Rickert RR, Carter HW: The gross, light mcroscopic and scanning electron microscopic appearance of the early lesions of Crohn's disease. Scanning Electron Microscopy 2:179–186, 1977.
50. Heatley RV, Bolton PM, Hughes LE, Owen EW: Mesenteric lymphatic obstruction in Crohn's disease. Digestion 20:307–313, 1980.
51. Lee RG, Epstein O, Jaurequi H, Sherlock S, Scheuer PJ: Granulomas in primary biliary cirrhosis: a prognostic feature. Gastroenterology 81:983–986, 1981.
52. Iliffe GD, Owen DA: Rectal biopsy in Crohn's disease. Dig Dis Sci 26:321–324, 1981.
53. Klein GL, Ament ME, Sparkes RS: Monozygotic twins with Crohn's disease: a case report. Gastroenterology 79:931–933, 1980.
54. Cave DR, Mitchell DN, Brooke BN: Experimental animal studies of the etiology and pathogenesis of Crohn's disease. Gastroenterology 69:618–624, 1975.
55. Cave DR, Mitchell DN, Brooke BN: Induction of granulomas in mice by Crohn's disease tissues. Gastroenterology 75:632–637, 1978.
56. Shafii A, Sopher S, Lev M, Das KM: An antibody against revertent forms of cell-wall-deficient bacterial variants in sera from patients with Crohn's disease. Lancet 8242:332–334, 1981.
57. Heatley RV, Bolton PM, Owen E, Jones-Williams W, Hughes LE: A search for a transmissible agent in Crohn's disease. Gut 16:528–532, 1975.
58. Phillpotts RJ, Hermon-Taylor J, Teich NM, Brooke BN: A search for persistent virus infection in Crohn's disease. Gut 21:202 207, 1980.
59. Antonius JI, Gump FE, Lattes R, Lepore M: A study of certain microscopic features in regional enteritis, and their possible prognostic significance. Gastroenterology 38:889–905, 1960.
60. Hayasaka H, Ishikura H, Takayama T: Acute regional ileitis due to *Anisakis* larvae. Int Surg 55:8–14, 1971.
61. Richman RH, Lewicki AM: Right ileocolitis secondary to anisakiasis. AJR 119:329–331, 1973.
62. Hildell J, Lindström C, Wenckert A: Radiographic appearances in Crohn's disease. I. Accuracy of radiographic methods. Acta Radiol (Diagn) 20:609–625, 1979.
63. Matsuura K, Nakata H, Takeda N, Nakata N, Shimoda Y: Innominate lines of the colon. Radiology 123:581–584, 1977.
64. Schmutz G, Kempf F: Frühveränderungen bei Crohnscher Kolitis im Doppelkontrast. RÖFO 132:237–242, 1980.
65. Laufer I: Air contrast studies of the colon in inflammatory bowel disease. CRC Crit Rev Diag Imag 9:421–447, 1977.
66. Persigehl M, Spieth W, Klose KC, Cen M: Feinreliefveränderungen des Kolons im Frühstadium der Colitis ulcerosa und Colitis granulomatosa. ROEFO 129:177–180, 1978.
67. Laufer I, Costopoulos L: Early lesions of Crohn's disease. AJR 130:307–311, 1978.
68. Simpkins KC: Aphthoid ulcers in Crohn's colitis. Clin Radiol 28:601–608, 1977.
69. Pringot J, Goncette L, Van Heuverzwyn R, Bodart P: The features of granulomatous colitis in double contrast radiography. J Belge Radiol 60:25–35, 1977.
70. Ghahremani GG, Port RB, Beachley MC: Pneumatosis coli in Crohn's disease. Am J Dig Dis 19:315–323, 1974.
71. Lingg G, Nebel G, Dihlmann W: Aphthoide Ulzerarönt-genologische Frühzeichen des morbus Crohn? ROEFO 133:138–141, 1980.
72. Max RJ, Kelvin FM: Nonspecificity of discrete colonic ulceration on double-contrast barium enema study. AJR 135:1265–1267, 1980.
73. Schmutz G, Zeller C, Baumann R, Schutz JF, Kempf F, Weil JP: Exploration radiologique en double contraste de la colite granulomateuse de Crohn. J Radiol 62:377–384, 1981.
74. Brunton FJ, Guyer PB: Diverticulum formation in Crohn's disease of the colon. Clin Radiol 30:39–44, 1979.
75. Hammerman AM Shatz BA, Sussman N: Radiographic characteristics of colonic 'mucosal bridges': sequelae of inflammatory bowel disease. Radiology 127:611–614, 1978.
76. Zegel HG, Laufer I: Filiform polyposis. Radiology 127:615–619, 1978.
77. Freeman AH, Berridge FR, Dick AP, Gleeson JA, Zeegen R: Pseudopolyposis in Crohn's disease. Br J Radiol 51:782–787, 1978.
78. Jones B, Abbruzzese AA: Obstructing giant pseudopolyps in granulomatous colitis. Gastrointest Radiol 3:437–438, 1978.
79. Joffe N: Localised giant pseudopolyposis secondary to ulcerative or granulomatous colitis. Clin Radiol 28:609–616, 1977.
80. Wills JS, Han SS: Localized giant pseudopolyposis complicating granulomatous ileocolitis. Radiology 122:320, 1977.
81. Ayre-Smith G: Localized giant pseudopolyposis of the colon in granulomatous colitis: a case report and review of the literature. Br J Radiol 50:916–917, 1977.
82. Goldberger LE, Neely HR, Stammer JL: Large mucosal bridges. An unusual roetgenographic manifestation of ulcerative colitis. Gastrointest Radiol 3:81–83, 1978.
83. Bartram CI, Herlinger H: Bowel wall thickness as a differentiating feature between ulcerative colitis and Crohn's disease of the colon. Clin Radiol 30:15–19, 1979.
84. Herlinger H: Angiography in Crohn's disease. The zoning sign revisited. Gastrointest Radiol 2:397–400, 1978.
85. Brahme F, Hildell J: Angiography in Crohn's disease revisited. AJR 126:941–951, 1976.
86. Nasr K, Morowitz DA, Anderson JGD, Kirsner JB: Free perforation in regional enteritis. Gut 10:206–208, 1969.
87. Janevicius RV, Bartolome JS, Schmitz RL: Acute free perforation as a presenting sign of regional enteritis. Case report and collective review of the literature. Am J Gastroenterol 74:143–149, 1980.
88. Genant HK, Mall JC, Wagonfeld JB, Vander Horst J, Lanzl LH: Skeletal demineralization and growth retardation in inflammatory bowel disease. Invest Radiol 11:541–549, 1976.
89. Enker WE, Block GE: Occult obstructive uropathy complicating Crohn's disease. Arch Surg 101:319–326, 1970.
90. Laufer I, Joffe N, Stolberg H: Unusual causes of gastrocolic fistula. Gastrointest Radiol 2:21–25, 1977.
91. Grieco MB, Bordan DL, Geiss AC, Beil AR Jr: Toxic megacolon complicating Crohn's colitis. Ann Surg 191:75–80, 1980.
92. Greene L, Kresch L, Held B: Acute toxic dilatation limited

to the ileum in Crohn's disease. Am J Dig Dis 17:439–446, 1972.
93. Koep L, Zuidema GD: The clinical significance of retroperitoneal fibrosis. Surgery 81:250–257, 1977.
94. Lightdale CJ, Sternberg SS, Posner G, Sherlock P: Carcinoma complicating Crohn's disease: report of seven cases and review of the literature. Am J Med 59:262–268, 1975.
95. Weedon DD, Shorter RG, Ilstrup DM, Huizenga KA, Taylor WF: Crohn's disease and cancer. N Engl J Med 289:1099–1103, 1973.
96. Zinkin LD, Brandwein C: Adenocarcinoma in Crohn's colitis. Dis Colon Rectum 23:115–117, 1980.
97. Gyde SN, Prior P, Macartney JC, Thompson H, Waterhouse JAH: Malignancy in Crohn's disease. Gut 21:1024–1029, 1980.
98. Greenstein AJ, Sachar D, Pucillo A, Kreel I, Geller S, Janowitz HD, Aufses A Jr: Cancer in Crohn's disease after diversionary surgery. A report of seven carcinomas occurring in excluded bowel. Am J Surg 135:86–90, 1978.
99. Traube J, Simpson S, Riddell RH, Levin B, Kirsner JB: Crohn's disease and adenocarcinoma of the bowel. Dig Dis Sci 25:939–944, 1980.
100. Craft CF, Mendelsohn G, Cooper HS, Yardley JH: Colonic 'precancer' in Crohn's disease. Gastroenterology 80:578–584, 1981.
101. Simpson S, Traube J, Riddell RH: The histologic appearance of dysplasia (precarcinomatous change) in Crohn's disease of the small and large intestine. Gastroenterology 81:492–501, 1981.
102. Valdes-Dapena A, Rudolph I, Hidayat A, Roth JLA, Laucks RB: Adenocarcinoma of the small bowel in association with regional enteritis — four new cases. Cancer 37:2938–2947, 1976.
103. Nesbit RR, Elbadawi NA, Morton JM, Cooper RA Jr: Carcinoma of the small bowel — a complication of regional enteritis. Cancer 37:2948–2959, 1976.
104. Floch HF, Slattery LR, Hazzi CG: Carcinoma of the small intestine in regional enteritis. Am J Gastroenterol 70:520–527, 1978.
105. Chang SF, Burrell MI, Belleza NA, Spiro HM: Borderlands in the diagnosis of regional enteritis. Trends in overdiagnosis and value of therapeutic trial. Gastrointest Radiol 3:67–72, 1978.
106. Kelvin FM, Oddson TA, Rice RP, Garbutt JT, Bradenham BP: Double contrast barium enema in Crohn's disease and ulcerative colitis. AJR 131:207–213, 1978.
107. Kirsner JB: Problems in the differentiation of ulcerative colitis and Crohn's disease of the colon: the need for repeated diagnostic evaluation. Gastroenterology 68:187–191, 1975.
108. Price AB: Overlap in the spectrum of non-specific inflammatory bowel disease–colitis indeterminate. J Clin Pathol 31:567–577, 1978.
109. Morson BC, Dawson IMP: Gastrointestinal Pathology, p. 549. Blackwell Scientific, Oxford, 1979.
110. Ferrucci JT, Ragsdale BD, Barrett PJ, Vickery AL, Dreyfuss JR: Double tracking of the sigmoid colon. Radiology 120:307–312, 1976.
111. Meyers MA, Alonso DR, Morson BC, Bartram C: Pathogenesis of diverticulitis complicating granulomatous colitis. Gastroenterology 74:24–31, 1978.
112. Berridge FR, Dick AP: Effect of Crohn's disease on colonic diverticula. Br J Radiol 49:926–929, 1976.

III.1.D. Cathartic colitis

It has been known for some time that the chronic use of various laxatives can result in irreversible changes in the bowel (1). Superficially, the changes resemble those seen in longstanding or burned-out ulcerative colitis although generally these conditions can be differentiated.

Laxative abuse has been called a type of Munchausen syndrome, with the patient surreptitiously abusing laxatives (2). The clinical findings can be confusing; alternating diarrhea and constipation are not unusual. Some of these patients tend to be emotionally labile.

Prolonged use of some cathartics results in systemic hypokalemia, possible steatorrhea (3), and severe cachexia (4). The findings in the colon are due to neuromuscular damage; this damage can either be segmental or involve the entire colon. The primary site and extent of involvement depends upon the type of laxative abused; overuse of anthraquinone laxatives generally results in the major damage being present primarily on the right side of the colon. Other laxatives produce their damage primarily on the left side.

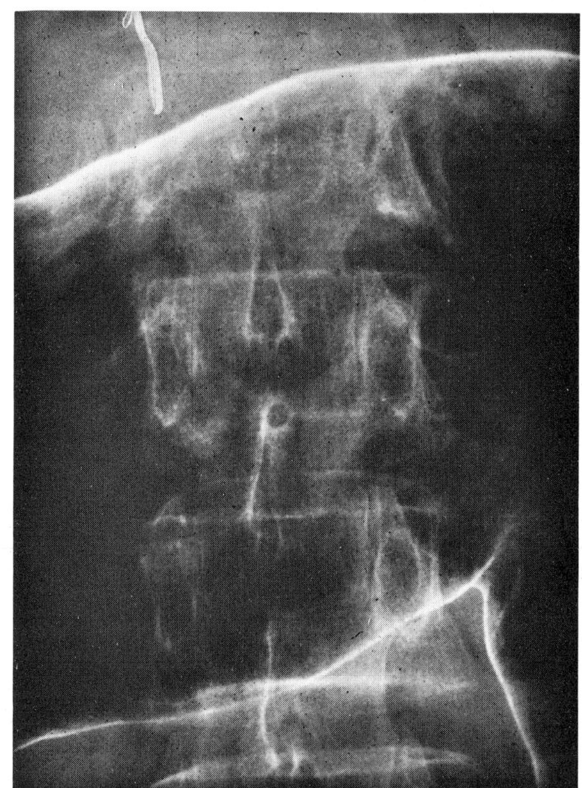

b

Pathological investigation of a cathartic colon reveals mucosal atrophy with thickening of the muscularis mucosa (5, 6). Melanin-like pigmentation is commonly seen. The submucosal nerve fibers can be severely damaged (7).

Radiographic examination reveals poor colon tonicity, a dilated colon, absent haustrations, and inconstant spasm (Fig. D.1). Prominent saccular outpouchings can be present (8). The ileocecal valve tends to be gaping with free ileal reflux. With chronic disease there is foreshortening of the colon. If the terminal ileum is involved it is similar to the backwash ileitis seen in ulcerative colitis. A coarse reticular pattern, similar to that seen with colon urticaria, is present in advanced disease (Fig. D.2) (9).

Distinguishing signs of this condition from ulcerative colitis are that the fine 'mucosal' pattern tends to be preserved, no ulcers are present, and the colon can be distended normally. The flexures are usually in their normal anatomic position unless with chronic disease the colon has become foreshortened. Most important, the rectum and sigmoid are either normal or only minimally involved, with

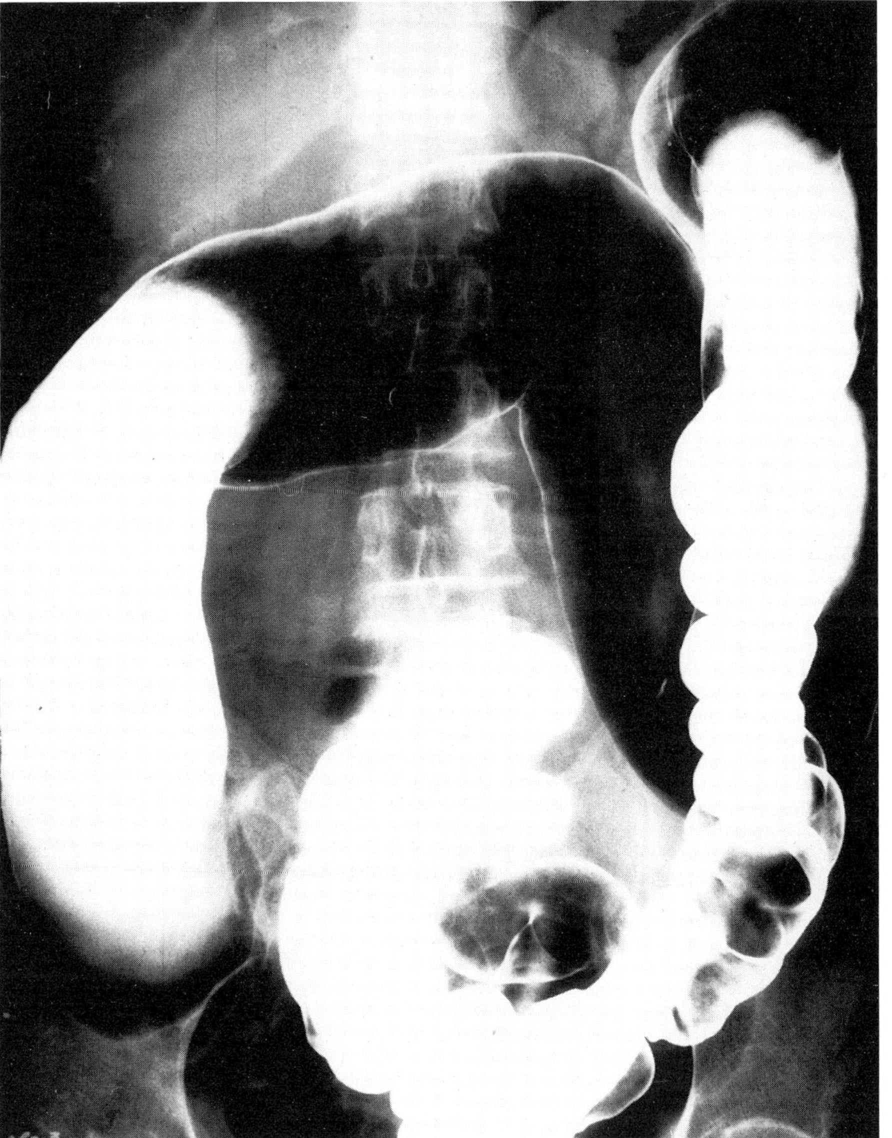

Fig. D.1. Cathartic colitis. (a) An ahaustral hypotonic colon is the end result in this patient with cathartic misuse. (b) The transverse colon reveals the marked atonicity present in this condition.

a

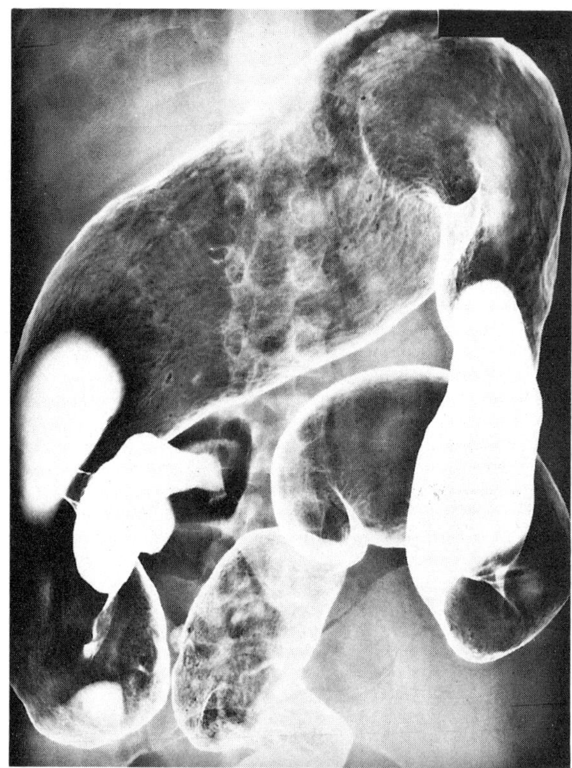

b

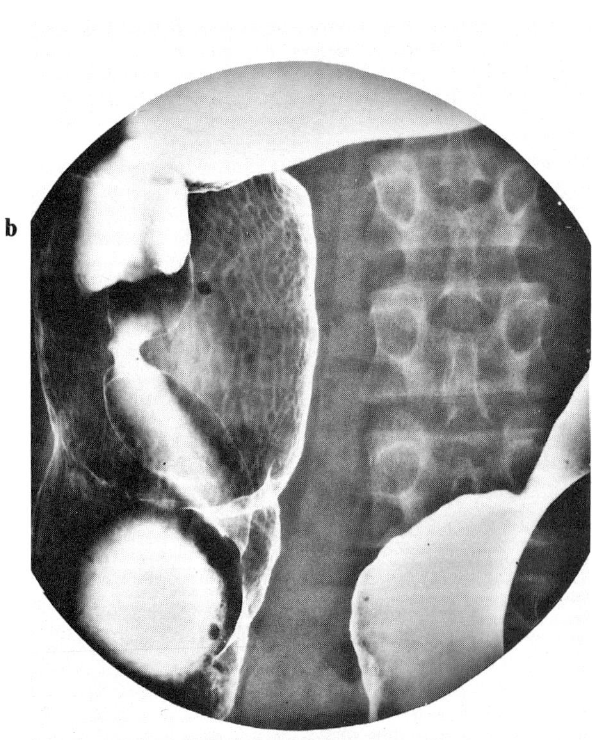

Fig. D.2. A coarse reticular pattern is present both in the (a) transverse colon and (b) right colon in this patient with chronic laxative abuse. (Courtesy of Drs. Delgoffe, Régent and Tréheux (9); copyright, Masson 1981.)

most of the abnormal changes being present proximally.

A post evacuation radiograph after a barium enema generally reveals considerable retained barium, reflecting the poor tonicity seen in this entity.

References

1. Heilbrun N, Bernstein C: Roentgen abnormalities of the large and small intestine associated with prolonged cathartic ingestion. Radiology 65:549–556, 1955.
2. Oster JR, Materson BJ, Rogers AI: Laxative abuse syndrome. Am J Gastroenterol 74:451–458, 1980.
3. Rawson MD: Cathartic colon. Lancet i:1121–1124, 1966.
4. Levine D, Goode AW, Wingate DL: Purgative abuse associated with reversible cachexia, hypogammaglobulinaemia, and finger clubbing. Lancet i:919–920, 1981.
5. Urso FP, Urso MJ, Lee CH: The cathartic colon: pathological findings and radiological/pathological correlation. Radiology 116:557–559, 1975.
6. Kim SK, Gerle RD, Rozanski R: Cathartic colitis. AJR 131:1079–1081, 1978.
7. Riemann JF, Schmidt H, Zimmermann W: The fine structure of colonic submucosal nerves in patients with chronic laxative abuse. Scand J Gastroenterol 15:761–768, 1980.
8. Marshak RH, Gerson A: Cathartic colon. Dig Dis Sci 5:724–727, 1960.
9. Delgoffe C, Régent D, Tréheux A: Images mucographiques de la colite aux laxatifs évoluée en technique double contraste. J Radiol 62:117–120, 1981.

III.1.E. Ulcerative colitis

a. Introduction

Although for some of the colitides a cause is known, the broad group of patients with nonspecific inflammation of the colon are still placed in the category of ulcerative colitis. What we now call ulcerative colitis probably was recognized by the ancient Greeks and Romans. The modern definition and associated name usually are accredited to Wilks and Moxon who first defined the disease in 1875 (1). A barium enema was used to study the abnormalities in 1912 (2).

Although there have been many theories about the cause of ulcerative colitis, the etiology is still not known. No pathogenic organisms have been established.

b. Clinical considerations

Ulcerative colitis is a disease primarily of young adults, although it may occasionally be seen in both extremes of age. There is no sex predilection.

Most patients present with abdominal pain, rectal bleeding and diarrhea. Considerable mucus can be present. The onset of the disease can be gradual or abrupt. The presenting symptom can simply be rectal bleeding, with diarrhea initially absent. At times, the patient has constipation during the early course of the disease but as the disease progresses, diarrhea appears. Similarly, with mild disease pain can be minimal or even absent, though as the disease progresses, pain does occur and tends to be crampy in nature. With extensive colon involvement the patient starts losing weight. In some patients the onset is sudden with high fever, pain, and a severe systemic toxic illness.

If one member of a family has ulcerative colitis, there is approximately a 17% chance of another member having the disease (3). Within any one family there may be some members with ulcerative colitis and others with regional enteritis. Many of these patients tend to be emotionally labile. The first attack may coincide with a period of stress.

These patients may be anemic from rectal bleeding. Although rare, there can be episodes of massive hemorrhage. Occasionally the first presentation of the disease is due to massive bleeding, with ulcerative colitis not being suspected initially in the differential diagnosis.

Clinically, the severity of an attack can be graded anywhere from mild to severe. The patient can have periods of active disease followed by remission, the disease can be chronic with periods of exacerbation, or there can be an acute fulminating course. The latter, while rare, is generally also the most severe form, with the most complications.

Patients with ulcerative colitis can have various systemic manifestations. It is speculative whether these manifestations are actually part of the basic disease or whether they simply represent complications induced by the colitis. A significant number of these patients have liver disease (4). The liver changes can range from fatty infiltration to pericholangitis, hepatomegaly, hepatitis, sclerosing cholangitis (5, 6), to carcinoma of the bile ducts (7, 8). In the general population bile duct carcinoma is seen in an older age group, while with ulcerative colitis bile duct carcinoma develops earlier. Usually, these patients have had ulcerative colitis for many years. Splenomegaly is not unusual. Although the data is incomplete, there may be some improvement in liver function after colectomy (4). Other conditions encountered with ulcerative colitis include sacroileitis, peripheral arthritis, and dermatitis (4, 9). Although the peripheral arthritis symptoms tend to parallel the course of ulcerative colitis, the sacroileitis tends not to be related to the severity of the ulcerative colitis. Other rarer conditions encountered are erythema nodosum, pyoderma gangrenosum, conjunctivitis, uveitis, venous thromboembolic disease, and amyloidosis leading to nephrotic syndrome (9). There also appears to be a higher incidence of renal calculi; in addition to unknown factors of the underlying disease, steroid therapy probably also contributes to calculi formation. An immunological condition may be responsible for some of the extracolonic manifestations. In some populations a high frequency of HLA antigens is associated with ulcerative colitis (10).

Many investigators believe that the only therapy for severe ulcerative colitis, or a cancer developing in a setting of ulcerative colitis, is total proctocolectomy. Colectomy with an ileorectal anastomosis results in residual disease in the rectum together with an associated risk of cancer (11), although this latter operation is preferred by some surgeons as a means, at least temporarily, to avoid an ileostomy, especially in a younger patient. Another incentive for temporarily retaining the rectum is that in males undergoing a total proctocolectomy there is a small but definite incidence of impotence.

Unlike patients with regional enteritis where an ileostomy may result in recurrent disease, patients with ulcerative colitis are cured after a colectomy. A continent ileostomy (Kock) is possible (12) with no danger of recurrent disease. Another procedure showing considerable promise is total colectomy with rectal mucosectomy and ileoanal anastomosis (13, 14).

c. *Pathology*

The sigmoidoscopic appearance in ulcerative colitis varies. Early in the disease the mucosa is friable and bleeds readily. Small, shallow ulcers gradually develop and with extension of disease the ulcers become confluent. The changes are usually most severe in the rectum. Skip areas are not seen. Swollen areas of mucosa produce an overall polypoid appearance.

Microscopic examination shows inflammation of varying severity. Inflammation at the mucosal crypt bases progresses to crypt abscesses. These abscesses can spread in the wall of the colon with sloughing of the overlying mucosa and resultant ulceration. Although crypt abscesses are characteristic of ulcerative colitis, they can also be seen in other entities, such as in regional enteritis and some of the infectious colitides.

The lymphatics are not as engorged as in regional enteritis and there are extensive capillaries in the reactive tissue. With chronic disease, there is muscularis mucosa hypertrophy. The appendix can be involved if there is disease in the cecum (15). Granulomas are not seen; if present, one should think of regional enteritis rather than ulcerative colitis. The bowel wall is generally not as thick as in regional enteritis (Fig. E.1).

With chronic disease there can be stenoses. During remission the ulcers may clear completely.

An irregular nodular pattern may represent dysplasia (16) or may simply reflect the underlying inflammation. Carcinoma appears to be closely related to adenomatous changes in the epithelium and to basal cell proliferation (17). It is doubtful that a macroscopic examination such as a barium enema will detect a sufficient number of these dysplastic changes to be clinically useful. There may be an increased risk of cancer in patients having such dysplasia-like lesions (18). The presence of these lesions is believed by some to be a possible indication for colectomy (18), although this field has not been adequately clarified. Dysplasia may be present at one time but may regress on a follow-up biopsy (19).

d. Radiology

It is believed that ulcerative colitis starts in the rectum and spreads proximally (Fig. E.2). Thus, to make a diagnosis of ulcerative colitis, the rectum should generally be involved, together with continuous disease in the adjacent colon. Unfortunately, a pancolitis will occasionally evolve into an abnormal appearing right colon with the rectosigmoid appearing normal (20). Similarly, use of steroid enemas may cause the rectum to appear normal (Figs. E.3 and 3.4). The overall length of involvement varies between rectal disease as one extreme and pancolitis as the other.

The extent of disease is difficult to gauge accurately. Colonoscopy has shown that radiology tends to underestimate the extent of the disease (21), while biopsies of 'normal' appearing mucosa through the colonoscope also show that visual colonoscopy underestimates the full length of involvement. Radiographically, if there is involvement from the hepatic flexure distally, then there probably is a pancolitis (22).

Although some authors have found the postevacuation film to be useful in ulcerative colitis, by the time the changes are visible on postevacuation films, the disease is no longer in its early stage. The difference between early ulcerative colitis and normal colon is too subtle to differentiate radiographically on either a single-contrast barium enema or on a postevacuation film and we do not advocate the routine use of postevacuation films for the early diagnosis of ulcerative colitis. The radiological changes of ulcerative colitis are best seen on a

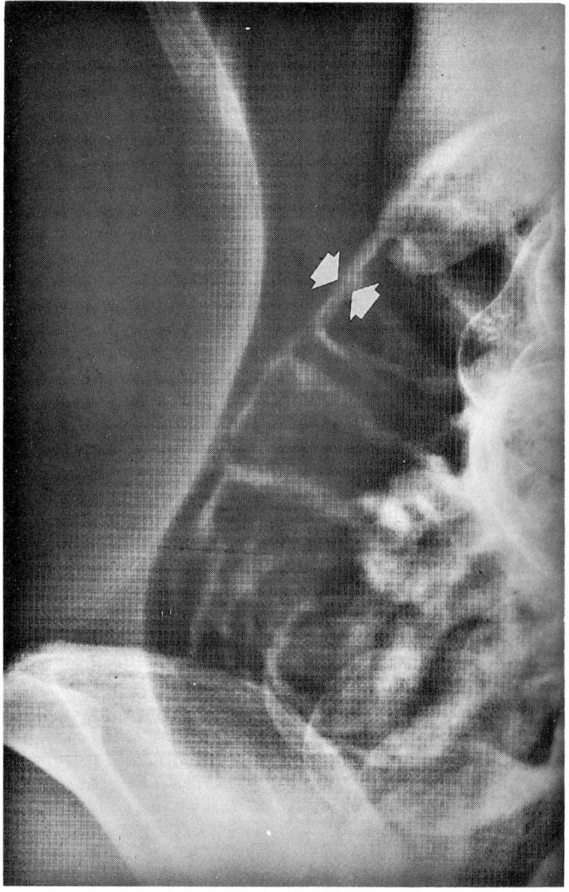

Fig. E.1. Pneumoperitoneum in a patient with ulcerative colitis. The wall of the ascending colon is outlined by gas in the lumen and in the peritoneal cavity (arrowheads); the wall thickness is normal.

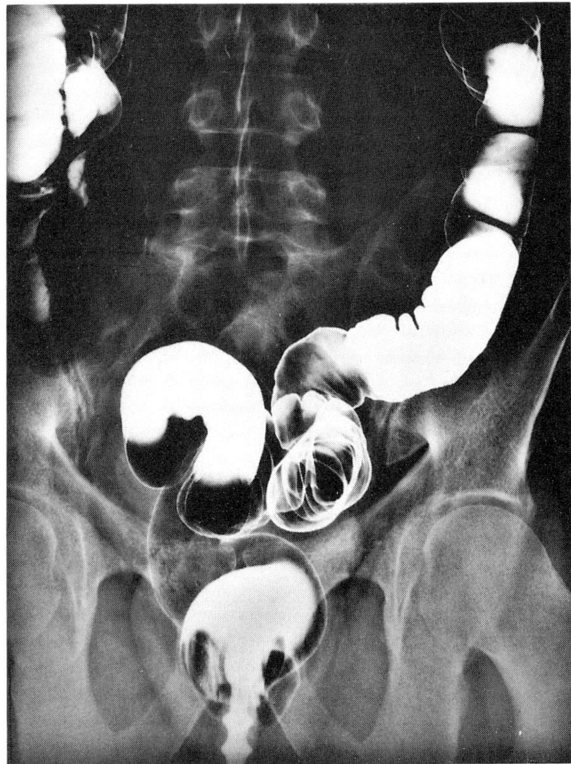

a

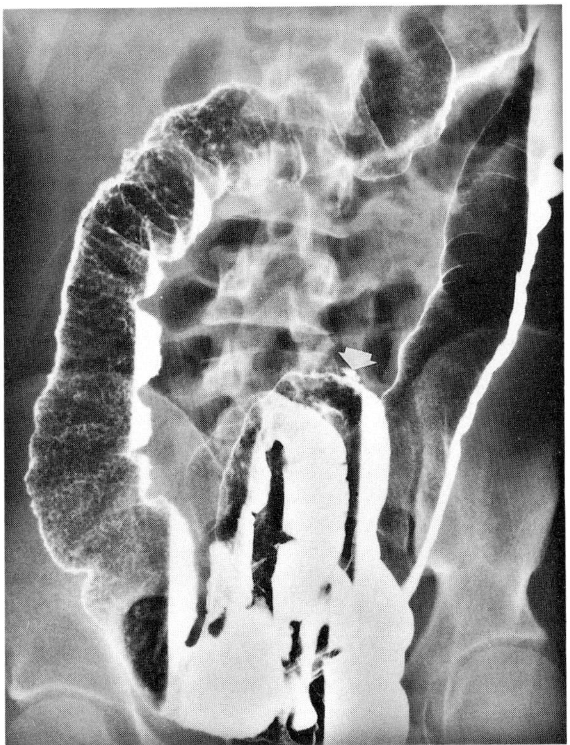

Fig. E.3. A pancolitis is present in this 19-year-old male. At this time the most severe ulcers were present in the right colon, with few ulcers apparent in the left colon. A linear ulcer is present in the sigmoid (arrowheads).

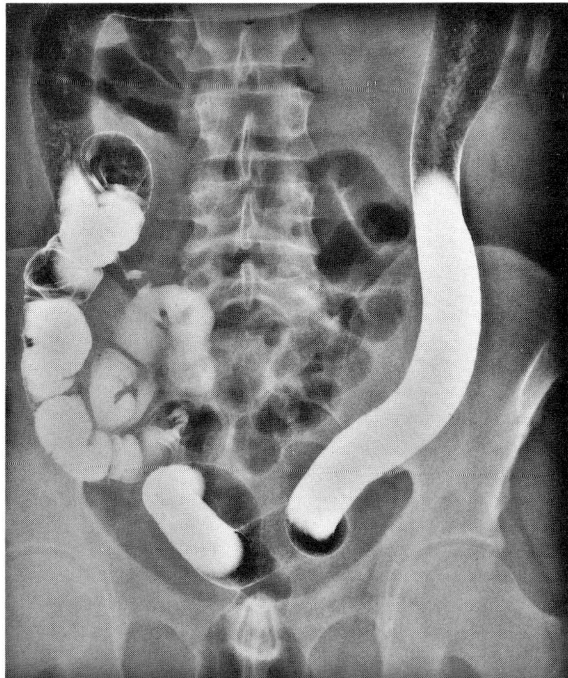

Fig. E.2. Development of ulcerative colitis. (a) The initial examination revealed barely perceptible ulcers limited to the rectum. (b) 16 months later a pancolitis is present. The colon is foreshortened, numerous shallow ulcers are scattered throughout, and the haustra are no longer present.

double-contrast barium enema with maximum distention of the colon (23–26).

The radiographic appearance in ulcerative colitis depends upon the phase of the disease. During the acute phase there may be marked colon spasm with accompanying difficulty in filling the entire colon. The use of a hypotonic agent, such as glucagon, usually results in sufficient colon relaxation to allow diagnosis (Fig. E.5).

In some patients with early disease diagnosed by rectal biopsy, a barium enema appears normal even in retrospect. The earliest radiographic change is a slight granular irregularity to the colon, a finding first described by Welin and Brahme (27). This 'grain of sand' appearance consists of fine punctate ulcers throughout the circumference of the colon (Figs. E.6 and E.7). When seen along the colon margin, these ulcers have a slightly serrated appearance. With more severe disease, there are deeper ulcers appearing as a coarser pattern (Fig. E.8). Intervening areas of mucosal regeneration

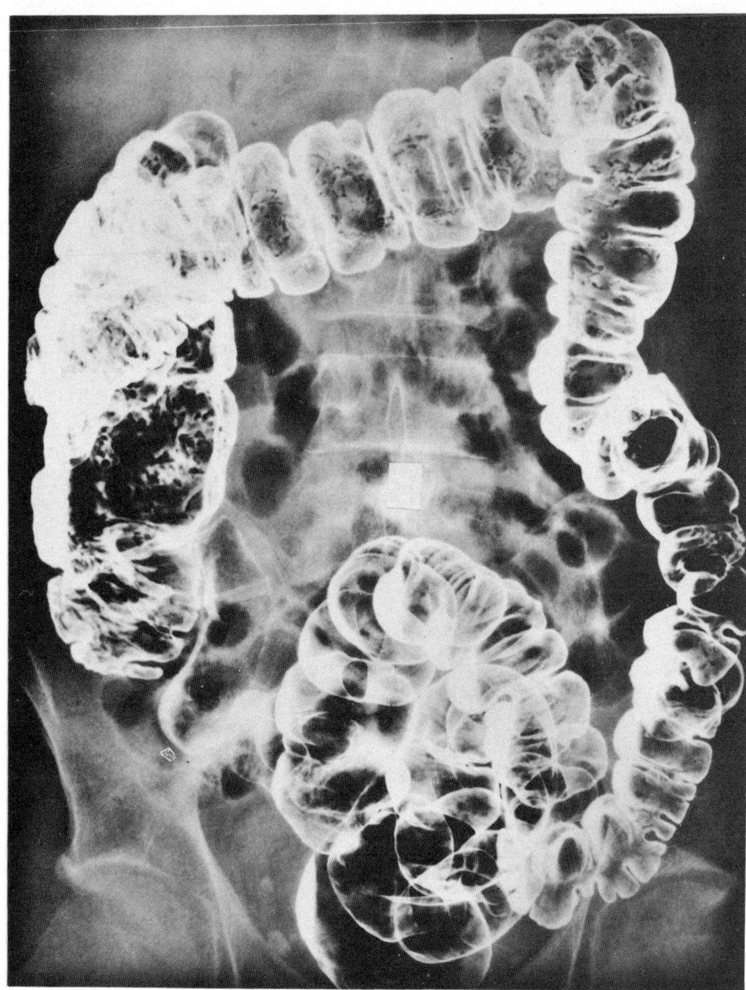

Fig. E.4. Both radiographically and sigmoidoscopically the rectum appeared normal in a patient with known ulcerative colitis. The only evidence of disease are numerous linear polyps scattered throughout the proximal portions of the colon.

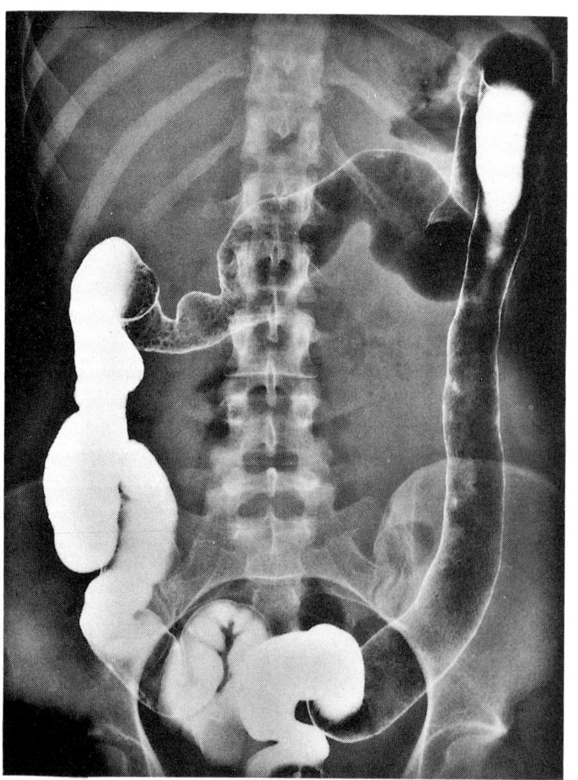

have a nodular pattern. With severe disease there are deep penetrating ulcers superimposed on an abnormal nodular pattern as a background. Isolated ulcers are not seen. The nodular and polypoid appearance throughout the involved portion of the colon is usually due to edematous residual mucosa and superimposed inflammation (Fig. E.9). These polyps may become quite large and mimic a neoplasm. Some authors use the term 'localized giant pseudopolyposis (28, 29) or 'filiform polyposis' (30) for these masses, which can be found both in ulcerative colitis and in regional enteritis. When prominent, these nodules can be seen on noncontrast radiographs of the abdomen as 'thumbprinting', an appearance similar to that seen in toxic megacolon (Fig. E.10). The nodules can present as discrete oval masses (Figs. E.11 and E.12) or they

Fig. E.5. 22-year-old music student with sudden onset of bloody diarrhea prior to her school examination. A pancolitis is present. The ascending and transverse portions of the colon are markedly spastic, the colon has an ahaustral appearance and there is considerable foreshortening.

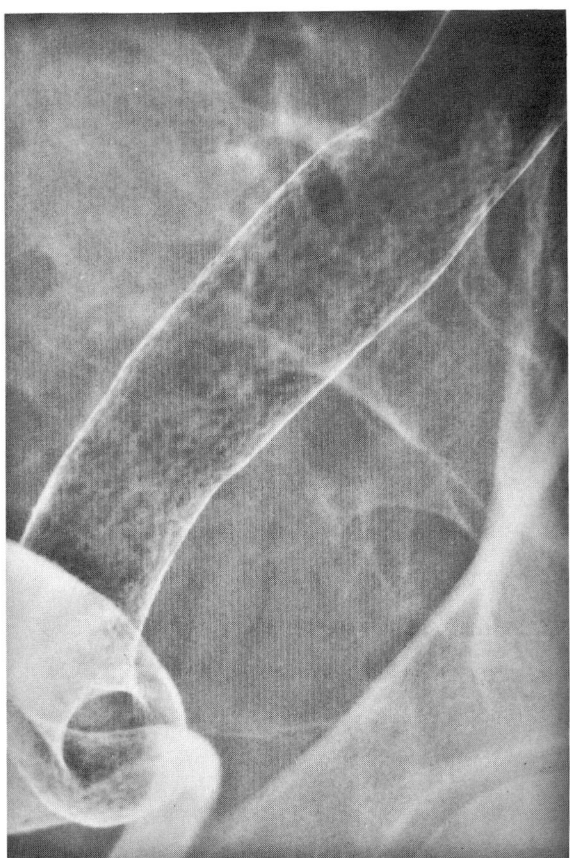

Fig. E.6. Ulcerative colitis. There is a fine 'grain of sand' appearance to the descending colon, representing many small ulcers scattered throughout.

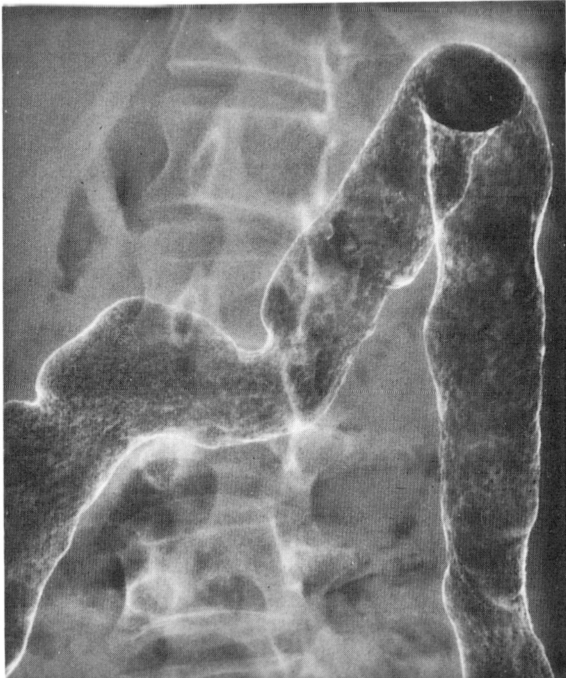

Fig. E.7. Ulcerative colitis. The ulcers are slightly deeper and more prominent than in the previous figure.

can appear as linear branching intraluminal masses (Figs. E.13 and E.14). When these polyps become undermined and are attached only at both ends, they have been called 'mucosal bridges' (31, 32). Whether a barium enema can be used to readily distinguish between mucosal bridges and filiform polyps remains to be seen.

With progression, deep ulcers develop throughout the involved segment. Some ulcers extend submucosally, parallel to the lumen and assume a flask-shaped 'collar-button' appearance. It is unusual, however, for these ulcers to extend through the serosa and result in fistulae. The submucosal extension is due to the relatively resistant muscular layers. By this time there is usually loss of haustration and obliteration of the valves of Houston (Fig. E.15). The loss of haustra may not be a permanent finding, because in the occasional patient with eventual remission the haustra may again reappear.

As the disease progresses there is further narrowing of the lumen and foreshortening of the colon, with either the sigmoid or the splenic flexture being considerably shorter than usual; the narrowed lumen may be due to either spasm or fibrosis (Fig. E.16). The result is a tubular and rigid appearance to the colon without the usual redundancies being present. Often noncontrast radiographs will show such a tubular colon outline (Fig. E.17). This appearance with chronic disease can be considered as the end stage and differentiation from other end stage colon inflammatory diseases can be difficult.

The entire bowel wall circumference is involved in a *symmetrical* fashion and the transition between normal and abnormal bowel is gradual. Regional enteritis presents with asymmetrical bowel involvement and the transition zone tends to be abrupt. Skip lesions do not occur with ulcerative colitis. With pancolitis the ileocecal valve is generally prominent and there is ready reflux into the terminal ileum through a patulous valve. The distal ileum can be hypotonic and the valvulae conniventes symmetrically effaced. Occasionally a polypoid appearance is seen in the terminal ileum (33). Currently, we are encountering such 'back-wash ileitis' less often. The changes in the ileum are invariably less pronounced than in the colon. Usually, only a short segment of the terminal ileum is involved.

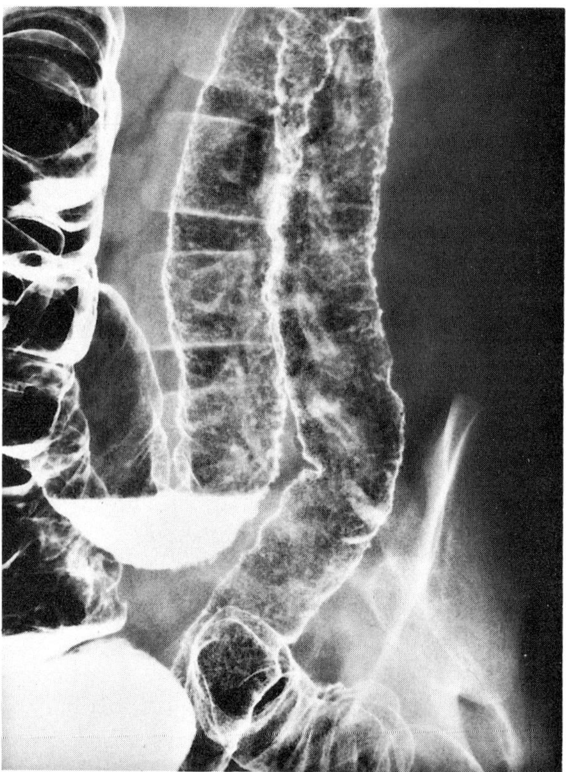

Fig. E.8. More advanced ulcerative colitis. Some of the ulcers are beginning to extend submucosally parallel to the lumen.

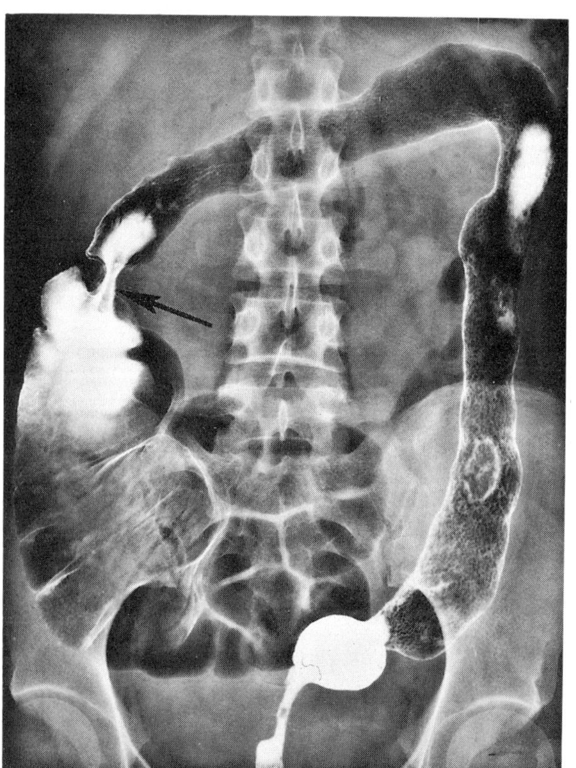

Most patients with severe disease have widening of the presacral space, best seen on the lateral rectal radiograph (Fig. E.18). The etiology of this widening is not known; in some patients it may be due to treatment with steroids, although some patients without any prior therapy but with active ulcerative colitis also have widening of the presacral space. It should be kept in mind that widening of the presacral space is not pathognomonic for ulcerative colitis but is also seen in many other diseases.

An occasional patient will undergo remission of the disease and the follow-up examination may appear completely normal radiographically. Such remissions are more common with initial disease

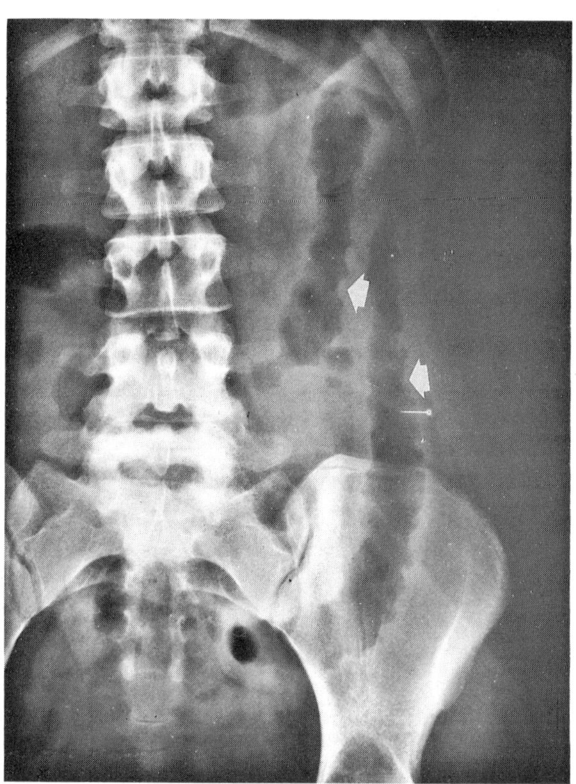

Fig. E.10. 22-year-old patient with severe ulcerative colitis. A radiograph of the abdomen shows 'thumbprinting' in the distal transverse and descending portions of the colon (arrowheads). The patient did not have toxic megacolon and the 'thumbprinting' was caused by inflammatory polyps.

Fig. E.9. 22-year-old female with 7 years of active ulcerative colitis. A stricture is present at the hepatic flexure (arrow). The rectosigmoid is markedly foreshortened and strictured. Nodules of varying size are scattered throughout the colon. No malignancy was found in the resected colon.

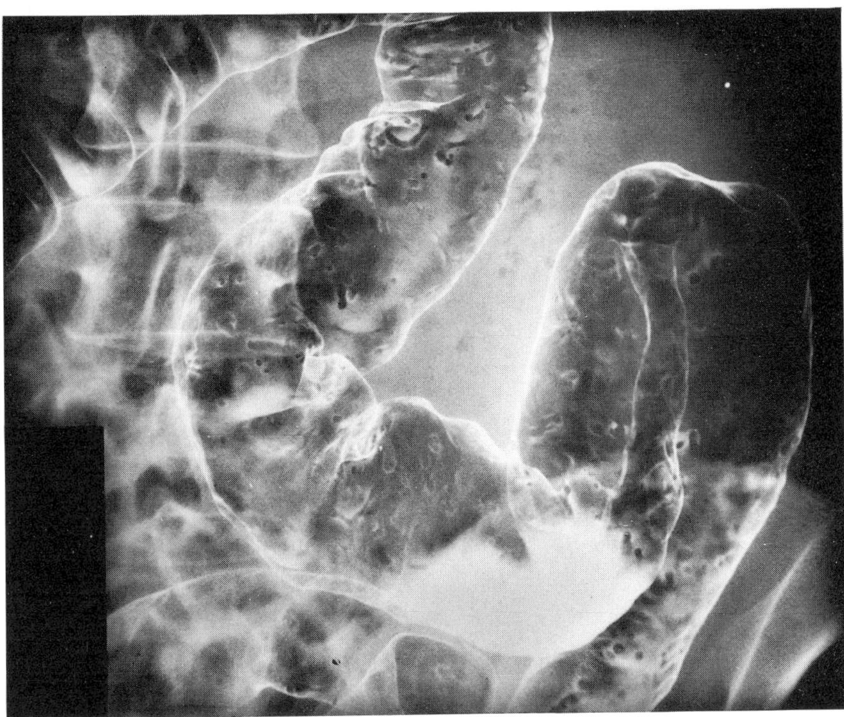

Fig. E.11. Well-defined discrete polyps are scattered throughout the colon in this patient with chronic ulcerative colitis. No ulcers are seen.

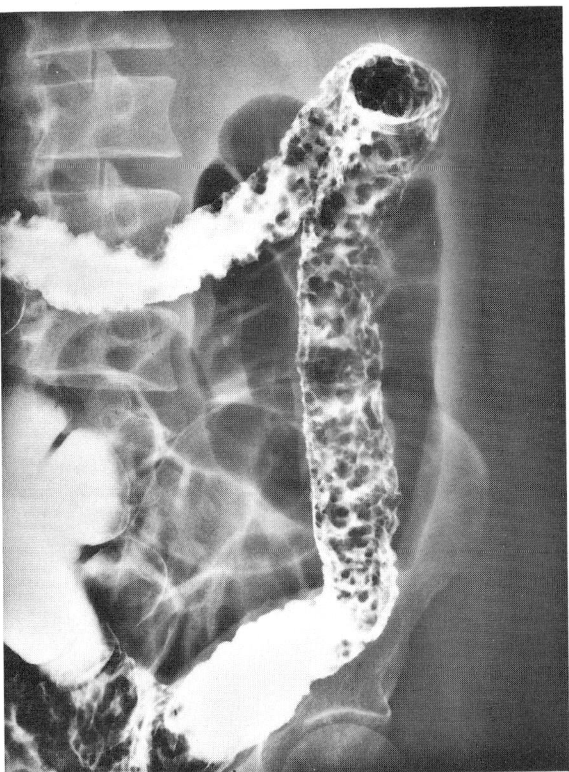

Fig. E.12. Severe polyposis in a patient with chronic ulcerative colitis. The polyps appear both linear and oval. The colon lumen is narrowed by these polyps.

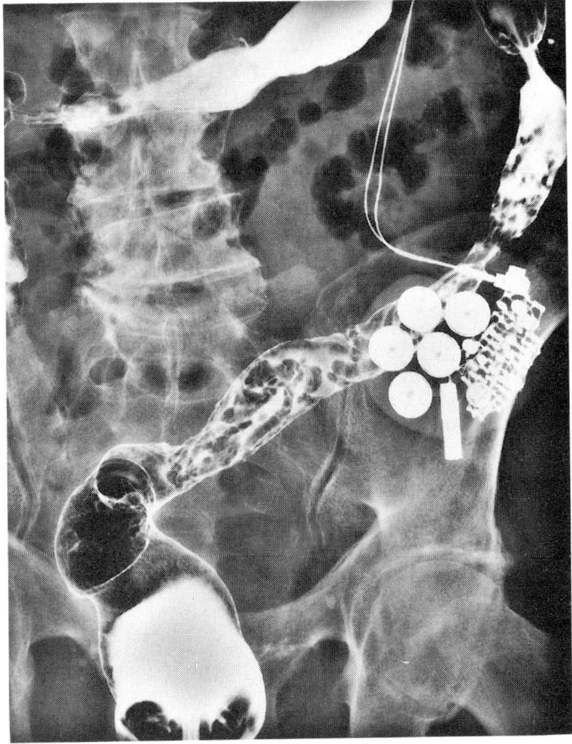

Fig. E.13. 71-year-old male with 50 years of active ulcerative colitis involving the distal half of the colon. Multiple linear branching intraluminal masses are present in the sigmoid colon. The subcutaneously implanted pacemaker is another sign of the patient's precarious health.

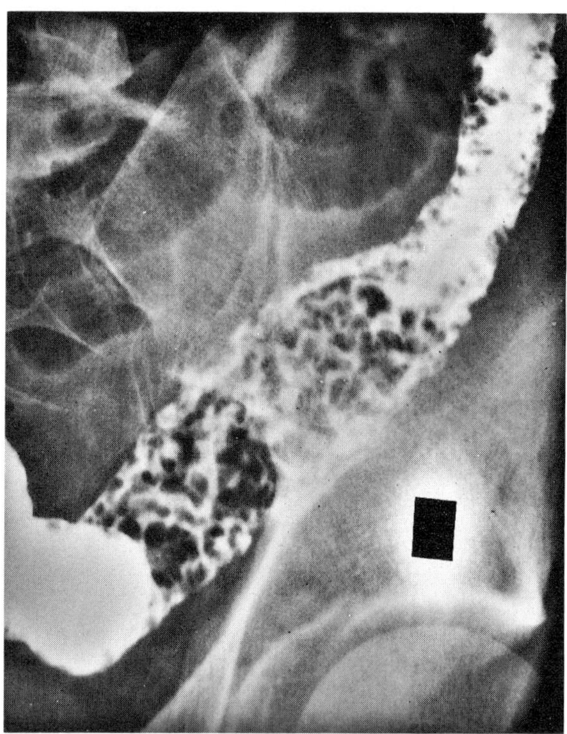

Fig. E.14. Multiple linear intraluminal masses and ulcers are present in the left colon. These inflammatory masses impinge upon the colon lumen.

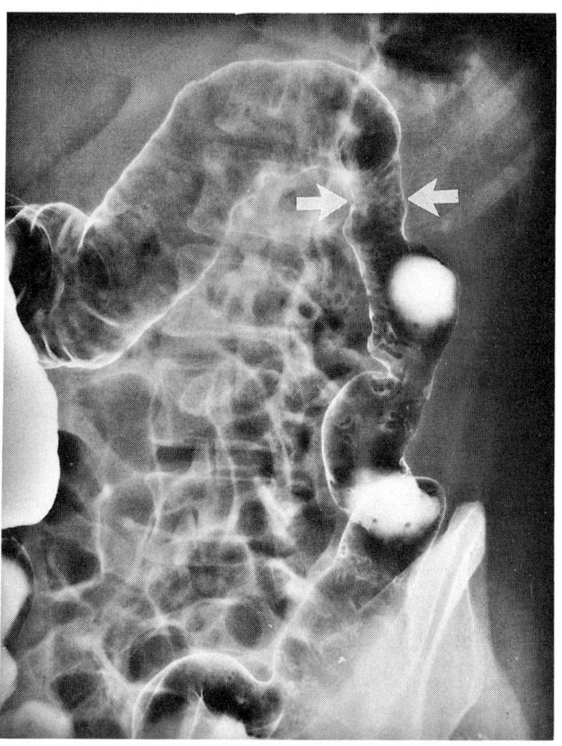

Fig. E.16. Chronic ulcerative colitis for 17 years. The haustra are obliterated, there is marked foreshortening of the colon, and a stricture has developed at the splenic flexure (arrows). Numerous linear inflammatory polyps are present in the descending colon.

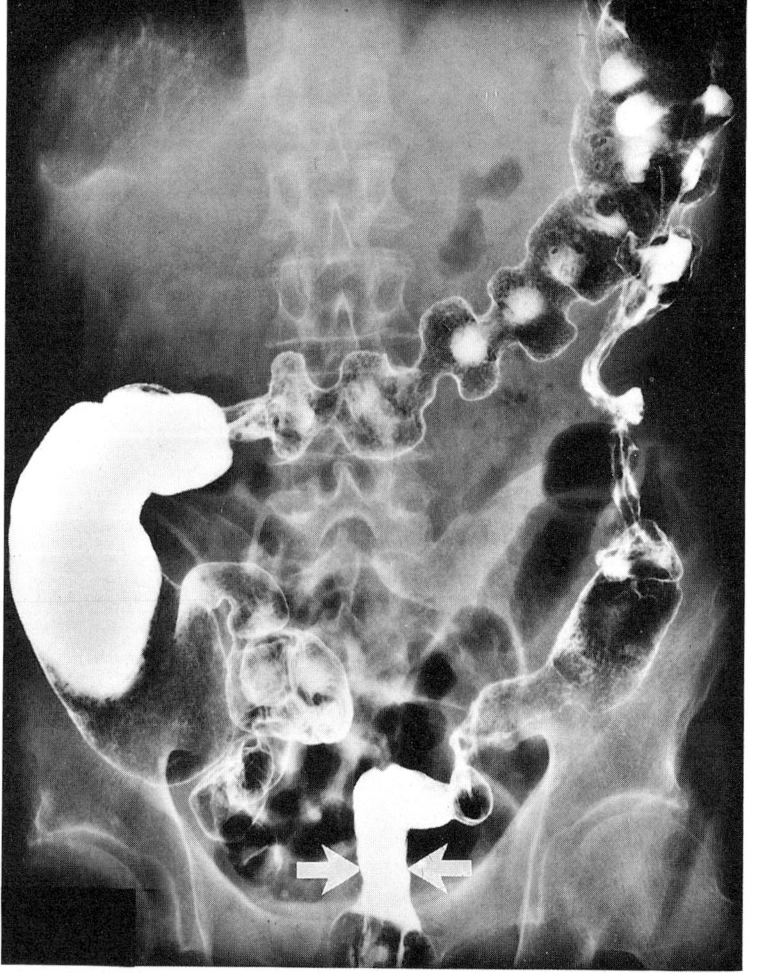

Fig. E.15. 80-year-old male with long-standing ulcerative colitis. A stricture involves the rectum (arrows). There is marked foreshortening of the sigmoid, fine ulcers are present throughout the colon, and extensive spasm is present. The valvulae conniventes in the terminal ileum are effaced, indicating a 'back-wash ileitis'. The resected colon revealed numerous adenomatous transformations and marked epithelial atypia.

limited to the distal colon rather than with pancolitis.

Angiography in a patient with ulcerative colitis reveals hypervascularity of the involved areas. The role of intraarterial steroid infusion in the therapy of ulcerative colitis remains to be established (34).

The splenomegaly seen in some patients with ulcerative colitis is puzzling; hypersplenism and portal hypertension may be present. Angiography shows increased splenic blood flow in these patients, with a resultant increase in portal vein pressure and increased portocaval shunts (35). These patients quite often have liver abnormalities, manifested as a mild type of cirrhosis. Whether the portal hypertension or the increased hepatic vascular resistance due to liver involvement comes first is not known. In either case, splenectomy cures the portal hypertension (35). Whether the liver abnormalities regress is not known. Likewise, it is not known whether splenectomy decreases the incidence of known liver disease in patients with ulcerative colitis.

e. Complications

Although strictures of the colon are more common in regional enteritis, they do occur with ulcerative colitis. The strictures are usually symmetrical and located in that portion of the colon most severely involved by the disease. Not all narrowed segments on a barium enema are strictures; there can be considerable spasm and what appears to be a strictured segment on one examination can be shown to have disappeared on a subsequent examination.

Earlier literature emphasized the increased incidence of colon carcinoma in patients with ulcerative colitis. It has been estimated that these patients have a five to ten times greater risk of developing colon carcinoma than the average population. At present, the incidence of cancer is believed to be lower and the average radiologist does not often encounter a carcinoma in a patient with ulcerative colitis. The reasons for the earlier greater reported incidence are probably twofold: 1) statistics in prior reports were based on surgical series where patients with more severe disease and disease of longer duration were encountered, and 2) there is currently a trend towards earlier surgical intervention.

The duration, severity and extent of active disease are probably the most important factors in determining whether carcinoma will develop (36). Patients with pancolitis have a higher incidence of cancer and develop the cancer earlier than patients with left-sided colitis only (37, 38). It is of interest that although almost all patients with ulcerative colitis have involvement of the rectum, the resultant cancers are scattered throughout the colon (39, 40). Both synchronous and metachronous colon carcinomas are more common in these patients than in the average population (40).

The etiology of carcinoma in ulcerative colitis is not known. Even in a bypassed segment there appears to be a higher incidence of carcinoma than expected normally. As an example, ileostomy and subtotal colectomy, leaving in place an excluded rectal stump, exposes the patient to a risk of developing cancer in the rectal stump (11).

There is also a higher incidence of scirrhous carcinoma developing in these patients. This type of carcinoma, commonly called linitis plastica of the colon, infiltrates submucosally and may leave the mucosa mostly intact. It can be difficult to distinguish between a benign stricture, an inflammatory polyp, and carcinoma (41) (Figs. E.19 and E.20). These carcinomata can be difficult to detect not only radiographically but also endoscopically (42). Colonoscopy can be used only distal to a stricture (Fig. E.21).

There is an increased association between ulcerative colitis and colon lyphoma (43) and leukemia (44), although the data so far is incomplete.

Marked acute dilatation of the colon, called toxic megacolon, is a dreaded complication of ulcerative colitis. Toxic megacolon as the initial presentation is occasionally encountered. Although the dilatation is usually seen in the transverse colon, any part of the colon can be involved and at times there is dilatation of the entire colon and rectum. Toxic megacolon almost always occurs on a setting of pancolitis. There can be an irregular outline to the colon wall, appearing as 'thumbprinting', although the 'thumbprinting' is not specific for toxic megacolon (Figs. E.22 and E.23). Involvement of other parts of the colon can be determined by prone or decubitus radiographs. The transverse colon involvement usually seen simply reflects retained gas rising to the highest part of the colon when the

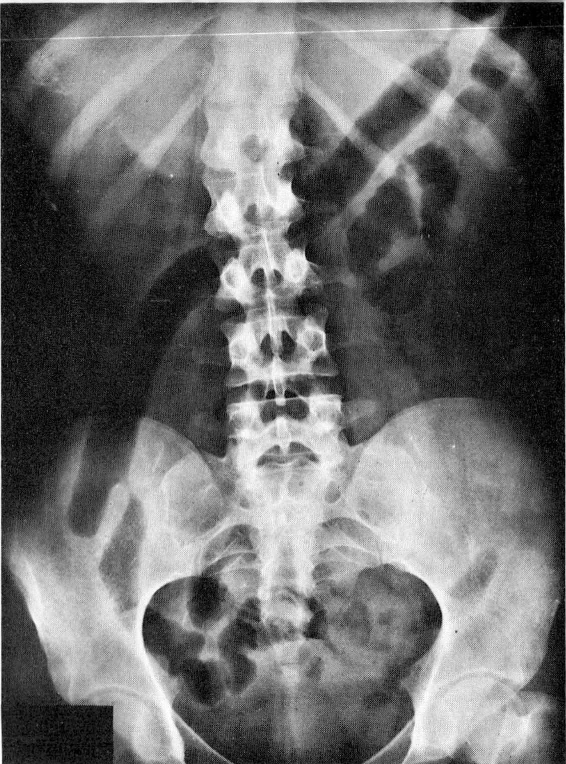

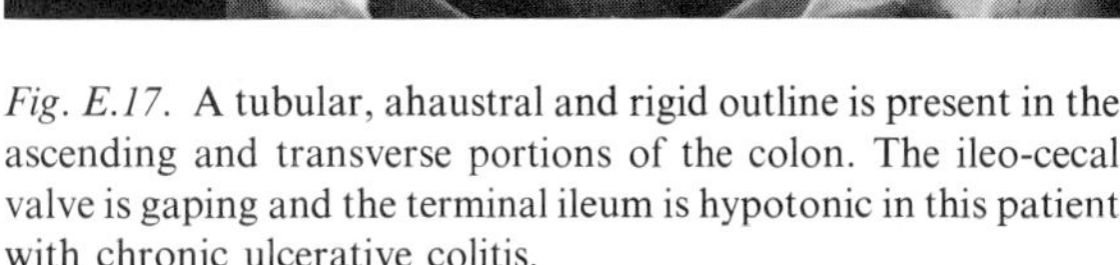

Fig. E.17. A tubular, ahaustral and rigid outline is present in the ascending and transverse portions of the colon. The ileo-cecal valve is gaping and the terminal ileum is hypotonic in this patient with chronic ulcerative colitis.

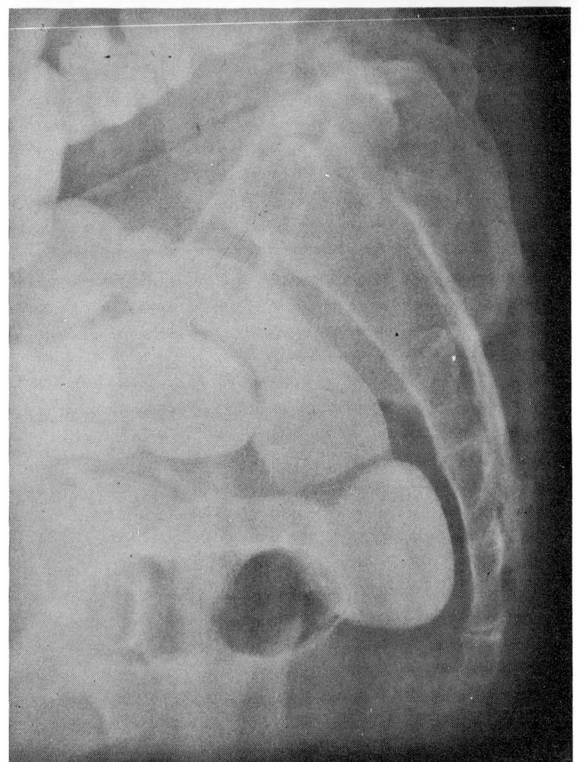

*Fig. E.18.***a**

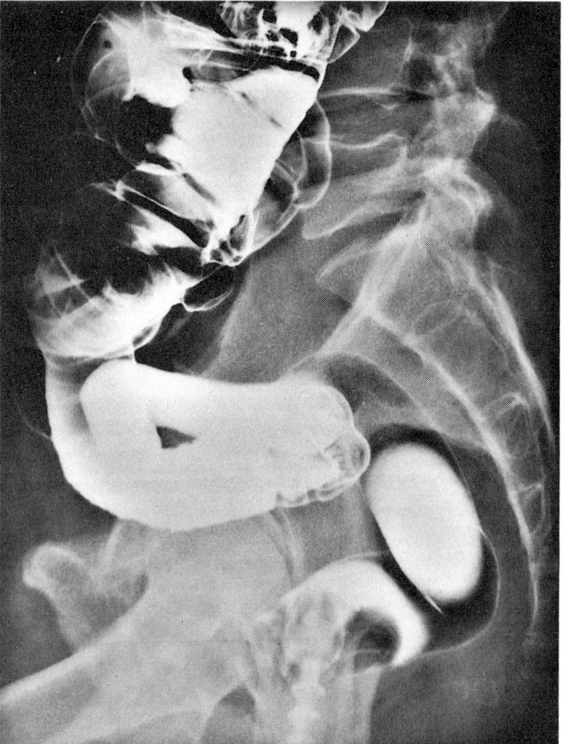

b

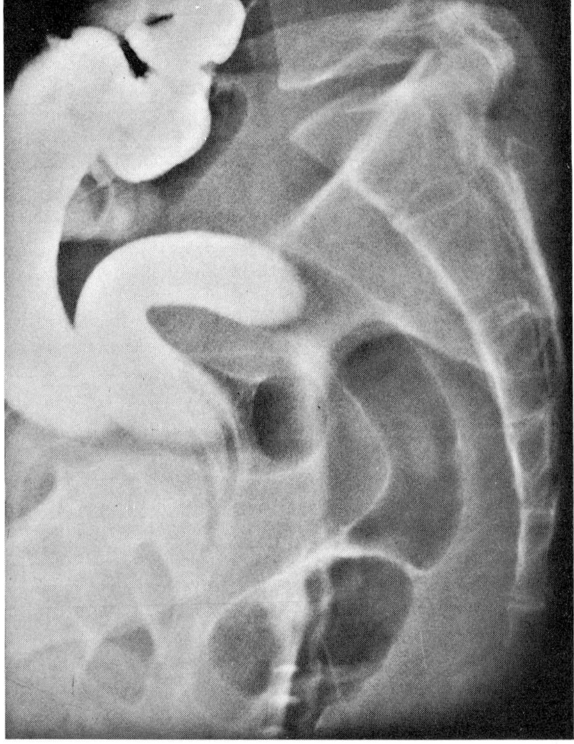

c

Fig. E.18. Widened presacral space in ulcerative colitis. (a) The initial single-contrast examination revealed a normal presacral space. The examination was considered normal although the patient was already symptomatic. (b) 17 months later there is a small but definite widening of the presacral space. The rectosigmoid had a fine granular pattern compatible with ulcerative colitis. (c) 16 months later the presacral space has widened considerably more, the sigmoid colon has foreshortened, and the colon lumen is narrowed.

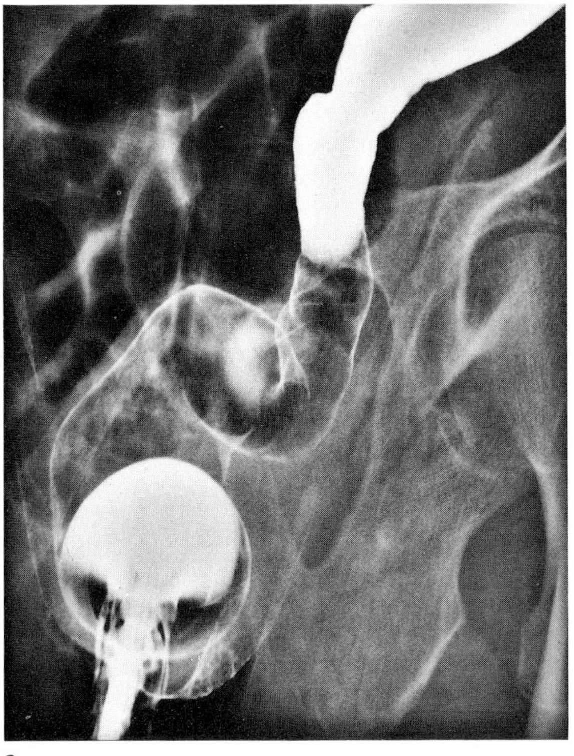
a

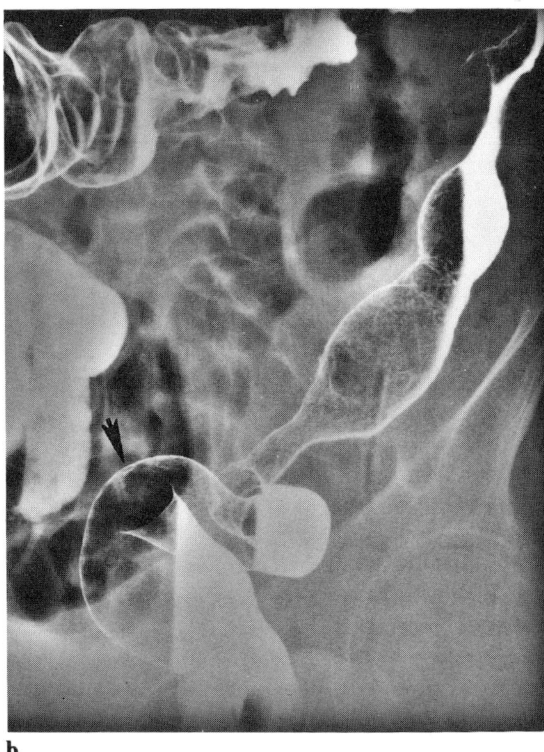
b

Fig. E.19. 80-year-old male with long-standing chronic ulcerative colitis involving entire colon. (a) Examination in 1975 reveals an ahaustral distal colon with sigmoid foreshortening and narrowing. (b) 20 months later there is further narrowing of the lumen and a small, sessile polyp is present in the sigmoid (arrowhead). (c) 3½ years later the stricture has progressed further and the sessile polyp has grown considerably (arrowheads). The polyp was a well-differentiated adenocarcinoma.

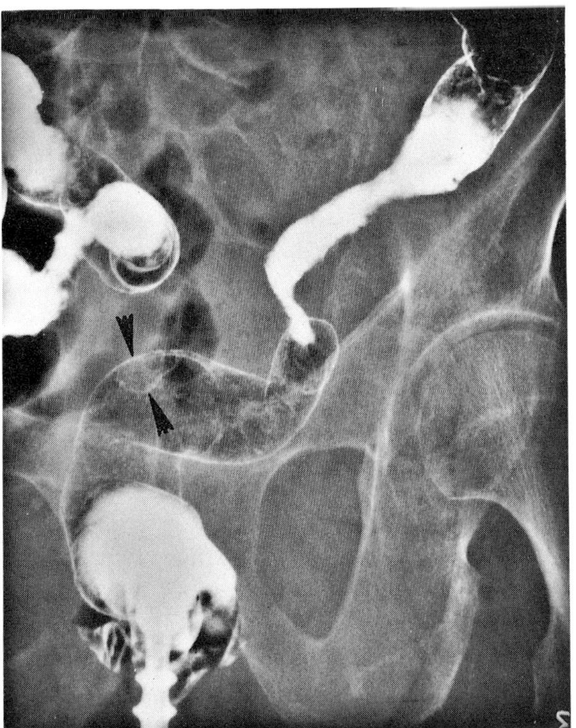
c

patient is supine (45).

Unfortunately, there have been reports of a barium enema precipitating toxic megacolon (46), although there has never been proof that such a relationship is anything but purely coincidental (47). If a patient is on the verge of developing toxic megacolon and is coming under medical management, it is not unnatural to consider a barium enema. If the patient then continues to progress to toxic megacolon, it is very tempting to ascribe such progression to thc barium enema.

The clinical or radiological suspicion of toxic megacolon is an absolute contraindication to the performance of any type of enema due to the high incidence of resultant perforation. Also, with a severe attack, no laxatives should be used for any reason. We delay the examination under these circumstances. Once the acute attack subsides, if an examination is indicated, it should be performed on an unprepared colon (25). Such an 'instant enema' will usually show the disease, although retained

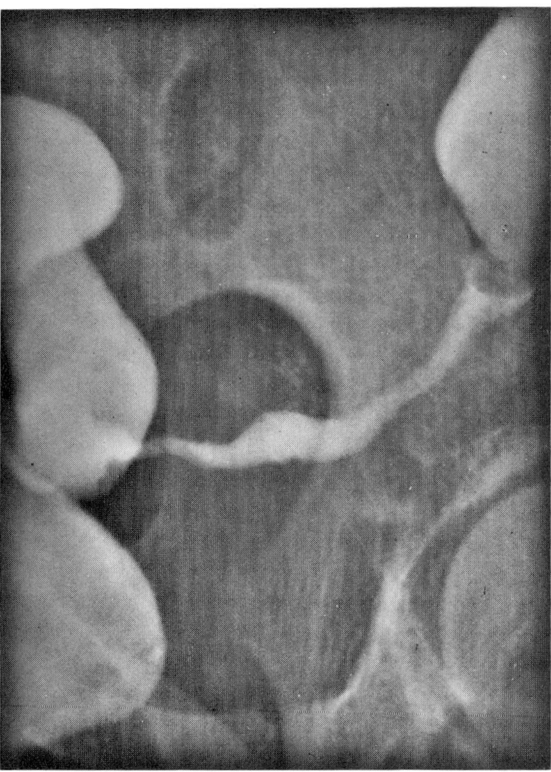

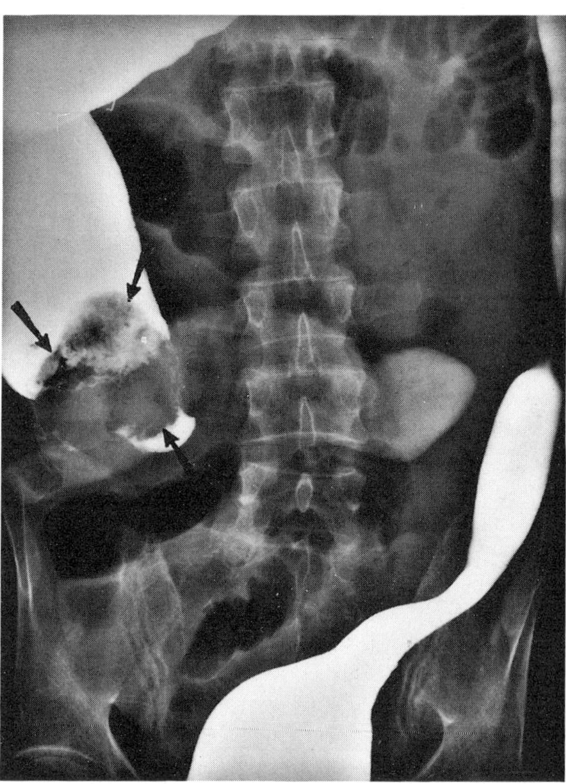

Fig. E.20. (a) This 26-year-old male had ulcerative colitis for 16 years. A stricture developed in the sigmoid colon. Although such long strictures in a 'normal' colon generally are benign, in a setting of ulcerative colitis they should be viewed with suspicion. This stricture was an adenocarcinoma. (b) 51-year-old male with long-standing ulcerative colitis and recent small bowel obstruction. A single-contrast barium enema was performed to locate the obstruction. A carcinoma fills almost the entire cecum (arrows). Some barium has refluxed proximal to the obstruction into dilated loops of small bowel.

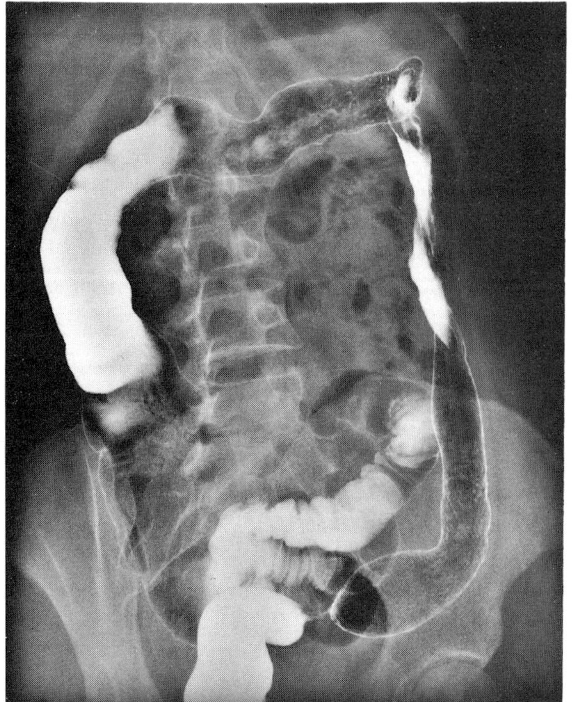

Fig. E.21. 27-year-old female with 10 years duration of ulcerative colitis. A pancolitis is present. Numerous fine ulcers are scattered throughout, the ahaustral colon is considerably foreshortened and a sigmoid stricture has developed. Colonoscopy and biopsy are not possible proximal to the stricture.

liquid residue will mask subtle radiographic changes.

Not all colon dilatations represent toxic megacolon; an obstructing carcinoma distally may mimic toxic megacolon (48).

With suspected toxic megacolon, we prefer following the patient with plain radiographs of the abdomen every 12 to 24 hours. Obviously, a horizontal beam radiograph should be included in each of these examinations. If there is both radiographic and clinical evidence of improvement, then medical therapy can be continued. Some advocate frequent rolling of the patient from the supine to prone position, together with insertion of a rectal tube, to decompress the colon (49). If after vigorous medical therapy, there is little or no clinical improvement

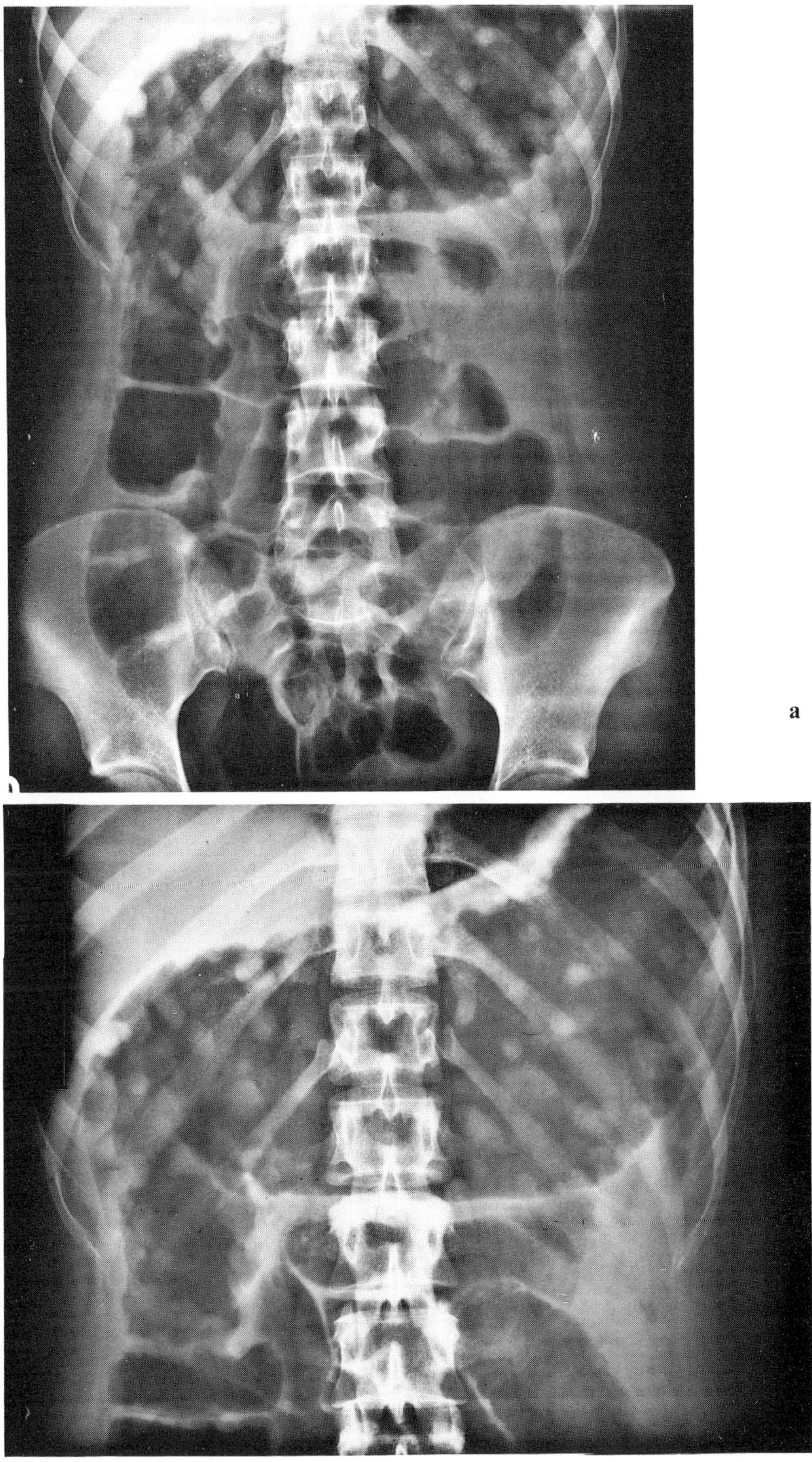

Fig. E.22. Toxic megacolon in a setting of ulcerative colitis. (a) The transverse colon is considerably dilated and numerous inflammatory polyps present as 'thumbprinting'. The small bowel is moderately dilated, probably secondary to peritoneal irritation. (b) Close-up appearance of the transverse colon 'thumbprinting'.

and radiographically the colon continues to show distension, surgery should be considered. Unfortunately, it is not uncommon to continue conservative medical therapy without any real evidence of improvement. An abdominal radiographic study may subsequently demonstrate free perforation. The perforation can be missed clinically because of the severe underlying disease and the first hint of perforation is seen on the radiographic examination. Occasionally, the perforation is retroperitoneal in location and gas tracks through the diaphragm into the chest and neck without any pneumoperitoneum being present (50).

A barium enema should be performed with caution in any patient with active ulcerative colitis. Both pneumoperitoneum and portal vein gas have been reported after a barium enema in patients with sufficiently acute colitis who have not yet developed toxic megacolon (51–53). Fortunately, such episodes are rare. Usually a full bowel preparation in patients with active disease is not necessary. Because of the disease few or no laxatives are needed. Usually there is little residue in the colon and a tap water enema may clear any remaining residue.

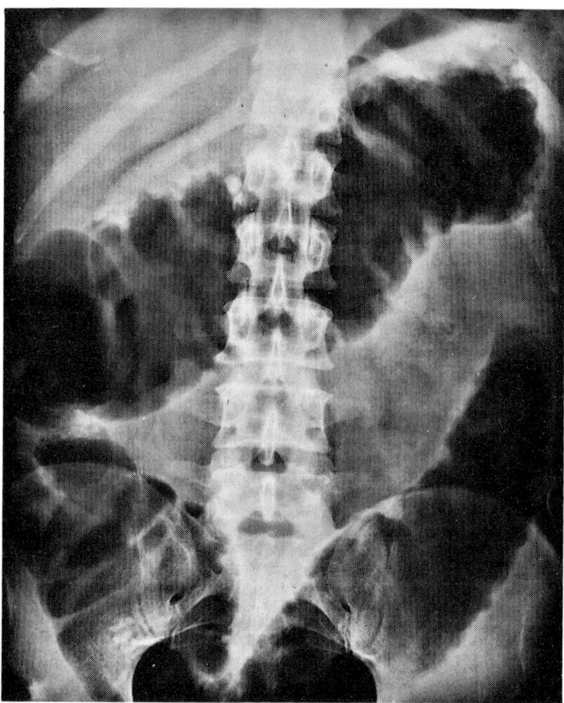

Fig. E.23. Toxic megacolon. The entire colon is considerably dilated. Numerous inflammatory polyps present as 'thumbprinting'. The overall appearance suggests impending perforation.

f. Differential diagnosis

The radiological appearance of pseudopolyposis in ulcerative colitis is mimicked by familial polyposis. In fact, at times, on a radiological basis alone, the differentiation can be impossible. In actual practice, however, this differentiation is readily made on the basis of the patient's history and clinical findings. Occasionally there is partial healing of ulcerative colitis with only inflammatory polyps being present. Here the past history of ulcerative colitis also allows one to differentiate ulcerative colitis from familial polyposis.

Regional enteritis is usually in the differential diagnosis, both clinically and radiologically. If the rectum is spared, if there is significant small bowel disease, or if there are skip areas of involvement in the colon, then presumably one is dealing with regional enteritis. Rectal bleeding is unusual in regional enteritis but almost always present in ulcerative colitis. If there are many small ulcers with a 'grain of sand' granular appearance, most likely the disease is ulcerative colitis (54). If there has been significant remission, it is more likely that the disease is ulcerative colitis. If one sees a deep fistula, regional enteritis rather than ulcerative colitis should be suspected. Further differentiation is discussed in the section on regional enteritis.

Patients with cathartic colitis have a long history of cathartic abuse. Infectious colitis can be confusing and differentiation on a bacteriological basis is necessary. Occasionally infection may be superimposed on ulcerative colitis (55). Ischemic colitis of a localized segment of the colon may appear similar to ulcerative colitis and with disease limited only to the rectum, differentiation can be difficult. More extensive disease involving the rectum and colon generally points to a nonischemic etiology because of the dual blood supply to this region. Unfortunately, ulcerative colitis can begin in the elderly (56) and can mimic ischemic colitis.

Although diverticulosis and regional enteritis may coexist, such an association between diverticulosis and ulcerative colitis is rare.

The final end point of many of the colitides is a narrow tube-like colon configuration. One can usually arrive at the correct diagnosis by correlating the radiological findings with the patient's history and clinical presentation. However, it should be kept in mind that occasionally one encounters a patient where considerable overlap exists and differentiation between some of the colitides may not be possible either by history, clinical findings, pathology, or by the radiographic appearance. Fortunately, in most radiologic practices, such patients are few.

Toxic megacolon is usually found in a setting of ulcerative colitis. Unfortunately, an occasional patient with fulminant regional enteritis or one of the other colitides may also present with toxic megacolon.

References

1. Wilks S, Moxon W: Lectures on Pathological Anatomy, Ed. 2, London, J & A Churchill, 1875.
2. Stierlin E: Zur Röntgendiagnostik der Colitis ulcerosa. Z Klin Med 75:486–493, 1912.
3. Singer HC, Anderson JGD, Frischer H, Kirsner JB: Familial aspects of inflammatory bowel disease. Gastroenterology 61:423–430, 1971.
4. Lupinetti M, Mehigan D, Cameron JL: Hepatobiliary complications of ulcerative colitis. Am J Surg 139:113–117, 1980.
5. Cello JP: Cholestasis in ulcerative colitis. Gastroenterology 73:357–374, 1977.
6. Schrumpf E, Elgjo K, Fausa O, Gjone E, Kolmannskog F, Ritland S: Sclerosing cholangitis in ulcerative colitis. Scand J Gastroenterol 15:689–697, 1980.
7. Ritchie JK, Allen RN, Macartney J, Thompson H, Hawley PR, Cooke WT: Biliary tract carcinoma associated with ulcerative colitis. Q J Med 43:263–279, 1974.
8. Williams SM, Harned RK: Bile duct carcinoma associated with chronic ulcerative colitis. Dis Colon Rectum 24.42–44, 1981.
9. Greenstein AJ, Janowitz HD, Sachar DB: The extra-intestinal complications of Crohn's disease and ulcerative colitis. Medicine 55:401–412, 1976.
10. Delpre G, Kadish U, Gazit E, Joshua H, Zamir R: HLA antigens in ulcerative colitis and Crohn's disease in Israel. Gastroenterology 78:1452–1457, 1980.
11. Kurtz LM, Flint GW, Platt N, Wise L: Carcinoma in the retained rectum after colectomy for ulcerative colitis. Dis Colon Rectum 23:346–350, 1980.
12. Thow GB, Castro AF, Beahrs OH, Goligher JC, Kock NG: Present status of the continent ileostomy. Dis Colon Rectum 19:189–212, 1976.
13. Telander RL, Perrault J: Total colectomy with rectal mucosectomy and ileoanal anastomosis for chronic ulcerative colitis in children and young adults. Mayo Clin Proc 55:420–424, 1980.
14. Utsunomiya J, Iwama T, Imajo M, Matsuo S, Sawai S, Yaegashi K, Hirayama R: Total colectomy, mucosal proctectomy, and ileoanal anastomosis. Dis Colon Rectum 23:459–466, 1980.
15. Jahadi MR, Shaw ML: The pathology of the appendix in ulcerative colitis. Dis Colon Rectum 19:345–349, 1976.
16. Frank PH, Riddell RH, Feczko PJ, Levin B: Radiological detection of colonic dysplasia (precarcinoma) in chronic ulcerative colitis. Gastrointest Radiol 3:209–219, 1978.
17. Riddell RH: The precarcinomatous phase of ulcerative colitis. Curr Top Pathol 63:179–219, 1976.
18. Blackstone MO, Riddell RH, Rogers BHG, Levin B: Dysplasia-associated lesion or mass (DALM) detected by colonoscopy in long-standing ulcerative colitis: an indication for colectomy. Gastroenterology 80:366–374, 1981.
19. Granqvist S, Gabrielsson N, Sundelin P, Thorgeirsson T: Precancerous lesions in the mucosa in ulcerative colitis. A radiographic, endoscopic, and histopathologic study. Scand J Gastroenterol 15:1–8, 1980.
20. Williams HJ Jr, Stephens DH, Carlson HC: Double-contrast radiography: colonic inflammatory disease. AJR 137:315–322, 1981.
21. Williams CB, Teague R: Colonoscopy. Gut 14:990–1003, 1973.
22. Bartram CI, Walmsley K: A radiological and pathological correlation of the mucosal changes in ulcerative colitis. Clin Radiol 29:323–328, 1978.
23. Laufer I: Air contrast studies of the colon in inflammatory bowel disease. CRC Crit Rev Diag Imag 9:421–447, 1977.
24. Fraser GM, Findlay JM: The double contrast enema in ulcerative and Crohn's colitis. Clin Radiol 27:103–112, 1976.
25. Bartram CI: Radiology in the current assessment of ulcerative colitis. Gastrointest Radiol 1:383–392, 1977.
26. Persigehl M, Spieth W, Klose KC, Cen M: Feinreliefveränderungen des Kolons im Frühstadium der Colitis ulcerosa und Colitis granulomatosa. ROEFO 129:177–180, 1978.
27. Welin S, Brahme F: The double contrast method in ulcerative colitis. Acta Radiol 55:257–271, 1961.
28. Joffe N: Localised giant pseudopolyposis secondary to ulcerative or granulomatous colitis. Clin Radiol 28:609–616, 1977.
29. Keating JW, Mindell HJ: Localised giant pseudopolyposis in ulcerative colitis. AJR 126:1178–1180, 1976.
30. Zegel HG, Laufer I: Filiform polyposis. Radiology 127:615–619, 1978.
31. Goldberger LE, Neely HR, Stammer JL: Large mucosal bridges. An unusual roentgenographic manifestation of ulcerative colitis. Gastrointest Radiol 3:81–83, 1978.
32. Hammerman AM, Shatz BA, Susman N: Radiographic characteristics of colonic 'mucosal bridges': sequelae of inflammatory bowel disease. Radiology 127:611–614, 1978.
33. Gardiner GA: 'Backwash ileitis' with pseudopolyposis. AJR 129:506–507, 1977.
34. Hiramatsu K, Asakura H, Baba S: Selective intraarterial steroid injection in ulcerative colitis. Acta Radiol Diagn 17:299–304, 1976.
35. Friman L: Splenomegaly, hyperkinetic splenic flow and portal hypertension in colitis. Acta Radiol Diagn 21:561–570, 1980.
36. Edwards FC, Truelove SC: The course and prognosis of ulcerative colitis. IV. Carcinoma of the colon. Gut 5:15–22, 1964.
37. Greenstein AJ, Sachar DB, Smith H, Pucillo A, Papatestas AE, Kreel I, Geller SA, Janowitz HD, Aufses AH Jr: Cancer in universal and left-sided ulcerative colitis: factors determining risk. Gastroenterology 77:290–294, 1979.
38. Kewenter J, Ahlman H, Hulten L: Cancer risk in extensive ulcerative colitis. Ann Surg 188:824–828, 1978.
39. Langman MJS: Epidemiology of cancer of the large intestine. Proc R Soc Med 59:132–134, 1966.
40. Fennessy JJ, Sparberg MB, Kirsner JB: Radiological findings in carcinoma of the colon complicating chronic ulcerative colitis. Gut 9:388–397, 1968.
41. James EM, Carlson HC: Chronic ulcerative colitis and colon cancer: can radiographic appearance predict survival

patterns? AJR 130:825–830, 1978.
42. Crowson TD, Ferrante WF, Gathright JB, Jr: Colonoscopy: inefficacy for early carcinoma detection in patients with ulcerative colitis. JAMA 236:2651–2652, 1976.
43. Wagonfeld JB, Platz CE, Fishman FL, Sibley RK, Kirsner JB: Multicentric colonic lymphoma complicating ulcerative colitis. Am J Dig Dis 22:502–508, 1977.
44. Fabry TL, Sachar DB, Janowitz HD: Acute myelogenous leukemia in patients with ulcerative colitis. J Clin Gastroenterol 2:225–227, 1980.
45. Kramer P, Wittenberg J: Colonic gas distribution in toxic megacolon. Gastroenterology 80:433–437, 1981.
46. Silverberg D, Rogers AG: Toxic megacolon in ulcerative colitis. Can Med Assoc J 90:357–363, 1964.
47. Goldberg HI: The barium enema and toxic megacolon: cause–effect relationship? Gastroenterology 68:617–618, 1975.
48. Greenstein AJ, Sachar DB, Pucillo A, Vassiliades G, Smith H, Kreel I, Geller SA, Janowitz HD, Aufses AH: Cancer in universal and left-sided ulcerative colitis: clinical and pathologic features. Mt. Sinai J Med NY 46:25–32, 1979.
49. Present DH, Wolfson D, Gelernt IM, Rubin PH, Bauer J, Chapman ML: The medical management of toxic megacolon: technique of decompression with favorable long term follow-up [Abstract]. Gastroenterology 80:1255, 1981.
50. Mogan GR, Sachar DB, Bauer J, Salky B, Janowitz HD: Toxic megacolon in ulcerative colitis complicated by pneumomediastinum: Report of two cases. Gastroenterology 79:559–562, 1980.
51. Weinstein GE, Weiner M, Schwartz M: Portal vein gas. Am J Gastroenterol 49:425–429, 1968.
52. Lazar HP: Survival following portal venous air embolization. Am J Dig Dis 10:259–264, 1965.
53. Kees CJ, Hester CL Jr: Portal vein gas following barium enema examination. Radiology 102:525–526, 1972.
54. Kelvin FM, Oddson TA, Rice RP, Garbutt JT, Bradenham BP: Double contrast barium enema in Crohn's disease and ulcerative colitis. AJR 131:207–213, 1978.
55. Mandal B: Ulcerative colitis and acute *Salmonella* infection. Br Med J 1:326, 1974.
56. Zeman R, Burrell M, Gold JA: Ulcerative colitis in the elderly. AJR 135:164–166, 1980.

III.1.F. Infectious colitis

a. Introduction

Although numerous bacteria, viruses, parasites, and other microbes have at one time or another infected man, only a small portion of these organisms are manifested by disease involving the colon. Discussed here are thus only those infections and related diseases which are primarily encountered by a radiologist while examining the colon.

Some patients with acute gastroenteritis have a self-limiting disease with no etiological agent being sought and identified. Likewise, although it is now generally believed that most cases of so-called 'traveler's diarrhea' are due to infection with a strain of *Escherichia coli* (1), the possible role of viruses is still not clear.

Table F.1. Bacterial enteric pathogens (2).

NONINVASIVE
Escherichia coli
Staphylococcus aureus
Clostridium perfringens
INVASIVE
Salmonella
Shigella
Campylobacter fetus

The bacterial pathogens can be divided into two groups (2): those non-invasive pathogens where no significant mucosal damage is produced and the invasive pathogens where mucosal damage can result in ulcers (Table F.1). Radiography of patients with infection with the noninvasive pathogens shows a nonspecific bowel gas pattern, a picture of adynamic ileus, or occasionally a pattern mimicking bowel obstruction. Both the small bowel and the colon can be considerably dilated with excessive amounts of fluid present within the lumen. In these bouts of gastroenteritis a barium enema is limited to the occasional patient where the diagnosis is in doubt, mechanical obstruction of the bowel is clinically suspected, or the disease has become chronic.

b. Bacterial colitides

Salmonella and shigella colitis. Throughout the centuries dysentery has had perhaps a greater influence on the course of history than any of the great wars or battles. In fact, the crowded and nonsanitary conditions existing in most wars, even in these so-called modern times, can lead to severe outbreaks of dysentery with both *Salmonella* and *Shigella* being implicated.

Both organisms, *Salmonella* and *Shigella*, exist throughout the world. Within tropical regions these diseases can spread in epidemic proportions. In the temperate zones there are generally explosive infections centered around a common supply or isolated infections with the disease spread both by contaminated food and water (3). Both infections can be spread by flies; there is no animal vector for the *Shigella* organism.

The incubation period for shigellosis is approximately two to three days while salmonellosis averages twelve hours. With both infections there is a sudden onset of fever, vomiting, and diarrhea, with blood and mucus present in the stool. The infections generally are more severe in children, although even adults can have a fatal outcome. There is an increased incidence of these infections in male homosexuals (4). The diagnosis can generally be established by appropriate cultures.

Both shigellosis and salmonellosis can develop into a chronic stage with intermittent exacerbation of the patient's symptoms. The asymptomatic carrier in salmonellosis has been well described both in the medical and in the lay literature.

In the colon, inflammation can vary from mild involvement of the superficial layers, bowel wall inflammation, necrosis, to pseudomembrane formation if the infection is sufficiently severe. Ulcers varying in depth can be present. The distal small bowel may also be involved by inflammation.

Contrast examination of the colon is generally of little use during the acute episode of salmonellosis because the patient cannot readily tolerate a barium enema examination. If a barium enema is performed, it shows a loss of haustration together with numerous ulcers scattered throughout the colon (Fig. F.1). The ulcers may extend intramurally in a 'collar button' appearance. In some patients the radiographic findings are indistinguishable from those seen in other colitides. Salmonellosis may involve only the small bowel where it is usually most evident in the distal ileum. Non-contrast radiographs of the abdomen in these patients reveal an adynamic ileus primarily involving the small bowel (5). Severe acute disease may result in toxic megacolon (6). Ileal perforation and pneumoperitoneum may be the end result (5).

Dysentery produced by infection with *Shigella* organisms is also due to acute inflammation. Subsequent necrosis results in ulcers of varying depths, with the distal colon usually being the most severely involved. Mild disease results in shallow ulcers, although sometimes no radiographic changes are present. There is a thickening of the colon wall, best seen as thickening of the plicae semi-lunaris. With progression of disease the ulcers become deeper, they assume a collar-button appearance, and a longer segment of colon is involved. Unlike salmonellosis, infection with *Shigella* generally does not lead to perforation. Chronic infection can mimic chronic ulcerative colitis.

The radiographic differential diagnosis of shigel-

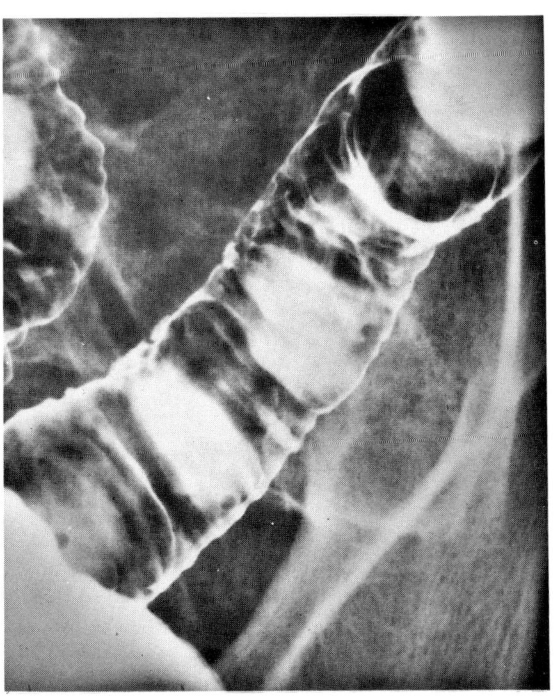
a

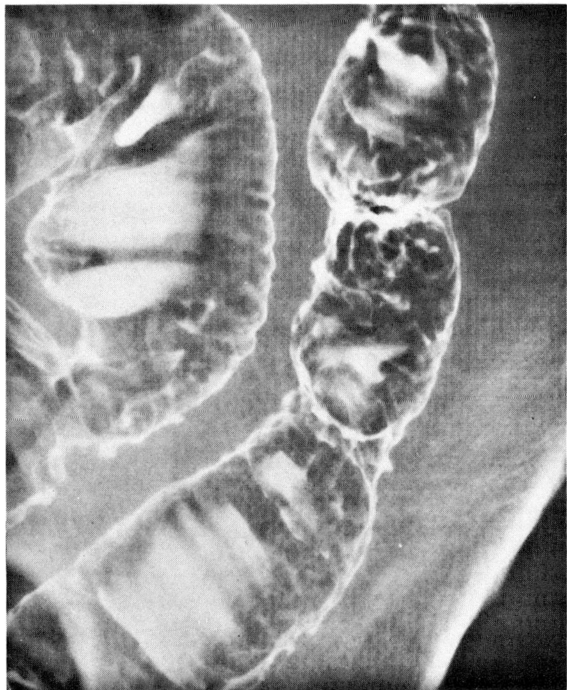
b

Fig. F.1. Salmonella colitis. Two views of the sigmoid colon reveal spasticity, in spite of glucagon, and numerous intramural ulcers scattered throughout.

losis and salmonellosis includes ulcerative colitis, regional enteritis, amebiasis, and pseudomembranous enterocolitis. More commonly ulcerative colitis and regional enteritis are diagnosed radiologically, while in reality the patient has *Shigella* or *Salmonella* colitis, than vice versa. Complicating the picture further, infection may coexist with ulcerative colitis (7).

If the colitis is due to infection by *Shigella* or *Salmonella*, a follow-up barium enema after the infection has cleared should be normal, unless there has been significant scarring from the prior infection.

Tuberculous colitis. Tuberculosis of the gastrointestinal tract may be either primary or secondary to pulmonary infestation. In the past, primary tuberculosis of the gastrointestinal tract was generally due to ingestion of infected milk. This source of infection has been essentially eradicated in the United States, although it still exists throughout a large portion of the world. Currently in the United States, gastrointestinal tuberculosis in patients who have not traveled outside the country is usually secondary to pulmonary tuberculosis. With the large influx of travelers and refugees from other countries, however, primary tuberculosis of the bowel is still not rare in the average radiological practice. Many of these latter patients have radiographically normal lungs. The etiology of the initial infection in these patients is speculative, but is probably due to direct ingestion of the tubercle organism.

Several reasons account for the marked decrease of intestinal tuberculosis. First, following the description of a nonspecific granulomatous disease involving the gastrointestinal tract by Crohn et al. in 1932 (8), it is believed that many patients previously labeled as having intestinal tuberculosis actually had regional enteritis. The second major reason for the decrease of intestinal tuberculosis has been pasteurization of milk. Currently, secondary tuberculosis of the bowel in the United States is generally believed to be from swallowed tubercle bacilli from the lungs.

Clinically, the patient may be either asymptomatic or may have various nonspecific complaints. Occasionally diarrhea is present but rectal hemorrhage is unusual.

Secondary tuberculosis of the gastrointestinal tract should be suspected in a patient with known tuberculosis of the pulmonary tract and abdominal symptoms. Cavitating lesions of the lungs appear to predispose to intestinal involvement by tuberculosis.

The definitive proof of colon tuberculosis is finding the tubercle bacillus, a finding not always achieved even with active disease. Unfortunately, in patients who have received anti-tuberculous therapy, no bacilli may be identified. At times, the diagnosis of colon tuberculosis must be made solely on an exclusion basis. A surgically resected specimen may eventually reveal the diagnosis only by animal inoculation.

The distal ileum and the right colon are involved in most of these patients, with the incidence decreasing both proximal and distal to the ileocecal valve region; the esophagus and rectum are thus least likely to be diseased. Usually there are no skip areas although in an occasional patient there can be involvement of the colon in a segmental fashion, simulating regional enteritis (9).

Although there have been many descriptions in the radiological literature of ileocolic tuberculosis, few signs are specific for this condition (10). One of the earliest described radiological signs was a spastic distal ileum, first described by Stierlin in 1911 (11). The terminal ileum can be narrowed and the folds thickened. Such a spastic segment may mimic the 'string sign' associated with regional enteritis. A small cecum with a narrow lumen is typical of advanced tuberculosis (12), with some authors using the term 'perityphlitis' to describe this appearance, although other inflammatory and ischemic conditions may result in a similar appearance. Bowel obstruction, especially in the distal ileum, may be present (13) and there may be a wide and gaping ileocecal valve.

A barium enema may reveal polyps, strictures, ulcers, or foreshortening of the colon. The tuberculous strictures tend to be short and nodular in outline (14). Ulcers are often present in the terminal ileum. Fistulae are rare but may occur (15); if one sees extensive fistulae the diagnosis of tuberculosis should be viewed with suspicion. Perforation is uncommon due to the thickened bowel wall.

Angiography in patients with ileocecal tuberculosis shows hypervascularity, thickened bowel wall, and an accentuated venous phase (16). The angiographic findings are very similar, if not identical, to regional enteritis, although hyperemic mesenteric lymph nodes appear to point towards tuberculosis (16).

Colon tuberculosis should be considered in the differential diagnosis of those patients who present with atypical regional enteritis or in patients who have been on anti-tuberculous medication. Since regional enteritis is also quite often centered on the ileocecal valve region, differential diagnosis between the two diseases can be difficult and in some patients the two diseases can be radiographically indistinguishable (9). Tuberculosis may mimic segmental regional enteritis (14, 17) (Fig. F.2a).

A distinguishing feature between regional enteritis and tuberculosis is the presence of anal lesions. These are rather common with regional enteritis and rare in tuberculous colitis. Similarly, internal fistulae are common in regional enteritis and are unusual in tuberculosis. Granulomata may be either present or absent in regional enteritis; if present, caseation is not seen. With tuberculosis, only tuberculous lymph nodes may reveal granulomata with central caseation, epithelioid cells, and Langhan's giant cells. Caseation may be mild or even absent after therapy.

It is not unusual for secondary tuberculosis of the bowel to involve the peritoneal cavity. Abdominal radiographs may reveal ascites and thickening of the small bowel wall. Obviously, at this stage of disease, the changes are nonspecific.

Appendicitis with a periappendiceal abscess can also deform the ileocecal region and mimic tuberculosis (Fig. F.2b). A periappendiceal mass may be present with both entities. In general, however, the clinical presentation of the patient allows for differentiation although in an occasional patient the two diseases may appear identical. Amebiasis may also result in similar findings. It is rare, however, to see amebiasis involve the small bowel.

An eccentric segment of abnormal colon generally should raise suspicion of either lymphoma or carcinoma. Lymphoma involving the ileocecal region is usually eccentric in location and quite often involves both the terminal ileum and a portion of the colon. Tuberculosis may mimic a cancer (18). Both carcinoma and tuberculosis can coexist, but there is little evidence to suggest any increased risk of developing carcinoma in patients with known bowel tuberculosis.

The differential diagnosis of enterocolic tuberculosis also includes infections such as South American blastomycosis, coccidioidomycosis, actinomycosis, histoplasmosis, and at times such diverse conditions as ischemia, radiation enteritis, and even sarcoidosis.

Yersinia colitis. An infectious agent identified more frequently is *Yersinia enterocolitica.* The clinical presentation may be similar to acute appendicitis or to regional enteritis (19, 20). Many of these patients are children and there are epidemic-like outbreaks of this infection within a community. It is usual to suspect the disease only after a normal appendix is found at surgery. The manifestations of this infection may be protean; as an example, a liver abscess may be a complication of this infection (21, 22). Presumably, some of the previously labelled 'acute typhlitis' patients and patients with 'cured' regional enteritis may in reality have been infected with this agent.

Yersinia colitis appears to be considerably less common in the United States than in Europe. A different and less virulent serotype may be involved in most attacks occurring in the United States. Most series have been reported from Europe and many American radiologists have seen only an isolated patient with this disease. A similar condition has been described in Japan after the ingestion of the fish tapeworm (23).

Radiographically, the disease tends to involve predominantly the terminal ileum and right colon (20). The valvulae conniventes in the ileum can be either thickened due to inflammation or destroyed. Linear and irregular ulcers and small nodules may be present (24). Aphthoid ulcers are occasionally seen. Overall, the disease most closely mimics regional enteritis (25). Usually the rectum is spared. When time allows, the disease can be confirmed by a rise in positive titers.

Campylobacter colitis. Colitis may be due to infection with *Campylobacter fetus* (subsp. *jejuni*). Whether this is an infection simply being identified correctly more often is not known; this organism is currently found as a common cause of infectious colitis in the temperate climate countries (26, 27). It

a

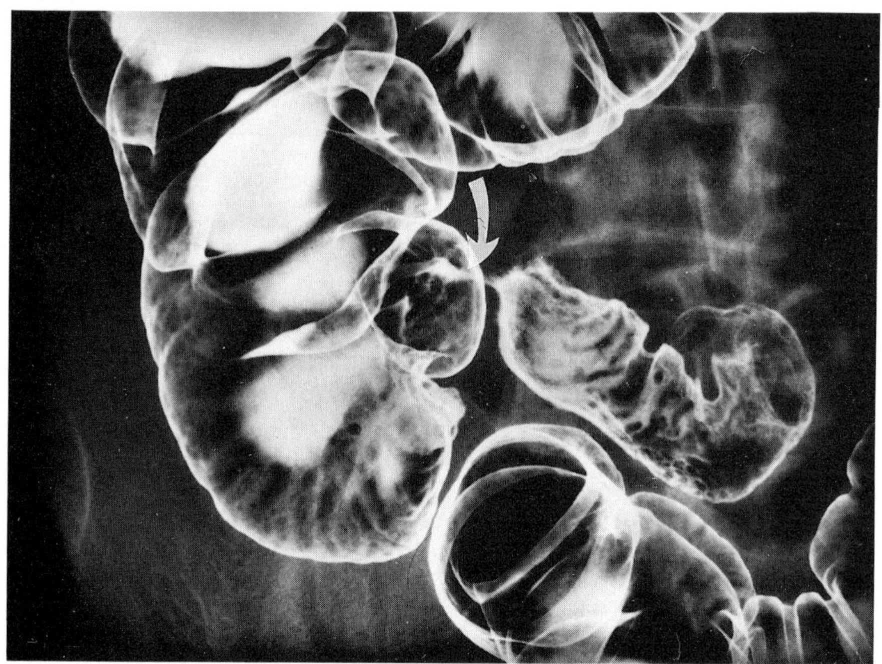

b

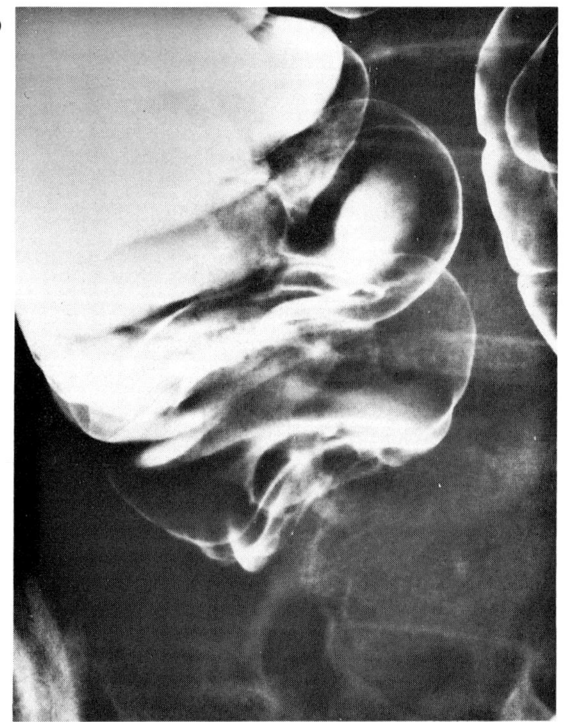

Fig. F.2. (a) Tuberculous ileocolitis. A sharply-defined stricture is present in the distal segment of the terminal ileum (arrow). Multiple inflammatory nodules are scattered in the ileum and cecum. The appearance is similar to that of regional enteritis. (b) Tuberculous colitis. This physician from Thailand gradually developed abdominal pain and a right lower quadrant mass. The appendix does not fill and a soft tissue mass indents the cecum. The appearance is identical to that seen with appendicitis and a periappendiceal abscess.

is more common than *Salmonella* or *Shigella* (28). The clinical features consist of the acute onset of pain, fever, and often bloody diarrhea (26, 29). Massive bleeding may occur and an arteriogram will reveal the site of extravasation (30). The radiographic and pathologic features are similar to those of other bacterial and ideopathic colitides (31, 32) (Fig. F.3). Identification is through bacteriologic and immunologic testing.

Post-antibiotic colitis. Occasionally encountered is a patient receiving antibiotics who subsequently develops severe diarrhea (33). This entity has been known as pseudomembranous enterocolitis, staphylococcal enterocolitis and as postoperative colitis (34). Pseudomembranous colitis is probably an inaccurate name because not all patients with this entity form a pseudomembrane and a pseudomembrane may be seen with some of the other colitides. Because this entity is usually, but not always, associated with antibiotic therapy, the term antibiotic colitis at least gives a hint of the association. Among other drugs, clindamycin (35–37) chloramphenicol, lincomycin (37–39), ampicillin (40), cephalosporins (41) and even penicillin (42) have been implicated. Ten percent of all patients taking clindamycin have been reported having such a colitis (43). The incidence of colitis appears not to be dose related. In addition to antibiotics, cancer chemotherapeutic agents can predispose patients to this entity (44). Rarely, no previous medication at all was given (45).

Generally, there is no prior history suggesting enterocolitic disease. Some of these patients may have had either pelvic or abdominal surgery and were subsequently placed on antibiotic coverage. Clinically, these patients can range from mild diarrhea to the other extreme of dehydration and shock. Although the colitis generally clears after discontinuing the offending antibiotic, in some patients the gastrointestinal signs not only do not abate, but become worse. Vancomycin (46, 47) and bacitracin (48) have been used with good response to treat some of these patients although the colitis may relapse once vancomycin is withdrawn (42, 44, 49).

It is believed that this condition results from an overgrowth of a cytotoxic strain of *Clostridium difficile* (50–53). *C. difficile* is readily cultured from the colon of affected patients. Some neonates may be asymptomatic carriers (54).

With severe involvement a membrane consisting of necrotic and inflammatory debris may form. Generally, the colon is more severely involved than the small bowel and at times the inflammation is limited to the colon. Abdominal radiographs reveal a 'tube-like' configuration of the colon, the bowel is hypotonic, and there is thickening of the transverse folds with narrowing of the haustra (55) (Fig. F.4). In the appropriate clinical setting, the correct diagnosis can be strongly suggested from abdominal radiographs without resort to contrast studies. In the occasional patient where the diagnosis is in doubt, a barium enema will reveal a shaggy and irregular contour (38) due to bowel wall edema, numerous ulcerations, and plaque-like masses (34) (Fig. F.5). There usually is generalized colon involvement.

Severe involvement results in peritoneal irritation and peritonitis, radiographically reflected as an adynamic ileus (56). The colon may assume an appearance similar to that seen with toxic megacolon. A pancolitis may be present (34). Generally, a finding on abdominal radiographs suggestive of toxic megacolon is a contraindication to the performance of any type of enema, including a barium enema. If there is any gas within the bowel wall, subsequent bowel perforation may be imminent.

Serial acute abdominal examinations are helpful in following the course of the disease and evaluating possible complications. Follow-up examination after resolution of the acute attack generally reveals a normal colon. In an occasional patient with a relatively severe attack, sequelae may include a stricture similar to the strictures seen with chronic ulcerative colitis.

Severe disease can result in vascular and lymphatic occlusion of the small vessels of the colon. The insult on the colon can thus be similar for both ischemic and postantibiotic colitis and it is not surprising that the radiographic appearance is similar for both (56). The radiological differential diagnosis also includes ulcerative colitis, regional enteritis, and the other infectious colitides. Yet, the patient's presentation, previous use of broad-spectrum antibiotics, and lack of any prior colon disease generally permits ready diagnosis of this entity.

Necrotizing enterocolitis. Although this entity is occasionally encountered in adults, it is a more common and serious disease in the neonate. The etiology remains unclear yet it is known that in order for necrotizing enterocolitis (NEC) to develop there generally must be associated mucosal damage. In adults, a necrotizing type of enteropathy is associated with leukemia, especially in a setting of chemotherapy. In infants, formula feeding has a higher association with this condition compared to breast feeding. There probably is some bacterial involvement although no specific pathogens have been implicated.

Clinically, the patients present with bloody diarrhea. The early radiographic signs of this entity are distended loops of bowel, poor definition of the bowel wall, scalloped bowel wall outline, and separation of bowel loops (57, 58). Adynamic ileus ensues. Radiographically the diagnosis is most often suspected when pneumatosis intestinalis develops, a condition commonly associated with NEC (59). The intramural gas is present in linear streaks or in well-defined oval collections and may be either in the small bowel or colon. Further complications include gas in the portal venous system and bowel perforation. A late complication is bowel stenosis (60–62), although there is some evidence that such a 'stricture' may eventually resolve (63). An enterocolic fistula is a rare complication (64). In general, the small bowel tends to be involved more often than the colon.

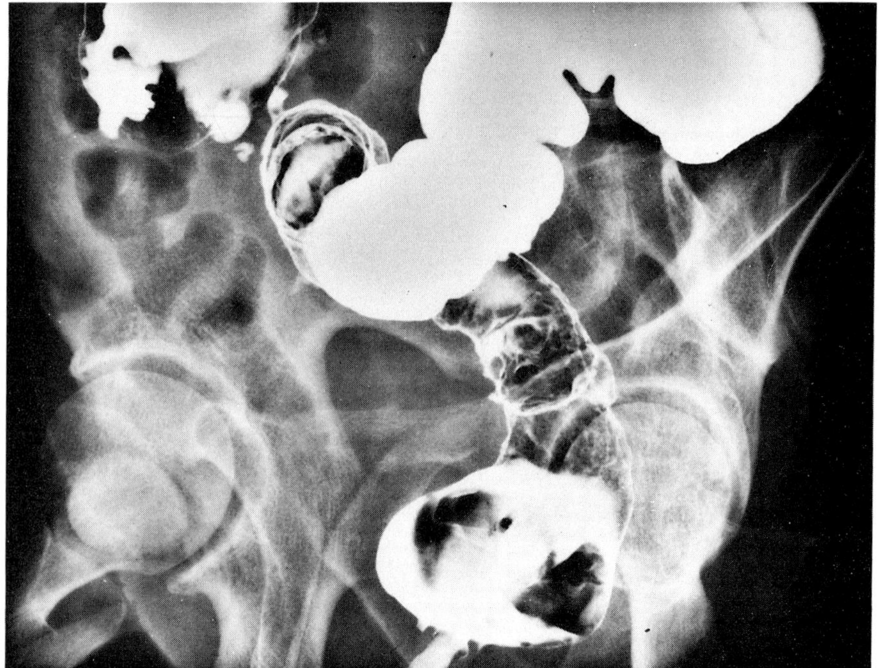

a

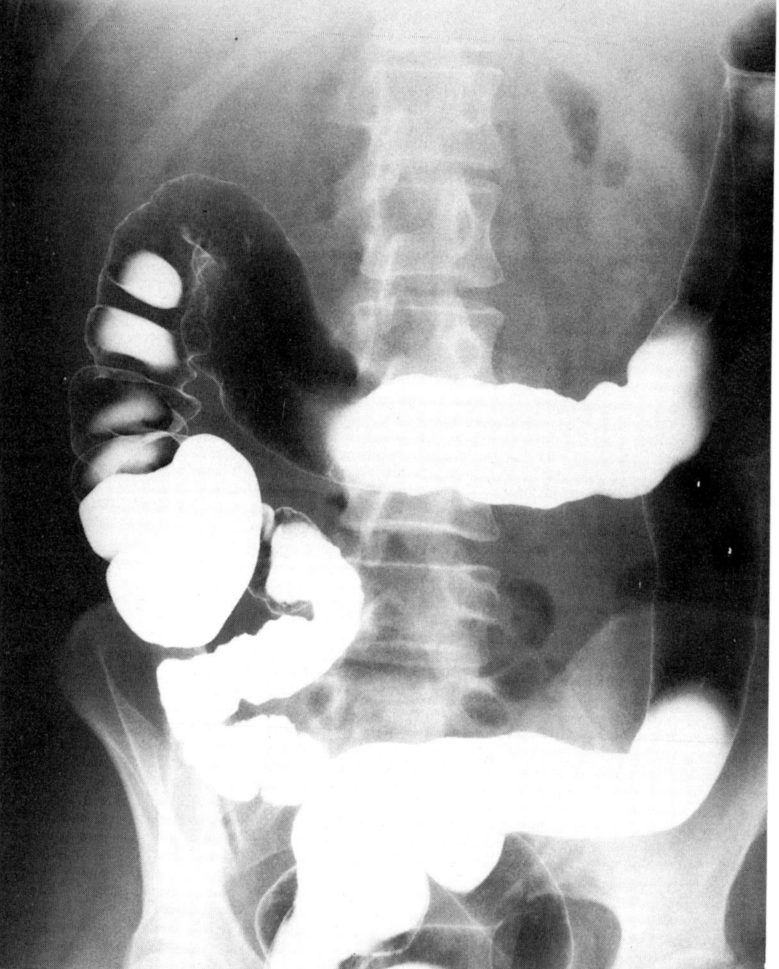

b

Fig. F.3.Campylobacter colitis. Numerous ulcers and flat polyps are scattered throughout the rectosigmoid. The bowel lumen is narrowed and the rectal valves destroyed. The remainder of the colon was normal. (b) Another patient with *Campylobacter* colitis shows involvement from the hepatic flexure distally. Small ulcerations are scattered throughout the involved area together with loss of haustra. The pattern is indistinguishable from ulcerative colitis. (Courtesy of Dr. Kollitz *et al.* (32), copyright 1981, Springer-Verlag.)

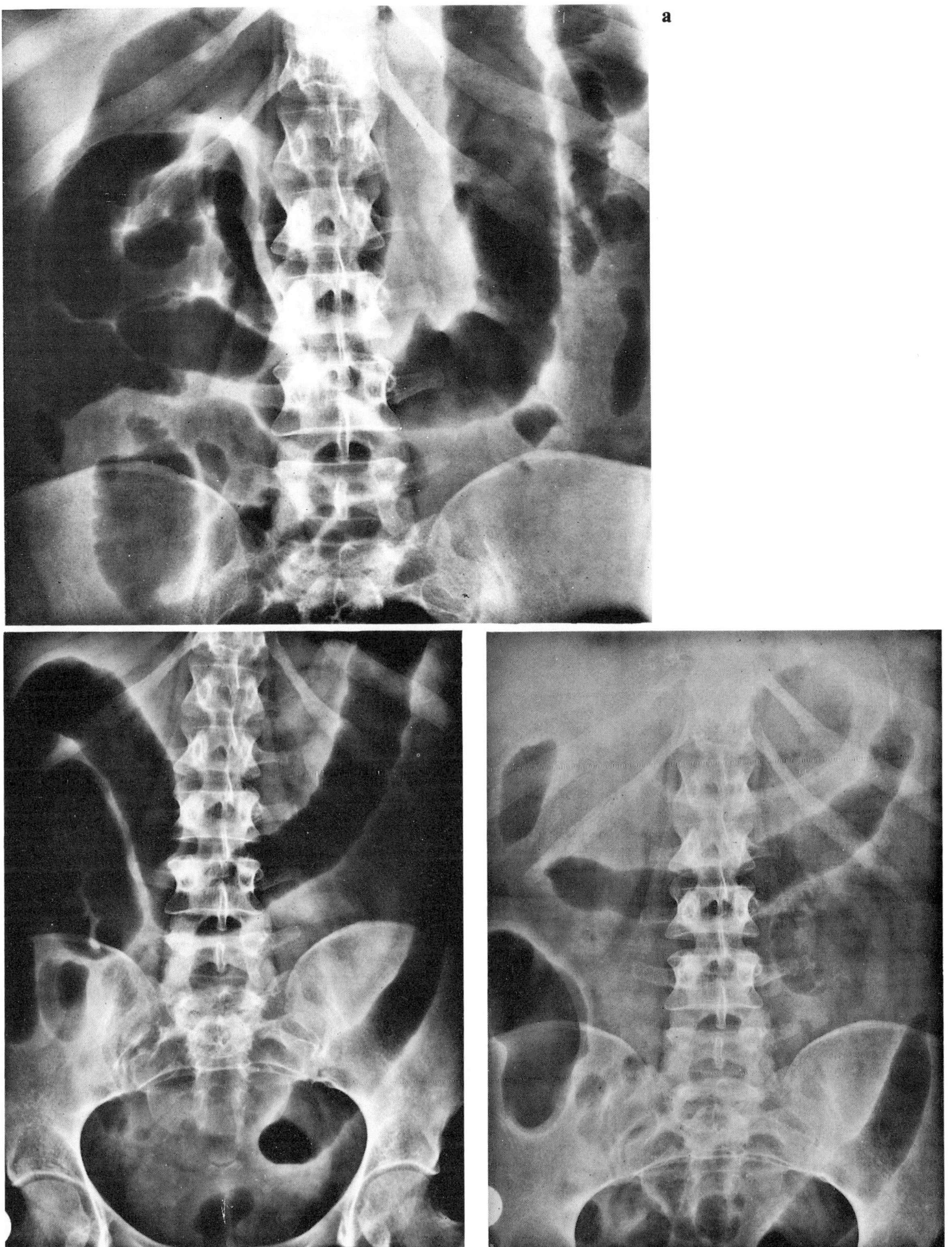

Fig. F.4. Antibiotic colitis. The patient had recently received several antibiotics, including clindamycin. She developed progressively severe diarrhea even when the antibiotics were stopped. (a) Shortly after the start of her symptoms there already is slight dilatation of the transverse colon with partial loss of haustra. (b) Two weeks later the haustra have been effaced and the colon has a 'tubelike' appearance. (c) Eventually the entire colon had a 'burned-out' colitis appearance. The patient recovered after a protracted illness.

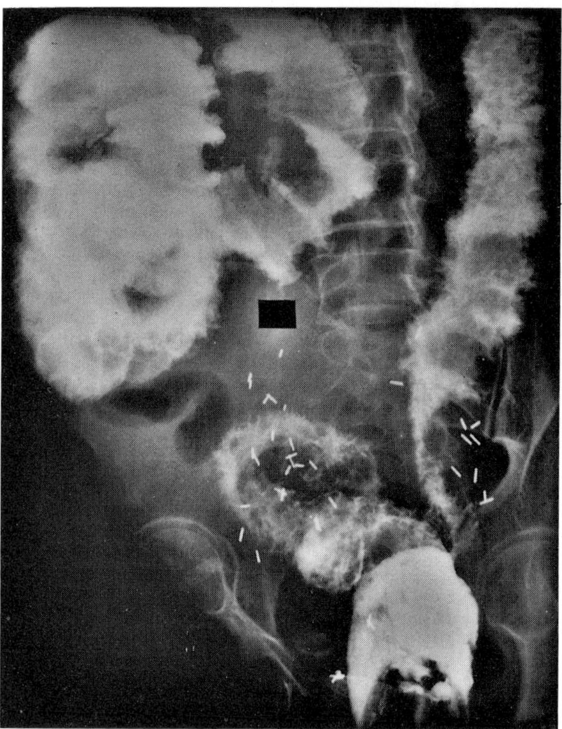

Fig. F.5. Antibiotic colitis. This 53-year-old female developed massive diarrhea two weeks after gynecological surgery. The shaggy outline due to edema, ulcers and intraluminal masses is evident throughout the colon and rectum.

A barium enema is probably not indicated and may actually be dangerous because of possible perforation if fulminant necrotising enterocolitis is present. Very early in the disease, however, an enema probably is safe (65), although little additional information is generally obtained.

Pneumatosis intestinalis in the neonate should suggest NEC, yet pneumatosis may also be due to ischemia, cardiothoracic disease, or it may even be seen in the absence of any disease.

c. Parasitic colitides

Amebiasis. Amebiasis is caused by infection with the protozoan *Entamoeba histolytica*. Although this disease is endemic worldwide, it is considerably more common in tropical climates.

There are several amoebas which are parasitic to man, but only the *Entamoeba histolytica* is pathogenic. The incidence of infestation with *E. histolytica* is greater than the incidence of the disease itself, with significant tissue invasion being necessary before clinical amebiasis is evident. Different strains of *E. histolytica* appear to vary in their degree of pathogenicity and the resultant infections also vary in their severity. In addition, pathogenicity can be influenced by certain bacteria in the colon.

The range of disease varies between the relatively asymptomatic chronic carrier and the patient with fulminant bloody diarrhea and a severe systemic illness. With chronic infestation, the patient can have few localizing symptoms. The infection can be limited to the colon, or it can be found in the liver or lungs. The cecum is the most common site of involvement in most populations, although rectosigmoid disease is not unusual. Other sites of involvement, such as the brain, are rare, but are occasionally encountered.

Amebiasis is contracted only if food or drink contaminated with viable cysts is ingested. The cysts pass to the small bowel, rupture, and the contained metacysts divide, forming trophozoites. The trophozoites invade the colon wall by lytic digestion and, together with associated bacteria such as *E. coli*, produce colon ulcers. The trophozoites within the colon wall feed upon the host and multiply. Any trophozoites discharged into the lumen gradually produce a surrounding cystic membrane, mature, and are excreted. Depending upon environmental conditions, viable cysts can survive for prolonged periods of time.

After invasion of the colon mucosa, the parasites multiply and spread in the submucosa, since muscle tissue tends to form a barrier to the initial spread of organisms. First, there are small ulcers in the involved area. Noncontrast radiographs are generally unrewarding. A barium enema performed at this point in the disease will reveal multiple small ulcers and edema, usually localized to one part of the colon (66, 67) (Fig. F.6). With severe involvement, the ulcers may deepen and extend in the wall of the colon, presenting with a ‘collar-button’ or flask-shaped appearance. Scattered areas of involvement may be present. Associated bacterial invasion of the ulcers results in further damage. With extensive invasion, the overlying mucosa sloughs, resulting in large confluent ulcers, with the ulcers eventually penetrating into the muscle layers to varying depths (Fig. F.7). Perforation and peritonitis are rare complications.

With chronic amebiasis, strictures or masses may develop, with the masses being caused by infection of amebic granulomas. These masses or amebomas, can be located anywhere in the colon, although the most common locations are the cecum and rectum. The strictures are usually symmetrical in appearance, smooth, and tend to be located at the flexures. They can be either long or short in length (Fig. F.8). The amebomas appear similar to neoplastic polyps and may be part of a stricture. Skip areas may be seen. The cecum can become narrowed and cone-shaped. Quite often the ileocecal valve is thickened and there is free reflux into the ileum. Generally, there is no gross involvement of the ileum. The considerable bowel wall thickening is due to inflammation and edema; the resulting radiographic appearance is that of 'thumbprinting'. Chronic disease may eventually lead to marked colon foreshortening, loss of haustra, and a smooth outline typical of end-stage appearance of the various colitides.

Toxic megacolon, consisting of dilatation and edema, may be precipitated by severe involvement of the colon. If such toxic dilatation is suspected, an acute abdominal examination should be obtained for confirmation; similar to a toxic megacolon due to the other colitides, a barium enema is a contraindication.

Especially in children, an ameboma may act as a lead point for intussuseption. Barium enema reduction of the intussuseption should reveal the underlying colitis.

At times, differentiation of an amebic stricture or ameboma from carcinoma is impossible. Few signs are reliable. If the diagnosis is suspected, clinical improvement with antiamebic medication may be

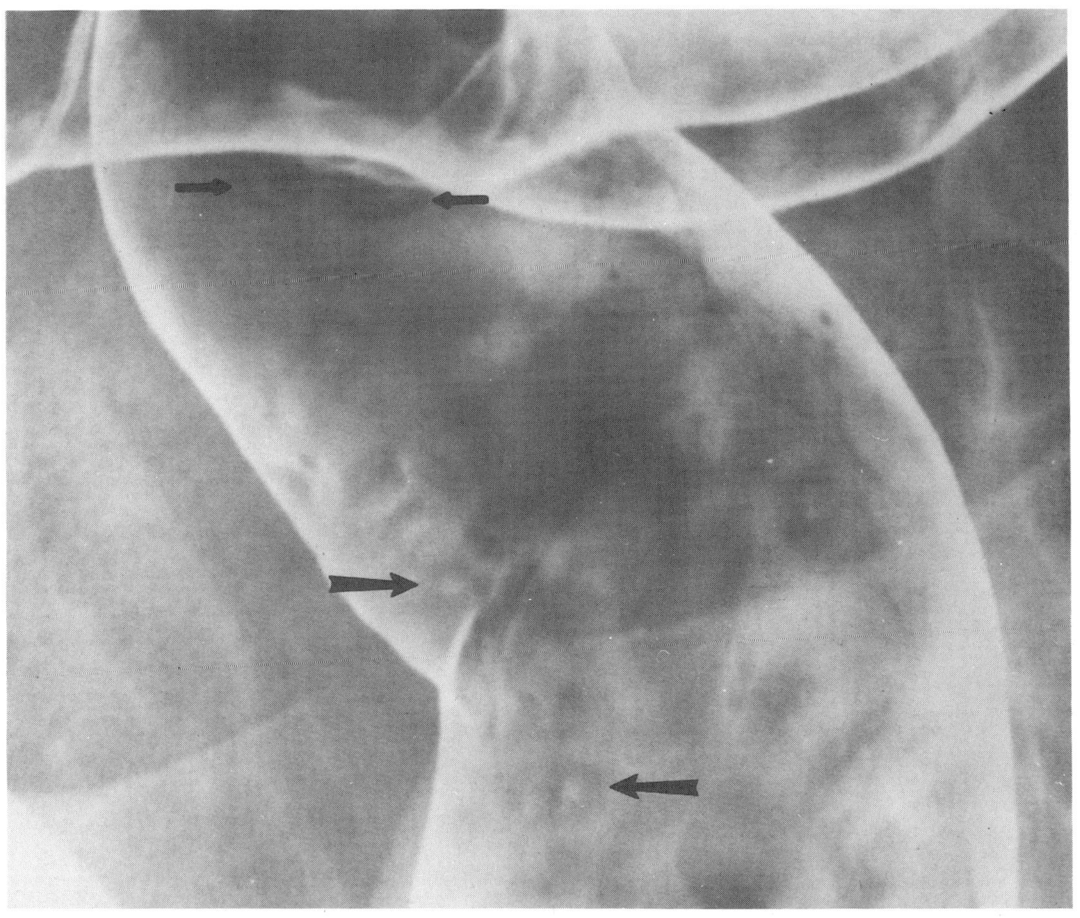

Fig. F.6. Amebic colitis. There are discrete rectosigmoid ulcers, with some appearing curvilinear (small arrows) and others having a typical aphthous appearance (large arrows). (Courtesy of Drs. R.J. Max and F.M. Kelvin (67), copyright 1980, ARRS.)

useful. Amebiasis can also be confused with regional enteritis or ulcerative colitis. In regional enteritis with extensive right colic disease the terminal ileum is usually also diseased; amebiasis tends to spare the ileum. Tuberculosis often involves the terminal ileum.

Complicating the picture is the occasional patient with amebiasis who also develops a carcinoma of the colon (68).

Amebiasis can be diagnosed by identifying the *E. histolytica* cysts in the stool, although the periodic absence of amebae in the stools may compound the difficulty of diagnosis (69). If time permits, several serological tests are available.

Schistosomiasis. Over 100 million people are infected by schistosomiasis, a disease already known to the ancient Egyptians (70). The morbidity and mortality from this infestation remain high in spite of medical advances.

The schistosomiases of importance are due to infection with *Schistosoma japonicum*, *S. mansoni* and *S. haematobium*, although other species may also produce infection. *S. mansoni*, which is widespread throughout the tropical world, is found in the United States mainland and Puerto Rico. *S. haematobium* is found primarily in Africa and southern parts of Asia, while *S. japonicum* occurs in eastern Asia.

These blood flukes live primarily in the venous system, with the portal venous system being primarily involved. The flukes mature in the portal venules, lay eggs, and the venules rupture into the bowel lumen. The eggs are excreted and start a new cycle of infestation, with snails acting as the intermediate host.

S. haematobium manifests primarily in the genitourinary tract. *S. mansoni* and *S. japonicum* involve the bowel and lungs.

The schistosoma eggs incite an inflammatory reaction which progresses to granuloma formation and eventual stricture. An arteritis can ensue. Clinically, the patients have bloody diarrhea and there may be systemic symptoms. Portal hypertension, hepatomegaly and splenomegaly may develop.

A barium enema during the acute phase of the disease reveals bowel wall edema and ulcers (Fig.

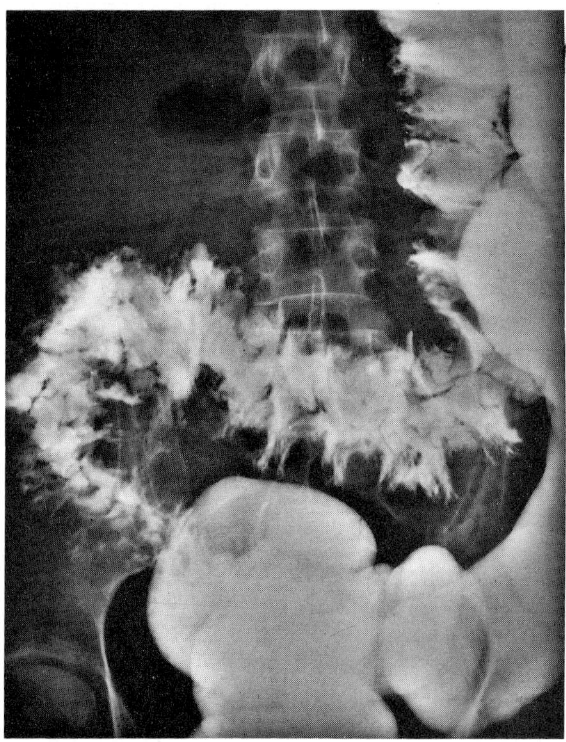

a

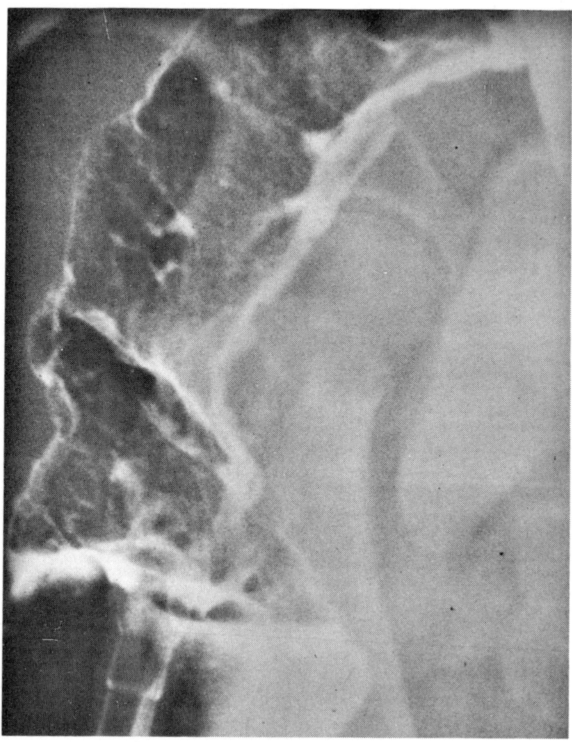

b

Fig. F.7. (a) Severe amebic colitis involving the right and transverse portions of the colon. Extensive ulcerations and inflammatory masses are present throughout the involved colon. (Courtesy of Dr. John Melmed, Soughton, MA.) (b) Rectal amebic colitis. Numerous inflammatory masses and scattered ulcers are present throughout the rectum. (Courtesy of Robert N. Berk, M.D., San Diego.)

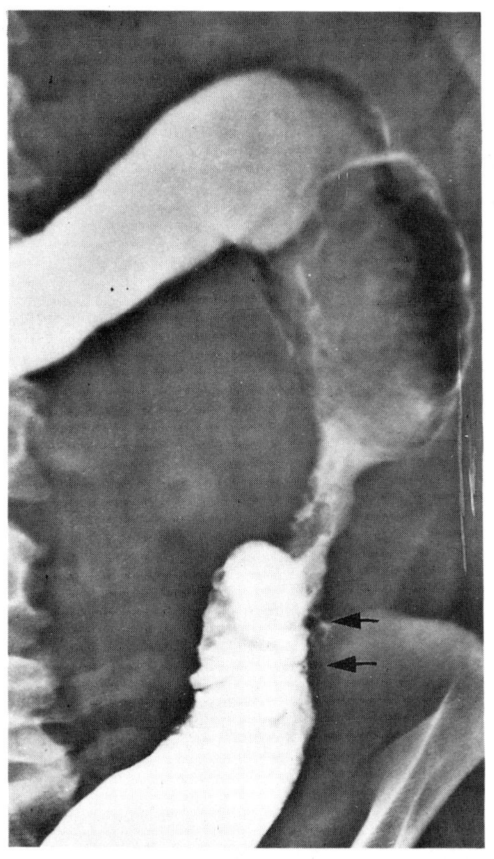

F.9). Inflammatory polyps of varying size containing schistosome eggs may develop (71). Although the entire colon can be involved, generally the greatest changes are in the rectosigmoid. Overall, the appearance is similar to ulcerative colitis. If inflammatory polyps predominate, one of the polyposis syndromes may be suspected. With chronic schistosomiasis calcifications may appear in the wall of the colon (71). There is a higher incidence of colon cancer in patients who have had long-standing chronic schistosomiasis (72, 73).

Overall, the radiographic findings are nonspecific. The appearance may be similar to regional enteritis, although fistulae are unusual in schistosomiasis.

Diagnosis is established by finding the parasite's eggs either in the stool or in samples of rectal biopsy.

Chagas' disease. Chagas' disease is caused by in-

Fig. F.8. (a) Amebic colitis. A relatively long stricture is present in the descending colon. The stricture has smooth proximal and distal margins. Several deep ulcers are present (arrowheads). (b) Cecal ameboma (arrows). A neoplastic polyp can have a similar appearance. (Courtesy of Robert N. Berk, M.D., San Diego.)

a

b

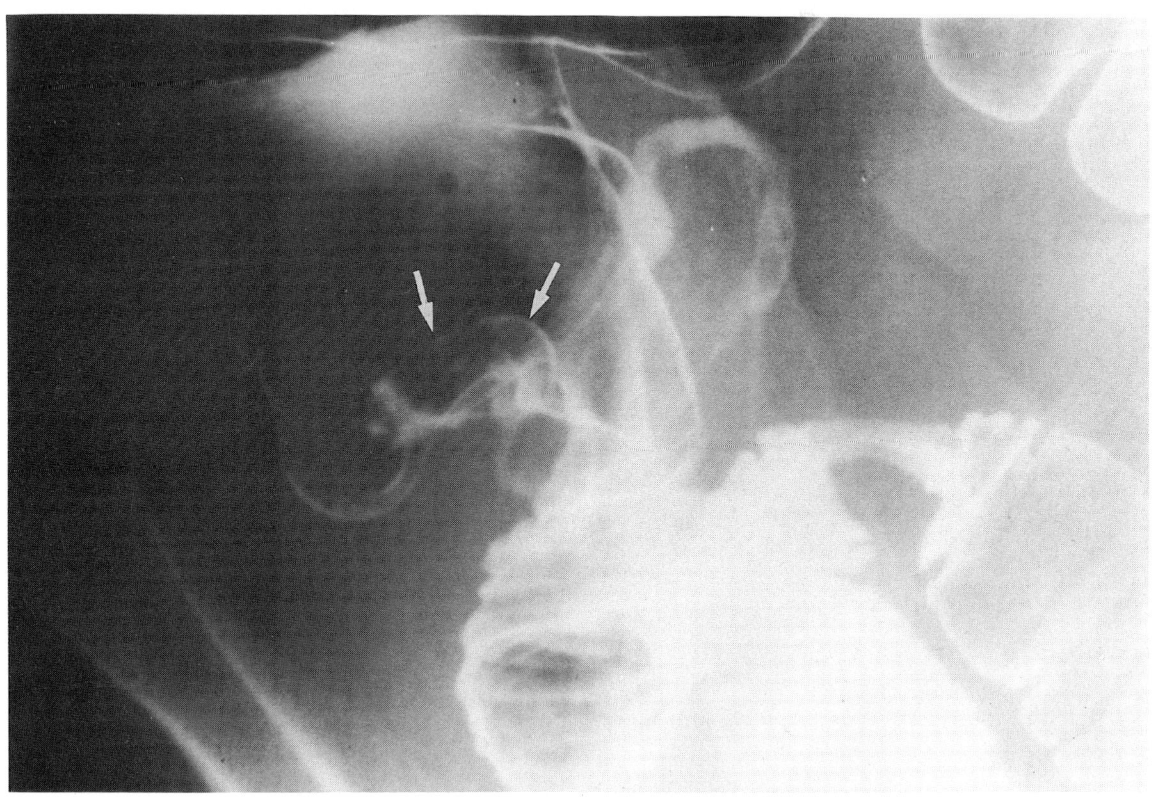

festation with the protozoan *Trypanosoma cruzi*. The protozoan is spread by the bite of the *Triatoma* bug. This disease is found in Central and South America where it is endemic and may occasionally be found in the southwestern United States.

Chagas' disease involves primarily the heart. Involvement of the autonomic nervous system of the gut with destruction of the ganglion cells results in bowel dilatation (74). These patients generally have chronic constipation.

The acute abdominal examination reveals a markedly dilated, stool filled colon. A barium enema shows marked colorectal dilatation throughout, the haustra may be effaced and, in general, there is poor tonicity. One should avoid overfilling the colon since undue barium retention may result. Superimposed inflammation due to stasis may result in ulceration. Acute perforation, due to stasis ulceration, may also occur (75). Characteristically the rectosigmoid shows greater involvement than the rest of the colon. Due to the resultant redundancy of the sigmoid, patients are prone to sigmoid volvulus (75).

The differential diagnosis includes a neoplasm with proximal dilatation and a stricture due to the various colitides. A technically adequate examination should show the rectosigmoid dilatation of Chagas' disease and exclude any organic lesion. There may be some confusion between Chagas' disease and Hirschsprung's disease, yet the appropriate geographical setting, the patient's age, and any possible esophageal involvement should allow ready differentiation between these two entities. Megacolon secondary to myxedema may occasionally be part of the differential diagnosis.

Trichuriasis. Infestation with the nematode *Trichuris trichiura* can result in colon involvement. This infection is encountered primarily in the warmer climates, including the southern portions of the United States. The adult whipworm, up to 5 cm in length, attaches to the mucosa and may result in rectal bleeding.

Typically, the cecum is involved and has a nonspecific pear-shaped appearance (76). Some patients will have a normal barium enema while others will show a nonspecific edema and a granular pattern. Rarely, an intraluminal mass will mimic a carcinoma (77). A double contrast examination may delineate the outline of numerous small worms attached to the colon wall (70, 78).

Diagnosis involves finding the characteristic eggs in the patient's stool.

Strongyloides colitis. The nematode *Strongyloides stercoralis* gains access through the skin, matures in the lungs, ascends the trachea and is swallowed, and may infiltrate into the bowel wall to lay eggs. Most infected patients are asymptomatic, although eosinophilia is generally present. Chronic debilitated patients and those who are immunosuppressed are especially at risk (79). Infection can result in tissue destruction, granuloma formation, and lymphatic obstruction.

A barium enema reveals changes similar to those seen in ulcerative colitis (80). Shallow ulcers are not unusual in the involved portions of bowel. Multiple such ulcers and shallow sinus tracts may be present. A small bowel examination may reveal similar involvement of the ileum (80). The radiographic changes are reversible after adequate medical therapy.

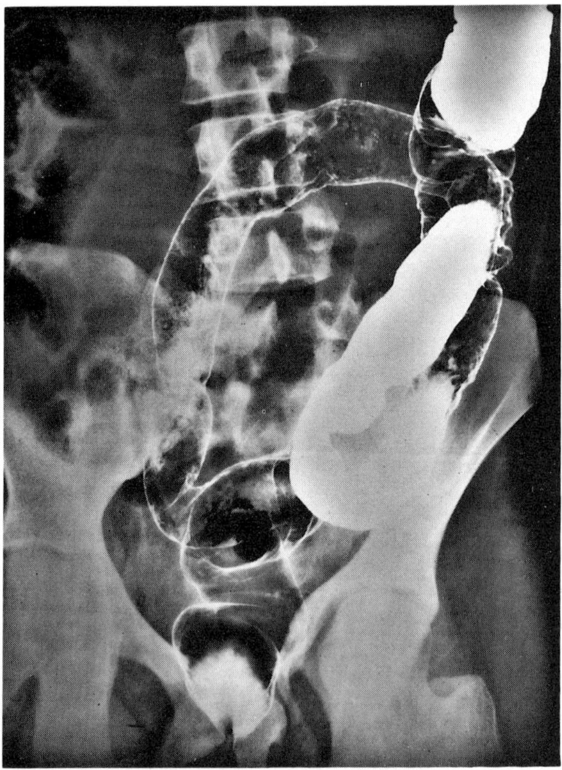

Fig. F.9. Schistosomiasis. There are multiple small ulcers and inflammatory polyps scattered throughout the distal colon. (Courtesy of Dr C. Bartram, London).

d. Fungal colitides

Histoplasmosis. Infection with *Histoplasma capsulatum* is relatively common throughout the major river basin areas of the United States. It is generally manifested as a pulmonary or cutaneous disease, with the gastrointestinal tract only occasionally being infiltrated. As with tuberculosis, there can be primary intestinal involvement mimicking colitis (81).

Clinically, the diagnosis of histoplasmosis is difficult. Often there is a setting of chronic illness. Massive hemorrhage, although unusual, may be the initial presentation. Likewise, perforation or obstruction may be rare complications. Both anemia and leukopenia may be present. If the rectum is involved, rectal biopsy may reveal the fungus (81). With systemic involvement, one may isolate the fungus from blood or lymph nodes. Any part of the intestinal tract may be involved, with involvement of the ileocecal region being common.

Quite often chest radiographs reveal evidence of disease. Abdominal radiographs can show typical histoplasma-like calcifications in the spleen. There may be hepatomegaly, splenomegaly, or both. Contrast studies of the colon and terminal ileum reveal thick folds, nodules or ulcers (82). The ulcers are shallow initially but may become deep in an occasional patient. The inflammatory nodules may progress to large intraluminal polyps or even encircling lesions mimicking carcinoma. Involvement of the ileocecal valve region can result in a large inflammatory mass mimicking a periappendiceal abscess, tuberculosis or a carcinoma (83). With chronic disease, there can be colon strictures suggesting regional enteritis, tuberculosis, or carcinoma.

Actinomycosis. Actinomyces israelii is an anaerobic saprophyte that can occasionally become pathogenic. The head and neck are most commonly involved, with the abdomen being the second most common site (84). With abdominal involvement the clinical findings are nonspecific and consist of vague abdominal pain and possibly diarrhea. An abdominal mass, especially in the right lower quadrant, may be palpable.

A barium enema reveals numerous strictures and fistulas, together with intra- and extraluminal masses (Fig. F.10). In particular, extensive intraabdominal fistulas should make one suspicious of actinomycosis. Most commonly the ileocecal region is involved.

The disease can mimic regional enteritis, diverticulitis, and occasionally amebiasis. Appendicitis may be suspected if the infection is located in the right lower quadrant. If there is a cutaneous fistula, the presence of a yellow-tinged discharge, consisting of so-called 'sulfur granules', can suggest the diagnosis.

Other fungal infections. South American blastomycosis, caused by *Paracoccidioides brasiliensis*, a mycotic infection, has two typical presentations; a cutaneous form involving the skin and oral mucosa, and a visceral form. The visceral form is common in Brazil and may also be encountered in patients from Central America. Usually the small bowel and right side of the colon are involved. The radiographic findings include stenotic segments, a contracted cecum, and a gaping ileocecal valve (85). Internal fistula may be present. Hepatosplenomegaly and abdominal masses may be palpable.

The differential diagnosis includes regional enteritis, actinomycosis, and occasionally tuberculosis and amebiasis. If there are cutaneous lesions present, the fungus can be readily identified from these.

North American blastomycosis, caused by *Blastomyces dermatidites*, does not involve the intestinal tract.

Other fungal diseases only rarely attack the intestinal tract. Nocardiosis has been reported to involve the appendix. Intestinal involvement tends to mimic amebiasis.

e. Venereal colitides

Lymphogranuloma venereum. This veneral disease is caused by *Chlamydia trachomatis*. It is present throughout the world, but is more commonly encountered in the tropics. Genitorectal lesions are common in women. These patients may have diarrhea, constipation, pain, or rectal hemorrhage. Eventually, as a stricture develops, the patients will complain of a change in bowel habits. Some patients develop significant strictures with few or no precedent symptoms. Sigmoidoscopy may show

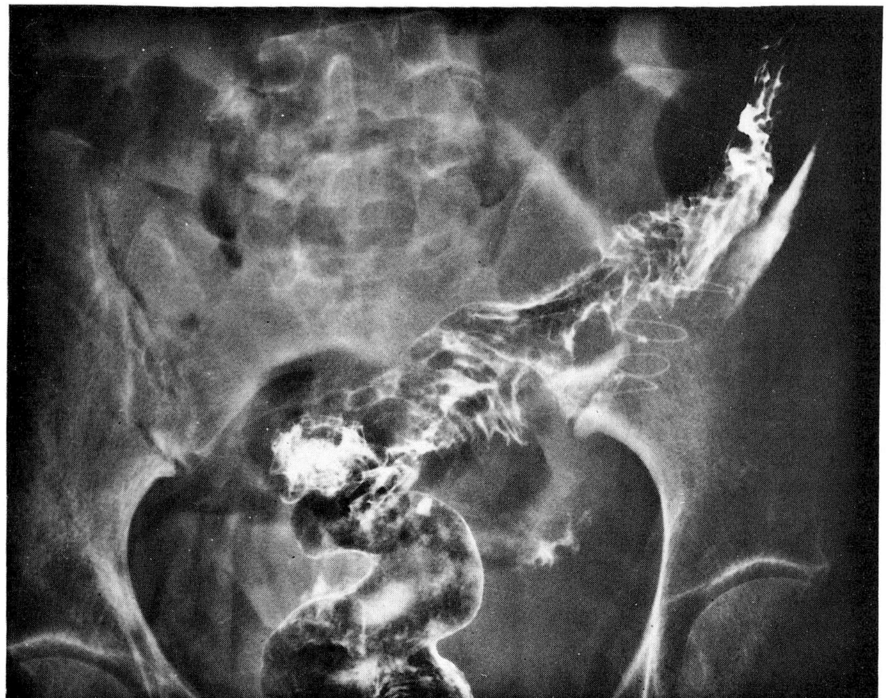

a

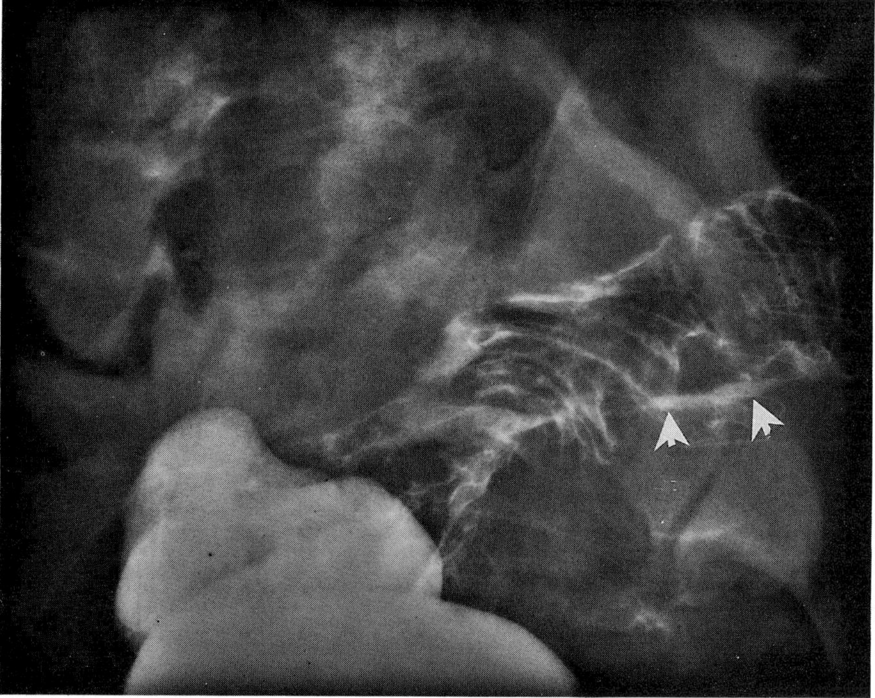

b

Fig. F.10. Colon actinomycosis in a 63-year-old woman. Previously she had cecal actinomycosis and now presented with a left lower quadrant mass and a colovesical fistula. (a) Frontal view shows marked sigmoid distortion. (b) A more distended sigmoid reveals that the colon folds are distorted and displaced, but not unduly destroyed. Several fistula are present (arrowheads). (c) Two months later the distortion and fistulas are still present. A stricture has now developed (arrowheads).

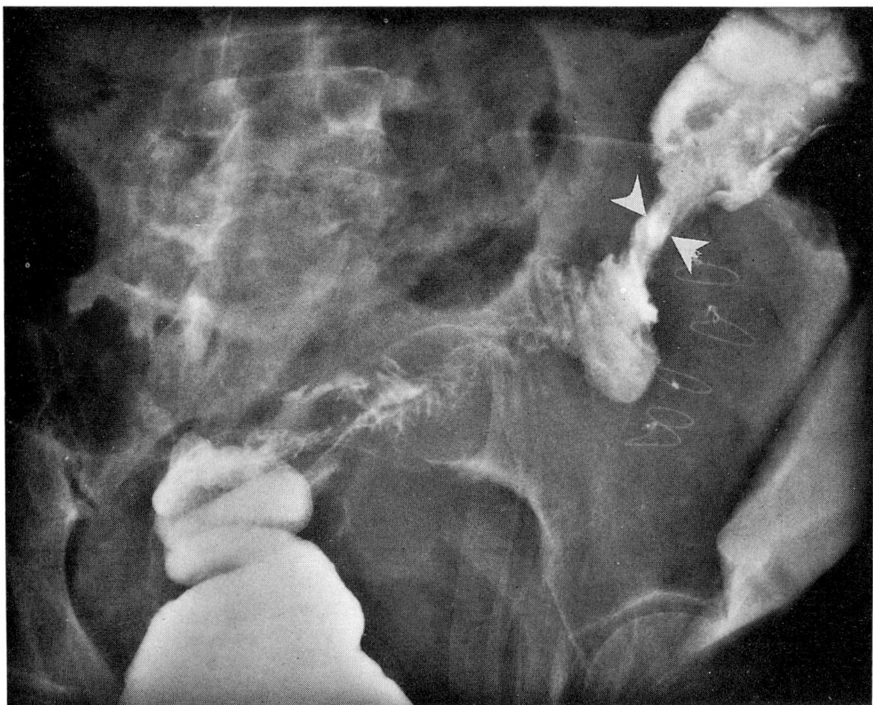

c

bleeding rectal ulcers; unfortunately, it may not be possible to perform sigmoidoscopy once a rectal stricture has developed. The colorectal findings are secondary to obstruction of lymphatics, bowel edema, and eventual fibrosis and stricture. Rectal biopsy may reveal granulomata.

The diagnosis can be suspected with the Frei antigen test or the complement fixation test, although the former may be relatively insensitive (86). Unfortunately, once the Frei test is positive it generally remains positive for the rest of the patient's life and thus simply indicates that the patient has or has had past infection. False negative and false positive results also occur. The complement fixation test is positive in approximately 80% of patients with this disease.

We believe that contrast studies of the colon should be performed in all patients suspected of harboring lymphogranuloma venereum of the rectum to document the extent of the disease. Shallow rectal ulcers are present initially. With progression, numerous ulcers of varying depth are scattered throughout the involved segment. Loss of haustra is common. The ulcers can develop into fistulous tracks to the perirectal soft tissues and vagina and such fistulas are common (87). With further progression, the rectum becomes narrowed, with the strictured segment being in the distal rectum or extending proximally to involve all of the rectum and part of the sigmoid. The proximal edge of the lesion is sharply defined. The presacral space may be widened considerably and with severe involvement the valves of Houston are destroyed. Although the involved areas are usually limited to the rectum and distal sigmoid, occasionally there may be skip lesions with essentially normal colon in between.

The presence of distal colorectal strictures, ulcers, or fistulas should raise suspicion of lymphogranuloma venereum. Regional enteritis or actinomycosis may be confused with this entity. Similar findings may also be seen in ulcerative colitis and tuberculosis. Unfortunately, biopsy may reveal granulomas in some of these conditions. Fistulas are rare with schistosomiasis and should exclude this disease from the differential. Radiation proctitis and stricture due to past surgical instrumentation can be excluded by history. Regional enteritis and ulcerative colitis should be suspected if the colon reveals extensive proximal involvement. With rectal involvement only, the diagnosis becomes more difficult and the history, laboratory findings, and biopsy must be used to differentiate among these conditions. Extensive pelvic inflammatory disease can also generally be excluded clinically. Endometriosis usually is asymmetrical in appearance and has a different clinical presentation.

An extensive infiltrating carcinoma may mimic lymphogranuloma venereum; further complicating this differential is the fact that carcinoma can arise in an area involved by lymphogranuloma venereum (88, 89).

Gonorrheal proctocolitis. Although gonorrheal proctocolitis can be seen in women with a primary urogenital infection (90), this condition in males is found mainly in homosexuals (91). Many infected patients may be asymptomatic, yet rectal bleeding and tenesmus may occur (92). During endoscopy there generally is ready friability and bleeding. If a barium enema is performed, the most severe changes are generally in the rectum. A barium enema is poorly tolerated by these patients due to the marked spasticity. Considerable edema and shallow ulcers may be present (Fig. F.11). Chronic infection can eventually lead to rectal stricture.

In homosexuals gonococcal infection may be superimposed on another infection already present in the rectum (4).

Syphilitic gummata of the rectum are rare (93); they can mimic a carcinoma in gross appearance.

f. Viral colitis

Viral enteritis generally involves the duodenum and small bowel. A biopsy of the colon in proven Norwalk-like virus and rotavirus infections has been normal (94).

There are occasional reports of colon involvement by herpes zoster. The patients may present with apparent colon obstruction (95) or adynamic ileus (96). The few radiographic descriptions of herpes infection mention sharply defined polygonal and angular polyps which may progress to small ulcers within a localized segment of the colon (97). These polyps appear identical to those seen with colon urticaria (98, 99); whether the end reaction in both entities is the same remains to be established. These sharply marginated polyps differ from the smoother appearing neoplastic or inflammatory polyps. In general, the colon changes of herpes tend to parallel the cutaneous manifestations.

Herpes zoster infection may result in 'apparent' distal colon obstruction; whether such an obstruction is anatomic in nature or due to spread of the virus to the sympathetic motor ganglia is not yet clear.

Cytomegalovirus infection has been associated with cecal ulcers (100). These infections have occurred in a setting of immunosuppression after renal transplantation. Cytomegalovirus infection has also been associated with pseudomembrane formation and a colitis similar to that seen with post-antibiotic colitis (101).

References

1. Rowe B: The role of *Escherichia coli* in gastroenteritis. Clin Gastroenterol 8:625–644, 1979.
2. Carpenter CCJ: Mechanisms of bacterial diarrheas. Am J Med 68:313–316, 1980.
3. Palmer SR, Jephcott AE, Rowland AJ, Sylvester DGH: Person-to-person spread of *Salmonella typhimurium* phage type 10 after a common-source outbreak. Lancet, i:881–884, 1981.
4. Sohn N, Robilotti JG: The gay bowel syndrome. A review of colonic and rectal conditions in two male homosexuals. Am J Gastroenterol 67:478–484, 1977.
5. Bohrer SP: Typhoid perforation of the ileum. Br J Radiol 39:37–41, 1966.

a

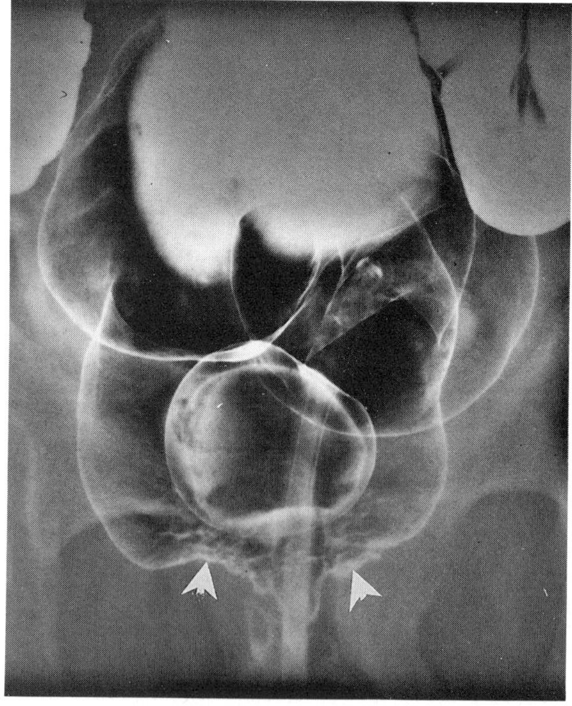

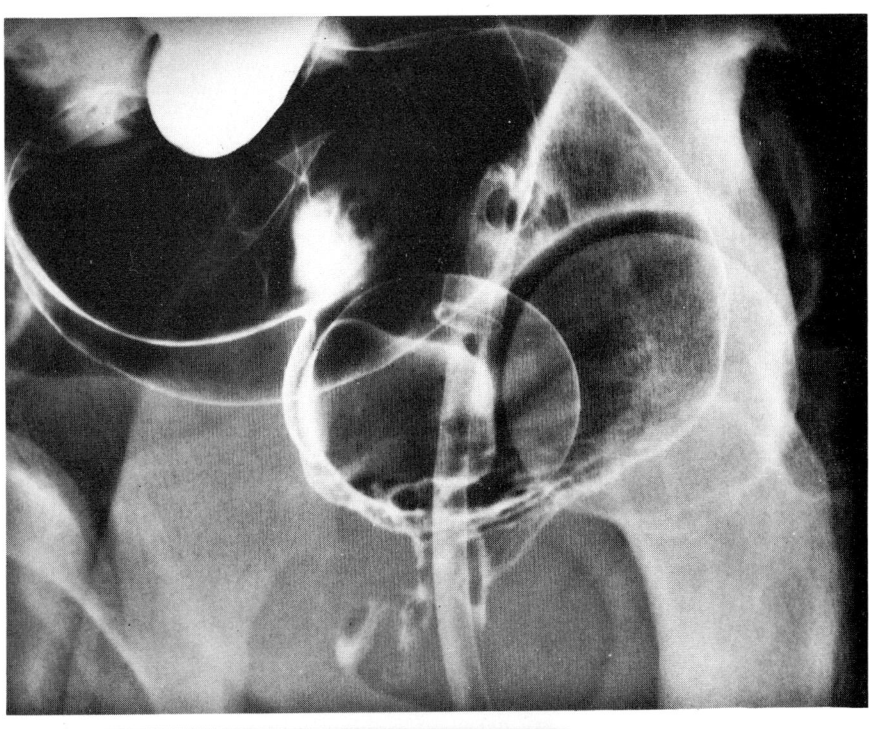

b

c

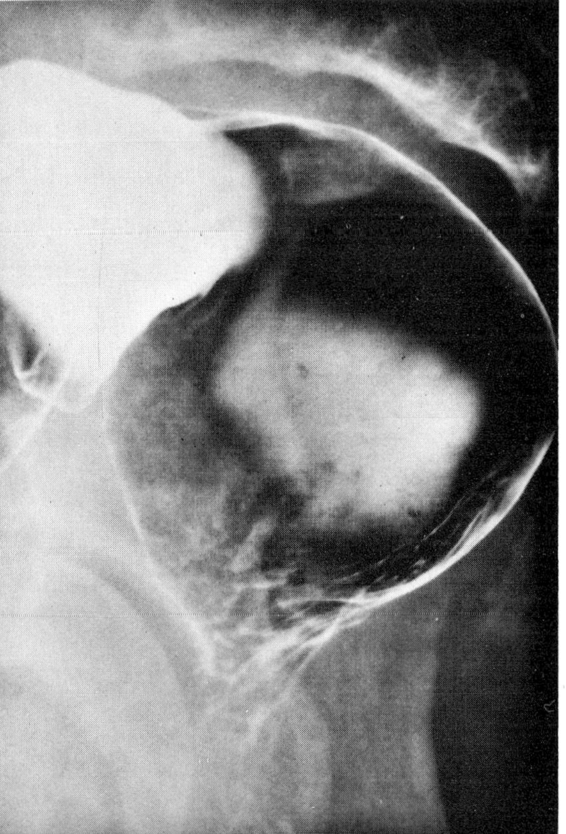

Fig. F.11. Gonococcal proctitis. (a) Frontal and (b) oblique views show multiple ulcers in the distal rectum (arrowheads). The diseased distal rectum was sharply marginated from the normal-appearing proximal bowel. An anal stricture necessitated use of a Foley catheter rather than a regular enema tip. (c) Lateral view after removing the Foley catheter shows the circumferential extent of the ulcers.

6. Schofield PF, Mandal BK, Ironside AG: Toxic dilatation of the colon in *Salmonella* colitis and inflammatory bowel disease. Br J Surg 66:5–8, 1979.
7. Dronfield MW, Fletcher J, Langman MJS: Coincident *Salmonella* infections and ulcerative colitis: problems of recognition and management. Br Med J 1:99–100, 1974.
8. Crohn BB, Ginzburg L, Oppenheimer GD: Regional ileitis. A pathologic and clinical entity. JAMA 99:1323–1329, 1932.
9. Carrera GF, Young S, Lewicki AM: Intestinal tuberculosis. Gastrointest Radiol 1:147–155, 1976.
10. Thoeni RF, Margulis AR: Gastrointestinal tuberculosis. Semin Roentgenol 14:283–294, 1979.
11. Stierlin E: Die Radiographie in der Diagnostik der Ileozoekaltuberculose und anderer Krankheiten des Dickdarms. Münch Med Wochenschr 1:1231–1235, 1911.
12. Anscombe AR, Keddie NC, Schofield PF: Caecal tuberculosis. Gut 8:337–343, 1967.
13. Vaidya MG, Sodhi JS: Gastrointestinal tract tuberculosis: a study of 102 cases including 55 hemicolectomies. Clin Radiol 29:189–195, 1978.
14. Balthazar EJ, Bryk D: Segmental tuberculosis of the distal colon: radiographic features in 7 cases. Gastrointest Radiol 5:75–80, 1980.
15. Patel MP, De I: Segmental tuberculosis of the colon with entero-colic fistula. Br J Radiol 45:150–152, 1972.
16. Herlinger H: Angiography in the diagnosis of ileocecal tuberculosis. Gastrointest Radiol 2:371–376, 1978.
17. Tishler JMA: Tuberculosis of the transverse colon. AJR 133:229–232, 1979.
18. King HC, Voss EC Jr: Tuberculosis of the cecum simulating carcinoma. Dis Colon Rectum 23:49–53, 1980.
19. Shrago G: *Yersinia enterocolitica* ileocolitis findings observed on barium examination. Br J Radiol 49:181–183, 1976.
20. van Wiechen PJ: Radiological changes in the distal part of the ileum in association with *Yersinia enterocolitica* infections. Radiol Clin Biol 43:242–253, 1974.
21. Capron J-P, Delamarre J, Delcenserie R, Gineston J-L, Dupas J-L, Lorriaux A: Liver abscess complicating *Yersinia pseudotuberculosis* ileitis. Gastronenterology 81:150–152, 1981.
22. Viteri AL, Howard PH, May JL, Ramesh GS, Roberts JW: Hepatic abscess due to *Yersinia enterocolitica* without bacteremia. Gastroenterology 81:592–593, 1981.
23. Hayasaka H, Ishikura H, Takayama T: Acute regional ileitis due to *Anisakis* larvae. Int Surg 55:8–14, 1971.
24. Vantrappen G, Agg HO, Ponette E, Geboes K, Bertrand P: Yersinia enteritis and enterocolitis: gastroenterological aspects. Gastroenterology 77:220–227, 1977.
25. Lachman R, Soong J, Wishon G, Maenza R, Hanelin L, St. Geme J: *Yersinia* colitis. Gastrointest Radiol 2:133–135, 1977.
26. Blaser MJ, Berkowitz ID, LaForce FM, Cravens J, Reller LB, Wang WLL: *Campylobacter* enteritis: clinical and epidemiologic features. Ann Intern Med 91:179–185, 1979.
27. Skirrow MB: *Campylobacter* enteritis: a 'new' disease. Br Med J 2:9–11, 1977.
28. Mensh RS, Brand MH, Troncale FJ: Campylobacter enterocolitis. J Clin Gastroenterol 3:147–151, 1981.
29. Drake AA, Gilchrist MJR, Washington JA Jr, Huizenga KA, VanScoy RE: Diarrhea due to *Campylobacter fetus* subspecies *jejuni*. A clinical review of 63 cases. Mayo Clin Proc 56:414–423, 1981.
30. Michalak DM, Perrault J, Gilchrist MJ, Dozois RR, Carney JA, Sheedy PF II: *Campylobacter fetus* ss. *jejuni:* A cause of massive lower gastrointestinal hemorrhage. Gastroenterology 79:742–745, 1980.
31. Blaser MJ, Parsons RB, Wang W-LL: Acute colitis caused by *Campylobacter fetus* ss. *jejuni*. Gastroenterology 78:448–453, 1980.
32. Kollitz JPM, Davis GB, Berk RN: *Campylobacter* colitis: A common infectious form of acute colitis. Gastrointest Radiol 6:227–229, 1981.
33. Groll A, Vlassembrouck MJ, Ramchand S, Valberg LS: Fulminating noninfective pseudomembranous colitis. Gastroenterology 58:88–95, 1970.
34. Stanley RJ, Tedesco FJ: Antibiotic-associated pseudomembranous colitis. CRC Crit Rev Clin Radiol 8:255–277, 1976.
35. Tedesco FJ: Clindamycin and colitis: a review. J Infect Dis 135:S95–S98, 1977.
36. Swartzberg JE, Maresca RM, Remington JS: Gastrointestinal side effects associated with clindamycin: 1000 consecutive patients. Arch Intern Med 136:876–879, 1976.
37. Gibson GE, Rowland R, Hecker R: Diarrhoea and colitis associated with antibiotic treatment. Aust NZ J Med 5:340–347, 1975.
38. Benner EJ, Tellman WH: Pseudomembranous colitis as a sequal to oral lincomycin therapy. Am J Gastroent 54:55–58, 1970.
39. Pittman FE, Pittman JC, Humphrey CD: Colitis following oral lincomycin therapy. Arch Intern Med 134:368–372, 1974.
40. Lusk RH, Fekety FR Jr, Silva J Jr, Bodendorfer T, Devine BJ, Kawanishi H, Korff L, Nakauchi D, Rogers S, Siskin SB: Gastrointestinal side effects of clindamycin and ampicillin therapy. J Infect Dis 135:S111–S119, 1977.
41. Newman RJ, McCollum CM: Pseudomembranous colitis due to cephradine. Br J Clin Pract 33:32–33, 1979.
42. Viscidi RP, Bartlett JG: Antibiotic-associated pseudomembranous colitis in children. Pediatrics 67:381–386, 1981.
43. Tedesco FJ, Barton RW, Alpers DH: Clindamycin-associated colitis: a prospective study. Ann Intern Med 81:429–433, 1974.
44. Fekety R, Kim K-H, Batts DH, Browne RA, Cudmore MA, Silva J Jr, Toshniwal R, Wilson KH: Studies on the epidemiology of antibiotic-associated *Clostridium difficile* colitis. Am J Clin Nutr 33:2527–2532, 1980.
45. Peikin SR, Galdibini J, Bartlett JG: Role of *Clostridium difficile* in a case of nonantibiotic-associated pseudomembranous colitis. Gastroenterology 79:948–951, 1980.
46. Tedesco F, Markham R, Gurwith M, Christie D, Bartlett JG: Oral vancomycin for antibiotic-associated pseudomembranous colitis. Lancet 2:226–228, 1978.
47. Tedesco FJ: Antibiotic-associated colitis — an abating enigma. J Clin Gastroenterol 3:221–224, 1981.
48. Tedesco FJ: Bacitracin therapy in antibiotic-associated pseudomembranous colitis. Dig Dis Sci 25:783–784, 1980.
49. Bartlett JG, Tedesco FJ, Shull S, Lowe B, Chang T: Symptomatic relapse after oral vancomycin therapy of antibiotic associated pseudomembranous colitis. Gastroenterology 78:431–434, 1980.
50. Bartlett JG, Chang TW, Gurwith M, Gorbach SL, Onderdonk AB: Antibiotic-associated pseudomembranous colitis due to toxin-producing clostridia. N Engl J Med 298:531–534, 1978.
51. Bartlett JG, Taylor NS, Chang TW, Dzink JA: Clinical and laboratory observations in *Clostridium difficile* colitis.

Am J Clin Nutr 33:2521–2526, 1980.
52. Dupont HL: Etiology of antibiotic-associated colitis. Gastroenterology 75:913–914, 1978.
53. Larson HE, Price AB, Honour P, Borriello SP: *Clostridium difficile* and the aetiology of pseudomembranous colitis. Lancet i:1063–1066, 1978.
54. Viscidi R, Willey S, Bartlett JG: Isolation rates and toxigenic potential of *Clostridium difficile* isolates from various patient populations. Gastroenterology 81:5–9, 1981.
55. Stanley RJ, Melson GL, Tedesco FJ, Saylor JL: Plain-film findings in severe pseudomembranous colitis. Radiology 118:7–11, 1976.
56. Ecker JA, Williams RG, McKittrick JE, Failing RM: Pseudomembranous enterocolitis — an unwelcome gastrointestinal complication of antibiotic therapy. Am J Gastroenterol 54:214–228, 1970.
57. Kogutt MS: Necrotizing enterocolitis of infancy. Early roentgen patterns as a guide to prompt diagnosis. Radiology 130:367–370, 1979.
58. Virjee J, Somers S, DeSa D, Stevenson G: Changing patterns of neonatal necrotizing enterocolitis. Gastrointest Radiol 4:169–175, 1979.
59. Kleinman P, Meyers MA, Abbott G, Kazam E: Necrotizing enterocolitis with pneumatosis intestinalis in systemic lupus erythematosus and polyarteritis. Radiology 121:595–598, 1976.
60. Costin BS, Singleton EB: Bowel stenosis as a late complication of acute necrotizing enterocolitis. Radiology 128:435–438, 1978.
61. Kosloske AM, Burstein J, Bartow SA: Intestinal obstruction due to colonic stricture following neonatal necrotizing enterocolitis. Ann Surg 192:202–207, 1980.
62. Virjee JP, Gill GJ, DeSa D, Somers S, Stevenson GW: Strictures and other late complications of neonatal necrotising enterocolitis. Clin Radiol 30:25–31, 1979.
63. Tonkin ILD, Bjelland JC, Hunter TB, Capp MP, Firor H, Ermocilla R: Spontaneous resolution of colonic strictures caused by necrotizing enterocolitis: therapeutic implications. AJR 130:1077–1081, 1978.
64. Paley RH, McCarten KM, Cleveland RH: Enterocolonic fistula as a late complication of necrotizing enterocolitis. AJR 132:898–900, 1979.
65. Leonidas JC, Bhan I, Leape LL: Barium enema in suspected necrotizing enterocolitis: is it ever indicated? Clin Radiol 31:587–590, 1980.
66. Cardozo JM, Kimura K, Stoopen M, Cervantes LF, Elizondo L, Churchill R, Moncada R: Radiology of invasive amebiasis of the colon. AJR 128:935–941, 1977.
67. Max RJ, Kelvin FM: Nonspecificity of discrete colonic ulceration on double-contrast barium enema study. AJR 134:1265–1267, 1980.
68. Camacho E: Amebic granuloma and its relationship to cancer of the cecum. Dis Colon Rectum 14:12–16, 1971.
69. Vajrabukka T, Dhitavat A, Kichananta B, Sukonthamand Y, Tanphiphat C, Vongviriyatham S: Fulminating amoebic colitis: a clinical evaluation. Br J Surg 66:630–632, 1979.
70. Reeder MM, Hamilton LC: Radiologic diagnosis of tropical diseases of the gastrointestinal tract. Radiol Clin North Am 7:57–81, 1969.
71. Lehman JS Jr, Farid Z, Bassily S, Kent DC: Colonic calcification and polyposis in schistosomiasis. Radiology 98:379–380, 1971.
72. Shindo K: Significance of *Schistosomiasis japonica* in the development of cancer of the large intestine: report of a case and review of the literature. Dis Colon Rectum 19:460–469, 1976.
73. Ming-Chai C, Pei-Yu C, Chi-Yuan C, Yi-Jen C, Fu-Pan W, Yang-Chuan T, Shun-Chuan C: Colorectal cancer and schistosomiasis. Lancet i:971–973, 1981.
74. Köberle F: Enteromegaly and cardiomegaly in Chagas' disease. Gut 4:399–405, 1963.
75. Ferreira-Santos R, Carril CF: Acquired megacolon in Chagas' disease. Dis Colon Rectum 7:353–363, 1964.
76. Manzano C, Thomas MA, Valenzuela C: Trichuriasis. Roentgenographic features and differential diagnosis with lymphoid hyperplasia. Pediatr Radiol 8:76–78, 1979.
77. Kojima Y, Sakuma H, Imuzi R, Nakagawara G, Miyazaki I, Yoshimura H: A case of granuloma of the ascending colon due to penetration of *Trichuris trichiura*. Gastroenterol Jpn 16:193–196, 1981.
78. Fischer RM, Cremin BJ: Rectal bleeding due to *Trichuris trichiura*. Br J Radiol 43:214–215, 1970.
79. Milder JE, Walzer PD, Kilgore G, Rutherford I, Klein M: Clinical features of *Strongyloides stercoralis* infection in an endemic area of the United States. Gastroenterology 80:1481–1488, 1981.
80. Drasin GF, Moss JP, Cheng SH: *Strongyloides stercoralis*: findings in four cases. Radiology 126:619–621, 1978.
81. Kirk ME, Lough J, Warner HA: Histoplasma colitis: an electron microscopic study. Gastroenterology 61:46–54, 1971.
82. Haws CC, Long RF, Caplan GE: *Histoplasma capsulatum* as a cause of ileocolitis. AJR 128:692–694, 1977.
83. Dietz MW: Ileocecal histoplasmosis. Radiology 91:285–289, 1968.
84. Sechas M, Christeas N, Balaroutsos C, Demertzis A, Skalkeas G: Actinomycosis of the colon: report of two cases. Dis Colon Rectum 15:366–369, 1972.
85. Avritchir Y, Perroni AA: Radiological manifestations of small intestinal South American blastomycosis. Radiology 127:607–609, 1978.
86. Schachter J, Smith DE, Dawson CR, Anderson WR, Deller JJ Jr, Hoke AW, Smartt WH, Meyer KF: Lymphogranuloma venereum. I. Comparison of the Frei test, complement fixation test, and isolation of the agent. J Infect Dis 120:372–375, 1969.
87. Annamunthodo H, Marryatt J: Barium studies in intestinal lymphogranuloma venereum. Br J Radiol 34:53–57, 1961.
88. Guzman L: Co-existence of chronic lymphogranuloma venereum and cancer. Radiology 41:151–156, 1943.
89. Levin I, Romano S, Steinberg M, Welsh RA: Lymphogranuloma venereum: rectal stricture and carcinoma. Dis Colon Rectum 7:129–134, 1964.
90. Olsen GA: Value of vaginal and rectal cultures in the diagnosis of gonorrhoea. Br J Vener Dis 47:102–106, 1971.
91. Klein EJ, Fisher LS, Chow AW, Guze LB: Anorectal gonococcal infection. Ann Intern Med 86:340–346, 1977.
92. Babb RR: Acute gonorrheal proctitis. Am J Gastroenterol 61:143–144, 1974.
93. Quinn TC, Lukehart SA, Goodell S, Mkrtichian E, Schuffler MD, Holmes KK: Rectal mass caused by *Treponema pallidum*: confirmation by immunofluorescent staining. Gastroenterology 82:135–139, 1982.
94. Blacklow NR, Cakor G: Viral gastroenteritis. N Engl J Med 304:397–406, 1981.
95. Kesner KM, Bar-Maor JA: Herpes zoster causing apparent low colonic obstruction. Dis Colon Rectum

22:503–504, 1979.

96. Johnson JN, Sells RA: Herpes zoster and paralytic ileus: a case report. Br J Surg 64:143–144, 1977.
97. Menuck LS, Brahme F, Amberg J, Sherr HP: Colonic changes of herpes zoster. AJR 127:273–276, 1976.
98. Berk RN, Millman SJ: Urticaria of the colon. Radiology 99:539–540, 1971.
99. Clemett AR, Fishbone G, Levine RJ, James AE, Janower M: Gastrointestinal lesions in mastocytosis. AJR 103:405–412, 1968.
100. Sutherland DER, Chan FY, Foucar E, Simmons RL, Howard RJ, Najarian JS: The bleeding cecal ulcer in transplant patients. Surgery 86:386–398, 1979.
101. Beaugrand M, Poynard T, Callard P, Ferrier JP, Bernades P, Molas G, Ferchal F, Perol Y: Recherche d'une infection à cytomégalovirus au cours des colites pseudo-membraneuses. Nouv Presse Med 10:1199–1203, 1981.

III.1.G. Radiation colitis

Radiation therapy to some malignant tumors can prolong patient survival. Unfortunately, simultaneous radiation to surrounding normal structures, such as the small bowel or colon, can result in significant damage. With pelvic radiation to the relatively common gynecological neoplasms, the adjacent ileum and colon can receive large doses of radiation. If the patient subsequently develops gastrointestinal complaints, the radiologist may be asked to differentiate between residuel neoplastic involvement and secondary radiation enterocolitis.

For some tumors, the radiation dose that can be administered is limited by the radiation sensitivity of adjacent bowel. Although there are ideosyncratic responses with serious injury occurring at relatively 'safe' radiation doses, generally little clinically significant symptomatology is expected with an externally administered dose of less than 4,000 rads. The severity of damage begins to increase with increasing dose. Tolerance to radiation is directly related to patient age (1). Most radiation enteritis patients become symptomatic within two years after the completion of therapy, although occasionally the damage manifests itself many years later.

The radiation damage to the colon can be divided into an acute and a chronic phase.

Acute radiation damage is manifested primarily by damage to the epithelium and to the capillaries. As the surface cells are destroyed, the underlying crypt cells begin to proliferate. Some mucosal damage can eventually heal, although if there has been sufficient radiation damage, necrosis and ulceration of the underlying structures occurs. The small vessels reveal swelling and proliferation of the endothelial cells with a resultant decrease in the lumen. Such an endarteritis, together with the subsequent ischemia, produces damage that will depend upon the radiation dose received by the involved tissue. If the colon is studied during this period, one sees ulcers and an irregular appearance resembling 'thumbprinting' (Fig. G.1).

Chronic damage consists of thickening of the vessel wall and gradual ischemia to the involved bowel. Significant chronic radiation injury generally manifests between six and eighteen months after therapy (2). The colon wall becomes edematous and thickened with extensive adhesions and fibrosis, together with muscle atrophy. The fibrosis can lead to stricture. In general, the changes secondary to radiation colitis are primarily from ischemia of the colon wall.

The radiographic changes of chronic radiation colitis range from ulcers, inflammatory polyps, stenotic segments, bowel wall rigidity, a 'tubelike' configuration to the colon, to elevation of the sigmoid colon out of the pelvis on postevacuation radiographs. Rectal involvement results in a narrowed tubular outline, similar to 'burned-out' colitis. The presacral space is often widened (3) (Fig. G.2). Long-term sequelae to small bowel irradiation likewise include a fixed, stenotic appearance (Fig. G.3). The most common appearance is that of a 'tubelike' narrowed segment with a smooth outline (Fig. G.4). The transition between abnormal and normal bowel is abrupt (Fig. G.5). Fistulae into the surrounding soft tissues, or a rectovesical or rectovaginal fistula can develop.

Angiography is of little use in evaluating radiation colitis. Occasionally, arterial stenosis or occlusion can be seen. The vasa recta tend to be tortuous and the involved bowel segment hypovascular (4). The veins can be irregular in outline and early draining veins are not uncommon (5). If new capillaries have formed, hypervascularity instead of hypovascularity is seen.

Generally, a past history of radiation, together with a typical appearance of radiation colitis, allows one ready diagnosis of this entity. Occasionally, the distinction from tumor, either primarily colic or serosal implantation, can be difficult. A large extrinsic mass or an asymmetrical

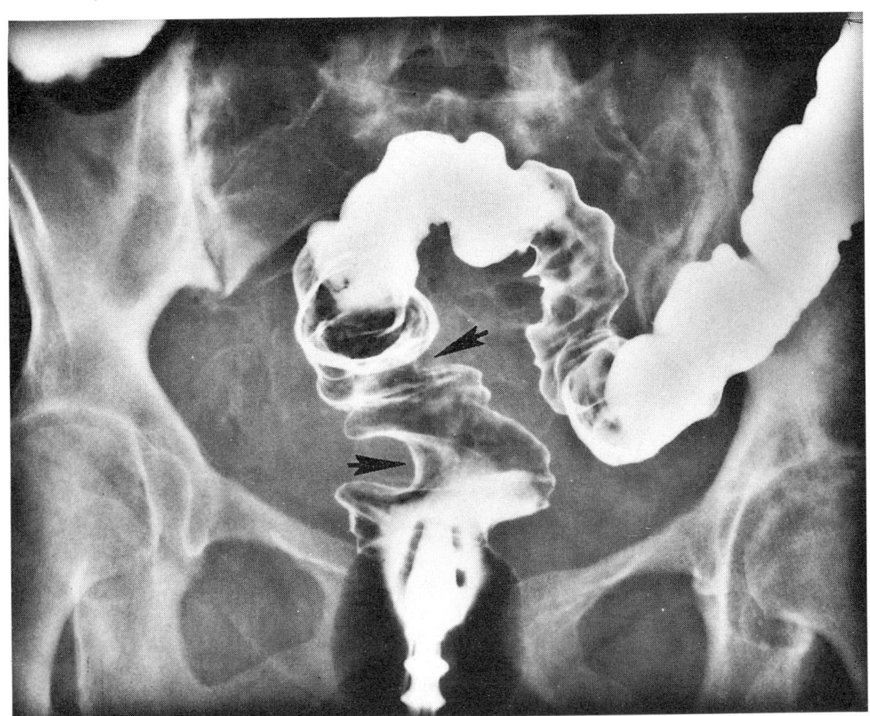

Fig. G.1. Shortly after radiation therapy the rectosigmoid is narrowed, the rectal valves thickened, and there is intramural thickening of the sigmoid colon (arrowheads). Colonoscopy revealed a friable mucosa. Nonspecific inflammation was present on the biopsy specimens.

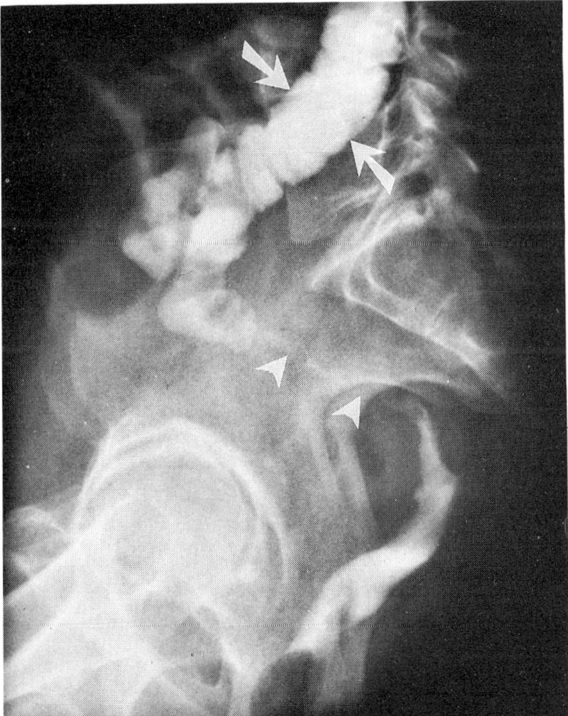

Fig. G.2. This 59-year-old patient had received pelvic irradiation and now presented with obstruction. A single-contrast barium enema was performed to locate the site of obstruction. The rectum is narrowed and the valves are obliterated. The rectosigmoid region is severely strictured (arrowheads). The presacral space is widened. The colon proximal to the stricture is not dilated (arrows), indicating that the major obstruction is not at the rectosigmoid. Further reflux identified an obstruction in the distal ileum.

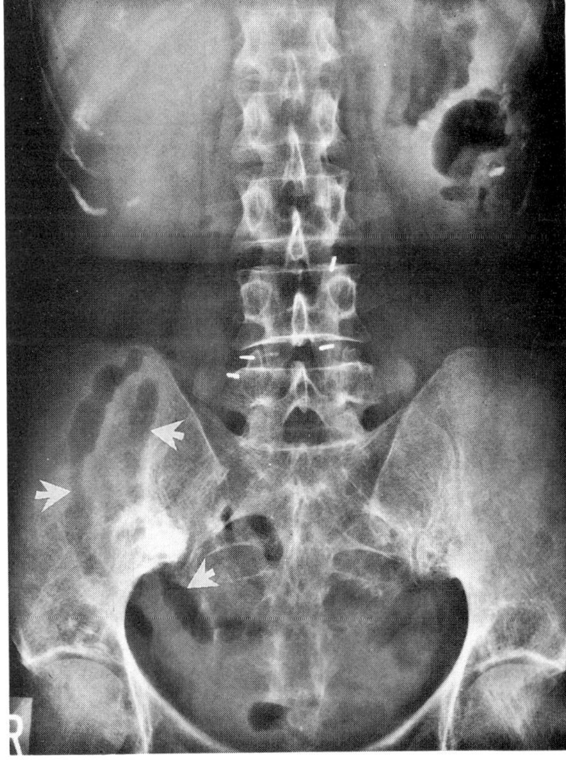

Fig. G.3. This patient received radiation therapy 20 years ago for fallopian tube adenocarcinoma. She has had intermittent small bowel obstruction. A stenotic, fixed loop of small bowel (arrowheads) has been a constant finding. Radiation changes are also present in the bones.

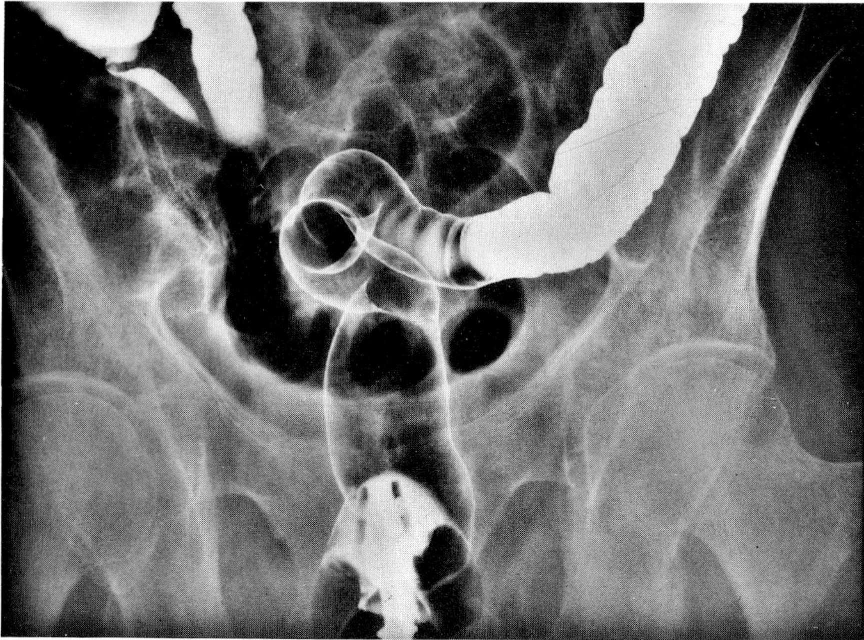

a

b

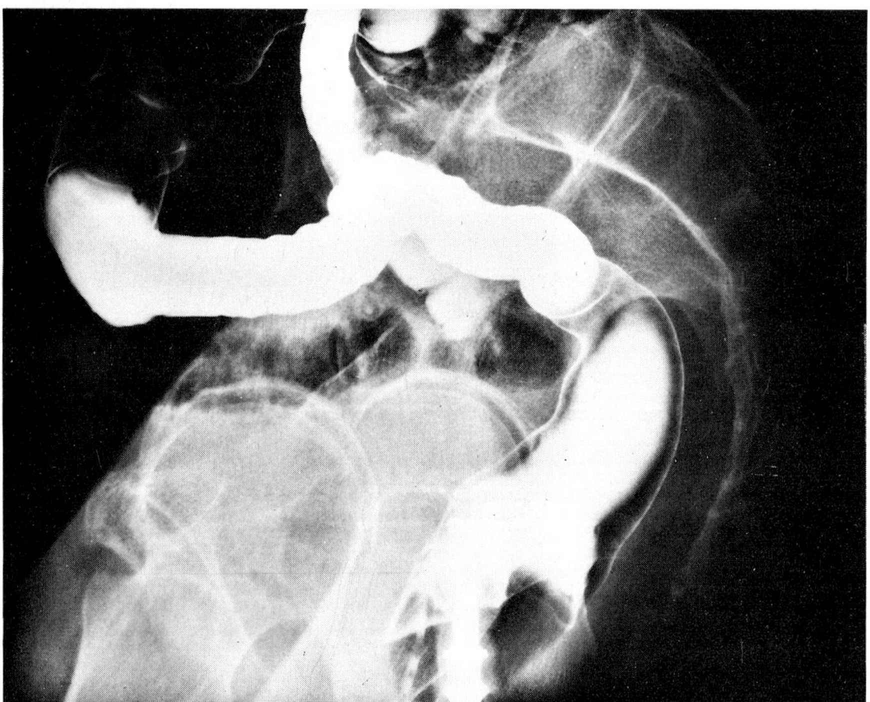

Fig. G.4. Radiation therapy was given to this 72-year-old patient with prostatic carcinoma. (a) Frontal and (b) lateral radiographs reveal considerable narrowing of the rectosigmoid lumen, obliteration of the rectal valves, and widening of the presacral space. No ulcers were present.

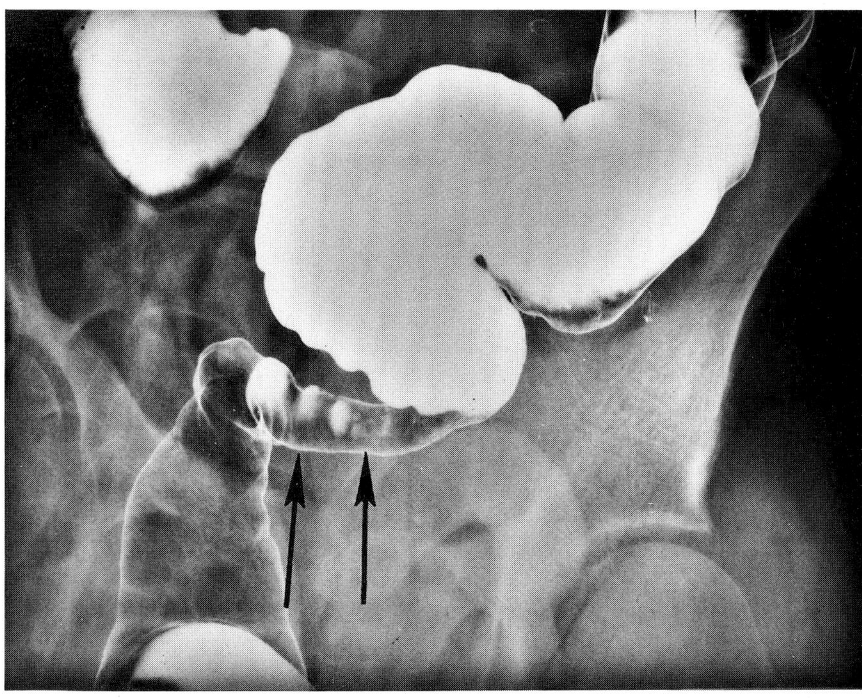

Fig. G.5. A stricture is present in the sigmoid (arrows). The junction between normal and abnormal bowel is abrupt, although the rectum is also involved by the radiation proctitis.

stricture generally implies tumor recurrence. Computerized tomography may be helpful in differentiating between the two conditions. If ulcers are present, radiation colitis may mimic some of the colitides. A previous examination can be very useful in narrowing the diagnosis to the actual condition present (3).

Both carcinoma and sarcoma can develop after radiation therapy. The average interval between radiation therapy and subsequent diagnosis of colorectal cancer is approximately 15 years, although an extreme range exists (6).

References

1. Jampolis S, Martin P, Schroder P, Horiot JC: Treatment tolerance and early complications with extended field irradiation in gynecological cancer. Br J Radiol 50:195–199, 1977.
2. Burg R, Abitbol A, Calanog A: Intestinal and anorectal complications of treatment for gynecologic malignancy. Dis Colon Rectum 22:459–465, 1979.
3. Meyer JE: Radiography of the distal colon and rectum after irradiation of carcinoma of the cervix. AJR 136:691–699, 1981.
4. Dencker H, Holmdahl KH, Lunderquist A, Olivecrona H, Tylen U: Mesenteric angiography in patients with radiation injury of the bowel after pelvis irradiation. AJR 114:476–481, 1972.
5. Sprayregen S, Glotzer P: Angiographic demonstration of radiation colitis. AJR 113:335–337, 1971.
6. Martins A, Sternberg SS, Attiyeh FF: Radiation-induced carcinoma of the rectum. Dis Colon Rectum 23:572–575, 1980.

III.2. DIVERTICULAR DISEASE

III.2.A. Introduction

The potential of diverticula as sites of infection was already pointed out by Cruveilhier in 1849 (1), yet diverticulitis was apparently regarded as a curiosity for many years thereafter. Although in the last century there were isolated reports describing colon diverticula, it was only after the introduction of the barium enema that it was shown that there exist asymptomatic patients with diverticulosis (2). The distinction between diverticulosis and diverticulitis was subsequently emphasized. Among leaders in devising a workable concept of diverticulosis was the radiologist Dr. Felix Fleischner, who together with others suggested that muscular dysfunction of the colon is of vital importance in the development of this entity (3).

'Diverticulosis' simply states that diverticula are present. 'Diverticulitis' is a clinically diagnosed entity due to inflammation of one or more diverticula. Diverticula are usually, but not always, present. Occasionally encountered is a typical clinical setting of diverticulitis, yet a barium enema shows none of the radiographic signs of diverticulitis. To avoid such confusion in trying to differentiate between diverticulosis and diverticulitis, the term, 'diverticular disease of the colon', is used by some investigators. This latter broad and non-specific term includes the early changes of colon muscular dysfunction, hypertrophy, subsequent diverticula formation, and later inflammation and other complications.

A surgeon may not appreciate the extent of diverticula formation because of considerable serosal fat. Since most diverticula fill readily with barium, the radiologist is in an excellent position to evaluate the size and extent of diverticulosis. The colonoscopist can also often identify diverticular communication with the colon lumen, although if the diverticular neck is narrow it can be readily missed. With a peridiverticular abscess the radiologist relies on secondary signs for a diagnosis, while a surgeon can readilly visualize such serosal extensions of the infection and inflammation.

III.2.B. Etiology and pathogenesis

It is surprising how little is known about the etiology and pathogenesis of both diverticulosis and diverticulitis. The clinical and radiographical distinction between diverticulosis and diverticulitis can be difficult. In some patients there is lack of correlation between pathological findings on post-mortem or surgical specimens and antecedent clinical symptoms (4, 5).

Diverticular disease is a disease of the affluent and industrialized nations (6), where the incidence appears to be increasing. The disease may be associated with a highly refined carbohydrate and low vegetable fiber diet (7) although such an association is being questioned. This disease is rare in rural Africa (8). It would seem that both racial factors and diet have an influence on the incidence of diverticulosis, since blacks in the United States have a higher incidence of diverticular disease as compared to blacks in Africa, yet diverticulosis in American blacks is still less common than in whites.

Diverticulosis may take up to 40 years to develop (6). The incidence of diverticular disease is the same in males and females. There is some suspicion that the incidence in the general population is increasing; however, part of this may be due to an overall older population group. There may be a predisposition to this entity in patients with collagen disease; Marfan's syndrome appears to be associated with both diverticulosis and diverticulitis in younger patients (9). The etiology may be due to the underlying generalized connective tissue disorder in these patients. Obesity probably is not related to diverticula formation.

The muscular layer of the colon consists of an internal circular layer and three external bunched longitudinal bands, the teniae coli. There is a potential weak spot in the wall of the colon where the supplying blood vessels pierce through the circular muscle layer and it is at these weak points that the colon mucosa herniates through the muscle. Since the vessels pass through the muscle layer along the mesenteric border of the colon, it is here that a longitudinal row of diverticula is most often seen. The vessels piercing the antimesenteric border are considerably smaller and as a result the incidence of diverticula here is less.

Since only the mucosa and portions of the submucosa herniate through the muscle layers, the resultant diverticula should be called pseudodiverticula or false diverticula; however, common usage generally refers to them simply as diverticula.

High intraluminal pressure may be produced by excessive muscle contracture. Pressure waves in excess of 30 cm of water have been found to be common in patients with diverticular disease both at rest and postprandially (10). Such excessive contracture, together with the potential weak spots in the wall of the colon, probably are the causes of diverticula formation (11).

The symptoms associated with diverticular disease do not necessarily imply inflammation; thickening of the colon muscle with no histological evidence of inflammation may be found in patients who have had considerable prior chronic symptoms (5). In these patients both the circular muscle and the taenia coli may be thickened. The muscle thickening probably is due to foreshortening of the bowel, rather than due to hypertrophy or hyperplasia (5). Little evidence exists that any abnormality in Auerbach's or Meissner's neural plexuses is present. There may be excess fat on the outside of the bowel wall, a finding of limited importance.

Cecal diverticulosis, unlike sigmoid diverticulosis, is usually associated with a normal musculature and is generally seen in a younger patient population.

With mucosal herniation through the muscle the overlying small artery becomes elevated. Thus, as a diverticulum enlarges, the wall of the overlying artery tends to stretch and weaken. In 1976, Meyers et al. (12, 13) showed that diverticular bleeding was caused by arterial rupture, with the rupture being into the diverticulum. Intimal thickening of the vessel suggests trauma as an etiologic factor. Although the incidence of *left* colon diverticula is more common, diverticular bleeding quite often originates from *right* colon diverticula (14–16).

Diverticulitis develops if there is spasm and obstruction in the neck of the involved diverticulum, leading to stasis. Such episodes are probably more common if the diverticulum has a narrow neck. Since the diverticulum represents mucosal herniation, the lack of muscle prevents contracture of the diverticulum and thus leads to further stasis. Spasm, inflammation, and edema lead to obstruction and eventual rupture into the surrounding soft tissues. Generally there is sufficient pericolic inflammation to limit the perforation; if not, generalized peritonitis results. With insufficient reaction a fistula may develop to an adjacent structure.

Although rare, diverticulitis developing in a bypassed and defunctionalized colon has been reported (17). Congenital diverticula of the colon are rare (4). There may be associated bone abnormalities.

III.2.C. Clinical considerations

Diverticulosis is unusual but not rare under the age of 30 years (18) with most patients being over 40 years old. The incidence increases with age (19). Occasionally encountered is a young patient with both clinical and radiographic evidence of diverticulitis (20).

The patients may complain of left lower quadrant pain or back pain. If diverticula are subsequently demonstrated, it is tempting to ascribe the patient's pain to diverticular disease, although the symptoms may be due to some other disease. Diverticulitis may also present with bleeding, fever, or signs of peritoneal irritation. With chronic disease, only mild signs may be present, such as tenderness on deep palpation in the left lower quadrant.

Clinically, the differential diagnosis of diverticular disease includes the irritable colon syndrome. This latter entity, known by numerous descriptive names (21), does not have any pathognomonic or confirmatory laboratory tests. There is an abnormal myoelectric pattern, abnormal motility in the colon (22) and the small bowel may also exhibit an abnormal motility pattern (23). The irritable colon syndrome is used by some to explain a patient's symptoms where diverticular disease has been excluded.

It is difficult to know whether the irritable colon syndrome is actually a disease entity or not. It is also pure speculation as to whether the irritable colon syndrome actually represents a prediverticular stage in patients who will subsequently develop diverticular disease.

The radiographic changes associated with the irritable bowel syndrome have been described in the past as consisting of spastic segments appearing as localized contractions, narrowing of the lumen, and crowding together of the haustra (24). However, in view of our newer but still rather limited knowledge of this entity, it is best to consider that even if such an entity does exist, there are no specific radiographic signs for this syndrome. We routinely examine patients with a clinical diagnosis of the irritable bowel syndrome; in an occasional patient there are radiographic changes characteristic of either regional enteritis or ulcerative colitis. In the vast majority of these patients, however, the colon examination is normal. We believe that the irritable bowel syndrome, at present, cannot be diagnosed by radiological studies. Radiology is useful only to diagnose or exclude more ominous diseases.

Especially in patients with rectal bleeding, one should not ascribe bleeding to diverticular disease until the rest of the bowel has been adequately studied. Too often the bleeding is coming from a neoplasm or even a Meckel's diverticulum which had been missed.

The results of therapy with supplemental dietary fiber in patients with symptomatic diverticular disease are controversial. One study found that the only result of supplemental dietary fiber was relief of constipation (25).

To a large extent, the surgical treatment of diverticulitis consists of treatment of complications. In general, no attempt is made to surgically treat the etiology of the condition, with surgery generally consisting of excision of the involved segment. Those operations that resect or exteriorize the perforated segment at the first operation, rather than simply by-pass it with a colostomy, appear to be associated with a lower mortality rate (26). The role of sigmoid myotomy in preventing further attacks remains to be established.

III.2.D. Radiology of diverticulosis

A barium enema is an excellent tool in the study of uncomplicated diverticular disease. With a full column barium enema, postevacuation films are often useful in defining the extent of diverticular disease; with a double contrast enema the filled views of the colon are most helpful because the involved segments are fully distended and transparent.

Although diverticula can be scattered throughout the colon, they are most common in the sigmoid. Descending colon diverticula occur next in frequency. Appendiceal diverticula are generally incidental findings. Rectal and anal diverticula, although rare, do occur (27, 28).

Occasionally diverticula may be identified on noncontrast radiographs, with gas-filled diverticula having a 'bubbly' pattern (29). However, a barium enema is usually necessary for their evaluation.

Thick circular folds, due to fibrosis, muscle hypertrophy, or muscle hypertonicity, can be readily identified on a double contrast barium enema. If no diverticula are present, some label the thickened folds as representing the prediverticular stage of diverticular disease. Such thickened folds may have a corrugated appearance on a barium enema and may narrow the lumen considerably.

Diverticula vary in size and shape. They can be minute or very large. The diverticular neck can be broad or narrow. In general, right colon diverticula tend to have a wider neck and are larger than those located in the sigmoid. The diverticulum can be smooth, irregular, or even bilobed, presenting with a 'diverticulum in a diverticulum' appearance. Frequently there is residue within a diverticulum, leading to an irregular appearance.

The clearest differentiation of a diverticulum from a polyp on a barium enema is its visualization outside of the lumen of the colon. If the diverticulum fills with barium obviously there is no diagnostic problem. At times there is difficulty in differentiating a diverticulum from a polyp when the diverticulum is visualized *en face*. Welin (30) found that in a diverticulum there is a sharp inner edge and the outer edge is blurred (Fig. D.1). In many patients such a radiographic differentiation between a diverticulum and a polyp can be made readily, although in an occasional patient the sharp or hazy barium outline cannot be adequately defined. In these patients only by appropriate patient positioning and subsequent outline of the diverticulum in profile can a true distinction be made between a diverticulum and a polyp (Fig. D.2). Thus, while Welin's sign is useful in many patients it is not pathognomonic.

It is not unusual to have a neoplasm in a portion of the colon extensively involved by diverticulosis. The distortion produced by diverticula can often hide even relatively large lesions. Extensive maneuvers, such as barium drainage, filming while an area is being distended, and optimal patient positioning are necessary to ensure that the area in question is fully covered. Thus, quite often radiographs in addition to the standard views are necessary.

Sometimes one examination reveals diverticula while a subsequent examination fails to demonstrate any diverticula. The difference can be due to different degrees of distension between two examinations, insufficient filling of the colon, or inspissated matter within a diverticulum. Small diverticula may reduce through the bowel wall muscle defect (4).

It is not unusual to see retained barium and feces in diverticula for days, weeks, or occasionally even months. To our knowledge, such prolonged re-

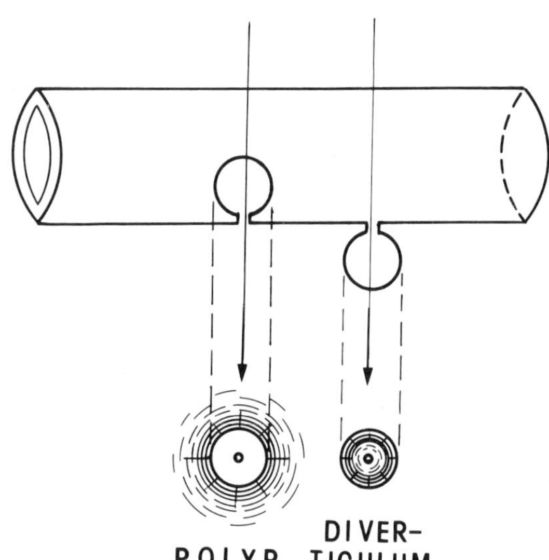

Fig. D.1. En face differentiation between a polyp and a diverticulum. A polyp has a sharp barium–polyp interface, with the barium gradually tapering off on the *outside*. Since the sharp barium–diverticular wall interface marks the outer border of the diverticular lumen, barium gradually tapers towards the *inside* of the image. (Adopted from ref. 30.)

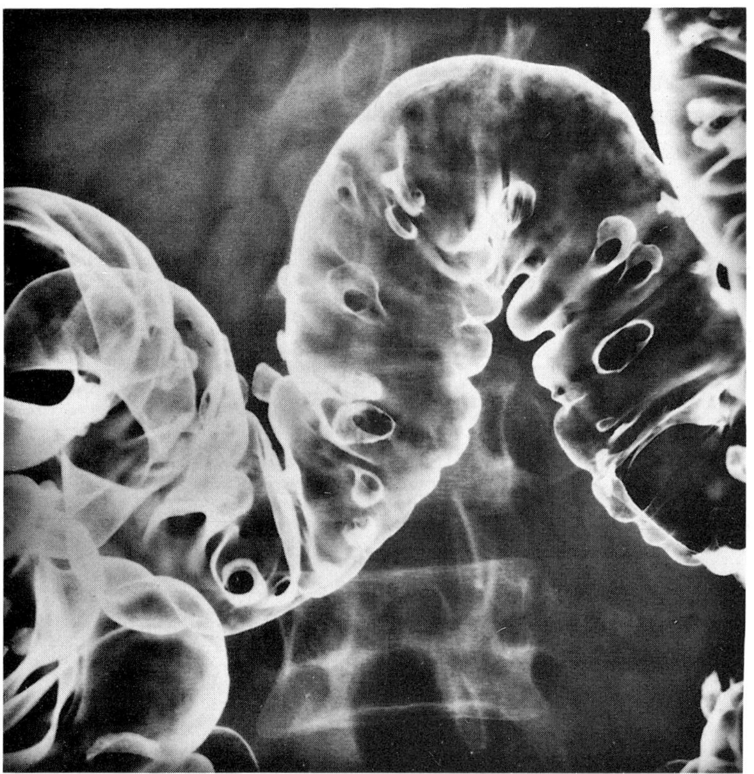

Fig. D.2. Diverticulosis. Numerous diverticula are seen both in profile and *en face*. Some are filled with barium while others are filled with air. The diverticular neck can be readily identified for some of the diverticula seen *en face*. The diverticula are aligned along linear rows corresponding to the weak points in the colon musculature.

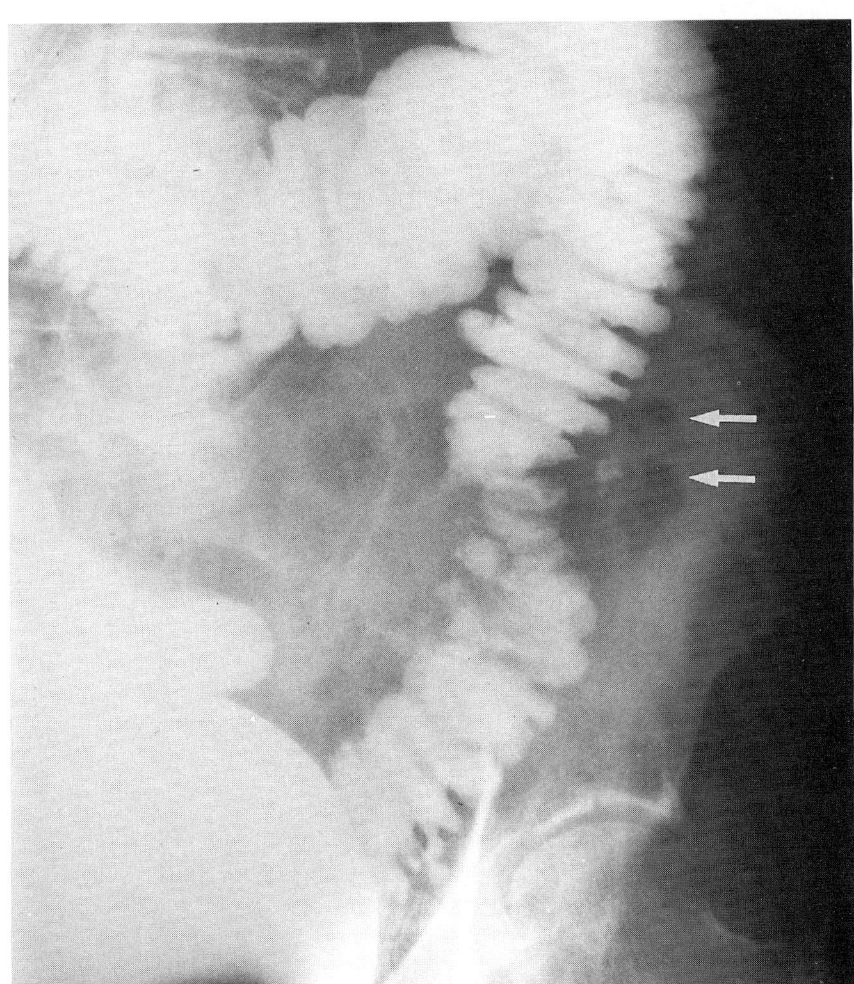

*Fig. D.3.***a.** For legend see page 202.

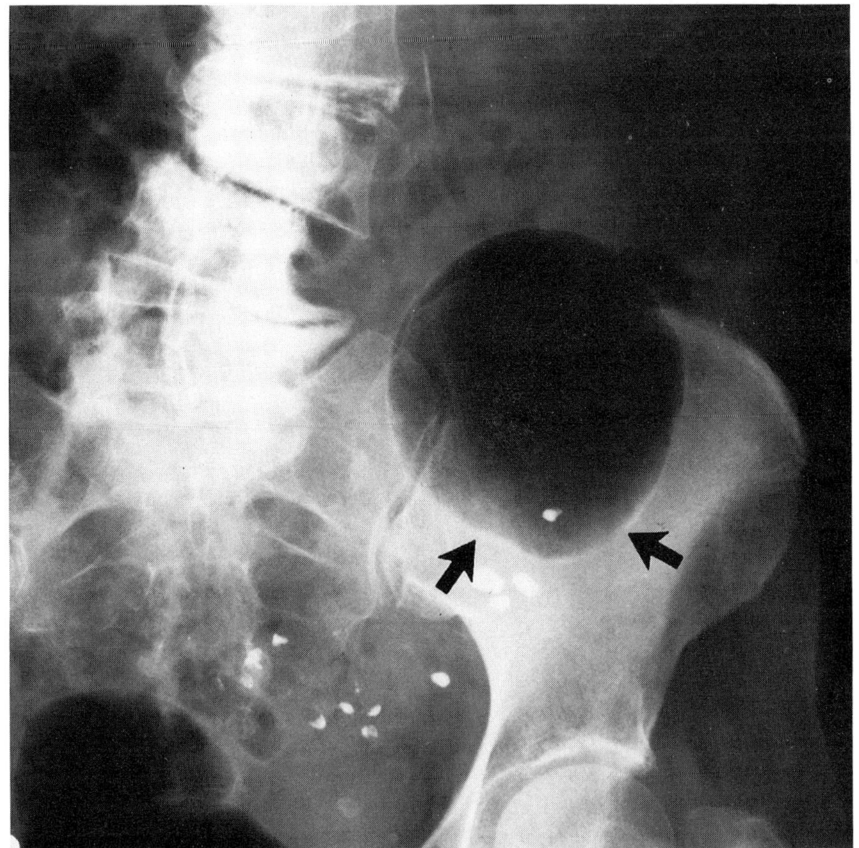

*Fig. D.3.***b.** For legend see page 202.

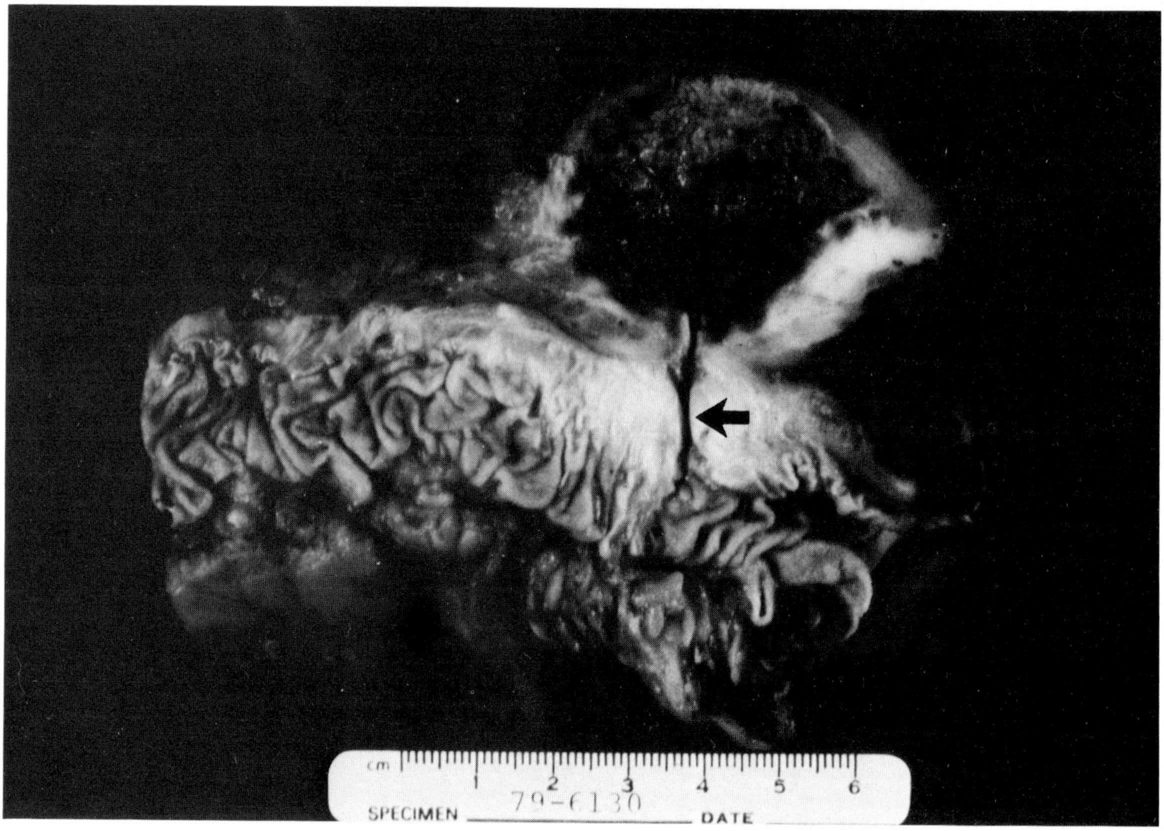

*Fig. D.3.*c

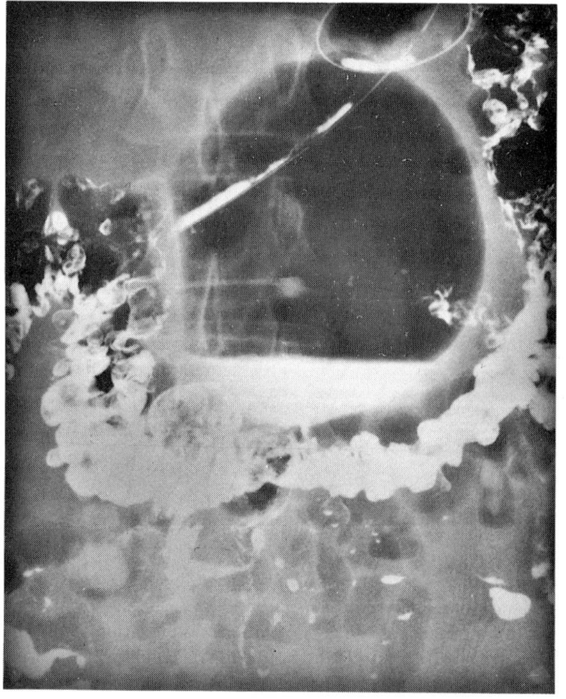

Fig. D.3. Giant colon diverticulum. (a) A barium enema revealed descending colon diverticula and small collections of gas adjacent to the colon (arrows). (b) Five months later a large gas-filled structure is present (arrows). Contrast outlines several smaller diverticula. (c) The resected specimen reveals a thick-walled cavity communicating with the colon through a narrow tract (arrow). (Courtesy of Dr. C.A. Muhletaler et al. (34), copyright Springer-Verlag, 1981.)

Fig. D.4. Giant diverticulum in the transverse colon. The radiograph was obtained six hours after the patient ingested barium. Some barium has accumulated in the diverticulum. (Courtesy of Dr. K.J. Wallers (35), copyright, British Institute of Radiology, 1981.)

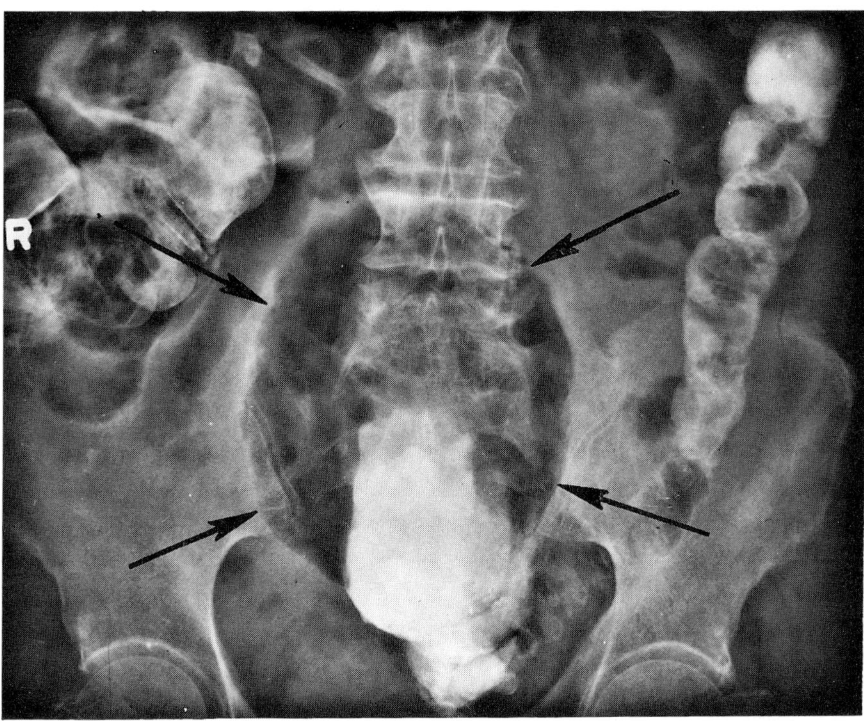

Fig. D.5. Giant colon diverticulum. A full-column barium enema shows contrast flowing into a large gas-filled structure (arrows). Subsequent views revealed this structure to be outside the colon.

tention does not lead to problems and is only an incidental finding.

Giant colonic diverticula are an interesting entity. These large cyst-like structures can be solitary or multiple and can be huge (31–33). Their pathogenesis is not entirely clear; most are acquired and probably represent a residual cavity formed as a complication of diverticulitis (34) (Fig. D.3). Most are in the sigmoid colon, with an occasional one being in other parts of the colon (35) (Fig. D.4). These diverticula can be confused with a redundant sigmoid loop (Fig. D.5), especially on a full column barium enema. The true nature is usually readily apparent on a double contrast examination. Complications encountered with these giant diverticula include perforation, abscess formation, and in a rare patient development of a carcinoma (33).

III.2.E Radiology of diverticulitis

A patient with a classic attack of acute diverticulitis is generally already hospitalized and receiving antibiotic therapy. Some degree of rebound tenderness is usually evident in the left lower quadrant, reflecting peritoneal irritation. During the acute episode these patients should be followed with acute abdominal examinations. These examinations will note any possible free perforation, colovesical fistula, or obstruction either in the colon or small bowel. A sigmoid peridiverticular abscess can involve a loop of adjacent small bowel and result in small bowel obstruction.

A barium enema is relatively contraindicated during the acute attack. The reasons are twofold. First, the laxatives used to clean out the colon may themselves be detrimental. These patients are generally managed by giving them nothing by mouth; the increased intraluminal fluid and increased tonicity produced by laxatives may lead to perforation. Second, almost invariably there is severe distortion and spasm at the site of diverticulitis, making differentiation between a peridiverticular abscess and a possible necrotic carcinoma difficult if not impossible. A barium enema on an unprepared colon tends to accentuate the difficulty in differentiating between a neoplasm and diverticulitis. A follow-up examination is almost always required to ensure that there is no underlying neoplasm. For these reasons, we perform a diagnostic enema in a patient during the acute episode of diverticulitis only if the patient's diagnosis is in doubt and the immediate subsequent management would be significantly altered if another cause for the patient's symptomatology was found. Practically, this means that a diagnostic enema is performed in that occasional patient where there is clinical and radiological suspicion of bowel obstruction, the patient has not responded adequately to hydration and antibiotics, and immediate surgical intervention is being considered. The greatest dilemma is presented by these patients; should one assume that they have acute diverticulitis and follow them radiographically as outlined above or should one assume that the patients have some other underlying disease? We try to individualize the examinations. For these patients we perform the examination using one of the water soluble iodinated contrast media, the patient has no preparation whatsoever (not even a tap water enema before the contrast study), and the purpose of the examination is to confirm or exclude obstruction or perforation (Fig. E.1). Under these circumstances it is obviously not possible to exclude other colon lesions such as superimposed neoplasms.

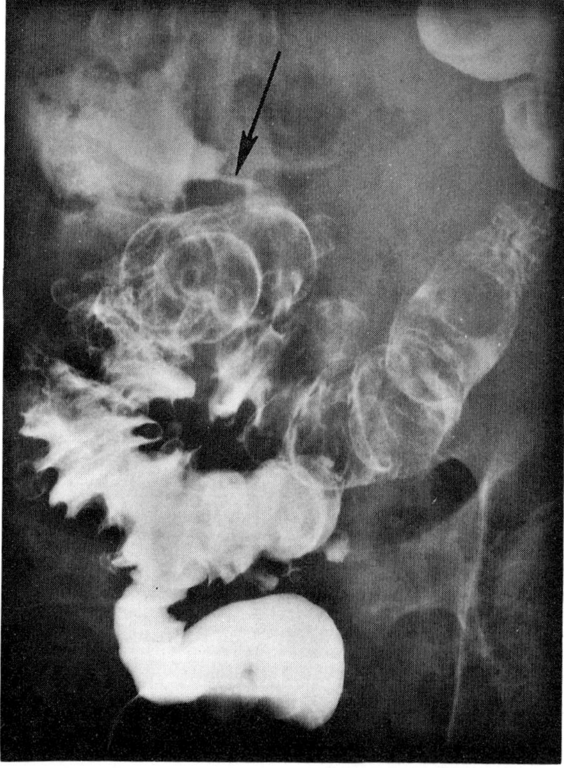

Fig. E.1. Sigmoid diverticulitis with perforation. A perforation (arrow) extends from the sigmoid into the peritoneal cavity. Impacted stool outlines most of the sigmoid. Gastrograffin was used for the enema and the examination was terminated when the perforation was seen. At surgery the same day an exudate surrounded the serosal side of the perforation, which was in an inflamed diverticulum.

There is an unsupported opinion among some physicians that in a patient with diverticulitis a double-contrast barium enema is more dangerous than a full-column barium enema. Diner et al. have shown that the intraluminal pressure with air contrast is *not* greater than that during a full column enema (36). There was no statistical difference in the pressure between the two examinations. The increased intraluminal pressures encountered with inflammatory disease are primarily due to spasm; a hypotonic agent generally helps prevent or reduce these episodes.

The vast majority of patients with acute diverticulitis do respond to medical management. Under these circumstances, we prefer to wait for a few weeks or a month and then perform a double-contrast barium enema to confirm the clinical diagnosis and exclude any other lesions (Fig. E.2).

We believe that there are only two relatively reliable signs of diverticulitis available to the radiologist. These are: (1) the presence of a fistula and (2) a peridiverticular abscess or inflammatory mass. A fistula should be readily seen and may be linear and intramural in location, similar to those seen in regional enteritis (37), or may be quite long. The abscess usually appears either as an adjacent soft tissue mass indenting the colon or the colon wall is fixed and infiltrated by the inflammation (Figs. E.3 and E.4). An abscess may communicate with the colon lumen through a fistulous tract. Generally the involved segment does not distend readily.

Although spasm is common in diverticulitis, we believe that spasm alone has little significance in the diagnosis. Spasm can be seen in patients with diverticulosis and in patients with a normal colon. Some authors have advocated the use of glucagon if there is spasm or apparent retrograde obstruction of the colon (38). We believe this is a moot point since we recommend routine premedication with glucagon prior to the barium enema. This hypotonic agent leads not only to more patient comfort, but also allows better distensibility of

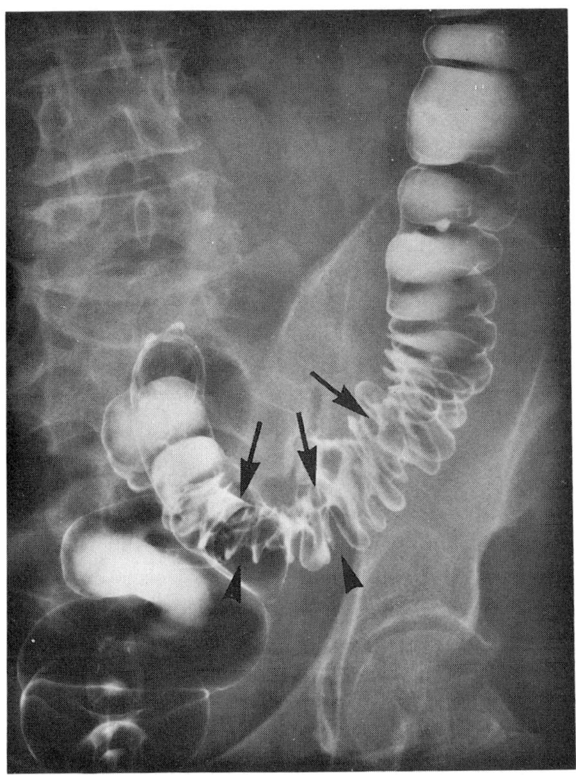

Fig. E.2. Chronic diverticulitis. This 66-year-old female has had intermittent left lower quadrant pain and tenderness for several months. A barium enema was performed after the most recent attack subsided after medical management. The sigmoid is distorted, with the folds thickened considerably (arrowheads). A long infiltrating mass is present along the mesenteric side of the sigmoid (arrows) tethering and distorting the residual diverticula, but not destroying them. A cancer this large should destroy some of the folds and the radiologist can predict with reasonable certainty that the lesion is due to diverticulitis and not neoplasm.

Fig. E.3. Diverticulitis. The angled sigmoid view shows best the diseased segment. A fistula extends inferiorly (arrowheads). The colic folds are thickened, infiltrated, and the diverticula are tethered. The infiltration involves almost the entire sigmoid. Surgery revealed inflammation, suppuration and fat necrosis of the pericolic tissues.

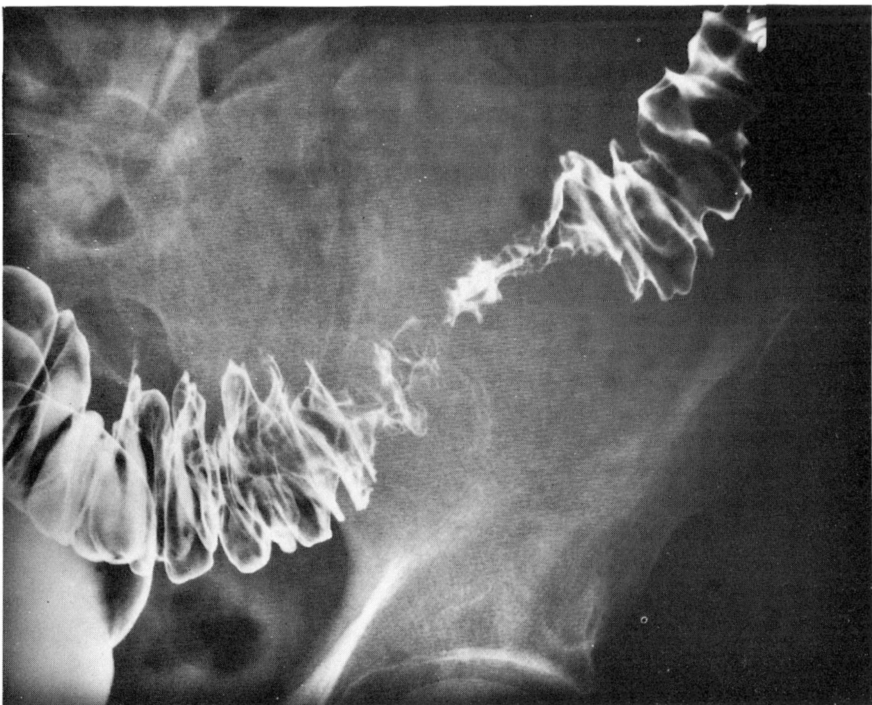

Fig. E.4. Diverticulitis. The involved segment did not distend throughout the examination. The colon folds are distorted but not destroyed. Some of the residual diverticula are tethered in appearance. The colon is circumferentially involved. The resected specimen showed acute and chronic diverticulitis.

inherently spastic areas, leading to better radiographic evaluation.

Theoretically, only one diverticulum is necessary for an attack of diverticulitis and the involved diverticulum is obliterated in the subsequent inflammatory reaction. Diverticulitis is thus possible even if a barium enema does not demonstrate any diverticula. On a statistical basis alone, however, the vast majority of patients with diverticulitis do have extensive diverticulosis. An abscess may or may not eventually communicate with the colon lumen. If it does communicate, a barium enema performed even after the acute attack has subsided may demonstrate the fistula. It can take months for these fistula to head. Another sequella of diverticulitis is intraabdominal adhesions (Fig. E.5).

The above description of diverticulitis applies primarily to the sigmoid colon. Diverticulitis of the rectum and the transverse colon is rare (39), while the incidence of diverticulitis of the descending colon is in between that of the transverse colon and the sigmoid. The rare rectal diverticulitis can be readily misdiagnosed as a necrotic carcinoma.

Althougy not common, diverticulitis of the cecum and ascending colon does occur (40). These patients tend to be younger than those with sigmoid diverticulitis (41). There is generally an intramural or extrinsic soft tissue mass with the mass usually being eccentric (Figs. E.6 and E.7). Diverticula may be present. There is generally little spasm of the adjacent colon and fistulas to the adjacent bowel are rare. The colon folds tend to be thickened. A paracolic abscess may develop (Fig. E.8). Unfortunately, other infections in the bowel, gallbladder, retroperitoneal structures and pelvic organs can also result in a pericolic abscess. Thus, the presence

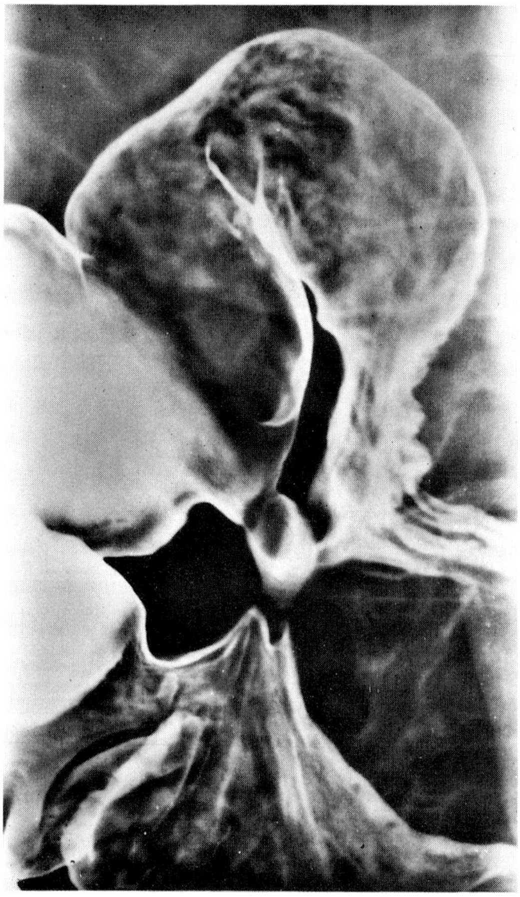

Fig. E.5. Intraabdominal adhesions between a diverticulum and an adjacent loop of bowel. The adhesions presumably are from prior inflammation.

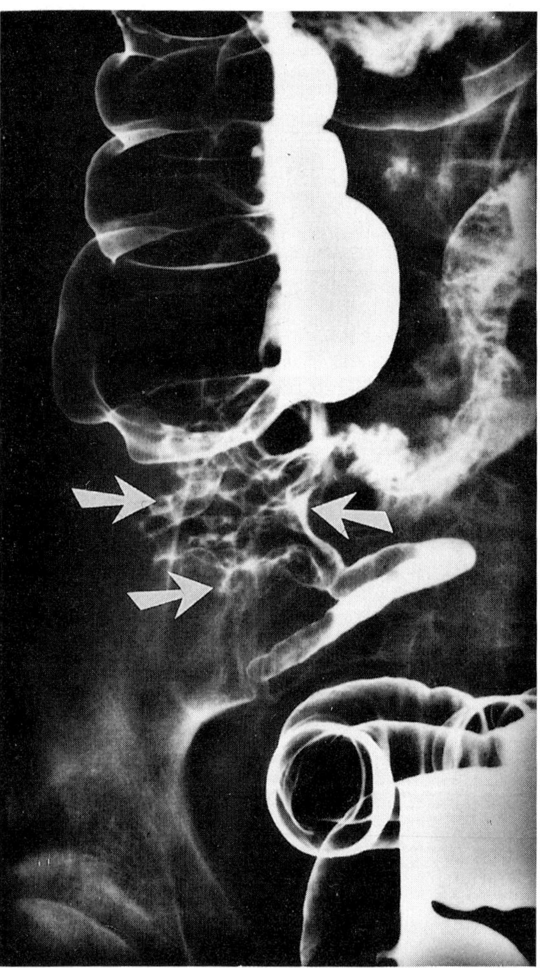

Fig. E.6. Cecal diverticulitis. There is an irregular infiltrating mass involving approximately half of the cecum (arrows). No diverticula were identified. The appendix fills readily.

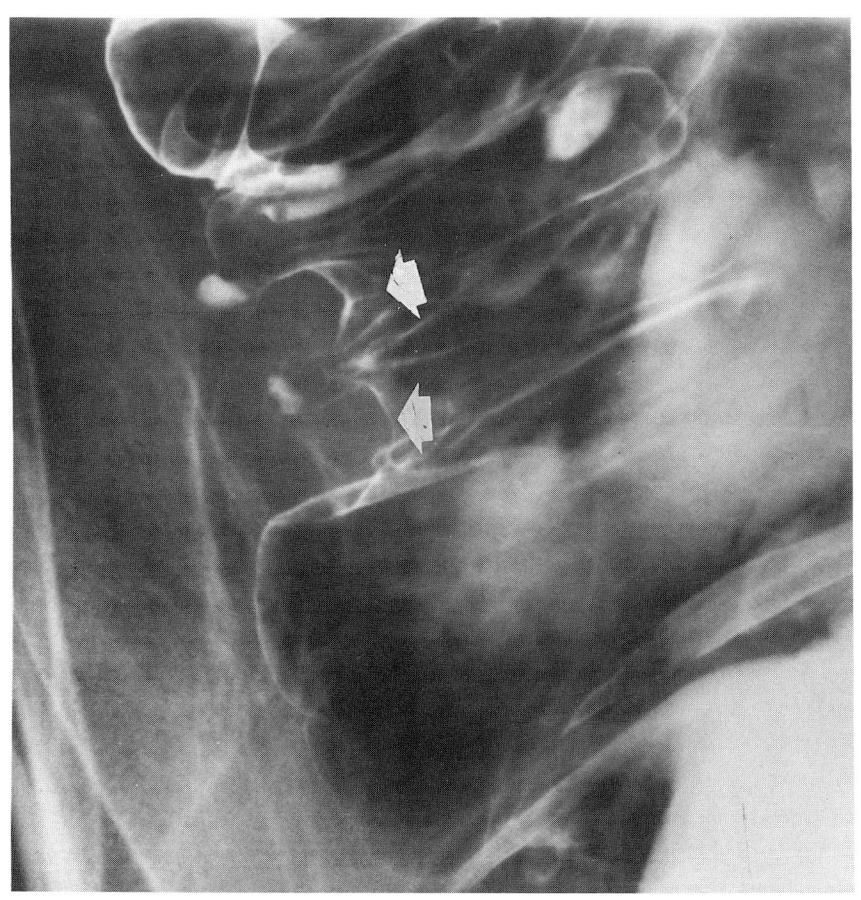

Fig. E.7. Right colic diverticulitis presenting as an intramural mass (arrowheads). Numerous diverticula are present throughout the area.

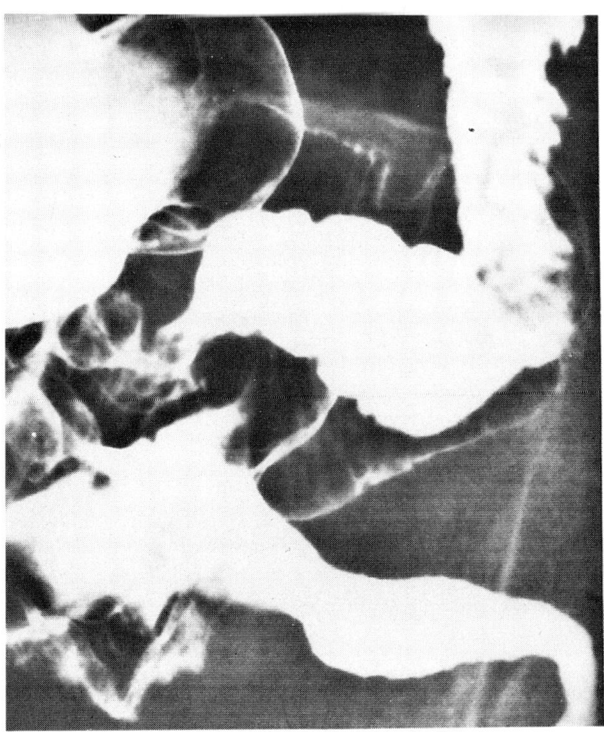

Fig. E.8. Cecal diverticulitis and pericolic abscess. The cecum is markedly narrowed, distorted, and infiltrated. A gaping ileocecal valve is present. The appendix fills readily. The patient underwent surgery because of persistent pain, a palpable right lower quadrant mass, and a radiographic appearance consistent with a neoplasm. The resected cecum revealed that virtually the entire cecum was inflamed. The abscess was along the lateral cecal wall.

of such an abscess is only of limited value in the differential diagnosis. Likewise, an intramural tumor quite often is in the radiological differential diagnosis.

III.2.F. Complications

a. Obstruction

One of the indications for surgery in patients with diverticulitis is intestinal obstruction, with the obstruction being either in the small bowel or in the colon. Occasionally, a patient develops a stenotic segment which can also eventually obstruct and require surgical intervention (Fig. F.1). When such a stricture is seen radiographically, carcinoma must be excluded (Fig. F.2). However, since diverticulitis generally involves the serosa or is intramural in location, leaving the mucosa and submucosa essentially intact, a double contrast barium enema can usually differentiate between these two entities. Not all narrowed segments represent stenoses; persistent spasm may mimic stenosis.

Occasionally complete *retrograde* obstruction is found in a patient who is otherwise not obstructed *antegrade*. In these patients the extent of the involved segment cannot readily be studied and it may be impossible to differentiate between diverticulitis and carcinoma (Fig. F.3).

Occasionally diverticulitis may result in ureteral obstruction (42) or may eventually lead to retroperitoneal fibrosis (43, 44). The association is nonspecific; other chronic inflammatory conditions may also lead to retroperitoneal fibrosis.

b. Perforation and fistula formation

The greatest risk in performing an enema during a bout of acute diverticulitis is colon perforation and resultant peritonitis (Fig. F.4). Although a peridiverticular abscess may perforate into the peritoneal cavity either spontaneously or during the barium enema, these tragic complications generally occur *early* in the acute attack before the abscess cavity is walled off. It is for this reason that a barium enema should be performed with extreme trepidation during the acute attack but is relatively safe later.

A peridiverticular abscess can either extend intraperitoneally or dissect along extraperitoneal tissue planes (Fig. F.5). Fistulas to adjacent organs

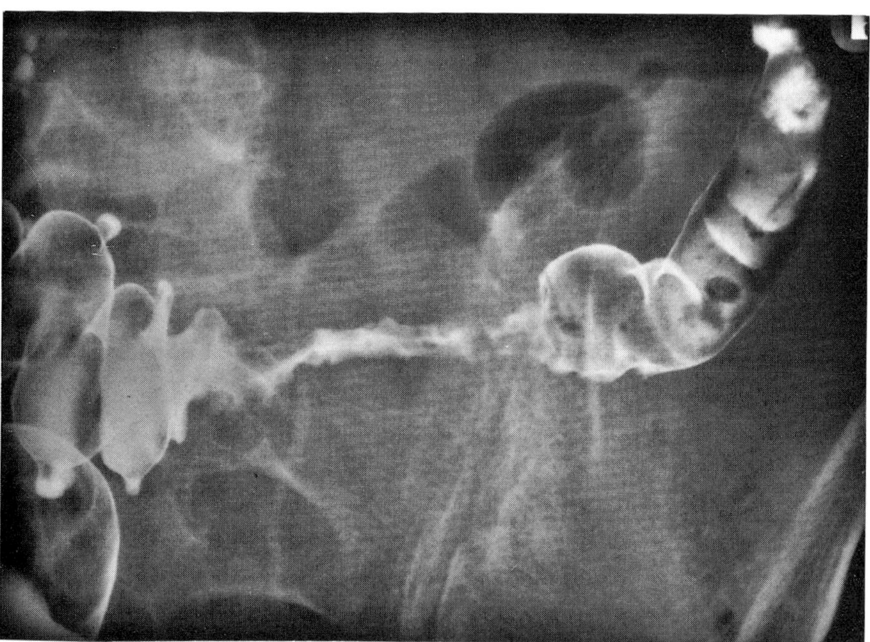

Fig. F.1. Sigmoid stenosis secondary to chronic diverticulitis. The long, tight stricture was beginning to obstruct. Differentiation from a carcinoma can be difficult once the stricture has advanced this far. The resected specimen revealed a bowel wall thickness averaging 5 cm in diameter.

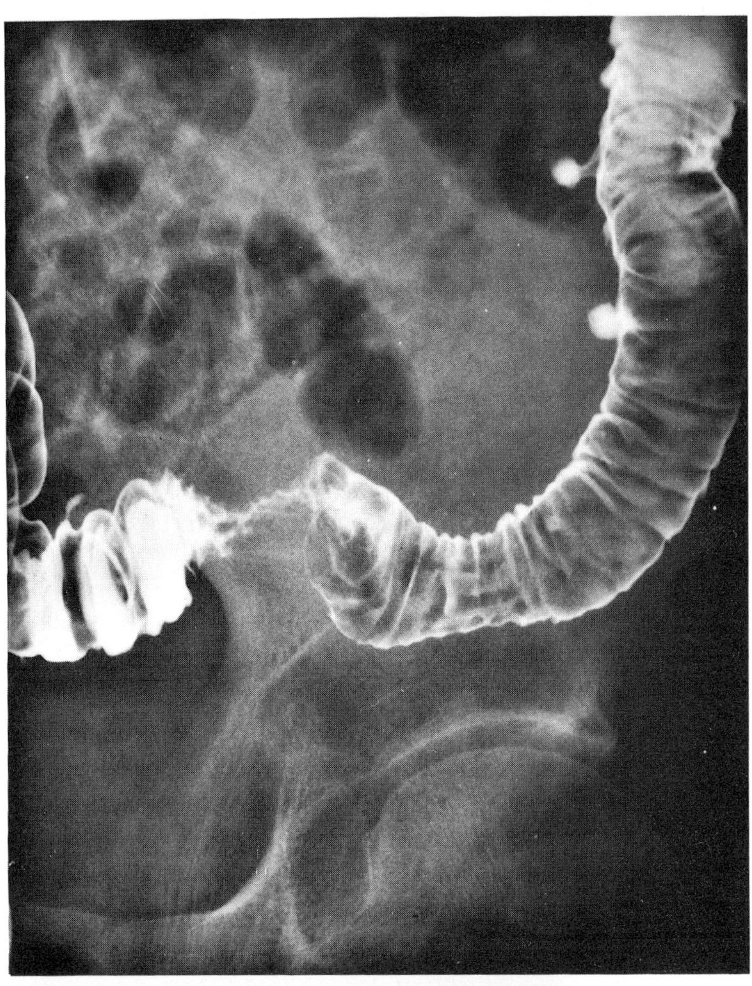

Fig. F.2. Diverticulitis with intramural abscess. The marked narrowing, sharp borders between normal and abnormal appearing bowel and marked distortion make differentiation from a carcinoma difficult. Endoscopy was not possible because of the narrowed lumen. The patient underwent sigmoid resection.

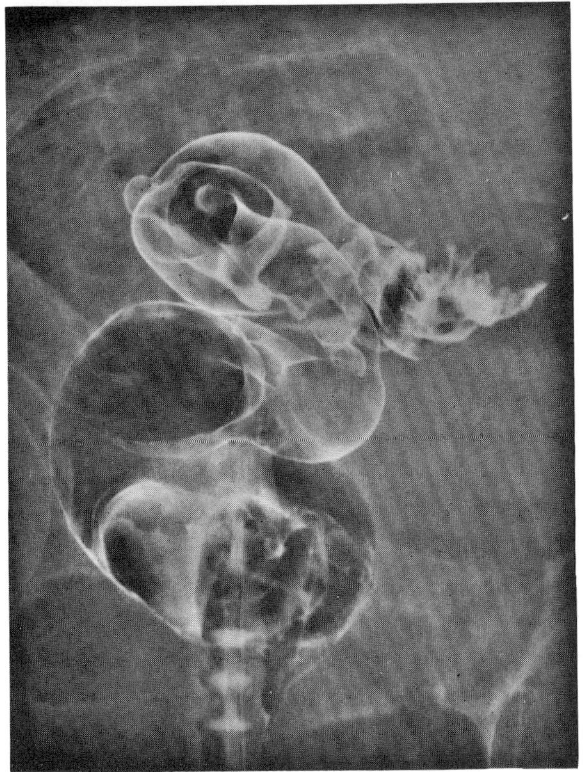

are well known to all radiologists performing barium enema examinations (Fig. F.6).

Most colovesical fistulas occur in men, while in women a colovaginal fistula is more common (Fig. F.7). The fistula may extend to an unusual location such as the hip, thigh, another loop of bowel, ureters, and even to the venous system or the epidural space (45). Diverticulitis only rarely leads to gas in the portal venous system (46). A colocutaneous fistula may be anyplace in the pelvic region, sometimes even presenting with subcutaneous emphysema (47). Most of these colocutaneous fistulas develop after surgery rather than arising spontaneously.

The easiest method of demonstrating these fistulas is to perform the appropriate fistulogram, cystogram or vaginogram using fluoroscopic con-

Fig. F.3. Sigmoid diverticulitis with complete retrograde obstruction. It is not possible to estimate the length of the obstructed segment nor to differentiate between diverticulitis and neoplasm. The distortion at the proximal end of the barium column may be produced by either entity. Resection revealed diverticulitis.

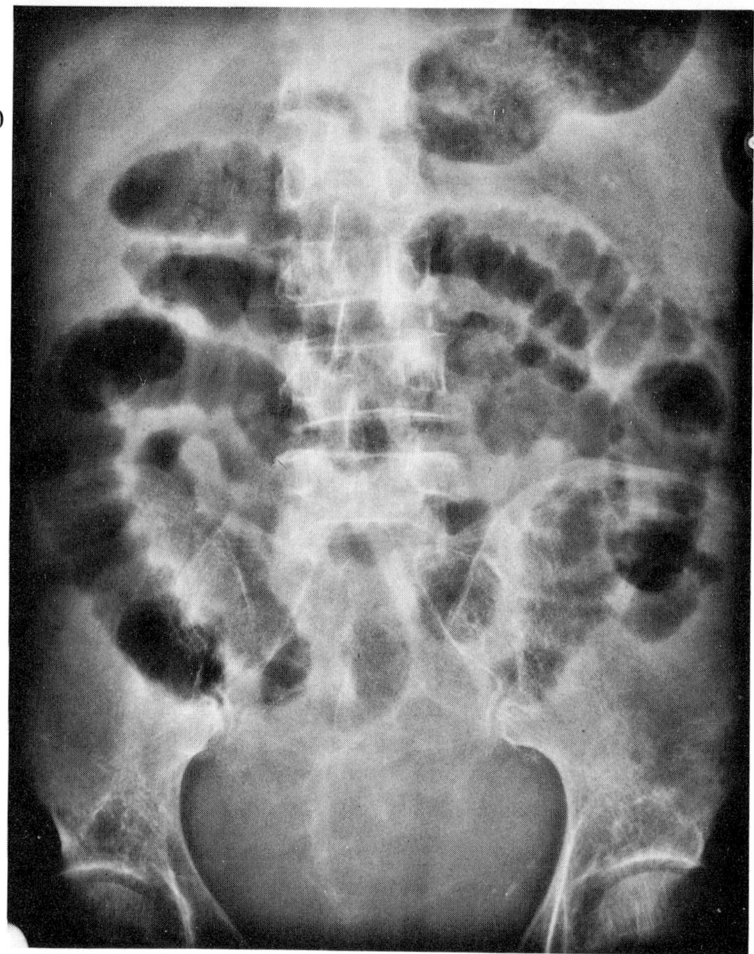

Fig. F.4. A 75-year-old female developed clinical signs of sigmoid diverticulitis. Her condition gradually deteriorated in spite of medical management. This radiograph, part of an acute abdominal examination, was obtained when she developed rebound tenderness. There are numerous dilated loops of small bowel floating centrally in the abdomen; the valvulae conniventes are thickened considerably, no colic gas can be identified, and a groundglass appearance to the abdomen is present. Pneumoperitoneum was not present on decubitus views. The radiographic picture is consistent with small bowel obstruction with superimposed peritonitis, presumably from ruptured diverticulitis. A barium enema is obviously contraindicated under these conditions. Surgery revealed bacterial peritonitis and a perforated sigmoid diverticulum. A toothpick was impacted at the site of perforation.

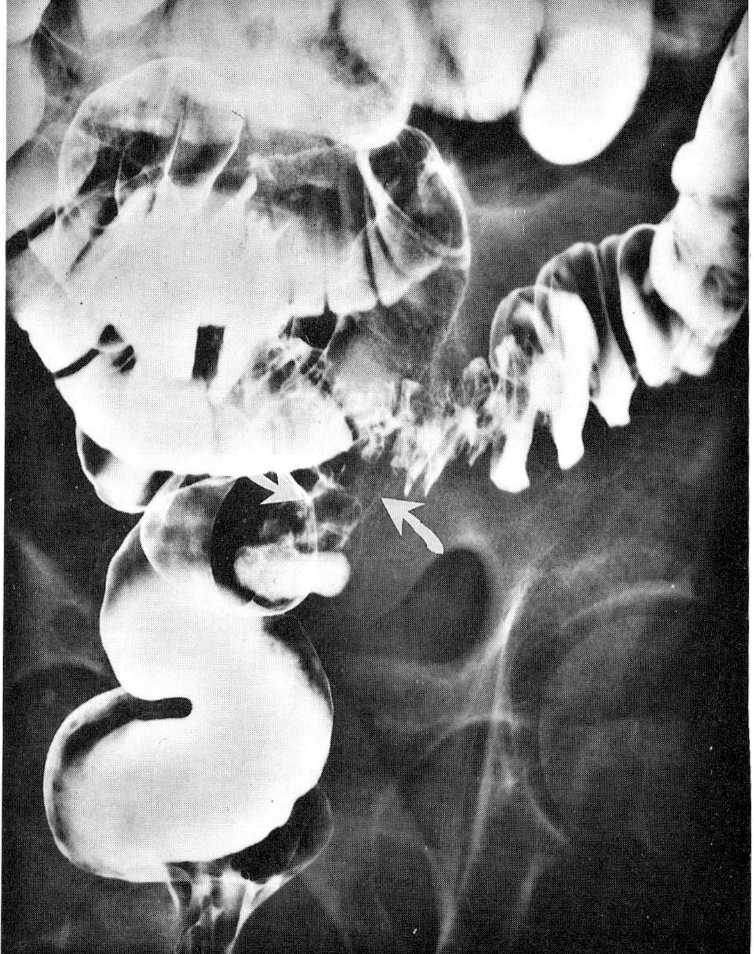

Fig. F.5. Sigmoid diverticulitis with perirectal abscess (arrows) in a 42-year-old female. There is marked infiltration and distortion of the sigmoid. An inflammatory mass is present along the mesenteric side. Fistulas connect the abscess to the bowel lumen.

trol and appropriate patient positioning. A barium enema is the next most useful examination, although in some patients even with a clinically obvious fistula the barium enema will not demonstrate any communication with the colon. In our experience, the least useful examination of all is an antegrade study of the small bowel and colon. Even if there is an obvious leak of contrast, generally the overlying loops of bowel hide the site of leakage, making evaluation difficult.

A fistula due to diverticulitis tends to heal slowly. If a small fistula is suspected but the contrast filled colon radiographs do not demonstrate one, postevacuation views in the anteroposterior and lateral projections may be helpful. The lateral projection, in particular, is useful with suspected colovesical or colovaginal fistulae.

c. Bleeding

Patients may present with melena or the bleeding may be massive and life-threatening. Usually there is little pain and the onset of bleeding may be abrupt. The massive diverticular bleeding is generally because of erosion of a vessel adjacent to a diverticulum (12, 13) and many of these patients do not have clinical evidence of diverticulitis (48). Lack of pain helps distinguish diverticular bleeding from ischemic colitis; in the latter condition pain is generally a prominent feature. Many of these patients are old, have arteriosclerotic cardiovascular disease, and the bleeding artery cannot constrict adequately.

One should be cautioned, however, that before bleeding is attributed to a diverticular source, other conditions causing gastrointestinal bleeding should be excluded.

Generally, colonoscopy is not useful in the presence of active bleeding. Likewise, a diagnostic barium enema cannot be performed, because the colon cannot be adequately cleansed of blood.

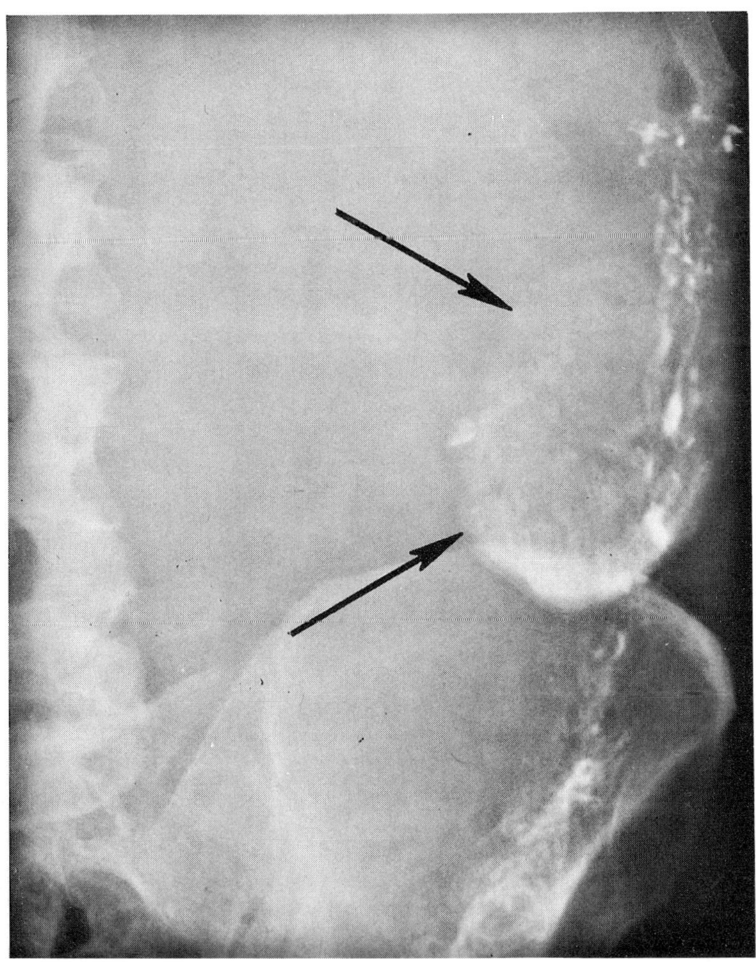

Fig. F.6. A postevacuation radiograph reveals barium in a cavity adjacent to the left kidney (arrows). The patient had diverticulitis with extraperitoneal perforation and developed an abscess in the left kidney.

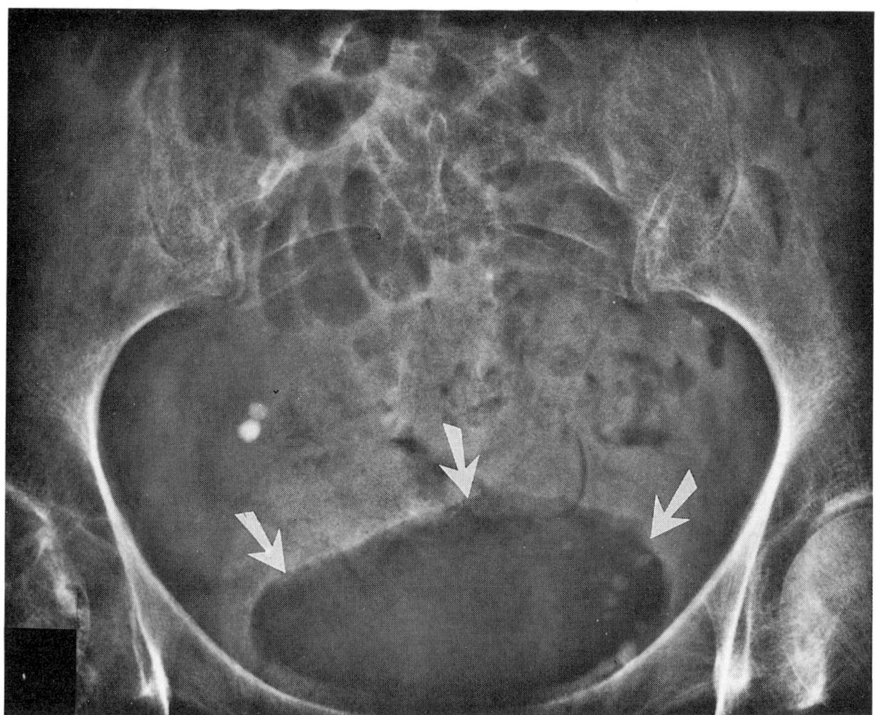

a

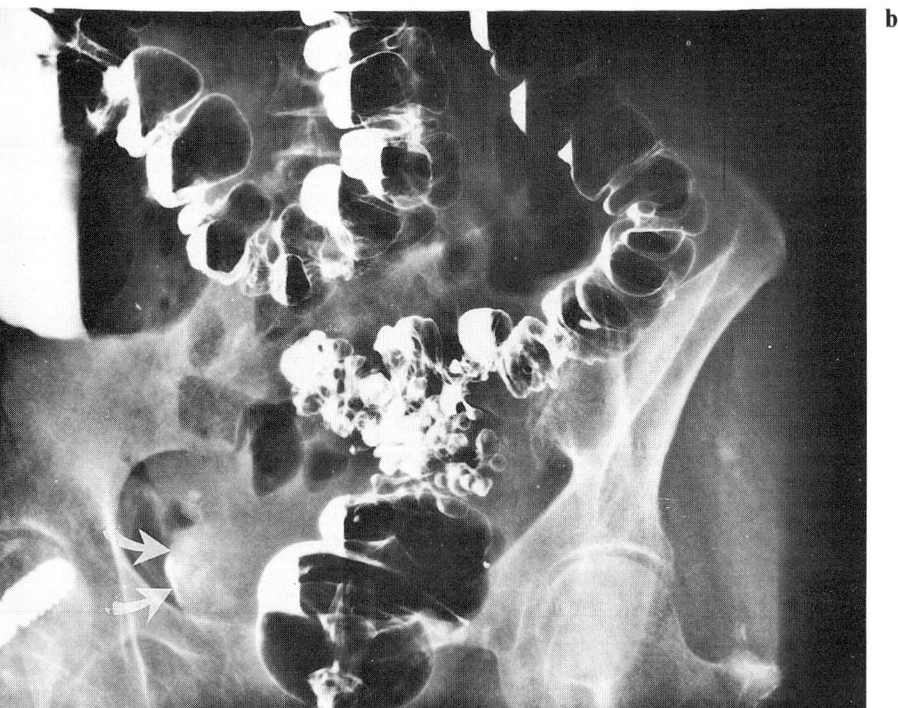

b

Fig. F.7. Colovesical fistula in a patient with pneumaturia. (a) An abdominal radiograph reveals gas in the bladder (arrows). (b) A barium enema the next day reveals marked spasm of the sigmoid, numerous diverticula, and barium in the bladder (arrowheads). No specific site of perforation could be identified.

A proposed approach in these patients has been a therapeutic barium enema (49, 50). However, it should be realized that some of the additives used in commercial barium sulfate products can delay blood clotting. The combination of blood and barium sulfate in a bleeding patient may result in an inhibition of blood clot formation (51).

The examinations of choice in the patient presenting with acute gastrointestinal bleeding are technetium-99 sulfur colloid scan and selective arteriography. It goes without saying that nuclear studies and arteriography should precede any barium study. If for some reason the patient has received barium prior to a needed arteriogram, saline enteroclysis of the bowel can clean out the majority of the barium present in the colon within several hours (52).

Angiography should include study of both the inferior mesenteric and the superior mesenteric artery. Bleeding at a rate greater than approximately 0.5 ml per minute is necessary for angiographic demonstration of the bleeding site and it is obvious that the greatest yield will be in those

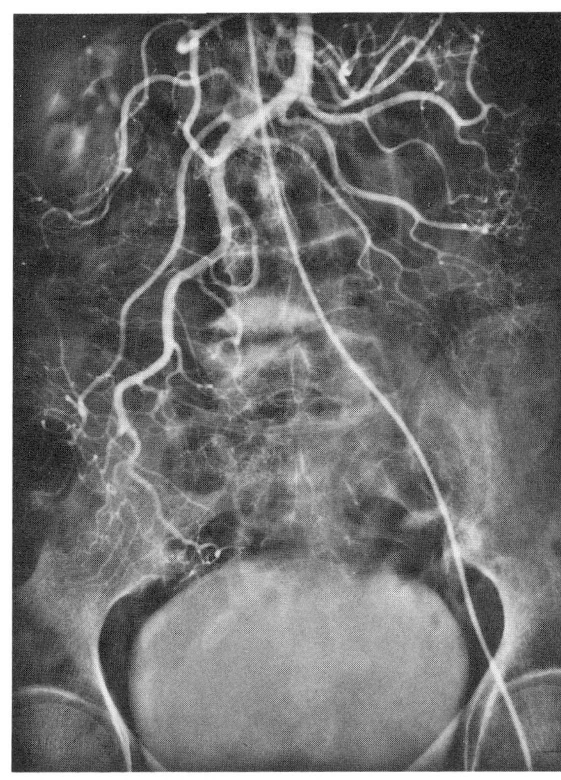

a

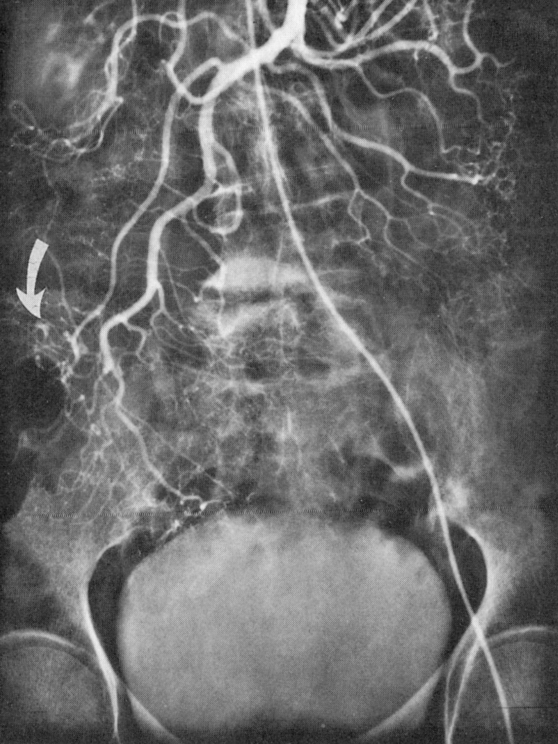

b

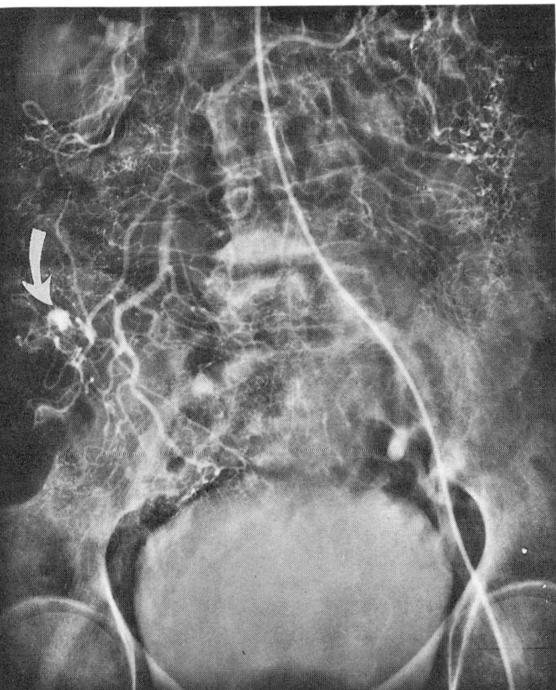

c

Fig. F.8. The patient developed massive lower gastrointestinal bleeding. (a) The arterial phase of a superior mesenteric artery injection shows no bleeding site. (b) Late arterial phase reveals beginning extravasation (arrow). (c) The extravasation into the right colon is better seen on delayed views (arrow). (Courtesy of Dr. O. Guttierrez, Rochester, New York.)

patients who are bleeding profusely during the angiogram. The extravasated contrast provides ready visualization of the bleeding site (Fig. F.8).

Once the site of bleeding is identified radiographically, vasopressin infusion into the feeding artery is relatively successful in stopping bleeding (14, 16, 53). Vasopressin is started at a rate of 0.2 units/ml/min. The dose can be increased, if necessary, to 0.3 units/ml/min but should eventually be tapered to 0.1 units/ml/min. Such therapy should control bleeding in most patients. The selective intraarterial infusion of vasopressin appears to be more effective than intravenous infusion (54).

If vasopressin does not control the bleeding in a high risk surgical patient, some angiographers recommend embolization (55). Some of the reluctance to perform embolization in the colon appears to be due to the relatively poor colon collateral supply. Although ischemic complications after embolization do occur (56, 57), in some patients this technique can be lifesaving.

III.2.G. Differential diagnosis

Most patients with diverticulosis and diverticulitis do not present any significant problems in differential diagnosis. With an incomplete radiographic examination or an examination performed on an emergency basis, missing an underlying carcinoma is always a possibility. The greatest value to the patient is served by performing an adequate barium enema. If such an examination is not possible, the referring physician should be made aware that differentiation between diverticulitis and carcinoma is not possible. The radiologist should always keep in mind that a carcinoma can also be present in an area involved with diverticulosis. Similarly, diverticulitis consisting either of an abscess or an inflammatory mass generally infiltrates the colon from the serosal side inward. Thus, in a subsequent barium enema the colon lumen may appear narrowed and distorted but the folds are usually not destroyed as happens with a primary colon car-

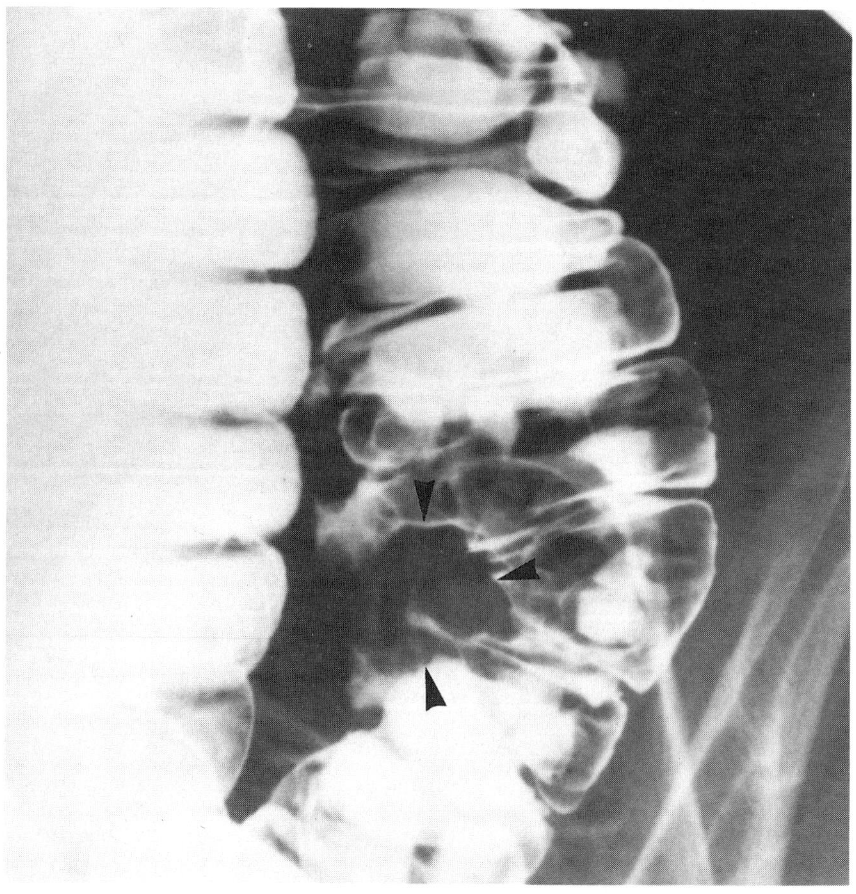

Fig. G.1. Chronic diverticulitis app[…] as a well-defined intramural mass (a[…] heads). There is little distortion […] adjacent bowel. Numerous divertic[…] present. The lesion closely mimi[…] intramural neoplasm.

cinoma. In an occasional patient diverticulitis can be confused with serosal metastases or an intramural neoplasm (Fig. G.1).

Likewise, some of the colitides may coexist with diverticular disease. In particular, regional enteritis and diverticulitis may coexist (58). From the radiographic appearance alone, occasionally it may not be possible to distinguish between these two diseases. A fistula may be due to regional enteritis, infection, or neoplasm.

In patients with right colon diverticulitis the disease tends to mimic appendicitis in its clinical presentation; yet on an barium enema the appendix fills readily. If there is inflammation of an appendiceal diverticulum with resultant diverticulitis, the patient may present clinically and radiologically with findings identical to appendicitis. To confuse the picture is sigmoid diverticulitis with a redundant sigmoid located in the right lower quadrant (59). In most of these patients a well-performed barium enema generally points to the true diagnosis.

Pelvic inflammatory disease is usually not part of the diagnostic differentiation, since this condition generally occurs in younger women. Similarly, the clinical presentation in patients with endometriosis generally leads one to the correct diagnosis.

References

1. Cruveilhier J: Traité d'Anatomie Pathologique Genérale, Vol 1, p 593. Baillière, Paris, 1849. Quoted in: Painter NS, Burkitt DP: Diverticular disease of the colon, a 20th century problem. Clinics Gastroenterol 4:3–21, 1975.
2. Spriggs EI, Marxer OA: Intestinal diverticula. Q J Med 19:1–35, 1925.
3. Fleischner FG: Diverticular disease of the colon: new observations and revised concepts. Gastroenterology 60:316–324, 1971.
4. Hughes LE: Postmortem survey of diverticular disease of the colon. I. Diverticulosis and diverticulitis. Gut 10:336–351, 1969.
5. Morson BC: The muscle abnormality in diverticular disease of the sigmoid colon. Br J Radiol 36:385–392, 1963.
6. Painter NS, Burkitt DP: Diverticular disease of the colon, a 20th century problem. Clin Gastroenterol 4:3–21, 1975.
7. Painter NS, Burkitt DP: Diverticular disease of the colon: a deficiency disease of western civilization. Br Med J 2:450–454, 1971.
8. Bohrer SP: Hiatus hernia and diverticulum in Nigeria. N Eng J Med 272:695, 1965.
9. Mielke JE, Becker KL, Gross JB: Diverticulitis of the colon in a young man with Marfan's syndrome. Gastroenterology 48:379–382, 1965.
10. Arfwidsson S: Pathogenesis of multiple diverticula of the sigmoid colon in diverticular disease. Acta Chir Scand, Suppl. 342:1–68, 1964.
11. Morson BC: Pathology of diverticular disease of the colon. Clin Gastroenterol 4:37–52, 1975.
12. Meyers MA, Alonso DR, Grey GF, Baer JW: Pathogenesis of bleeding colonic diverticulosis. Gastroenterology 71:577–583, 1976.
13. Meyers MA, Alonso DR, Baer JW: Pathogenesis of massively bleeding colonic diverticulosis: new observations. AJR 127:901–908, 1976.
14. Athanasoulis CA, Baum S, Rösch J, Waldman AC, Ring EJ, Smith JC Jr, Sugarbaker E, Wood W: Mesenteric arterial infusions of vasopressin for hemorrhage from colonic diverticulosis. Am J Surg 129:212–216, 1975.
15. Patel HD, Chawla K, Chawla SK, Soterakis J, LoPresti PA: Massive rectal hemorrhage from right-sided colonic diverticula. Am J Gastroenterol 66:76–78, 1976.
16. Baum S, Athanasoulis CA, Waldman AC: Angiographic diagnosis and control of large bowel bleeding. Dis Colon Rectum 17:447–453, 1974.
17. Desechalliers JP, Galmiche JP, Denis P, Teniere P, Testart J, Colin R: Diverticulitis in a patient with a 47-year defunctionalized colon. Dig Dis Sci 26:187–190, 1981.
18. Homer MJ, Danford RO: Acute diverticulitis in the young adult. Radiology 125:623–626, 1977.
19. Parks TG: Natural history of diverticular disease of the colon. Clin Gastroenterol 4:53–69, 1975.
20. Evans WE, Dawson RG: Diverticulitis in the young adult. Am Surg 36:518–521, 1970.
21. Fielding JF: The irritable bowel syndrome. Clin Gastroenterol 6:607–622, 1977.
22. Burns TW: Colonic motility in the irritable bowel syndrome. Arch Intern Med 140:247–251, 1980.
23. Thompson DG, Laidlow JM, Wingate DL: Abnormal small bowel motility demonstrated by radiotelemetry in a patient with irritable colon. Lancet ii:1321–1323, 1979.
24. Lumsden K, Chaudhary NA, Truelove SC: The irritable colon syndrome. Clin Radiol 14:54–63, 1963.
25. Ornstein MH, Littlewood ER, McLean Baird L, Fowler J, North WRS, Cox AG: Are fibre supplements really necessary in diverticular disease of the colon? A controlled clinical trial. Br Med J 282:1353–1356, 1981.
26. Greif JM, Fried G, McSherry CK: Surgical treatment of perforated diverticulitis of the sigmoid colon. Dis Colon Rectum 23:483–487, 1980.
27. Walstad PM: Sahibzada AR: Diverticula of the rectum. Am J Surg 116:937–939, 1968.
28. Töterman S, Ahovuo J, Möller C, Nickels J: Divertikelbildung am Afterkanal. ROEFO 131:223–224, 1979.
29. Russin LD: Plain film recognition of air within colonic diverticula. AJR 134:176–177, 1980.
30. Welin S: Über die röntgenologische Untersuchung des Dickdarmes mit der Doppelkontrastmethode. Die Malmömodifikation. Radiologe 2:87–100, 1962.
31. Moss AA: Giant sigmoid diverticulum: clinical and radiographic features. Am J Dig Dis 20:676–683, 1975.
32. Johns ER, Hartley MG: Giant gas filled cysts of the sigmoid colon: a report of two cases. Br J Radiol 49:930–931, 1976.
33. Kricun R, Stasik JJ, Reither RD, Dex WJ: Giant colonic diverticulum. AJR 135:507–512, 1980.
34. Muhletaler CA, Berger JL, Robinette CL Jr: Pathogenesis of giant colonic diverticula. Gastrointest Radiol 6:217–222, 1981.
35. Wallers KJ: Giant diverticulum arising from the transverse colon of a patient with diverticulosis. Br J Radiol 54:683–684, 1981.
36. Diner WC, Patel G, Texter EC Jr, Baker ML, Tune JM, Hightower MD: Intraluminal pressure measurements

during barium enema. Full column vs. air contrast. AJR 137:217–221, 1981.

37. Ferrucci JT Jr, Ragsdale BD, Barrett PJ, Vickery AL Jr, Dreyfuss JR: Double tracking in the sigmoid colon. Radiology 120:307–312, 1976.
38. Ferrucci JT, Farooq J, Seidler R: Muscle spasm in sigmoid diverticulosis: evaluation of retrograde colon obstruction by hypotonic barium enema. J Can Assoc Radiol 25:269–274, 1974.
39. Kent SJS: Diverticulitis of the transverse colon. Br Med J 2:219, 1973.
40. Beranbaum SL, Zausner J, Lane B: Diverticular disease of the right colon. AJR 115:334–348, 1972.
41. Norfray JF, Givens JD, Sparberg MS, Dwyer RM: Cecal diverticulitis in young patients. Gastrointest Radiol 5:379–382, 1980.
42. Siminovitch JMP, Fazio VW: Obstructive uropathy secondary to sigmoid diverticulitis. Dis Colon Rectum 23: 504–507, 1980.
43. Harbrecht PJ, Ahmad W, Fry DE, Amin M: Occult diverticulitis a cause of retroperitoneal fibrosis. Dis Colon Rectum 23:255–257, 1980.
44. Koep L, Zuidema GD: The clinical significance of retroperitoneal fibrosis. Surgery 81:250–257, 1977.
45. Smith HJ, Berk RN, Janes JO, Clayton RS, Williams JL: Unusual fistulae due to colonic diverticulitis. Gastrointest Radiol 2:387–392, 1978.
46. Graham GA, Bernstein RB, Gronner AT: Gas in the portal and inferior mesenteric veins caused by diverticulitis of the sigmoid colon. Report of a case with survival. Radiology 114:601–602, 1975.
47. Lipsit ER, Lewicki AM: Subcutaneous emphysema of the abdominal wall from diverticulitis with necrotizing fasciitis. Gastrointest Radiol 4:89–92, 1979.
48. Gennaro AR, Rosemond GP: Colonic diverticula and hemorrhage. Dis Colon Rectum 16:409–415, 1973.
49. Adams JT: The barium enema as treatment for massive diverticular bleeding. Dis Colon Rectum 17:439–441, 1974.
50. Adams JT: Therapeutic barium enema for massive diverticular bleeding. Arch Surg 101:457–460, 1970.
51. Miller RE, Skucas J, Violante MR, Shapiro ME: The effect of barium on blood in the gastrointestinal tract. Radiology 117:527–530, 1975.
52. Skucas J, Cutcliff W, Fischer HW: Whole-gut irrigation in preparation for barium enema examination. Radiology 112:303–305, 1976.
53. Baum S, Rösch J, Dotter CT, Ring EJ, Athanasoulis C, Waltman AC, Courey WR: Selective mesenteric arterial infusions in the management of massive diverticular hemorrhage. N Engl J Med 288:1269–1272, 1973.
54. Davis GB, Bookstein JJ, Coel MN: Advantage of intraarterial over intravenous vasopressin infusion in gastrointestinal hemorrhage. AJR 128:733–735, 1977.
55. Bookstein JJ, Naderi MJ, Walter JF: Transcatheter embolization for lower gastrointestinal bleeding. Radiology, 127:345–349, 1978.
56. Mitty HA, Efremidis S, Keller RJ: Colonic stricture after transcatheter embolization for diverticular bleeding. AJR., 133:519–521, 1979.
57. Shenoy SS, Satchidanand S, Wesp EW: Colonic ischemic necrosis following therapeutic embolization. Gastrointest. Radiol., 6:235–237, 1981.
58. Marshak RH, Janowitz HD, Present DH: Granulomatous colitis in association with diverticula. N Eng J Med, 283:1080–1084, 1970.
59. Assa J, Zoireff L, Iuchtman M: Perforation of the sigmoid colon simulating acute appendicitis. Isr J Med Sci 16:646–648, 1980.

III.3 TUMORS

III.3.A. Introduction

Both benign and malignant tumors of the colon are relatively common. In the past authors have maintained a clear distinction between the benign and malignant tumors. This distinction, however, has become less clear during the last several years, with emphasis currently being placed on the malignant potential of some of the benign neoplasms.

Some physicians use the term 'polyp' synonymously with a benign neoplasm. Yet, this term is only descriptive of the gross appearance of a lesion and a 'polyp' can be benign, malignant, or inflammatory in origin. We and others use the term 'polyp' purely as a descriptive radiological term for the typical intraluminal lesion, regardless whether it is neoplastic, hyperplastic, or inflammatory. With such a definition of a polyp, there is no such thing as a pseudopolyp.

Most colon polyps are benign. The relative incidence of the various types of polyps varies considerably depending upon the particular study. Some investigators believe that polyps smaller than 5 mm are primarily hyperplastic (1, 2), while others have found that 37–60% of polyps smaller than 5 mm are neoplastic in origin and thus possible precursors of a carcinoma (3, 4).

The pathogenesis of adenomata in nonfamilial colon polyposis is not known. It is believed that adenomata originate from the basal cells (5). Microscopic adenomata appear to be closely associated with lymphoid follicles (5). In most populations the relative incidence of carcinoma is directly proportional to the incidence of adenomata (6). Although the incidence of adenomata is about equally distributed throughout the colon, in general, carcinomata tend to be more common in the distal portion of the colon.

An adenoma can have a predominantly tubular (glandular) pattern or it can be villous (frond-like) in appearance. Likewise, an adenoma can exhibit a spectrum of changes anywhere in between these two extremes. Morson uses the terms tubular, villous, and intermediate to classify these adenomata (7). Others have called the intermediate type as tubovillous, villotubular, and semipapillary. Although some believe that the tubular adenomatous polyps tend to be smooth while the villous tend to have a frond-like appearance, there is considerable overlap in the radiographic appearance and the radiologist cannot predict with any reasonable certainty the microscopic appearance of a particular polyp (Fig. A.1). The overlap in the radiographic appearance is especially evident with small polyps, where both benign and malignant lesions tend to be smooth (8, 9). Similar findings are seen with induced colon cancer in animals; the tumors were invariably smooth when small and gradually became irregular in outline as they grew (10).

Little controversy exists as to whether benign adenomata can become malignant; sufficient evidence has been accumulated by Morson and others to show that an adenoma can transform and is a precursor to an adenocarcinoma (11). While the lesion is small, it is benign but with growth carcinomatous transformation occurs. One study over a 25-year period followed thousands of patients by annual proctosigmoidoscopic examination and removal of all visualized polyps (12). These patients developed a significantly lower incidence of carcinomata within the region examined than that predicted in a similar patient population group who did not have removal of the tumors. Within the patient population studied, the incidence of cancer in the *remaining* portion of the colon, not visualized by proctosigmoidoscopy, was similar to that predicted in a general patient population.

Not all adenomata have an equal statistical

Table A.1 The incidence of carcinoma within an adenomatous polyp.

Investigator	Reference	Date	Polyp size		
			<1 cm	1–2 cm	>2 cm
Muto et al.	16	1980	7%	30%	68%
Shinya and Wolff	14	1979	0.5	4.6	11
Day and Morson	11	1978	1.3	9.5	46
Watanabe et al.	45	1979	14	12	50

incidence of carcinomatous transformation. Predominantly tubular appearing adenomata have a lower frequency of transformation than predominantly villous adenomata (13, 14). Rarely, a carcinoma can probably also arise from previously 'normal' colon mucosa; study of normal-appearing mucosa surrounding a proven carcinoma has revealed abnormal histochemical changes (15) and such mucosa may be more prone to undergo carcinomatous transformation. It is not unusual for the radiologist to see a central large carcinoma surrounded by separate and discrete carcinomatous nodules. These nodules have been described as 'satellite tumors'.

Whether an adenoma is likely to contain a focus of carcinoma depends primarily on the size of the polyp (Table A.1). The different incidence noted by various investigators probably reflects different patient population groups studied and the definition of the entity of 'carcinoma'. If noninvasive intramucosal 'carcinomata' are included, the incidence of carcinoma is higher (14). There is a suggestion that adenomata in females have a higher malignant potential than in males (16).

Initially a carcinoma is limited entirely to the mucosa. Such an in-situ or intramucosal cancer

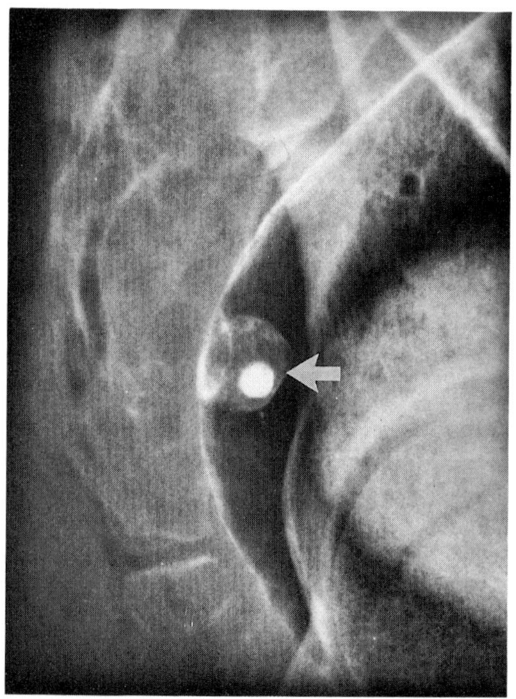

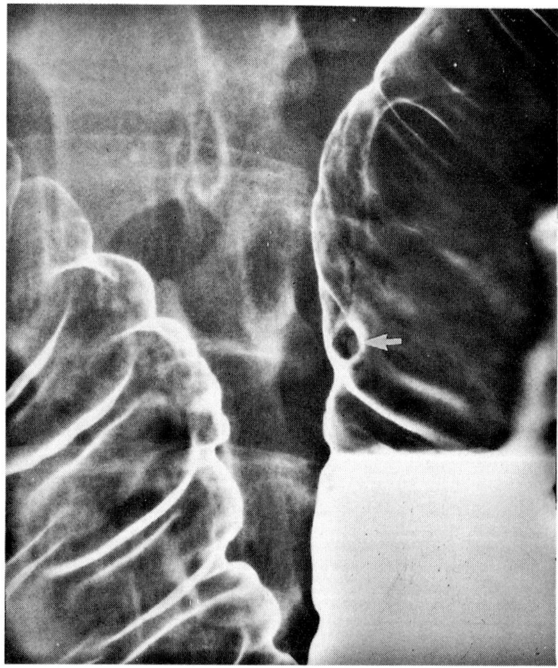

Fig. A.1. (a) Rectal villous adenoma (arrow). The lesion is completely smooth. A drop of barium hangs as a stalactite from the tumor. A similar appearance can be seen with other benign and malignant tumors. (b) Small, smooth transverse colon adenoma (arrow). Small intramural tumors can have a similar appearance. (c) Small, descending colon adenocarcinoma (arrow). No distinguishing characteristics can be identified. (From Skucas et al. (9); copyright RSNA, 1981.) (d) Small and smooth rectal polyp. It was a villous adenoma with carcinomatous transformation.

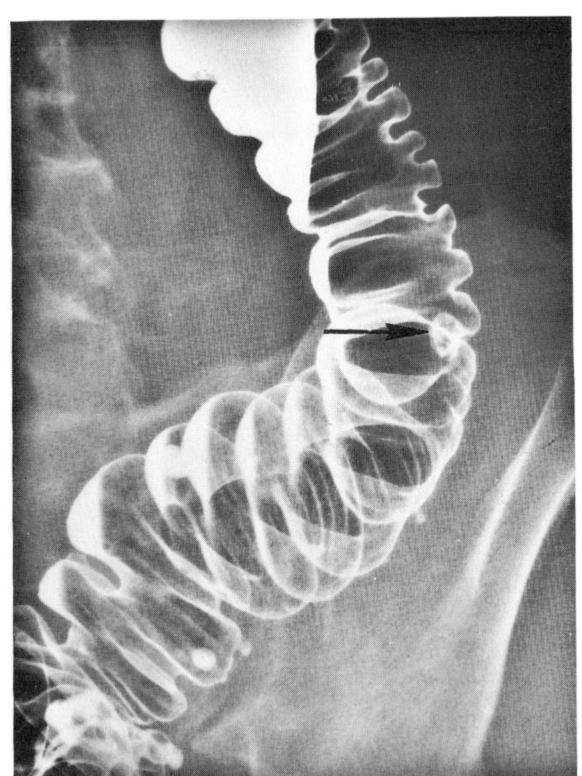

c

does not metastasize because there are no lymphatics more superficial than the muscularis mucosae (17) and such a lesion is thus of limited significance. Only when the cancer invades through the muscularis mucosa into the submucosa is there the possibility of lymphatic metastasis.

Tumor spread is partly related to size. One investigator found no deep invasion in polyps smaller than 1.0 cm (18), while another found no metastases in cancers smaller than 1.5 cm in diameter, but 23% of cancers 1.5–2.9 cm in diameter already had regional lymph node metastases (19). Yet examples of very small adenomatous polyps containing a focus of adenocarcinoma *and* lymphatic invasion are occasionally reported (20).

With growth, a carcinoma overwhelms any adjacent benign tumor tissue. In Morson's series (21), when a rectal cancer had not spread beyond the submucosa, 57% of these tumors still contained

d

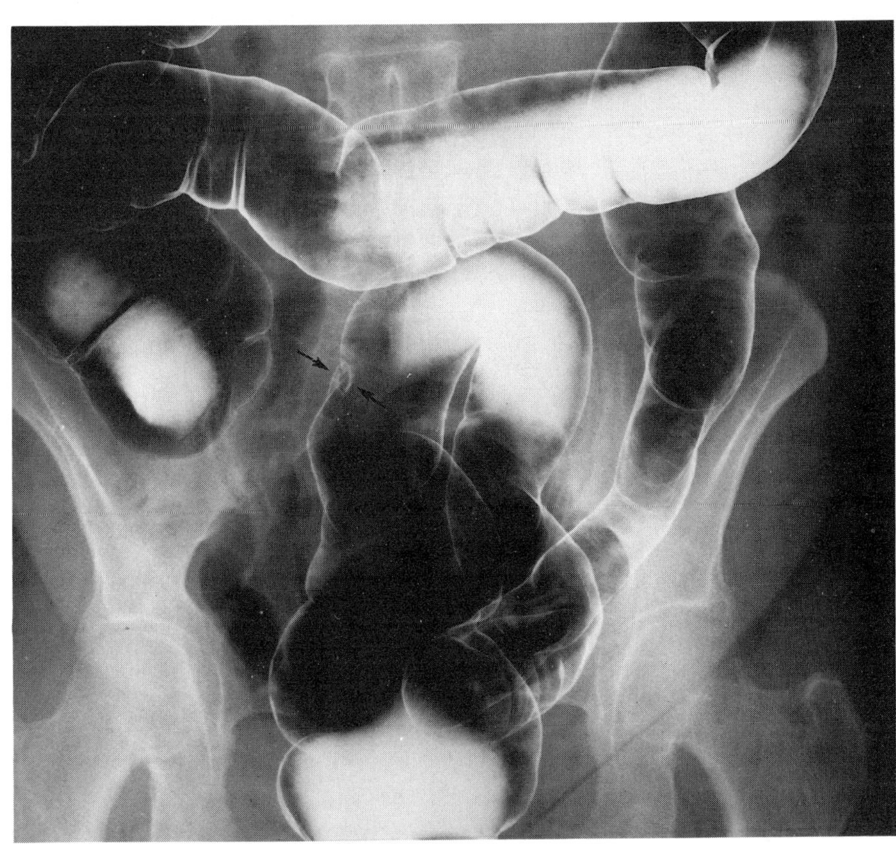

adenomatous tissues. When the cancer had spread to involve the remaining bowel wall, an adenomatous component was seen in only 18% of patients. If the tumor had spread to the extramural tissues, a benign component was found in only 8% of the patients. Other investigators have confirmed such an inverse relationship between the amount of adenomatous tissue present and the degree of carcinomatous involvement (22).

Pedunculated polyps seen on colonoscopy or sigmoidoscopy should be removed completely whenever possible (Fig. A.2). Malignancy is not uncommon in pedunculated polyps (18) (Fig. A.3). Biopsy of a polyp presents several problems to the pathologist. It is difficult for the pathologist to orient a small biopsy specimen to the residual polyp. Even multiple biopsies are of limited reliability in the histological classification of a polyp (23). Biopsies also give a significant incidence of false negative results in the detection of invasive cancer (23). The biopsy may be through an area which is completely benign and thus miss a carcinomatous focus in an adjacent site. Any large irregular lesion, even with a benign biopsy, should be viewed with suspicion.

The question should be raised as to whether *all* colon adenomatous polyps would eventually become carcinomatous; the data so far are incomplete because most visualized polyps are promptly removed. Morson has followed four patients with adenomatous polyps of the rectum (11). Three of the four eventually developed a carcinoma, with the time interval from initial polyp detection to carcinomatous transformation ranging from 5 to 13 years. Realistically, some adenomatous polyps probably never become malignant during a patient's lifetime. It may take 5 years, and possibly considerably longer, to develop fully the adenoma–carcinoma sequence (11).

There is an increased incidence of synchronous colon cancers (7, 11, 24–26) (Figs. A.4–A.6). The reason for such synchronous cancers is not clear. There is also a higher incidence of cancer in those patients who do have a known benign colon neoplasm and vice versa (27) (Fig. A.7). The incidence of

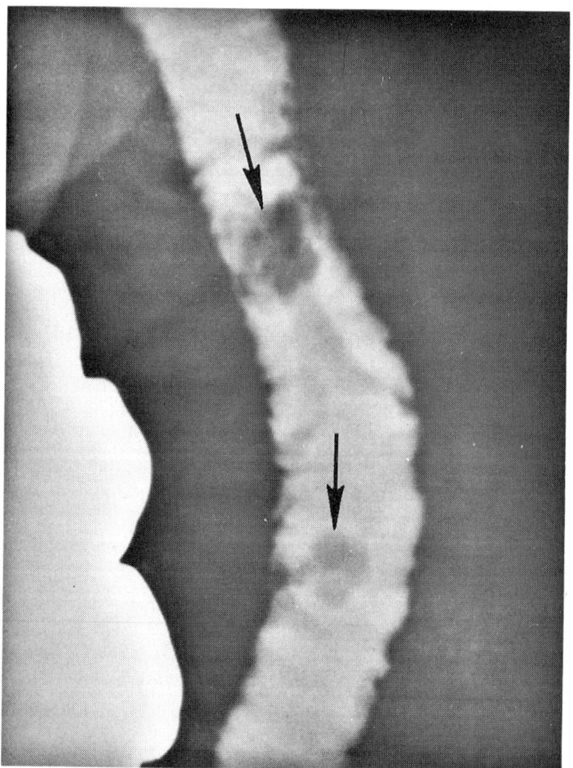
a

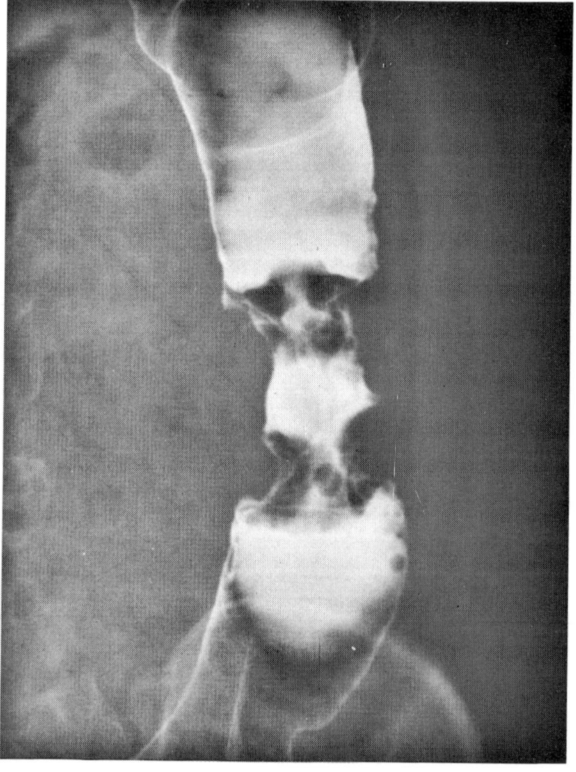
b

Fig. A.2. (a) Several pedunculated polyps (arrows) were seen. The patient was then lost to follow-up. (b) Two and one-half years later a circumferential carcinoma has developed at the same site. No evidence of the pedunculated polyps could be found.

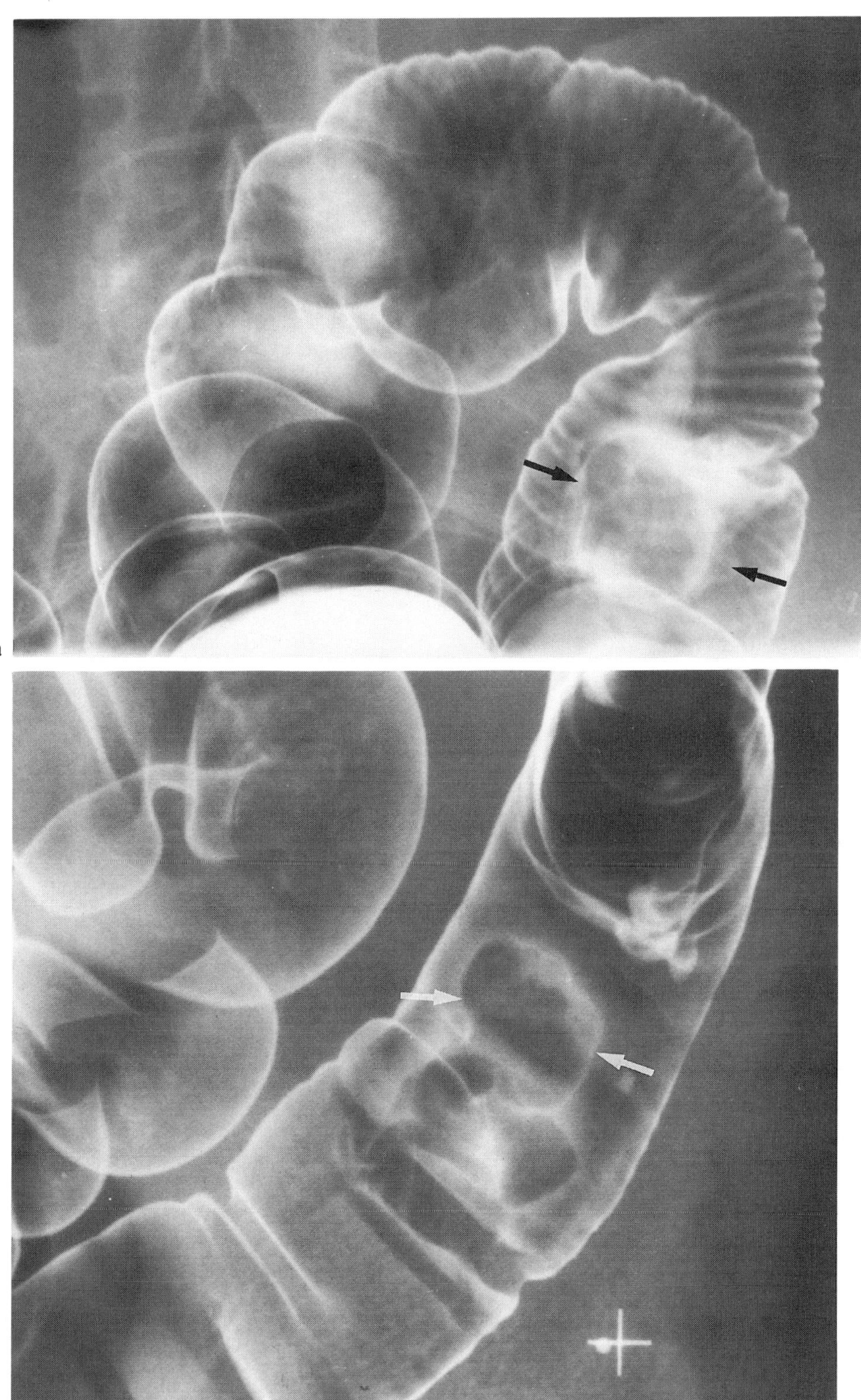

Fig. A.3. (a) Pedunculated, slightly lobulated sigmoid adenocarcinoma (arrows). There was invasion of the stalk. (From Skucas et al. (8); copyright RSNA, 1982.) (b) Well-differentiated adenocarcinoma arising in a pedunculated adenoma (arrows). The carcinoma had extended to the superficial part of the stalk.

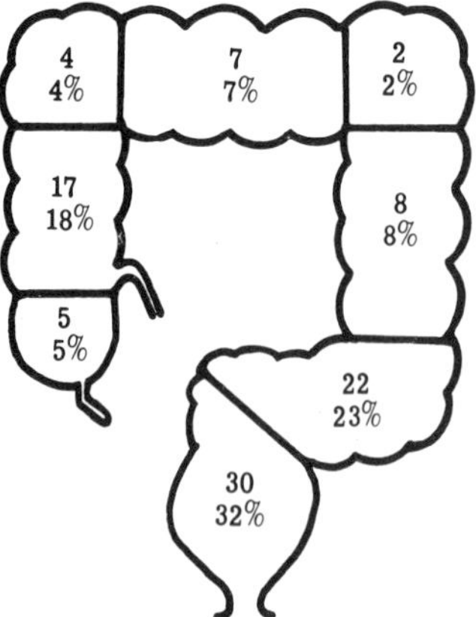

Fig. A.4. The location of a synchronous carcinoma in 95 patients. Sixty percent of these cancers occurred in adjacent colon segments while 40% were distally located. (From Miller and Lehman (63); copyright 1976, AMA.)

carcinoma in these patients varies with the size of the benign polyp and the underlying histology (13, 28, 29). Some have reported an incidence of 20–40% of multiple polyps, consisting of both benign or malignant synchronous tumors (13, 30). Whenever one colon or rectal tumor is found, the entire colon must be studied to exclude other lesions (26).

There are distinct cancer families and some colon cancers appear to be inherited (31–33). Some patients with colon cancer also develop other neoplasms. Warthin described a family with hereditary colon and uterine cancer (34), while Muir et al. reported hereditary association of skin tumors and multiple gastrointestinal cancers (35). In general, if a patient already has one cancer, there is an increased incidence of a new cancer developing in another organ (Fig. A.8). Similarly, if a patient already has had one colon cancer, the chances of later developing a second colon cancer (metachronous cancer) are greater than in the general population. Another way of looking at the risk of developing a metachronous cancer, with one known colon cancer there is a 2–5% chance of the patient developing a second subsequent colon cancer, with the incidence depending upon the follow-up time period (28, 36) (Fig. A.9). An initial cecal cancer appears to be associated with a higher incidence of a second colon cancer (37).

Considerable evidence has accumulated to show

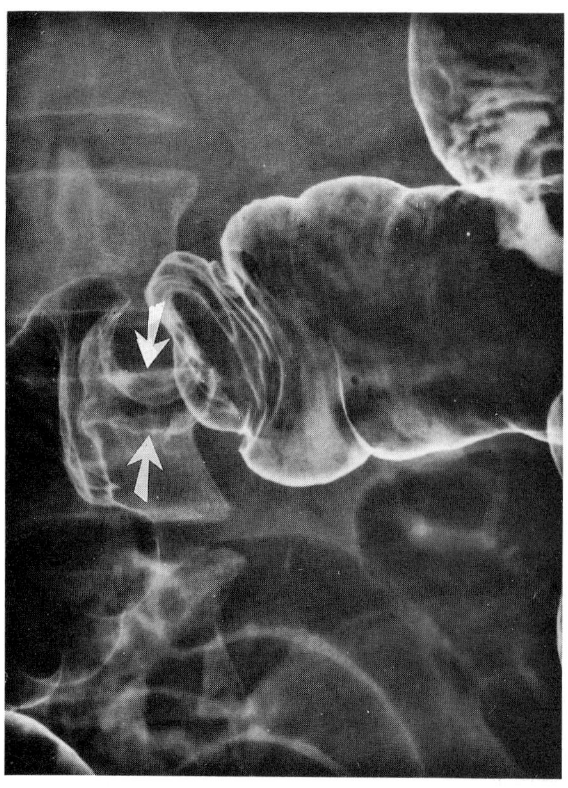
a

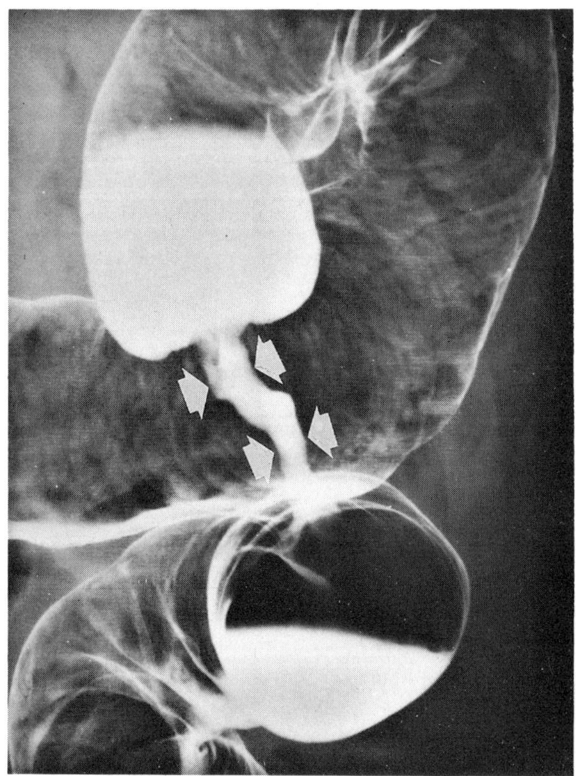

Fig. A.5. Two synchronous adenocarcinomata. (a) The proximal circumferential cancer is in the transverse colon (arrows), while (b) the more distal one, likewise circumferential, is in the descending colon (arrowheads).

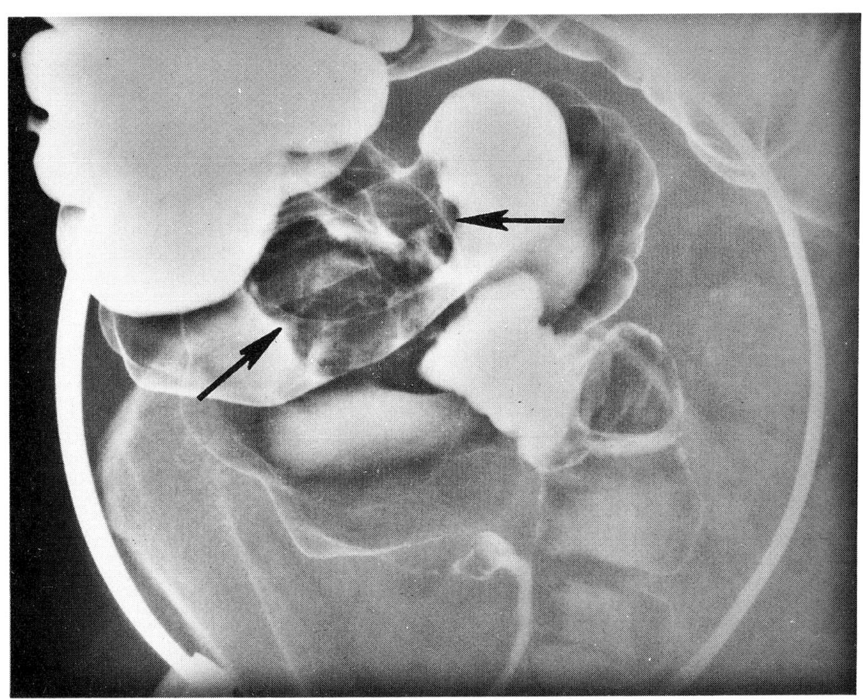

a

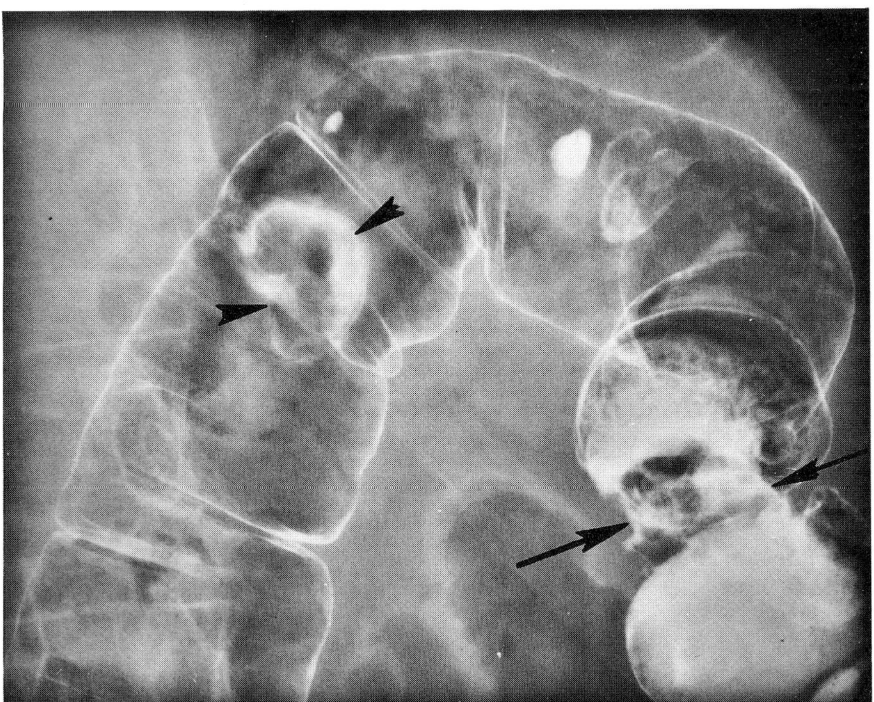

b

Fig. A.6. 70-year-old male with multiple synchronous colon tumors. (a) A sessile invasive carcinoma abuts the ileocecal valve (arrows). (b) A circumferential carcinoma is present in the descending colon (arrows). A villous adenoma can be seen in the transverse colon (arrowheads). The patient also had several other villous adenomata scattered throughout the colon.

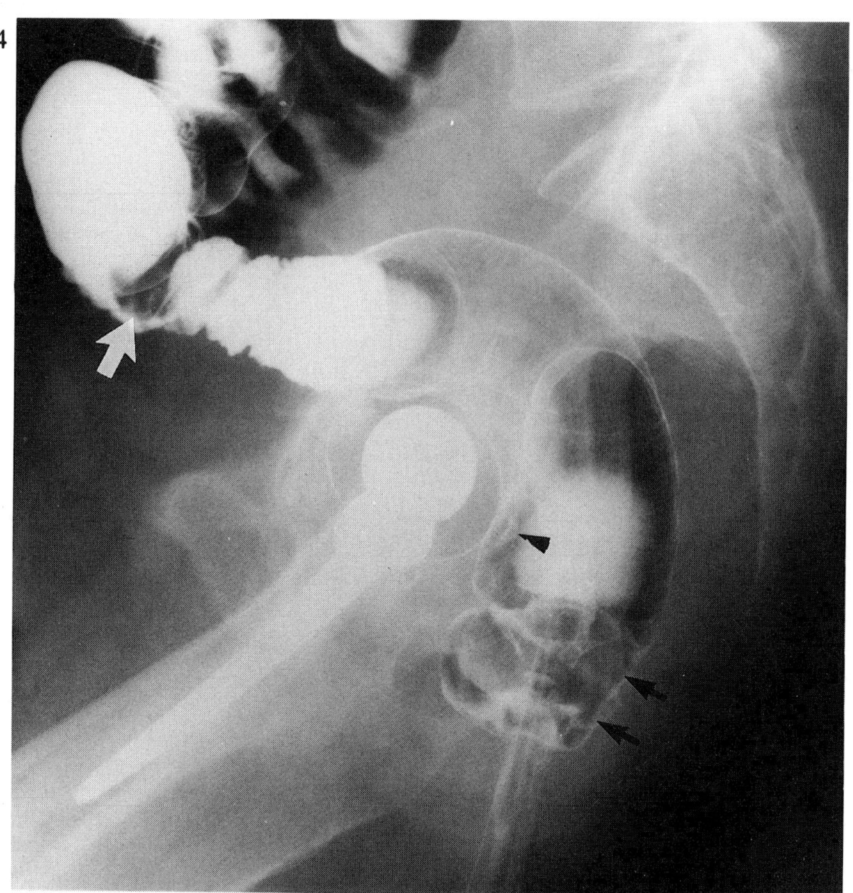

Fig. A.7. 69-year-old male with distal rectal adenocarcinoma (arrows), mid-rectal adenoma (arrowhead) and another sigmoid adenoma (white arrow).

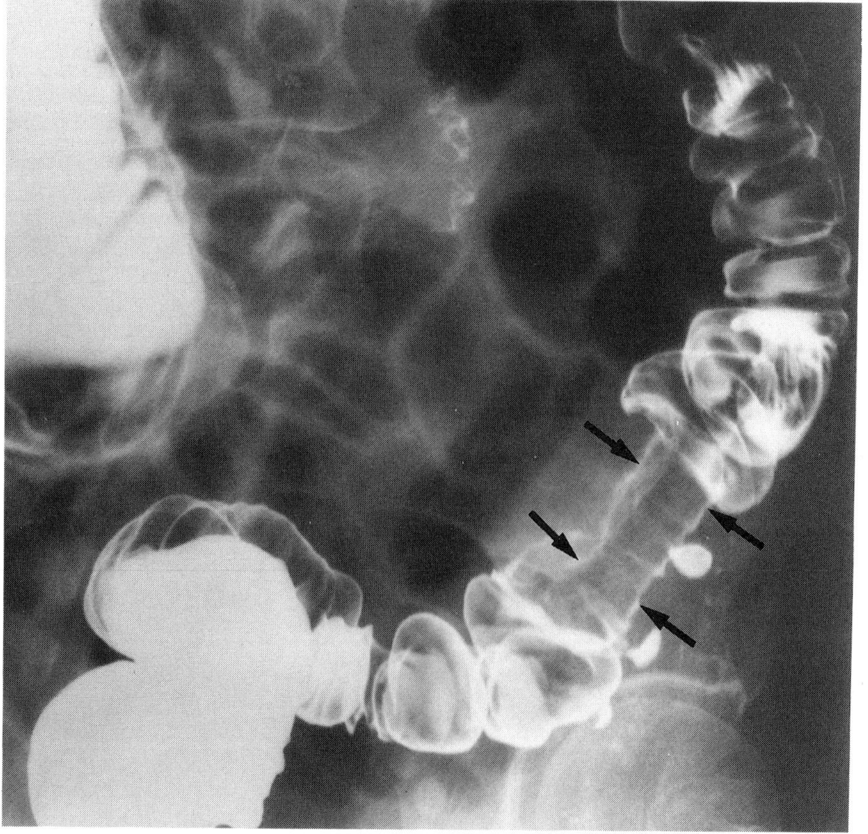

Fig. A.8. An 84-year-old male was found to have an adenocarcinoma of the sigmoid (arrows). Lymph node metastasis was present. In addition to this lesion he has had another adenocarcinoma and a left renal hypernephroma.

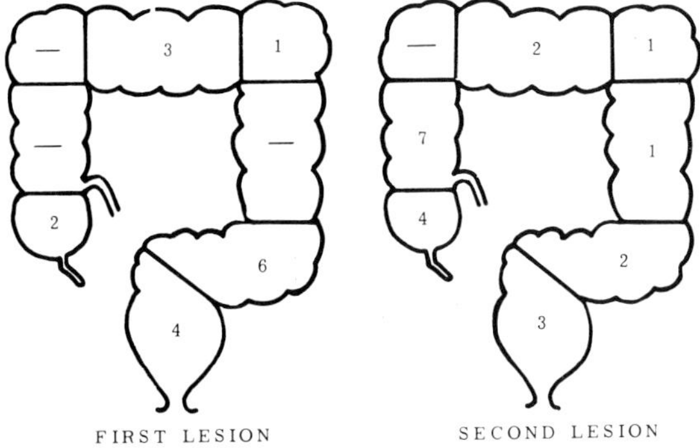

Fig. A.9. Location of second tumor in 16 patients who subsequently developed a second metachronous carcinoma.

that a double-contrast barium enema is superior to a single contrast examination in detecting colon polyps (38, 39) (Table A.2). One group reported a polyp incidence rate of 3.4% when performing single contrast examinations; after changing to double-contrast, the polyp incidence rose to 11.6% (40). The single contrast barium enema likewise has a relatively high false positive rate (41, 42). One study found the double contrast barium enema sensitivity to be 96% and specificity 94% (43). The potential sensitivity with a technically adequate study is believed to be 99% (44).

Numerous studies have been published comparing the diagnostic accuracy of colonoscopy and a barium enema (Table A.3). In general, the missed rate for barium enema decreases as the size of the lesion increases. Most studies are difficult to place in a proper perspective because:

a. Most studies have been retrospective.
b. The colon cleansing regimens have not been comparable.
c. Some have used a single contrast rather than a double-contrast barium enema.
d. The expertise of the respective examiners has not been comparable.
e. Often the colonoscopist knew the radiographic finding.
f. Many used colonoscopy as the final standard, ignoring lesions missed during colonoscopy.

References

1. Lane N, Kaplan H, Pascal RR: Minute adenomatous and hyperplastic polyps of the colon: Divergent patterns of epithelial growth with specific associated mesenchymal changes. Gastroenterology 60:537–551, 1971.
2. Ott DJ, Gelfand DW: Colorectal tumors: Pathology and detection. AJR 131:691–695, 1978.
3. Grinqvist S, Gabrielsson N, Sundelin P: Diminutive colonic polyps—clinical significance and management. Endoscopy 1:36–42, 1979.

Table A.2. Relative accuracy role in polyp detection. Single-contrast versus double-contrast barium enema.

Reference	Year	Polyp miss rate Single-contrast (%)	Double-contrast (%)	Comments
46,47	1974	82	22	<1.0 cm
		23	2	>1.0 cm
48	1974	17	—	61% were <0.5 cm
41	1975	42	—	>0.5 cm
		14		>1.0 cm
49	1975	37	—	>0.5 cm
50	1976	56	—	
51	1977	45	12	all sizes
52	1978	25	—	>0.5 cm
53	1979	42	—	Dukes' A&B
		9	—	Dukes' C&D
54, 55	1980	—	8	>0.5 cm (63% were between 0.5 and 1.0 cm)
56	1981	—	9	Dukes' A&B
			4	Dukes' C&D
43	1981		4	all sizes

Table A.3. Relative accuracy rate in polyp detection. Double-contrast barium enema versus colonoscopy.

Reference	Year	Polyp miss rate		Comments
		Double-contrast (%)	Colonoscopy (%)	
46, 47	1974	22	?	<1.0 cm
		2	?	>1.0 cm
57	1976	0	9	
58	1976	26 (? D-C)	?	? size of polyps
59	1977	34 (? D-C)	?	
60	1977	54	0	<1.0 cm
		15	12	>1.0 cm (Mix of S-C** and D-C)
61	1977	39	9	<1.0 cm
		18	3	>1.0 cm
51	1977	12	12***	all sizes
54, 55	1980	8	?	>0.5 cm
56	1981	9	?	Dukes' A and B
		4	?	Dukes' C and D
62	1981	9	14	rectum only
43	1981	4	?	all sizes

* D-C: Double-contrast barium enema.
** S-C: Single-contrast barium enema.
*** Includes 10% not seen because the area in question could not be reached by the colonoscope.

4. Estrada RG, Spjut HJ: Hyperplastic polyps of the large bowel. Am J Surg Path 4:127–133, 1980.
5. Oohara T, Ogino A, Tohma H: Microscopic adenoma in nonpolyposis coli: incidence and relation to basal cells and lymphoid follicles. Dis Colon Rectum 24:120–126, 1981.
6. Restrepo C, Correa P, Duque E, Cuello C: Polyps in a low-risk colonic cancer population in Columbia, South America. Dis Colon Rectum 24:29–36, 1981.
7. Morson B: The polyp–cancer sequence in the large bowel. Proc R Soc Med 67:451–457, 1974.
8. Skucas J, Spataro RF, Cannucciari DP: The radiographic features of small colon cancers. Radiology 143:335–340, 1982.
9. Skucas J, Spataro RF, Cannucciari DP: The radiologic appearance of small colon carcinomas. Radiographics 1:66–72, 1981.
10. Skucas J, Gluckman JB, Fowler EH, Turner MD, Narisawa T: Radiological evaluation of rat colonic tumors. Invest Radiol 13:34–39, 1978.
11. Day DW, Morson BC: The adenoma–carcinoma sequence. In: Morson BC (ed) The Pathogenesis of Colorectal Cancer, pp 58–71. WB Saunders, Philadelphia, 1978.
12. Gilbertsen VA: Proctosigmoidoscopy and polypectomy in reducing the incidence of rectal cancer. Cancer 34:936–939, 1974.
13. Muto T, Bussey HJR, Morson BC: The evolution of cancer of the colon and rectum. Cancer 36:2251–2270, 1975.
14. Shinya H, Wolff WI: Morphology, anatomic distribution and cancer potential of colonic polyps. An analysis of 7000 polyps endoscopically removed. Ann Surg 190:679–683, 1979.
15. Dawson PA, Filipe MI: An ultrastructural and histochemical study of the mucous membrane adjacent to and remote from carcinoma of the colon. Cancer 37:2388–2398, 1976.
16. Muto T, Kamiya J, Sawada T, Kusuma S, Itai Y, Ikenaga T, Yamashiro M, Hino Y, Yamaguchi S: Colonoscopic polypectomy in diagnosis and treatment of early carcinoma of the large intestine. Dis Colon Rectum 23:68–75, 1980.
17. Fenoglio CM, Kaye GI, Lane N: Distribution of human colonic lymphatics in normal, hyperplastic and adenomatous tissue. Gastroenterology 64:51–66, 1973.
18. Gabrielsson N, Granqvist S, Ohlsen H, Sundelin P: Malignancy of colonic polyps. Diagnosis and management. Acta Radiol Diagn 19:479–495, 1978.
19. Grinnell RS: The chance of cancer and lymphatic metastasis in small colon tumors discovered on X-ray examination. Ann Surg 159:132–138, 1964.
20. Blundell CR, Earnest DL: A caution concerning conservative management of colonic polyps containing invasive carcinoma. Gastrointest Endosc 26:54–55, 1980.
21. Morson BC: Factors influencing the prognosis of early cancer of the rectum. Proc R Soc Med 59:607–608, 1966.
22. Lane N, Fenoglio CM: The adenoma–carcinoma sequence in the stomach and colon. I. Observations on the adenoma as precursor to ordinary large bowel carcinoma. Gastrointest Radiol 1:111–119, 1976.
23. Pugliese V, Gatteschi B, Aste H, Nicolo G, Munizzi F, Giacchero A, Bruzzi P: Value of multiple forceps biopsies in assessing the malignant potential of colonic polyps. Tumori 67:57–62, 1981.
24. Abrams JS, Reines HD: Increasing incidence of right-sided lesions in colorectal cancer. Am J Surg 137:522–526, 1979.
25. Heald RJ, Bussey HJR: Clinical experiences at St. Mark's Hospital with multiple synchronous cancers of the colon and rectum. Dis Colon Rectum 18:6–10, 1975.
26. Ekelund GR, Pihl B: Multiple carcinomas of the colon and rectum. Cancer 33:1630–1634, 1974.
27. Chandler ER, Morris CR: Synchronous and asynchronous

carcinoma of the colon. Tex Med 71:60–66, 1975.
28. Morson BC: Evolution of cancer of the colon and rectum. Cancer 34:845–849, 1974.
29. Morson BC: Genesis of colorectal cancer. Clin Gastroenterol 5:505–525, 1976.
30. Bussey HJR: Multiple adenomas and carcinomas. In: Morson BC (ed) The Pathogenesis of Colorectal Cancer, p 73. WB Saunders, Philadelphia, 1978.
31. Lovett E: Family studies in cancer of the colon and rectum. Br J Surg 63: 13–18, 1976.
32. Anderson DE: Familial cancer and cancer families. Semin Oncol 5:11–16, 1978.
33. Kussin SZ, Lipkin M, Winawer SJ: Inherited colon cancer: clinical implications. Am J Gastroenterol 72:448–457, 1979.
34. Warthin AS: Heredity with reference to carcinoma. Arch Intern Med 12:546–555, 1913.
35. Muir EG, Yates-Bell AJ, Barlow KA: Multiple primary carcinomata of the colon, duodenum and larynx associated with keratoacanthoma of the face. Br J Surg 54:191–195, 1967.
36. Schottenfeld D, Berg JW, Vitsky B: Incidence of multiple primary cancers. II. Index cancers arising in the stomach and lower digestive system. J Natl Cancer Inst 43:77–86, 1969.
37. Chait MM, Lipkin M: Genetic and pathogenetic influences in the development of large bowel neoplasia. In: Enker WE (ed) Carcinoma of the Colon and Rectum, p 345. Year Book Medical, Chicago, 1978.
38. Laufer I: The double-contrast enema: myths and misconceptions. Gastrointest Radiol 1:19–31, 1976.
39. Gelfand DW, Ott DJ: Single vs. double-contrast gastrointestinal studies: critical analysis of reported statistics. AJR 137:523–528, 1981.
40. Marti R, Descombes P, Delamarre J, Dupas J-L, Capron J-P, Trinez G: Intérêt de la radiographie en double contraste dans le dépistage des polypes rectocoliques. Arch Fr Mal App Dig 65:197–200, 1976.
41. Wolff WI, Shinya H, Geffen A, Ozoktay S, DeBeer R: Comparison of colonoscopy and the contrast enema in five hundred patients with colorectal disease. Am J Surg 129:181–186, 1975.
42. Knutson CO, Williams HC, Max MH: Detection of intracolonic lesion by barium contrast enema. The importance of adequate colon preparation to diagnostic accuracy. JAMA 242:2206–2208, 1979.
43. Martin F, Ribet A, Escourron J, Delpu J, Klepping C, Bernier JJ, Soullard J, Marti R, Nisard A, Bader J-P, Sarles H, Sahel J, Bonfils S, Vilotte J, Grenier J, Loygue J: Étude multicentrique prospective sur la détection des polypes et des cancers rectocoliques dans une population d'hospitalisés et de consultants. Gastroenterol Clin Biol 5:58–66, 1981.
44. Kelvin FM, Gardiner R, Vas W, Stevenson GW: Colorectal carcinoma missed on double contrast barium enema study: a problem in perception. AJR 137:307–313, 1981.
45. Watanabe H, Numazawa M, Shoji K, Hiwatashi N, Goto Y: Diagnosis of early cancer of the colon and rectum. Tohoku J Exp Med 129:183–195, 1979.
46. Williams CB, Hunt RH, Loose H, Riddell RH, Sakai Y, Swarbrick ET: Colonoscopy in the management of colon polyps. D Br J Surg 61:673–682, 1974.
47. Loose HWC, Williams CB: Barium enema versus colonoscopy. Proc R Soc Med 67:1033–1036, 1974.
48. Sugarbaker PH, Vineyard GC, Lewicki AM, Pinkus GA, Warhol MJ, Moore FD: Colonoscopy in the management of diseases of the colon and rectum. Surg Gynecol Obstet 139:341–349, 1974.
49. Welch CE, Hedberg SE: Polypoid Lesions of the Gastrointestinal Tract, 2nd edn, pp 22–45. WB Saunders, Philadelphia 1975.
50. Coller JA, Corman ML, Veidenheimer MC: Colonic polypoid disease: need for total colonoscopy. Am J Surg 131:490–494, 1976.
51. Thoeni RF, Menuck L: Comparison of barium enema and colonoscopy in the detection of small colonic polyps. Radiology 124:631–635, 1977.
52. Tedesco FJ, Wayne JD, Raskin JB, Morris SJ, Greenwald RA: Colonoscopic evaluation of rectal bleeding. A study of 304 patients. Ann Intern Med 89:907–909, 1978.
53. Gilbertsen VA, Williams SE, Schuman L, McHugh R: Colonoscopy in the detection of carcinoma of the intestine. Surg Gynecol Obstet 149:877–878, 1979.
54. Ott DJ, Gelfand DW, Wu WC, Kerr RM: Sensitivity of double-contrast barium enema: emphasis on polyp detection. AJR 135:327–330, 1980.
55. Ott DJ, Gelfand DW, Ramquist NA: Causes of error in gastrointestinal radiology. II. Barium enema examination. Gastrointest Radiol 5:99–105, 1980.
56. Thorpe CD, Grayson DJ Jr, Wingfield PB: Detection of carcinoma of the colon and rectum by air contrast enema. Surg Gynecol Obstet 152:307–309, 1981.
57. Laufer I, Smith NCW, Mullens JE: The radiological demonstration of colorectal polyps undetected by endoscopy. Gastroenterology 70:167–170, 1976.
58. Swarbrick ET, Hunt RH, Fevre DI, Williams CB. Colonoscopy for unexplained rectal bleeding. Gut 17:823, 1976.
59. Hunt RH: Rectal bleeding. Clin Gastroenterol 7:719–740, 1978.
60. Leinicke JL, Dodds WJ, Hogan WJ, Stewart ET: A comparison of colonoscopy and roentgenography for detecting polypoid lesions of the colon. Gastrointest Radiol 2:125–128, 1977.
61. Hogan WJ, Stewart ET, Geenen JE, Dodds WJ, Bjork JT, Leinicke JA: A prospective comparison of the accuracy of colonoscopy vs. air–barium contrast exam for detection of colonic polypoid lesions [Abstract]. Gastrointest Endosc 23:230, 1977.
62. Evers K, Laufer I, Gordon RL, Kressel HY, Herlinger H, Gohel VK: Double-contrast enema examination for detection of rectal carcinoma. Radiology 140:635–639, 1981.
63. Miller RE, Lehman G: The barium enema. Is it obsolete? JAMA 235:2842–2844, 1976.

III.3.B. Benign tumors

a. Introduction

The reported incidence of colon polyps depends considerably upon the method employed in their detection. In any series the detection rate depends upon the patient population group selected and upon the care with which the colon is examined. In one series, colon polyps were grossly visible in almost 40% of all adult autopsies (1). However, in this same series, 50% were less than 0.5 cm in diameter and 84% were smaller than 1.0 cm. More than one-half of all patients with one polyp had at least one additional polyp. A large series using double-contrast barium enema examinations at Malmö, Sweden, detected colon polyps in 12.5% of all adult patients examined (2). A corresponding autopsy series performed at the same institution at approximately the same time also revealed an incidence of 12.5% colon polyps (3). In Malmö, almost all patients that died in hospitals underwent autopsy and it is thus apparent that the double-contrast barium enema detected polyps at essentially the same frequency as the autopsy series. In a collection of international investigators, a double-contrast barium enema likewise revealed a polyp detection rate of 10 to 13% (4).

b. Clinical considerations

A suprising number of benign colon tumors are discovered by chance during a barium enema, sigmoidoscopy, or colonoscopy. Even in retrospect there may not by any symptoms referable to the polyp. When present, the most common clinical sign of a polyp is bleeding. If the bleeding is slow, the patient may simply present with guaiac positive stool or anemia. With significant bleeding from a right colon polyp, melena or hematochezia is seen, while a profusely bleeding distal colon polyp presents with hematochezia. Some polyps produce excessive mucus.

Although an adenoma containing primarily a villous structure can be associated with hypokalemia, diarrhea and other systemic symptoms, we find such presentations rare. The vast majority of villous adenomata, even with a typical radiographic appearance, are not associated with any unusual signs or symptoms, with the exception of the occasional ulcerated one that bleeds. Some of these villous polyps are soft, deform and can readily be missed on rectal examination.

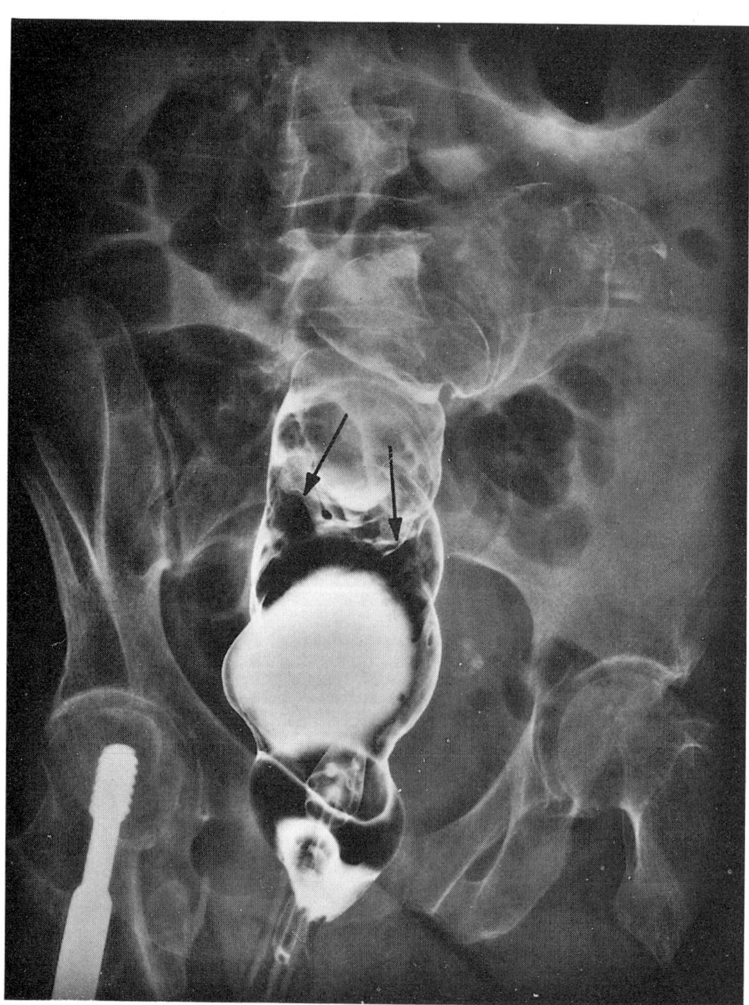

Fig. B.1. Sigmoid polyp acting as the lead point for an intussusception (arrows). No antegrade obstruction was present.

A polyp can act as a lead point for an intussusception (Fig. B.1). Most of these intussusceptions originate in the cecum. One should be suspicious of cecal polyps resulting in intussusception, because the vast majority of these polyps are adenocarcinomata, with lymphoma being a poor second finding. These intussusceptions can be a transient phenomenon, with the patient simply presenting with intermittent right lower quadrant pain.

It is unusual for a benign colon polyp to obstruct. Generally, by the time the polyp has grown to such a size that it produces even partial obstruction, there already is malignant degeneration.

c. Radiology of benign polyps

Although there are many ways of describing a colon polyp, from a radiologist's viewpoint, classification into categories of sessile and pedunculated polyps is useful. A sessile polyp has a broad base and a stalk cannot be readily identified. When a sessile polyp is viewed en face, the polyp will have a round or an oval appearance. A pedunculated polyp has a broad head and a neck which is more narrow than the head. The appearance of a pedunculated polyp will vary depending upon the length of the stalk; a short and relatively broad stalk results in an appearance similar to that of a sessile polyp. When the polyp has a long stalk, it can move back and forth during the examination. The en face appearance of a pedunculated polyp consists of two concentric circles, with the inner circle representing an outline of the stalk and the outer circle representing the actual head of the polyp. When seen in profile, both the head of the polyp and the stalk should be readily identifiable (Fig. B.2).

The most difficult areas for identifying polyps are the sigmoid, flexures, cecum, and any overlapping loops of bowel. In particular, utmost care must be taken to unravel the sigmoid colon; it is the most difficult portion of the colon to examine by any method, including colonoscopy. It is not unusual to find a polyp buried in an area severely involved with diverticulosis. Multiple polyps can be present (Fig. B.3).

If the colon cannot be adequately cleansed, it is easy to confuse retained fecal material with polyps. Undigested corn kernels, in particular, can mimic polyps (5). Sometimes it is possible to exclude other entities by appropriate patient positioning. Both decubitus and upright positions are by far the most helpful in such a differentiation because a polyp will have limited mobility while retained stool will gravitate toward the most dependent position.

Air bubbles can be confused with polyps. Here again, positioning the patient either in an upright or decubitus position generally allows ready differentiation. Small air bubbles commonly have a characteristic round or oval appearance and are surrounded by a thin and gradually diminishing density of barium (6). Multiple small satellite bubbles are frequently present.

Mucus strands generally have a long linear appearance, and change their shape and configuration depending upon patient positioning. Adequate colon cleansing should reduce the amount of mucus present.

When seen *en face*, a polyp can be confused with a diverticulum. If there is retained barium within the diverticulum, the differentiation is obviously easy (Fig. B.4). The most reliable way to differentiate a polyp from a diverticulum not filled with barium is to view the lesion in profile. If the fluoroscopist can show that the lesion extends outside of the colon lumen, then it must be a diverticulum and not a polyp, while if the lesion cannot be shown to extend outside of the colon lumen even by rotating the patient 360°, then one can generally assume that the lesion is a polyp.

Pressure applied over both a diverticulum and a polyp can change their shape. Palpation can occasionally be used to differentiate between a polyp and retained fecal material.

d. Adenoma

An adenoma is a benign neoplasm arising from bowel epithelium. Most adenomata tend to grow intraluminally rather than intramurally, thus presenting as a mass within the lumen. They can be sessile or pedunculated (Fig. B.5). Their size can vary from barely visible to large and irregular masses occupying a considerable volume in the clon lumen (Fig. B.6). Though the smaller adenomata tend to be smooth, with growth they acquire a lobulated outline. In general, however, a polyp with an irregular outline has a greater chance of being malignant than benign. Unfortunately, many small adenocarcinomata are completely smooth in

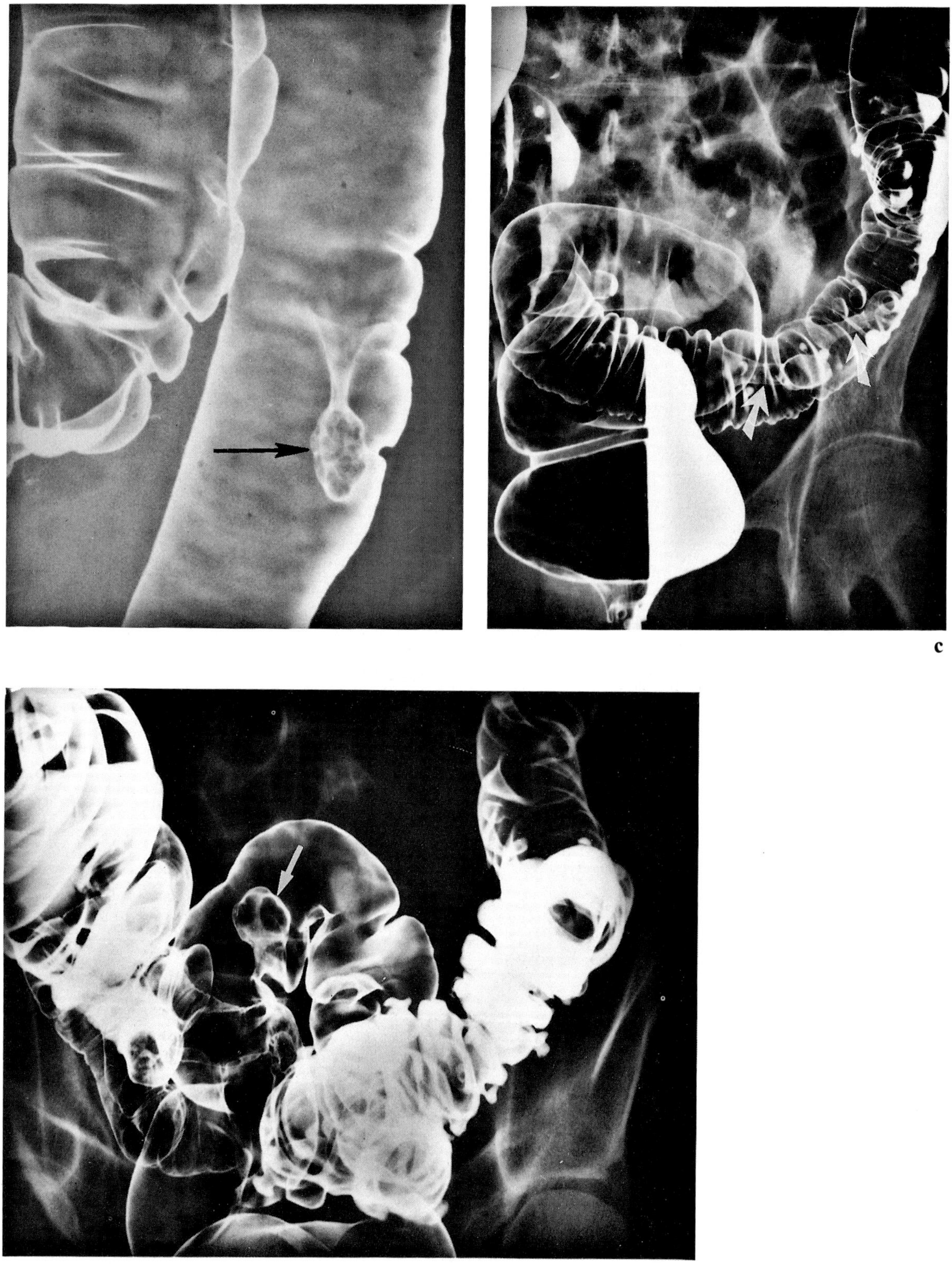

a

c

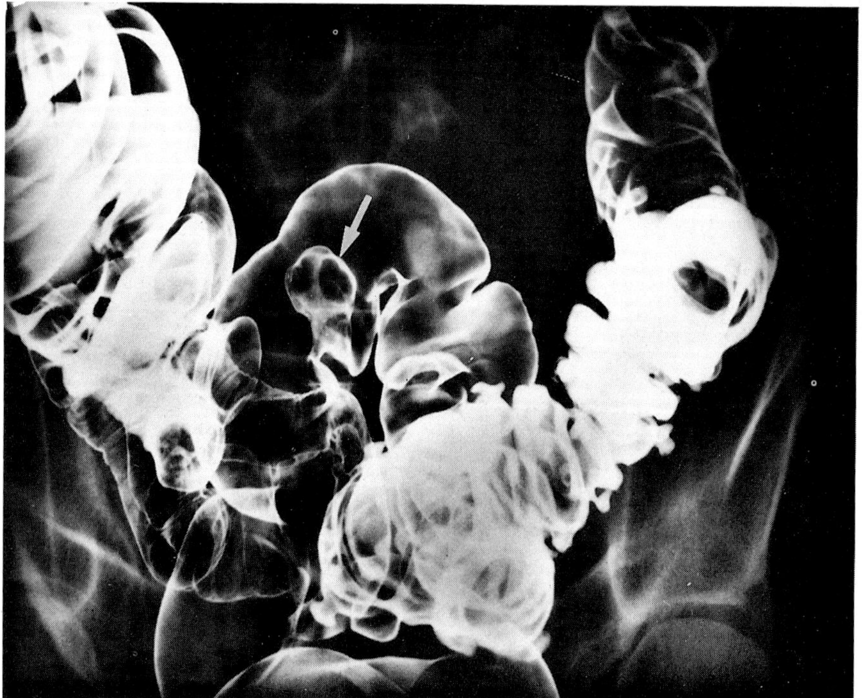

b

Fig. B.2. (a) Adenomatous pedunculated polyp (arrow). The polyp is on a relatively long stalk. (b) Another pedunculated polyp (arrow). These polyps have a similar appearance. (c) Two polyps on long pedicles (arrows) in sigmoid colon. Both polyps were adenomata.

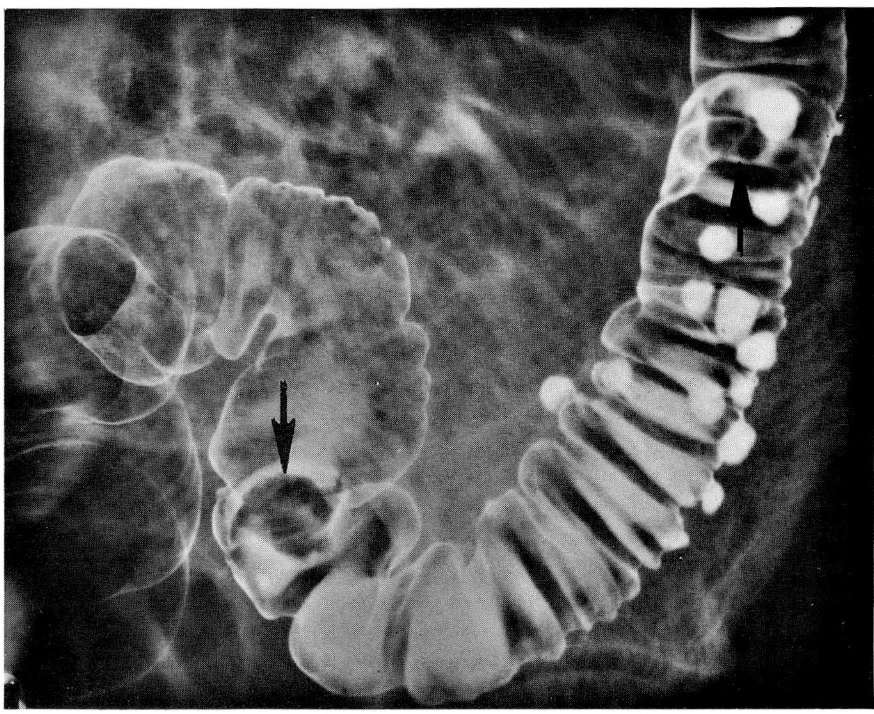

Fig. B.3. Two adenomata (arrows) in sigmoid colon. Numerous diverticula surround the polyps.

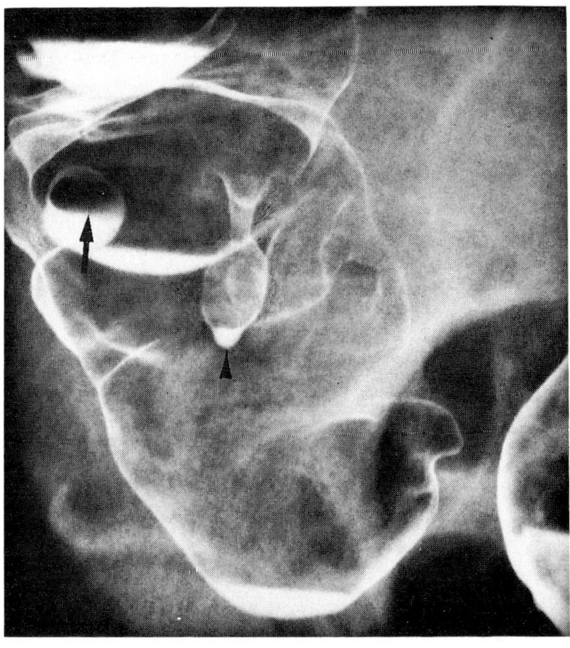

Fig. B.4. With the patient upright, an air–fluid level is present in a right colic diverticulum (arrow). An adjacent pedunculated polyp has a drop of barium clinging to the head of the polyp (arrowhead).

outline. It is impressive that, for the same size and shape, the incidence of malignancy in a rectal polyp tends to be greater than in a polyp elsewhere in the colon.

To evaluate whether a polyp is benign or malignant, the major criterion is size. Likewise, if there has been growth in the size of a polyp between two serial examinations, a malignancy should be suspected. Just because a lesion has grown, however, does not mean that there is a malignancy present because even adenomatous polyps grow in size. Although both skin and lung cancer exhibit an essentially geometric growth rate, there is evidence to suggest that colon malignancies do not always follow such a geometric progression (7).

At times a polyp may indent and retract the colon wall at the base of the polyp. This sign is best found by looking at the polyp in profile. Such an indentation at the base should be viewed with suspicion for malignancy, although an adenoma or inflammatory polyp can occasionally have an apparent retracted base depending on the geometry and angle of radiographic exposure (Fig. B.7).

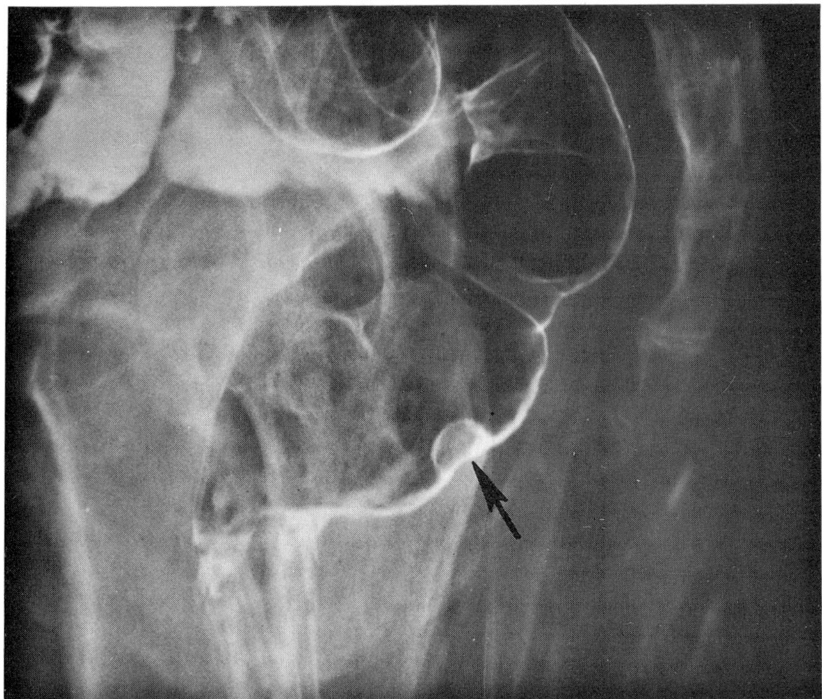

a

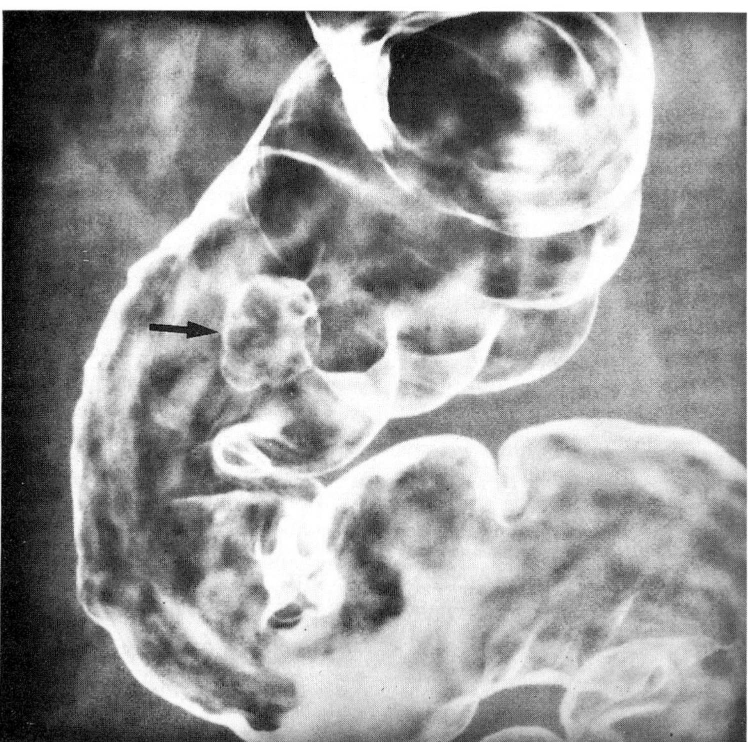

b

Fig. B.5. (a) Sesile rectal polyp (arrow). The polyp was an adenoma. It was not detected on initial endoscopic examination. (b) A small adenoma with a slightly irregular outline (arrow). (c) Irregular sessile polyp (arrow). It was an adenoma. (d) Larger, more irregular outline of an adenoma in the transverse colon (arrow).

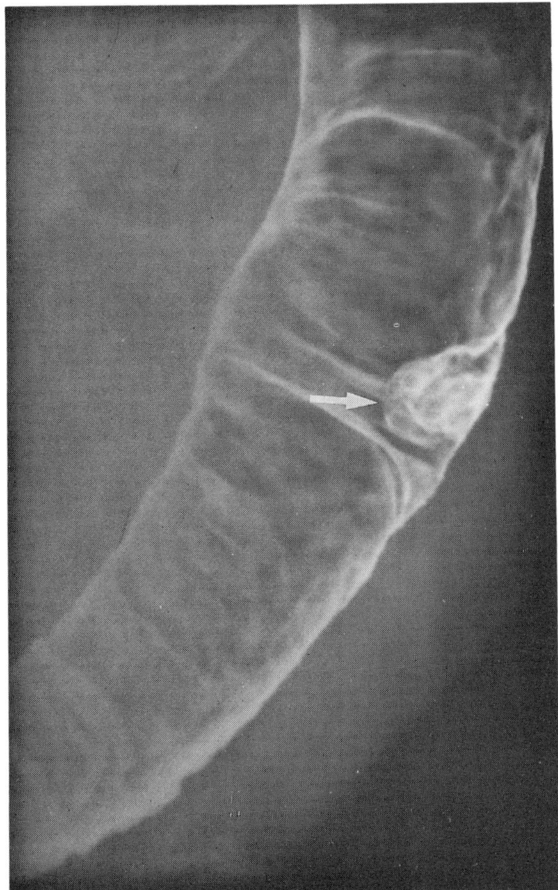

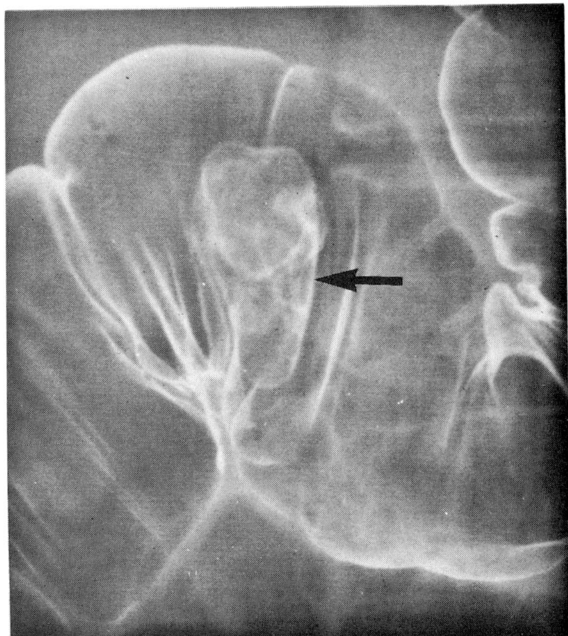

*Fig. B.5.***d.**

*Fig. B.5.***c.**

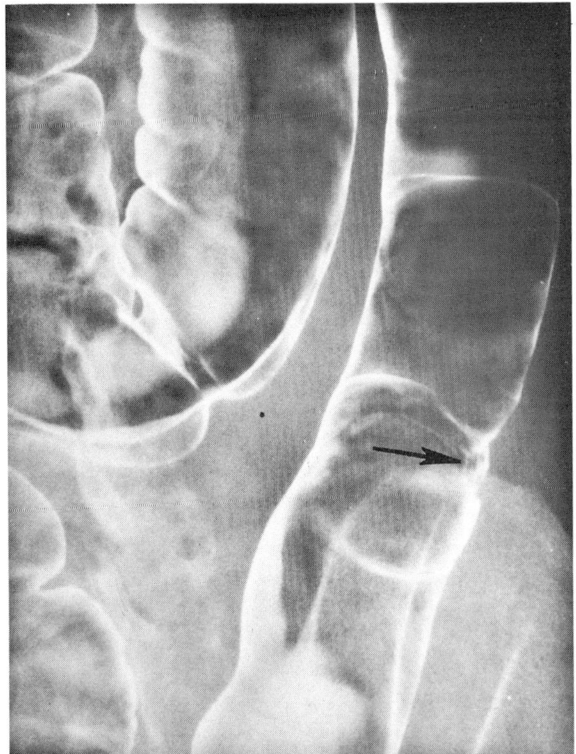

Fig. B.6. Small *irregular* descending colon polyp. It was an adenoma. (From Skucas et al. (95); copyright, RSNA, 1981.)

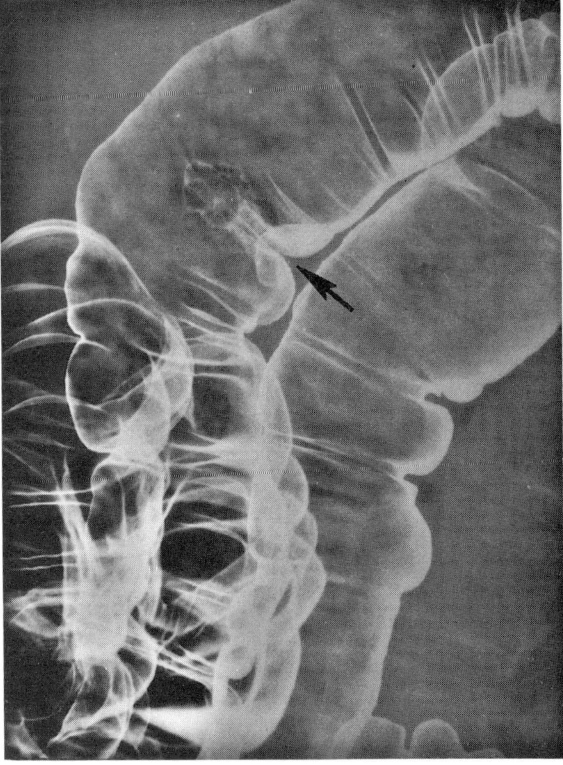

Fig. B.7. Retraction at the base of a pedunculated polyp (arrow). The polyp was an adenoma.

Many villous adenomata are either smooth or slightly irregular in outline and cannot be distinguished from tubular adenomata (Fig. B.8). A villous adenoma can be either sessile or pedunculated, although most eventually do have a wide base (Fig. B.9). A large villous adenoma can have an irregular and frond-like appearance, which is characteristic of these lesions (8) (Fig. B.10). Barium caught between the fronds produces this fine reticular pattern. Unfortunately, only approximately one-third of all villous adenomata exhibit these characteristic findings, with lesions in the proximal portion of the colon having the least likelihood of having such a characteristic appearance (9) (Fig. B.11).

Adenomata which contain primarily a villous structure have a high propensity for carcinomatous transformation. Such a change is more common with the larger tumors and quite often the malignancy is not apparent on a barium enema, the polyp having an overall relatively benign appearance (10) (Fig. B.12). A villous adenoma can likewise be associated with other gastrointestinal neoplasms.

e. Lipoma

A prominent ileocecal valve is usually caused by accumulations of fat or lipomatosis. Generally both the superior and inferior lips are equally involved. Such lipomatosis is considered to be of no significance and a moderately enlarged and relatively symmetrical valve can be assumed to be a normal variant.

A lipoma has a capsule while lipomatosis is unencapsulated. Lipomata are relatively common benign colon tumors and occur more often in the right side of the colon. They are the most common ileocecal valve tumor encountered and are generally confined to one lip of the valve (Fig. B.13). Histology reveals a capsule with diffuse fatty infiltration throughout. Unfortunately, the histological findings cannot be seen radiographically and the radiologist must rely on gross appearance. Because lipomata are intramural and encapsulated they tend to have a smooth and sessile appearance (Fig. B.14). Rarely are they pedunculated. They can ulcerate, intussuscept or bleed. Occasionally, with palpation a lipoma will change shape, thus suggesting the diagnosis, because most other polyps are not as soft (11). Lipomata can be small or large. Multiple lipomata can be present (12–14).

The differentiation of a lipoma from a malignant neoplasm is difficult. In general, symmetrical enlargement of both lips of the ileocecal valve is caused by valve lipomatosis. A smooth, pliable tumor of one lip usually represents a lipoma. If there is any irregularity of the lesion's surface, biopsy should be considered to help exclude a carcinoma.

A tap water enema has been suggested as an aid in diagnosing a lipoma (15). Because a lipoma consists primarily of fat, during a water enema the fat-containing polyp should be more lucent than the surrounding soft tissues and the intraluminal water and thus be readily apparent. Although this diagnostic test is described in many radiological textbooks, it has been helpful in only isolated and anecdotal instances. To our knowledge, a water enema combined with computerized tomography (CT) has not been described as an aid in diagnosis, although the increased contrast range available with CT makes this modality theoretically possible for the larger lesions.

a

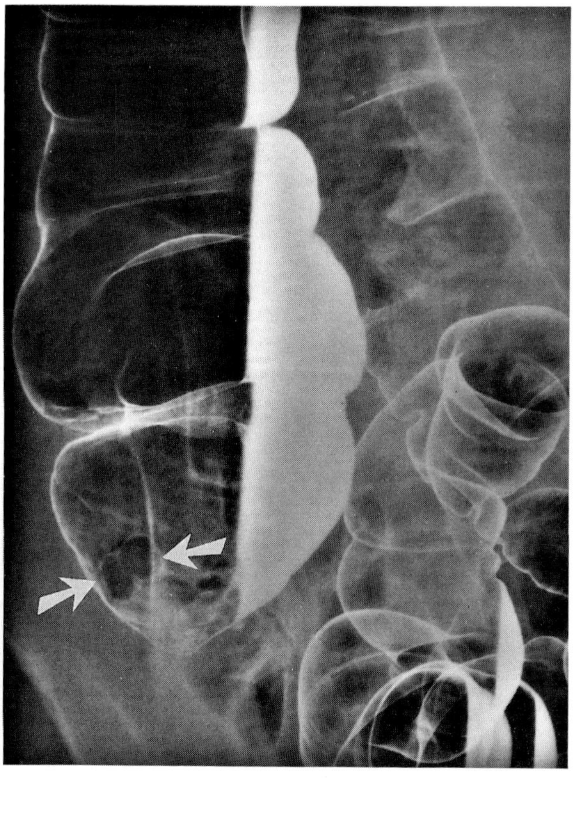

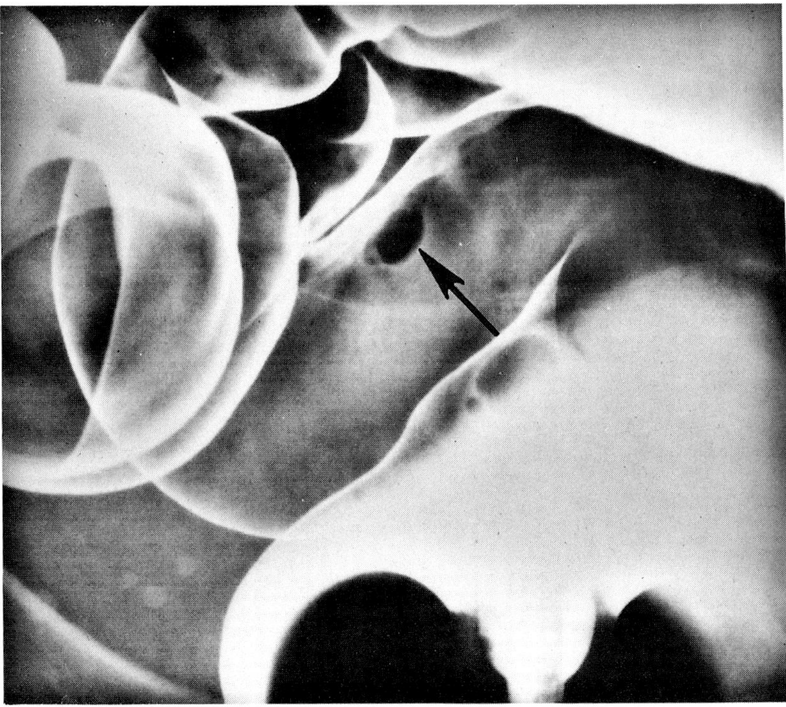

b

c

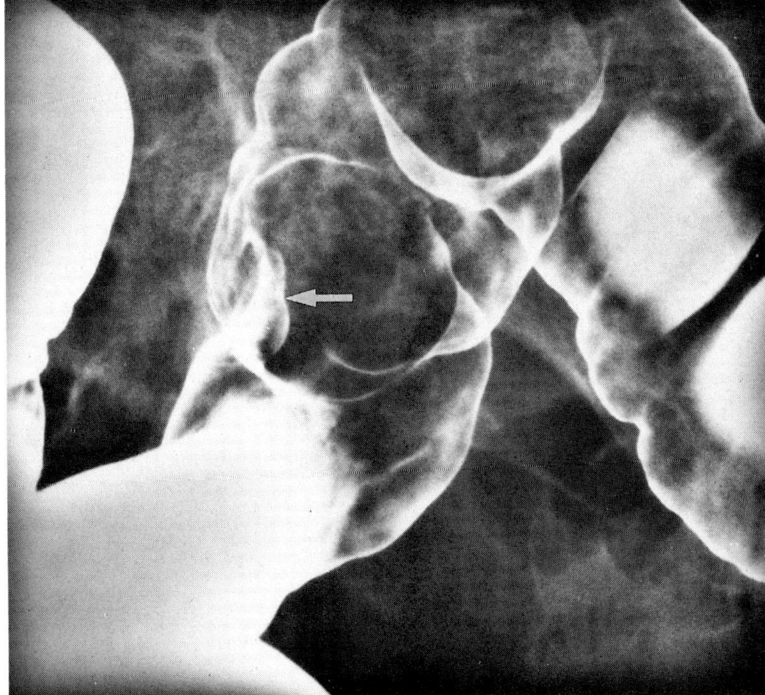

Fig. B.8. (a) Cecal villous adenoma (arrows). The bi-lobed tumor has a relatively smooth outline and there is nothing in its appearance suggesting a villous composition. (b) Small rectal villous adenoma (arrow). The lesion is smooth in outline. (c) Small sigmoid villous adenoma (arrow). The polyp has a broad base and is slightly irregular in outline. The appearance is nonspecific.

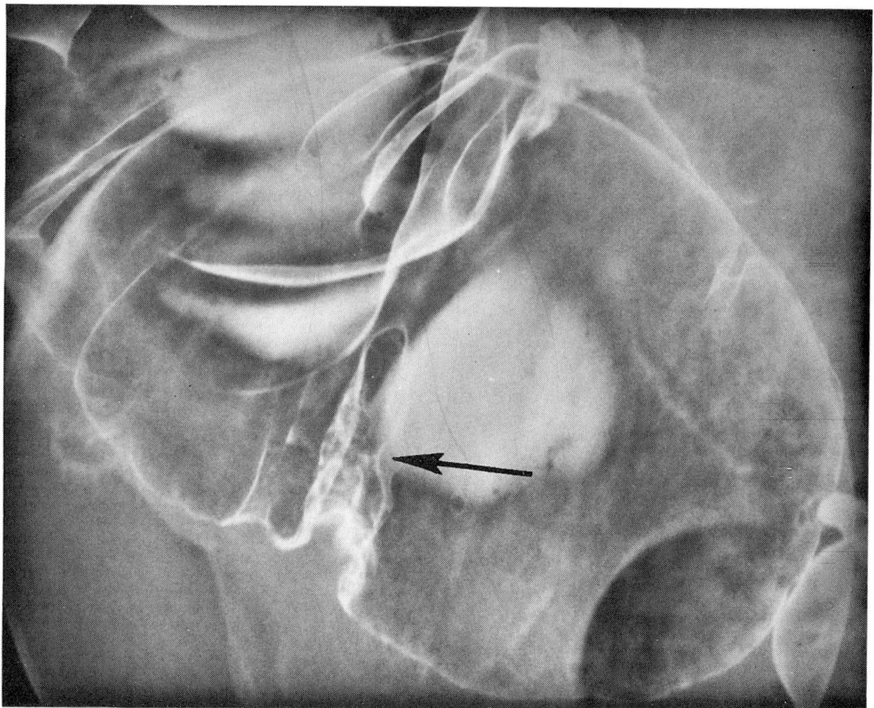

a

b

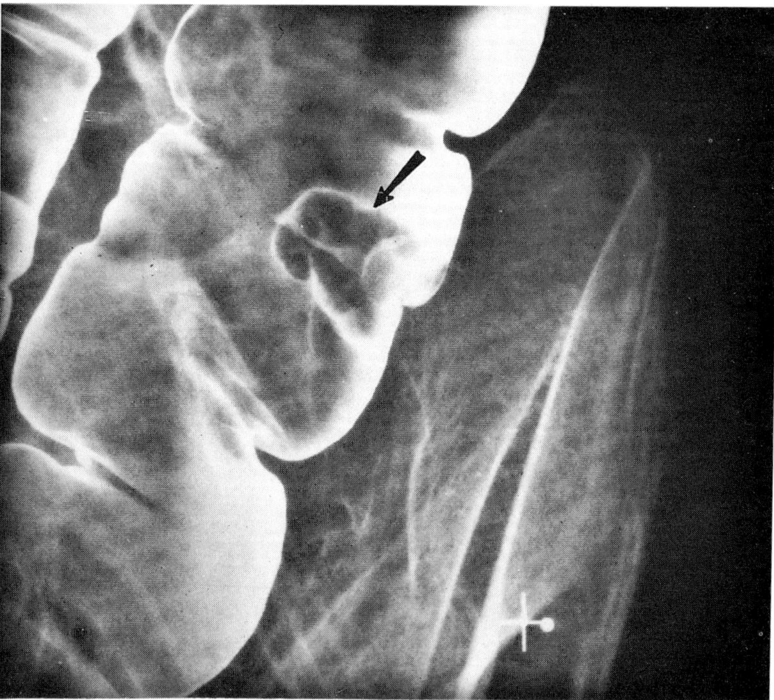

Fig. B.9. (a) Cecal villous adenoma (arrow). Although this tumor has an irregular outline, nothing distinguishes it from a tubular adenoma or a carcinoma. (b) Pedunculated sigmoid villous adenoma (arrow). A poorly-defined frond-like outline is beginning to form.

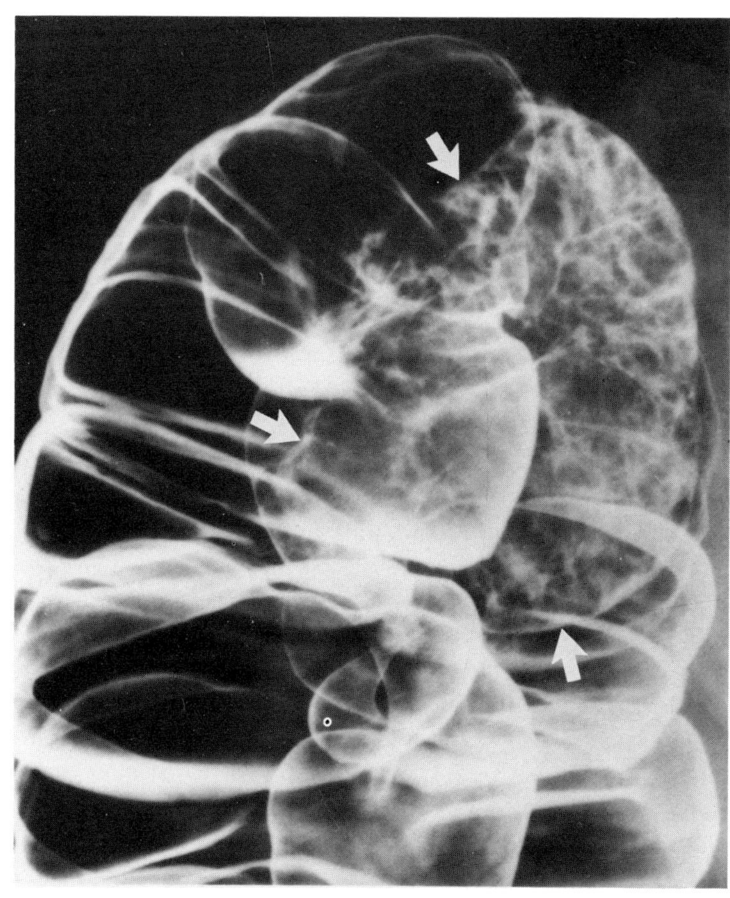

Fig. B.10. Typical frond-like irregular appearance of a large villous adenoma (arrows). Such a picture is characteristic for these tumors.

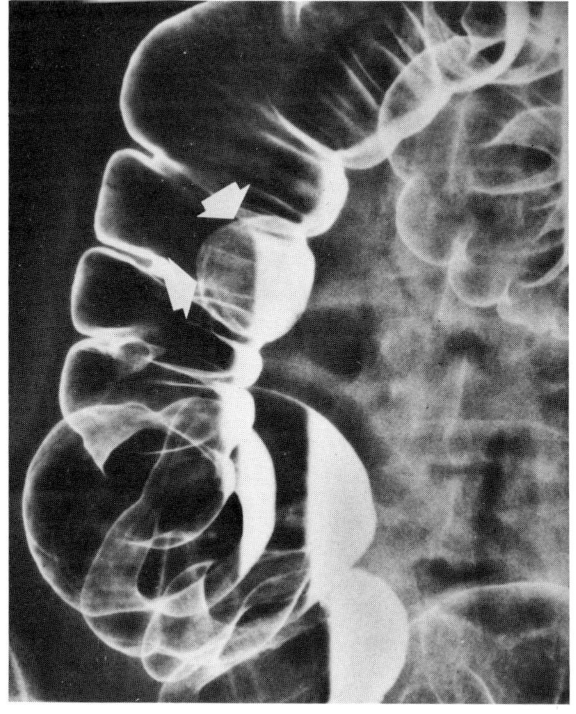

f. Hyperplastic polyp

These polyps have also been called metaplastic, a term preferred by some pathologists to emphasize their benign and non-neoplastic condition (16). Occasionally an adenomatous component is present (17). These polyps are most common in the rectum, are small and, as with most small polyps, have a smooth radiographic outline. Radiographically, they are indistinguishable from a neoplastic polyp (Fig. B.15).

A patient with hundreds of large hyperplastic polyps throughout the colon has been reported (18).

g. Hamartoma

A hamartoma is an inborn error in development and consists of an abnormal mixture of tissues. Morson distinguishes hamartomata from neoplasms (19). Hamartomata consist of fat, fibrous,

Fig. B.11. Smooth, sesile, 3 cm in diameter ascending colon polyp (arrowheads). It was a villous adenoma.

muscle, bone or other mesenchymal tissues. The diagnosis should be made only if two or more mesenchymal elements are present.

A barium enema cannot differentiate a hamartoma from any other colon polyp. Angiography, performed in an occasional patient, can reveal either a hypervascular (20) or a hypovascular pattern (21).

Hamartomatous polyps are encountered in juvenile polyposis, Peutz-Jegher syndrome, and Cronkhite-Canada syndrome. An isolated hamartoma is also sometimes encountered.

h. Carcinoid

This tumor was first mentioned by Langhans in 1867 (22) and further described by Lubarsch in 1888 (23). Although it can be found in various organs, by far the vast majority of carcinoid tumors originate in the gastrointestinal tract. The appendix is the most common site, followed by the ileum and the rectum (24). Carcinoids are somewhat uncommon in the remainder of the colon, although the larger carcinoids are generally found in the colon rather than the rectum. The vast majority of these tumors behave as if benign, yet some do metastasize. There appears to be an increased association with other gastrointestinal neoplasms (25).

Most appendiceal carcinoids are found in young and middle-aged adults, while colon carcinoids are seen in older individuals. These tumors arise from enterochromaffin cells, previously called Kulchitsky cells and argentaffin cells. The cells are neural in origin and are located in the crypts of Lieberkühn. The vast majority of these tumors are discovered incidentally in the submucosa of resected bowel specimens.

The primary tumor, as well as a metastatic focus, liberates hormones resulting in the classic signs of the syndrome which consist of cutaneous flushing, diarrhea, abdominal pain, together with other cardiac and respiratory symptoms. The typical syndrome is more often due to ileal rather than colon carcinoid. Rectal carcinoids tend to be less aggressive than those in the rest of the colon (24). Also, the carcinoid syndrome is less common with rectal lesions.

Appendiceal carcinoids, which exhibit a considerably lower malignant potential than colon carcinoids, are discussed further in the chapter on appendiceal disease.

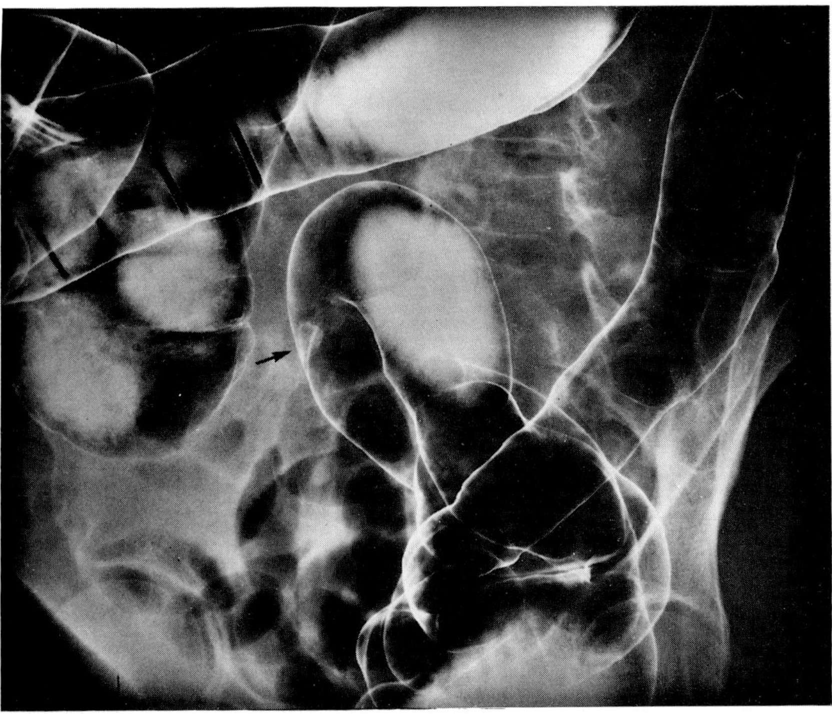

Fig. B.12. Small smooth-appearing villous adenoma (arrow). An adenocarcinoma had already developed in this polyp.

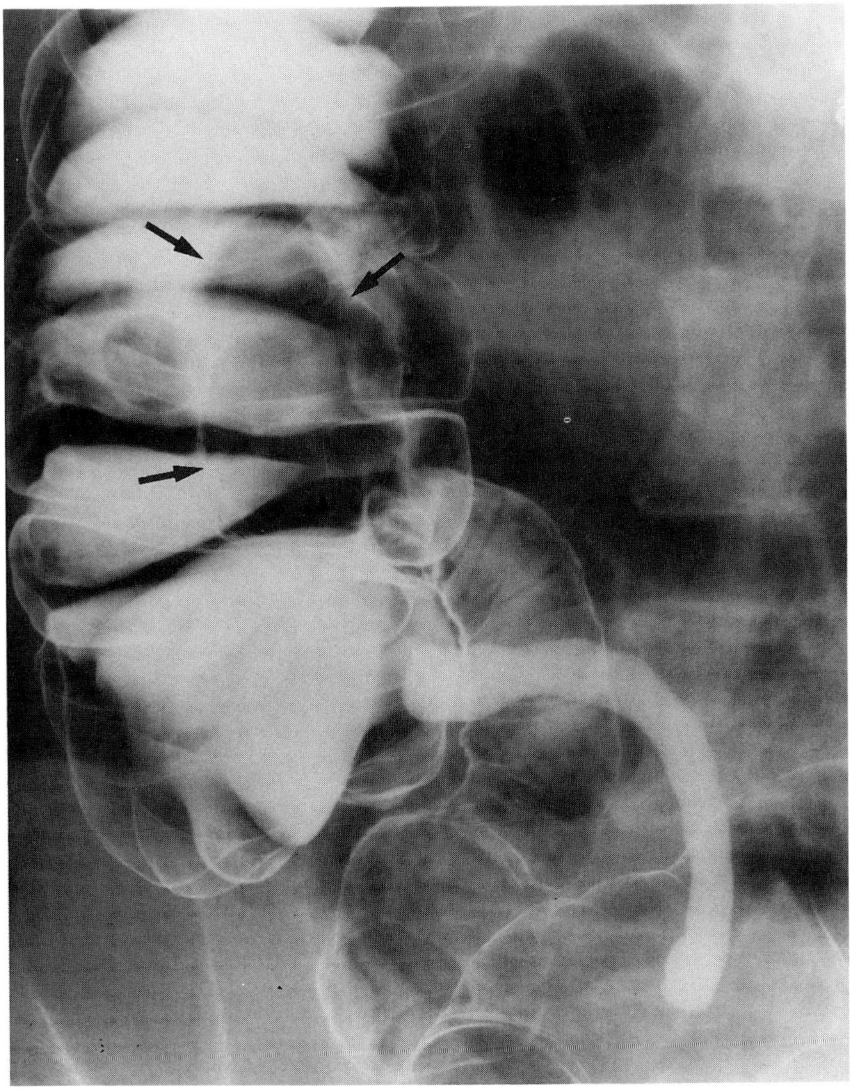

a

b

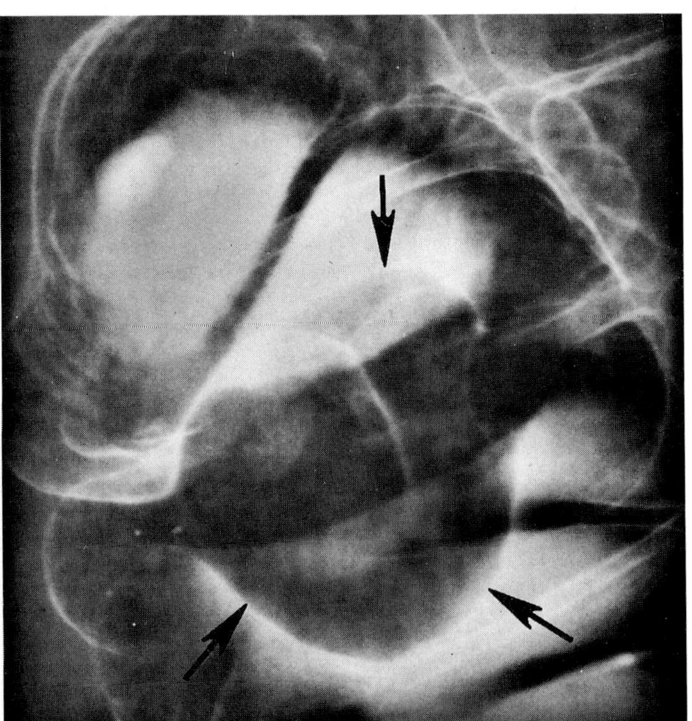

Fig. B.13. (a) Lipoma arising from the superior lip of the ileocecal valve (arrows). The lipoma is smooth in outline and not well defined, a characteristic of intramural tumors. (b) A large ileocecal valve lipoma (arrows).

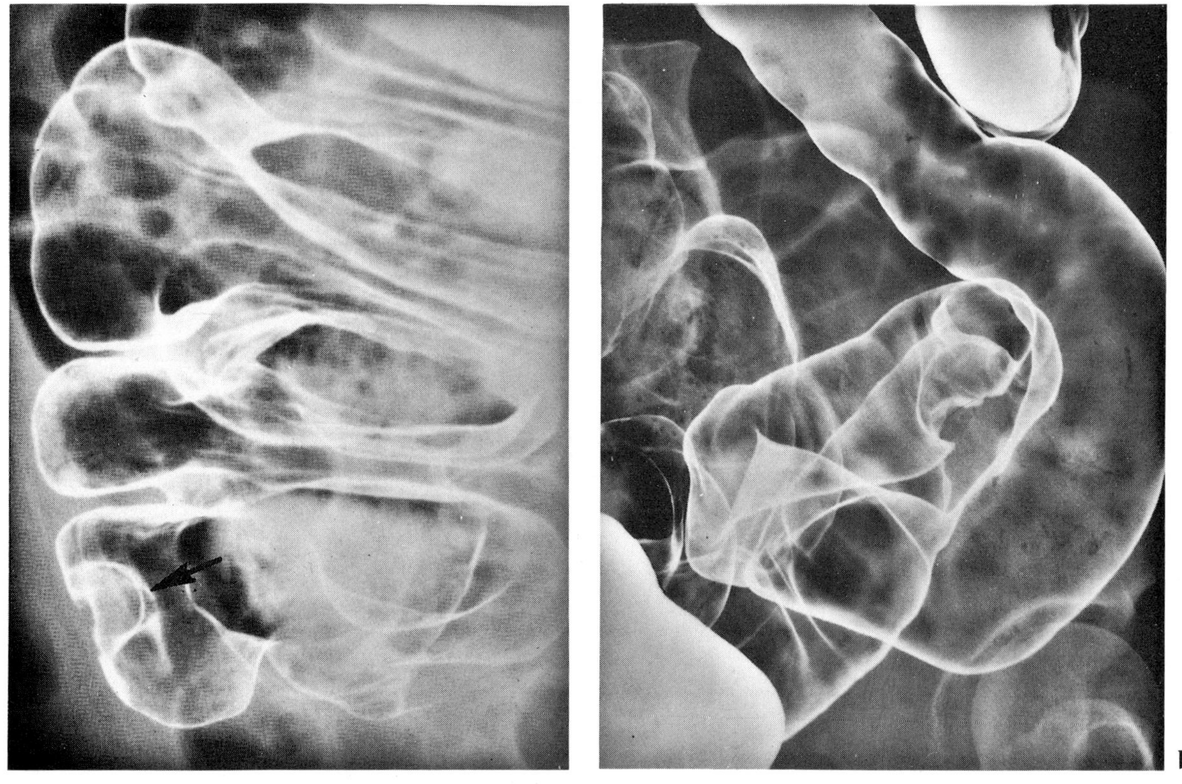

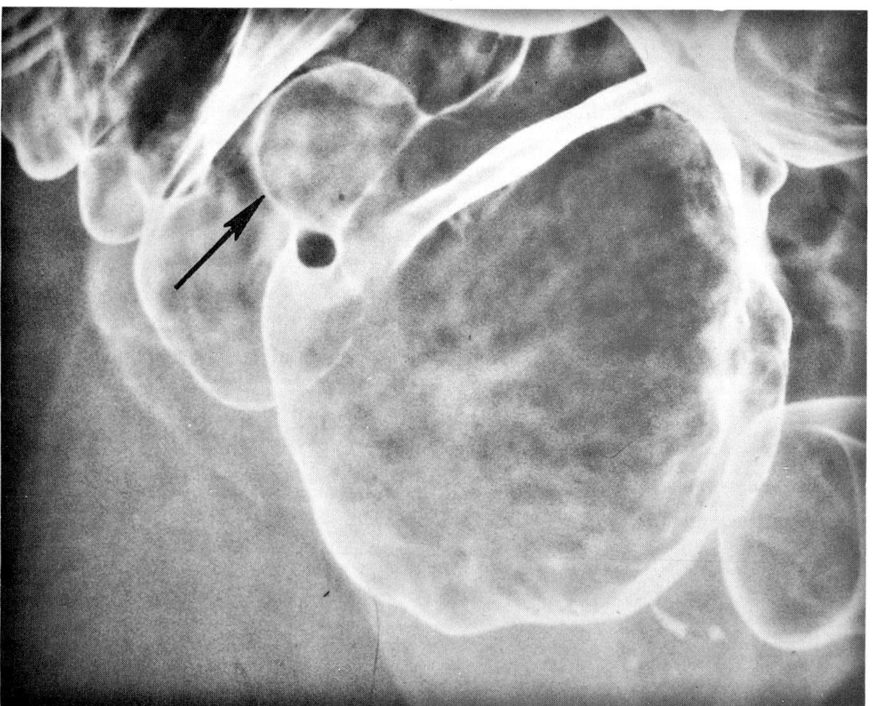

Fig. B.14. (a) Small cecal lipoma (arrow). The appearance is similar to other small neoplasms. (c) Cecal lipoma (arrow). The lesion is smooth in outline and typical for a lipoma. (b) A larger lipoma. The smooth outline suggests an intramural tumor.

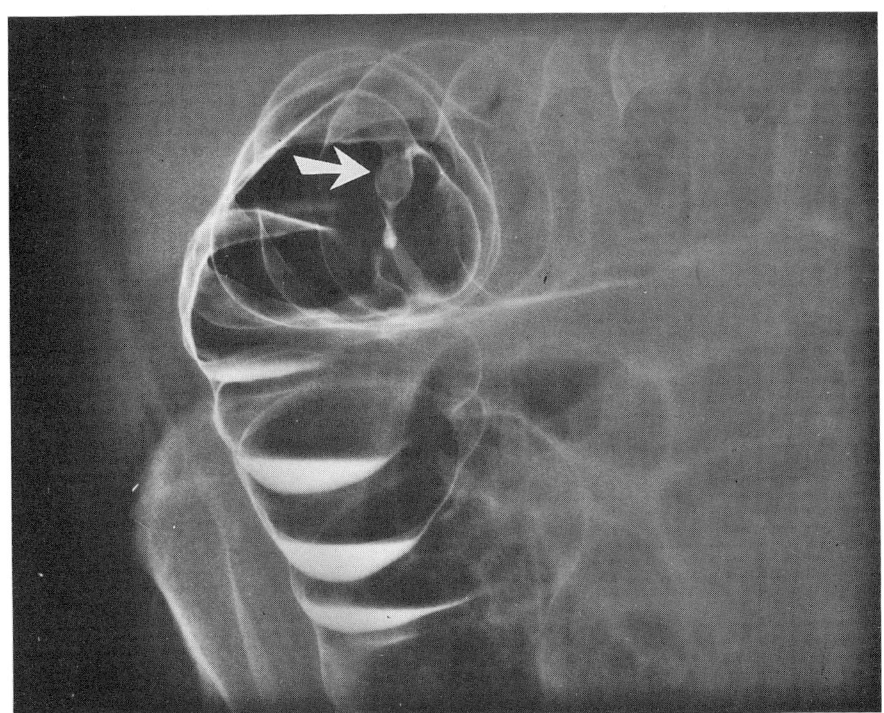

a

b

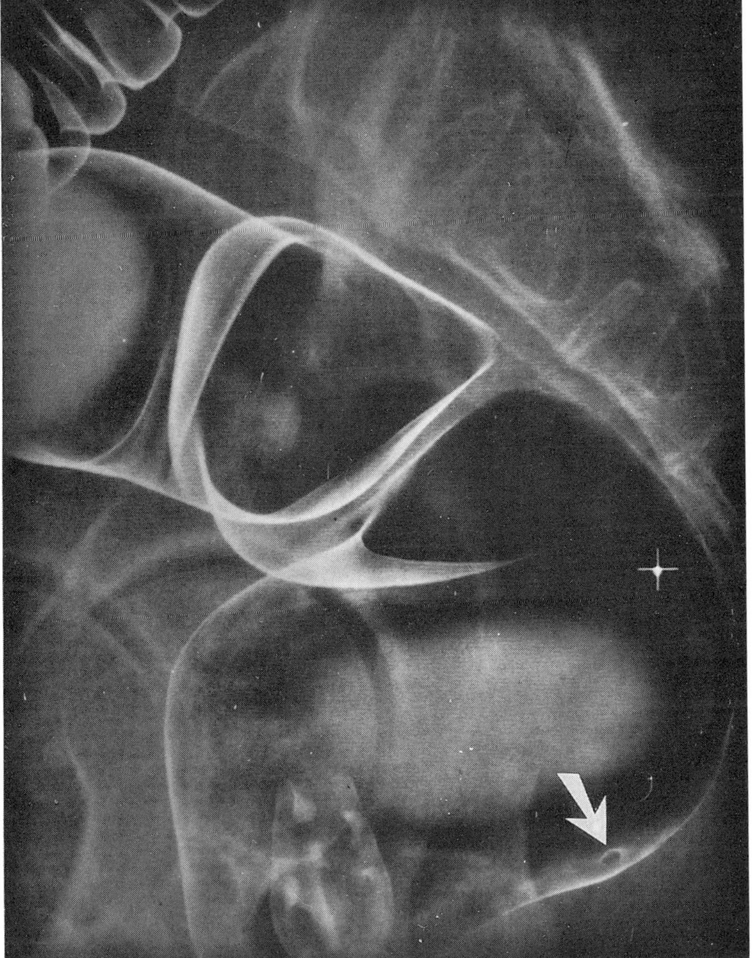

Fig. B.15. (a) Hyperplastic polyp (arrow). A drop of barium is suspended from the polyp. The polyp is smooth in outline and is similar in appearance to a neoplastic polyp. (b) Rectal hyperplastic polyp (arrow). The appearance is similar to the adenoma illustrated in Fig. B.5 (a).

Metastasis tends to depend upon the size of the primary tumor, with most small primary lesions rarely exhibiting malignant characteristics. It is not unusual, however, for a patient to seek medical attention when liver metastases and the characteristic clinical picture are already present.

Radiographically most carcinoids are sessile or infiltrating, with only an occasional pedunculated carcinoid being encountered. When small, most are smooth in outline, although with growth and invasion they tend to become irregular (26). Thus the larger lesions can mimic an adenocarcinoma (27). Occasionally a large extraserosal mass will be present. Colon carcinoids do not calcify.

Carcinoid metastasis to bone can show either an osteoblastic or a mixed pattern (26).

Whenever a carcinoid is suspected clinically, angiography is very useful in locating the primary tumor and in evaluating possible metastases (28). Staining at the tumor site is seen, the involved arteries and veins tend to be narrowed or obstructed, and there can be retraction of vessels because of a desmoplastic reaction, resulting in foreshortening of the mesentery. Liver metastases tend to be hypervascular.

i. Other miscellaneous polyps

Small polyps are occasionally encountered at the site of anastomosis after resection (Fig. B.16). If multiple, these polyps tend to be arranged in a row, as if they were 'man-made' (Fig. B.17). Generally the true nature of such 'suture granuloma' is readily recognized. The granuloma can persist for years with some eventually disappearing (29) (Fig. B.18). Similarly, an inverted appendiceal stump appears as a sessile polyp (Fig. B.19). The polyp is more prominent shortly after surgery when edema is still present.

Some of the initial descriptions of smooth muscle tumors still hold true today (30). They can have a variety of shapes. A 'dumb-bell' appearance, consisting of part of the lesion intraluminally and part growing outside the serosa, is not uncommon. These tumors can ulcerate and bleed. Although neither size nor shape predicts possible malignant potential, the larger lesions are associated with a higher incidence of malignancy (31). Whenever one encounters a large bulky tumor with extensive central ulceration, one should suggest a leiomyosarcoma. When a leiomyoma is small and located close to the lumen it will appear similar to other small polyps (Fig. B.20).

Other benign colon polyps are rare. A large inflammatory polyp may occasionally simulate a neoplasm (32). A neoplasm of fibrous or neurogenic origin, even if seen, has no distinguishing radiographic features but simply presents as an intramural lesion. Lymphangiomas (also called cystic hygromas) are rare in the colon (33). Most vascular malformations are flat and are not seen on a barium enema, but are recognized primarily on vascular studies. Their diagnosis is discussed further in the section on vascular disorders of the colon.

j. Polyposis syndromes

The word 'polyposis' has a similar connotation to the word 'polyp'. 'Polyposis' is a descriptive term for the radiographic appearance of multiple polyps. These polyps can be malignant or benign, neoplastic or inflammatory. Radiographically, some of the

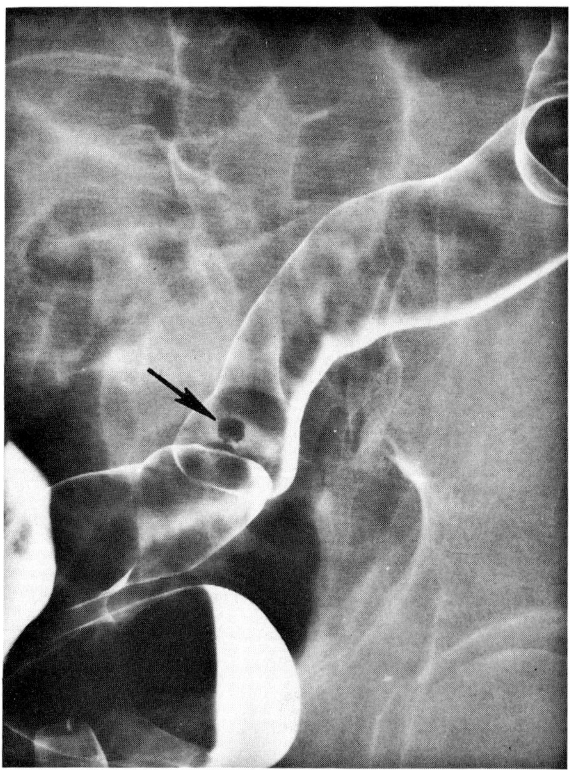

Fig. B.16. A single sessile polyp (arrow) is present adjacent to a colocolic anastomosis. The polyp represented a suture granuloma.

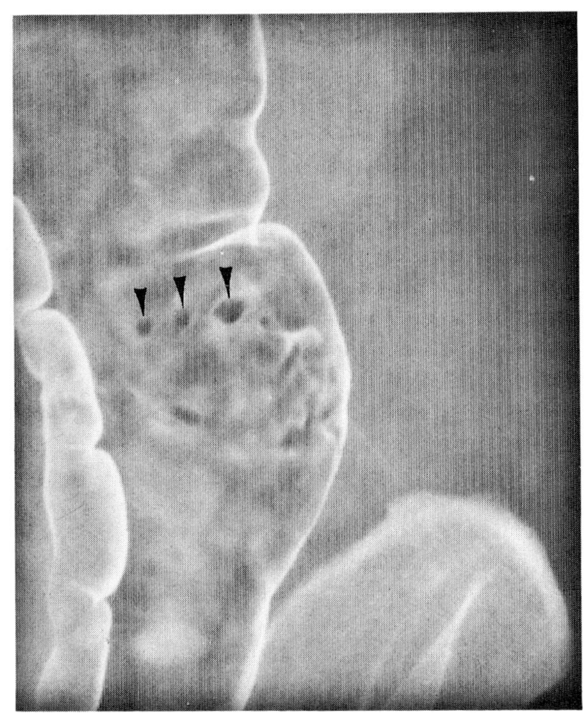

a

Fig. B.17. (a) Several polyps are arranged in a row close to a previous colocolic anastomosis (arrowheads). They represented suture granulomata. (b) Four peripheral and one centrally located polyps at the base of the cecum (arrowheads). The patient has had an appendectomy. Because of the symmetrical outline it is believed the peripheral polyps represent suture granulomata and the central polyp the appendiceal stump. (From Skucas et al. (95); copyright, RSNA, 1981.)

colitides mimic the polyposis syndromes (Table B.1).

Polyposis syndromes are relatively rare. Some, such as familial polyposis, are associated with the eventual development of cancer in almost 100% of patients. In others, although the risk of cancer is not as high, it is still greater than in the general population.

Polyposis syndromes represent a group of primarily inherited conditions, with most showing non-sex linked autosomal dominant traits having varying degrees of penetrance (34). Roughly half of the children of these patients can be expected to manifest the syndrome. In some patients the polyps are barely recognizable on a barium enema, while in others they are obvious. De novo appearance, with no family history of polyposis, is not unusual.

Historically these syndromes are classified into specific entities, but it should be kept in mind that, at least with some of them, there are varying degrees of overlap and some patients cannot be placed into a specific syndrome (Table B.2). The past literature described familial polyposis as a disease of the colon only; currently, emphasis is on the increased incidence of hyperplastic and adenomatous polyps in the stomach (35–40), duodenum (39, 41), and small bowel (39, 42). There is some evidence that

b

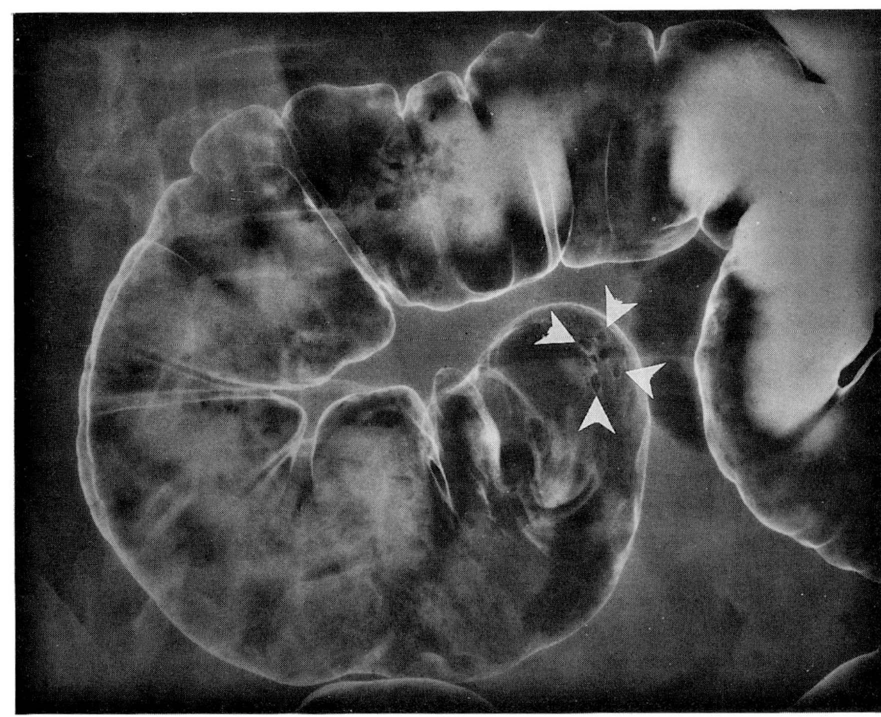

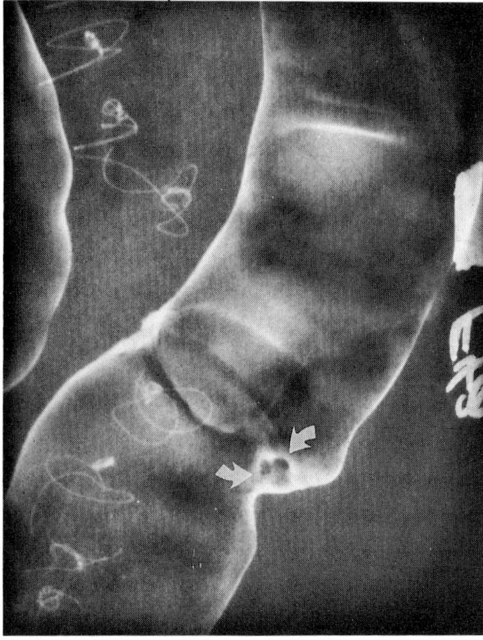

a

b

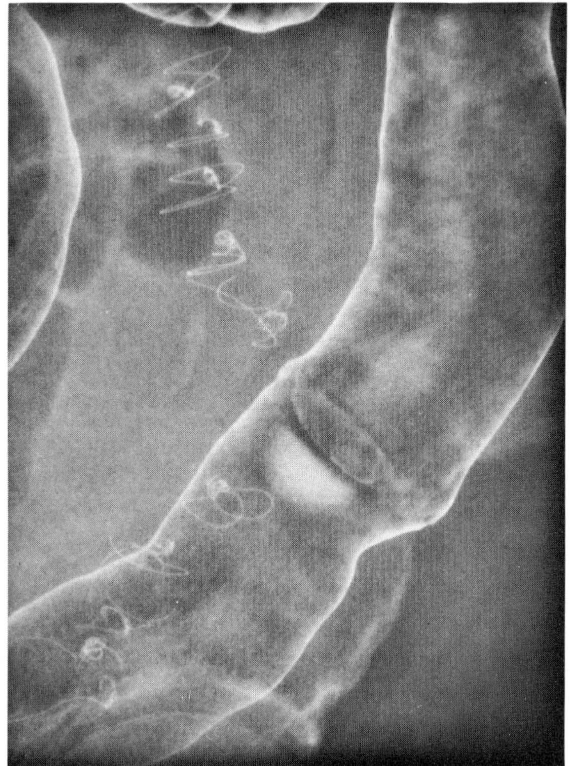

Fig. B.18. (a) Two small polyps are present at the site of a colocolic anastomosis (arrowheads), representing suture granulomata. (b) Nine months later the polyps have disappeared. Such change with time is typical of these suture granuloma.

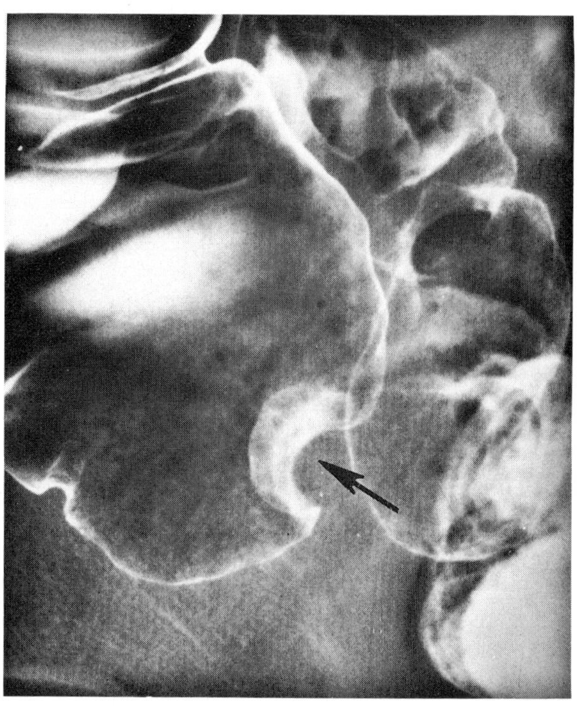

Fig. B.19. Inverted appendiceal stump (arrow). The patient had an appendectomy one year previously. The polyp is somewhat more prominent than usually seen.

ileal adenomata can develop after colon resection (42). All of these studies point out the difficulty of attempting to distinguish between familial polyposis and Gardner's syndrome. The difference may simply be a different expressivity of the same condition (39). One division is to use the term 'familial polyposis' if the lesions are limited to the colon and 'Gardner's syndrome' if there are extracolic manifestations; yet such an arbitrary division is not fully adequate. As an example of overlapping, it has been shown by careful investigation that 93% of patients with familial polyposis have radiopaque lesions in the mandible (43). Some investigators simply refer to all of these patients as having 'familial polyposis'. The subdivision in this text into familial polyposis and Gardner's syndrome is purely arbitrary. Future research may change the classification further.

A double contrast barium enema readily confirms or excludes the presence of colon involvement. If the colon is involved, both the upper gastrointestinal tract and the small bowel should be studied for additional polyps. If Gardner's syndrome is clinically suspected, appropriate skeletal radiographs should be obtained.

The literature is replete with various 'syndromes' consisting of colon lesions in association with some extracolic manifestation. As an example, there are associations of skin tumors and bowel neoplasms (Muir's syndrome) (44), skin and colon lipomata together with epiploic lipomatosis (12), extracolic adenomata and colon carcinomata, multiple hamartomata, and many others. Most are probably variants of the syndromes discussed here; occasionally one does not fit any pattern and because of limited reports cannot be classified adequately. As an example, if the colon is carpeted with hundreds of polyps in an 80-year-old patient who up to then had been asymptomatic, is this familial polyposis (45)? If this patient develops a periampullary carcinoma, is this then Gardner's syndrome?

A patient with multiple adenomatous polyps generally has less than 10 polyps present. A patient with polyposis generally has 100 or more polyps. It is unusual to encounter a patient with 10–100 polyps in the colon (excluding lymphoid hyperplasia); the occasional patient in this latter group probably should be labelled as having 'multiple adenomata'.

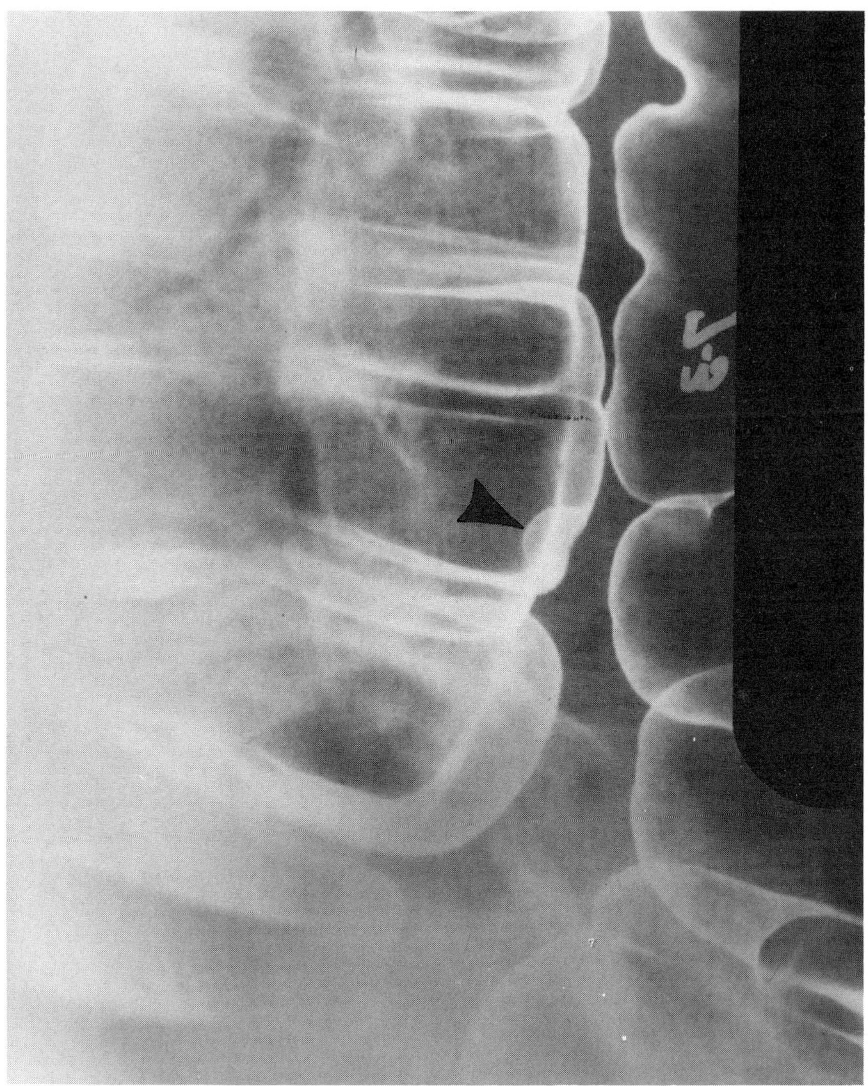

Fig. B.20. Small leiomyoma (arrowhead). The polyp was readily 'shelled out' by the surgeon when the patient underwent a cholecystectomy.

Familial polyposis. Multiple colon polyps were already mentioned in nineteenth century publications (46) and by 1890 it was known that there was an associated high incidence of cancer (47). Since then the hereditary nature of the condition has become firmy established.

Table B.1. Multiple colon polyps.

Normal
Lymphoid 'hyperplasia'
Inflammatory or infectious
Ulcerative colitis
Regional enteritis
Infectious colitis
Amebiasis
Schistosomiasis
Post-antibiotic colitis
Herpes colitis
Hamartomatous
Peutz-Jeghers' syndrome
Juvenile polyposis
Chronkhite-Canada syndrome
Hemangiomatosis
Neoplastic
Familial polyposis
Gardner's syndrome
Turcot's syndrome
Neurofibromatosis
Lipomatosis (may be hamartomatous)
Multiple adenomata
Lymphoma
Synchronous carcinomata
Metastases
Hemangiomatosis
Miscellaneous
Colon urticaria
Pneumatosis cystoides intestinalis
Lymphangiectasis
Ischemic colitis

Familial polyposis is transmitted as an autosomal dominant trait, with the incidence being about equal in men and women. The incidence is estimated to be approximately one in 8,000–10,000 births. There is considerable variation in the penetrance of the syndrome (48). About one-third of these patients have no family history of polyposis and one must postulate that the polyposis arose through spontaneous mutation, although thorough investigation of several generations may reveal existence of the syndrome. Intermarriage between related members may be denied in some families.

A colitis-type clinical picture, with diarrhea and bloody stool, is not unusual. Bleeding should be viewed with alarm and malignant degeneration suspected. Intussusception is unusual in these patients.

The polyps are adenomata. Because the incidence of eventual carcinomatous transformation approaches 100%, a vigorous diagnostic and therapeutic approach is recommended not only in the afflicted patients but also in asymptomatic related family members. Unfortunately, it is not unusual to diagnose the condition only when the patient already has cancer. A barium enema in asymptomatic family members of an afflicted patient yields approximately a 10% incidence of cancer (49).

Diagnosis can be readily made with a double contrast barium enema (Fig. B.21). The differential diagnosis, however, includes the other polyposis syndromes and a biopsy should be performed. Radiographically these polyps can be sessile, pe-

Table B.2. Multiple polyposis syndromes.

Syndrome	Predominant type of polyp	Usual location	Other abnormalities	Inheritance	Malignant potential
Familial polyposis	Adenoma	Colon	—	Autosomal dominant	Very common
Gardner's	Adenoma	Colon	Osteoma Fibroma, etc.	Autosomal dominant	Very common
Turcot's	Adenoma	Colon	Glioma	Autosomal recessive	May be increased
Peutz-Jeghers'	Hamartoma	Small bowel	Pigmentation	Autosomal dominant	Above average
Juvenile polyposis	Hamartoma	Throughout bowel	—	Autosomal dominant	May be increased
Chronkhite-Canada	Hamartoma	Throughout bowel	Alopecia Dystrophy	Not familial	None

dunculated, or both. The polyps can be essentially the same size or they can vary in size (Fig. B.22). Some individuals have thousands of small polyps scattered throughout, while others have fewer large polyps. Having one hundred polyps is generally regarded as the lower cut-off point for familial polyposis.

The polyps are generally not seen before the age of ten and thus a screening barium enema in children below this age will not be fruitful even if there is a family history of familial polyposis. The polyps generally appear after puberty and most patients begin to exhibit the syndrome when in their late teens or early twenties (Fig. B.23).

Superficially, familial polyposis and the other polyposis syndromes can have a radiographic appearance similar to regional enteritis. The sites of involvement, clinical history, and lack of ulcers generally allows ready diagnosis. The colon foreshortening and loss of haustration seen with the colitides are absent in the polyposis syndromes. In an occassional younger patient, lymphonodular hyperplasia is in the differential diagnosis, although it is unusual for the polyposis syndromes to present with the small round or oval intramural-appearing polyps as seen in lymphonodular hyperplasia. If in doubt, biopsy or a follow-up barium enema in several years should be diagnostic.

The only effective therapy for familial polyposis is a total proctocolectomy with an ileostomy. Because some of these patients are young adults who have minimal symptoms, some physicians believe that a total proctocolectomy is too harsh for initial therapy (50). They believe that surgery should be delayed for a few years, with a double-contrast barium enema or colonoscopy almost yearly, but once the polyps increase in size surgery is a necessity. Some surgeons advocate an initial colectomy with an ileorectal anastomosis, together with fulguration of any existing rectal polyps, followed by a subsequent proctectomy ten or so years later. The rationale is to preserve rectal function initially, but because the incidence of malignancy increases with time in the residual rectal pouch, the rectum should eventually be resected. As long as the rectum is in place, fulguration of all visualized polyps in the rectum should be performed serially during the patient's lifetime. Unfortunately, even with serial sigmoidoscopy and removal of all visualized polyps, there is still an increased incidence of rectal cancer. The incidence of malignancy increases with time with a rate of 30% to 50% being reported in patients followed for several decades (51, 52).

Following surgery, there appears to be a higher incidence of intestinal obstruction in these patients than in the average population (53), although the rate of obstruction is still considerably lower than encountered in Gardner's syndrome. Fibrous tissue formation in familial polyposis, if excessive, can merge with Gardner's syndrome.

An occasional complication of total proctocolectomy in males is impotence, another reason some surgeons prefer to perform the resection in two stages, delaying resection of the rectum until later in life.

It has been suggested that ascorbic acid ingestion may decrease the incidence of polyps in the remaining rectum after a colectomy and ileorectal anastomosis (54). The results are still uncertain. Occasionally there is spontaneous regression of rectal polyps after a colectomy (50).

Gardner's syndrome. The initial descriptions by Gardner in 1951 and 1953 (55, 56), and subsequent follow-up in 1962 (57) portrayed intestinal polyposis, osteomata, fibromata, and epidermoid cysts. In retrospect, an example of Gardner's syndrome probably was already described in 1912 (58). Others later described skin pigmentation (59), mesenchymal tumors (60), mesenteric fibrosis (61), gastric and small bowel polyps (38, 62, 63), benign and malignant neoplasms of the periampullary region of the duodenum (45, 61, 64, 65) and thyroid (66) and other abnormalities. The osteomata can be anywhere in the skeleton, with a distinctive feature being mandibular and sinus osteomata, consisting of dense sclerotic bone. Localized cortical thickening of the long bones is not uncommon. Many of the soft tissue tumors are located close to the skin and are readily palpable. The associated soft tissue and bone tumors occur at an earlier age than the bowel polyps (59, 67).

If Gardner's syndrome is defined as consisting of colon polyposis together with extracolic manifestations, then the incidence of this syndrome is somewhat less than that of familial polyposis, with the estimated incidence being approximately 1 in 14,000 births (68). Because there is a variable

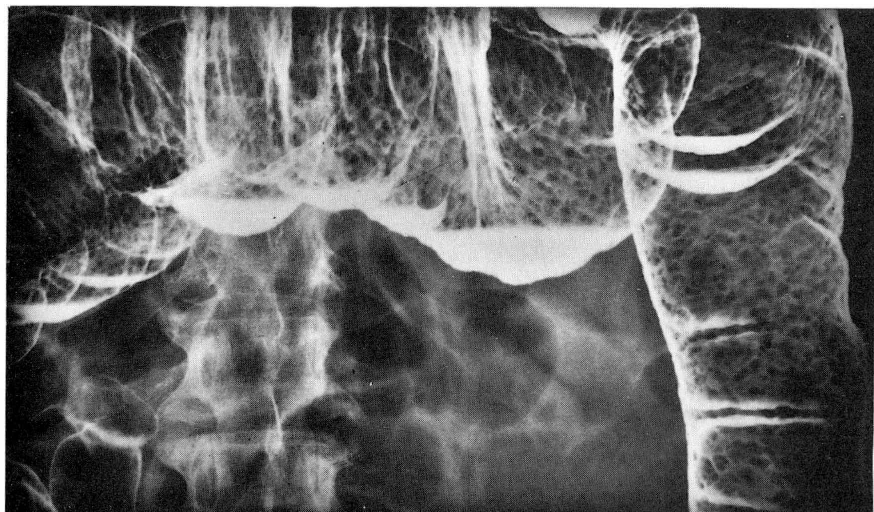

a

b

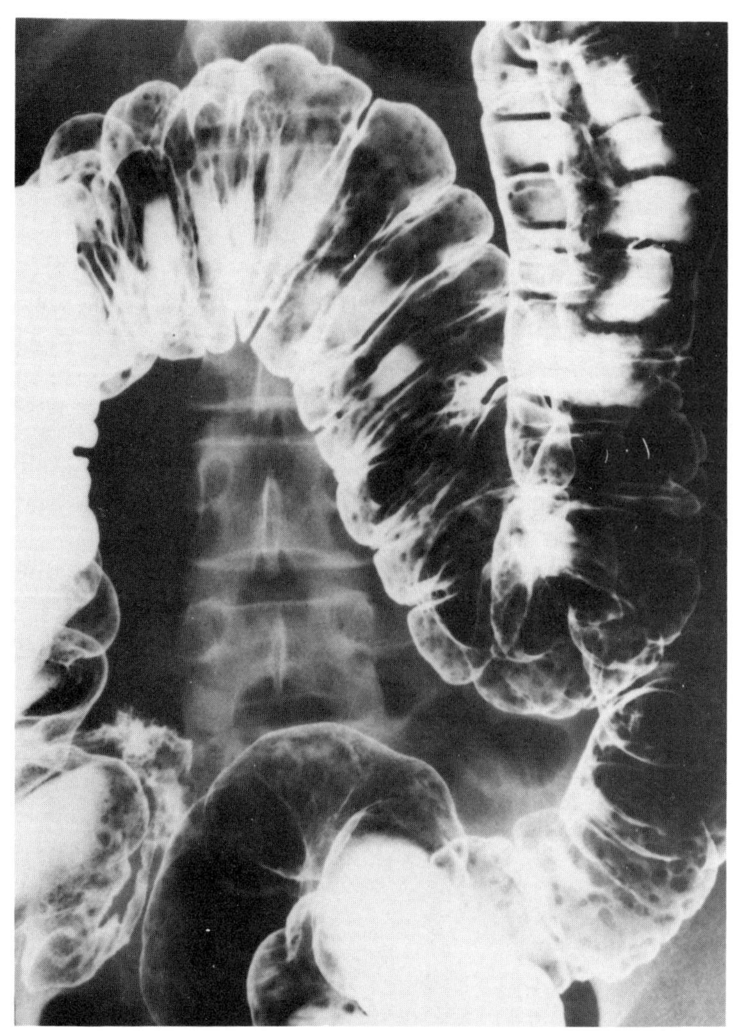

Fig. B.21. (a) Familial polyposis. The colon is studed with numerous polyps in this 52-year-old male. (b) Familial polyposis. This 16-year-old female exhibits fewer polyps than the previous patient. (c) Familial polyposis. Considerably more polyps are present in the transverse colon than in the sigmoid in a 43-year-óld female. Resection revealed approximately 700 polyps scattered throughout the colon.

penetrance, patients can have variable manifestations of any of the components. The number of polyps present likewise varies considerably. The polyp distribution, age of onset, growth and malignant potential are identical to familial polyposis. Histologically the polyps are adenomata and are indistinguishable from those seen in familial polyposis. If these patients are followed long enough without resection, probably all of them will develop a carcinoma.

Total colectomy and a permanent ileostomy is the procedure of choice. A two-stage operation is employed less often in these patients with extracolic manifestations, because post-operatively the patients with Gardner's syndrome have a higher incidence of retroperitoneal and intraaabdominal fibrosis (61, 64). The fibrosis can mimic a fibrosarcoma (69).

Polyps in the stomach, duodenum, or small bowel are generally not resected because they are usually multiple and the patient can end up with a short -bowel syndrome. The exceptions are bleeding polyps, polyps acting as lead points for an intussusception, or suspected malignancy.

c

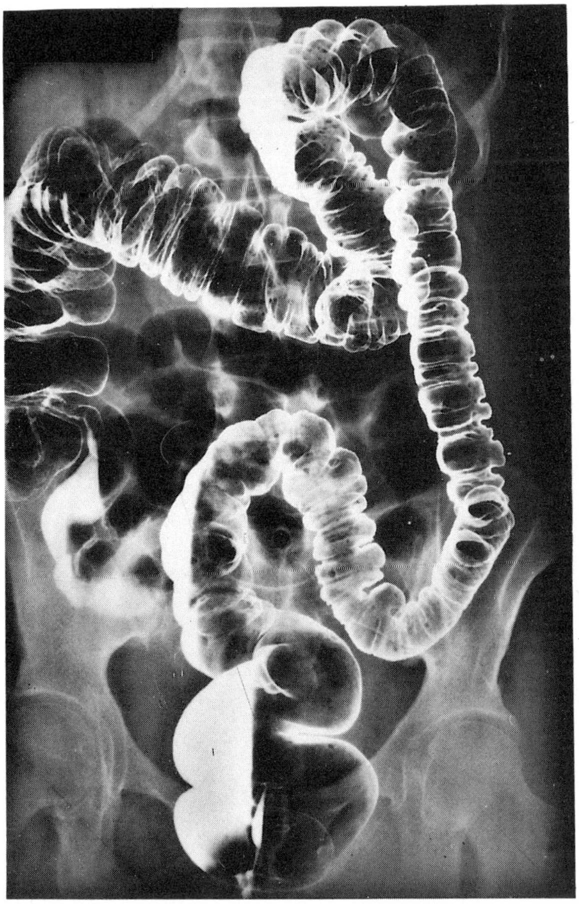

Turcot's syndrome. Turcot's syndrome is an extremely rare and interesting condition consisting of colon polyposis and brain gliomata (70–72). Only a few families have been reported so far. It is suspected that the syndrome is transmitted as an autosomal recessive trait. Turcot's syndrome may simply represent another manifestation of Gardner's syndrome The colon polyps are primarily adenomata similar to familial polyposis and Gardner's syndrome, but there appears to be an earlier age of onset of malignant degeneration. In the reported patients, death has been the result of the brain tumors, although in one of the five original patients reported by Turcot et al. (70) there already were two colon adenocarcinomata present.

There appears to be an association of colon adenomatous polyposis and multiple endocrine adenomatosis (73). Whether this condition belongs in the same category as Turcot's syndrome remains to be established.

Peutz-Jeghers' syndrome. In 1921, the Dutch physician, Peutz, described familial mucocutaneous pigmentation and intestinal polyposis (74). In 1949, Jeghers et al. (75) collected a number of such cases, both from the literature and from personal observations, and this entity has since been called the Peutz-Jeghers' syndrome.

The mucocutaneous pigmentation should alert the physician to this syndrome, because the vast majority of patients have some degree of pigmentation either on the lips or the buccal mucosa (49, 67). The pigmentation is usually already present in childhood and consists of melanin presenting as brown or black macules on the skin, lips or buccal mucosa. The pigmentation can be sparse or extensive.

This syndrome is inherited as an autosomal dominant trait, but de novo presentations do occur. The polyps, located throughout the gastrointestinal tract, are hamartomata; occasionally there is involvement of the urinary (76) or upper respiratory tracts (77). While most of the other polyposis syndromes have the greatest incidence of polyps in the colon, the small bowel is the site of greatest involvement in patients with Peutz-Jeghers' syndrome.

A barium enema generally reveals far fewer polyps than seen with familial polyposis. Smaller polyps tend to be sessile while the larger ones are pedunculated. The polyps vary in size and often have a lobulated appearance (78).

These hamartomatous polyps tend to be hypovascular during angiography, similar to most adenomatous polyps (20).

Polyp biopsy should establish the diagnosis. Once the diagnosis is known, the role of radiology is to document the extent of polyposis and/or exclude whether any complications develop.

Because the polyps are hamartomatous in origin, theoretically there should not be an increased risk of cancer. The incidence of cancer, however, is still slightly greater than in the average patient population (48, 49, 62, 78, 79), leading to speculation that the underlying bowel mucosa in these patients is abnormal. Because of this relatively low incidence of cancer, most surgeons do not advocate a prophylactic colectomy. Surgery is individualized for the complications of this syndrome, namely bleeding, intussusception, or obstruction. Occasionally a polyp may slough off.

Juvenile polyps. Juvenile polyps are not neoplastic in origin but represent hamartomata of the lamina propria (48). Such multiple polyps are common. There is an autosomal dominant inheritance trait for some of these patients, while others exhibit non-familial features (48, 80). About 20% of these patients have other associated congenital abnormalities (48). Although clinically and radiologically there can be overlap with familial polyposis, the number of polyps in juvenile polyposis is usually considerably less and the age is lower. There is occasional association of juvenile polyposis with adenomatous polyps (81, 82). Such an entity can be

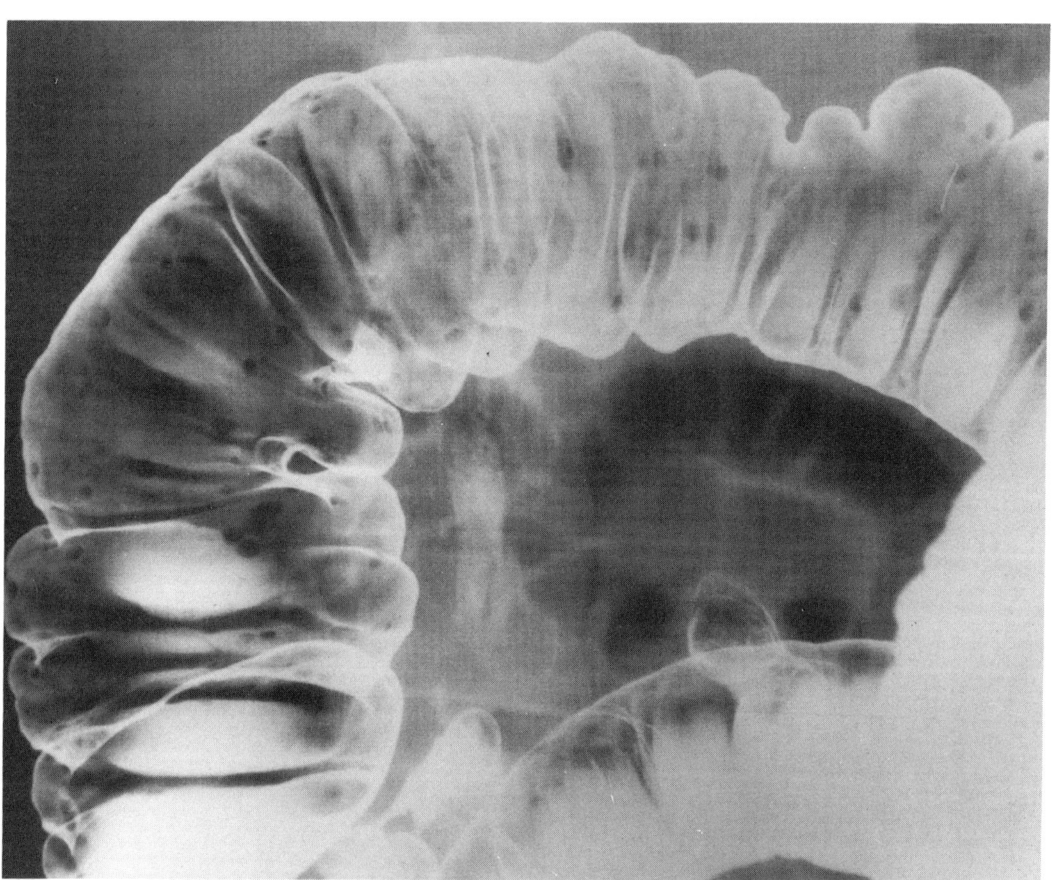

Fig. B.22. Familial polyposis. Although most of the polyps are the same size, some are considerably larger (arrowhead).

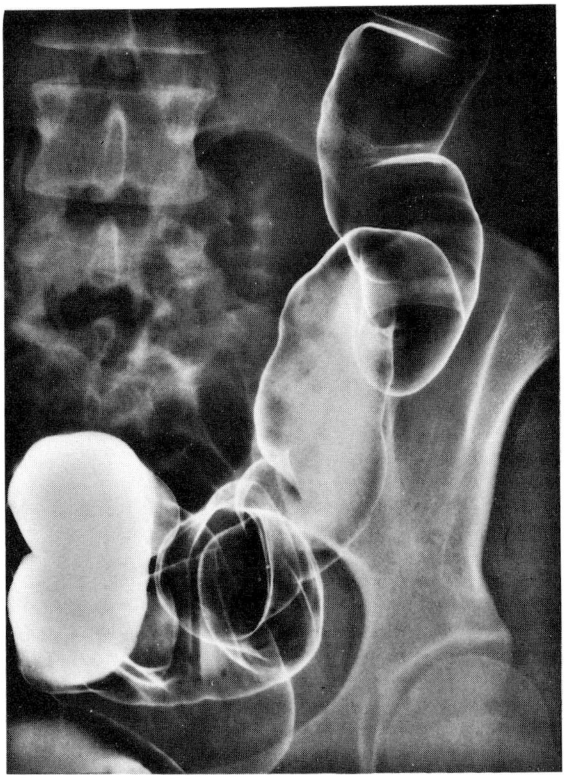

a

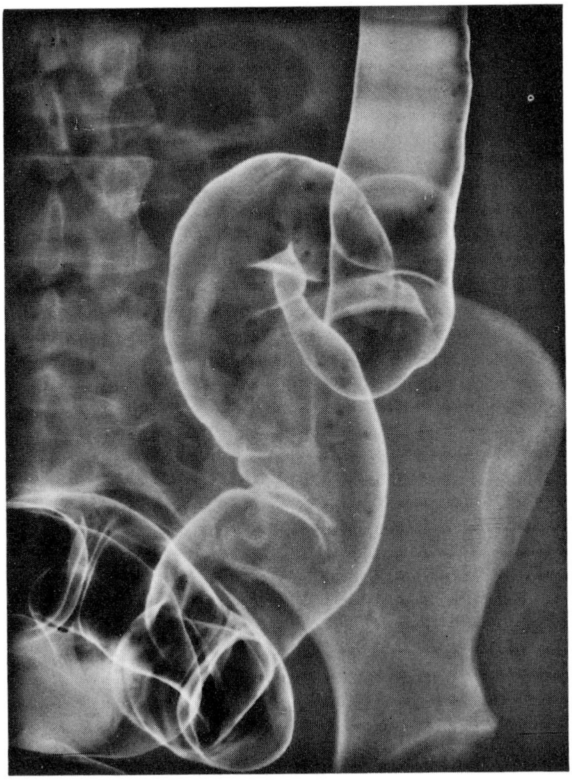

b

c

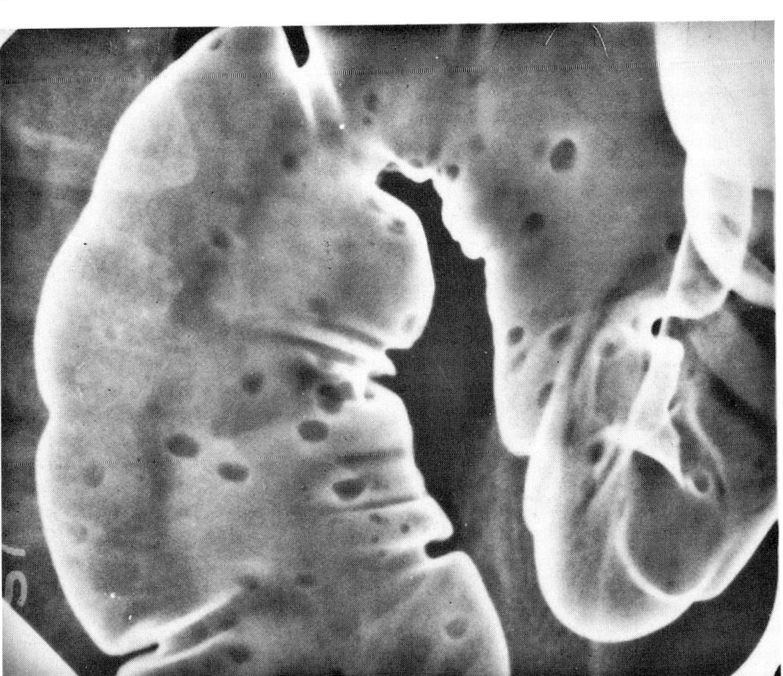

Fig. B.23. (a) 19-year-old female with a family history of colon cancer. The polyps are poorly defined. (b) One year later multiple polyps are clearly identified. (c) Four years later the polyps have increased considerably in size.

premalignant. The polyps are usually present in childhood. They are most common in the distal colon, but also found in the upper gastrointestinal tract and the small bowel (49, 67, 83).

The polyps contain multiple mucin-filled cysts and connective tissue, with considerably more connective tissue present than in adenomatous polyps. Because of the cystic nature of these lesions they have also been called retention polyps (80). Any inflammatory cells seen are probably secondary to surrounding inflammation and do not represent the primary pathogenesis of these polyps, although some authors refer to them as inflammatory polyps. There are rare reports of ossification within these polyps (84, 85). On colonoscopy they tend to appear bright red.

Of interest is an increased risk of carcinoma of the gastrointestinal tract and pancreas in the kindred of individuals with juvenile polyposis (80, 86). Some of these patients have a higher incidence of colon cancer than the general patient population (83, 86). To explain this higher incidence of cancer, a pathogenetic sequence consisting of focal mucosal hyperplasia evolving into hyperplastic polyps has been proposed. These polyps become inflamed and form juvenile polyps with subsequent epithelial atypia leading to adenoma formation and later carcinomatous transformation (83).

These patients usually present with gastrointestinal bleeding, obstruction, or intussusception. Because these polyps can be pedunculated, they can twist, necrose and undergo autoamputation. Thus, the number of polyps tends to decrease with age.

A double contrast barium enema, together with a study of the upper gastrointestinal tract and the small bowel, suggests this condition in the appropriate age group. Radiographically these polyps are generally smooth and most are less than 1 cm in diameter. They can be either sessile or pedunculated, solitary or multiple. When multiple it is unusual to see more than several polyps. In the occasional patient in whom angiography is performed because of bleeding one sees hypervascularity and early venous drainage (21). Biopsy is necessary to confirm the pathological nature of these polyps.

A rare picture of severe bloody diarrhea and anemia appearing in children less than one year of age has been associated with juvenile polyposis (87). The outcome in these severely involved patients is invariably fatal. At times there are associated abnormalities consisting of intracranial cysts or macrocephaly (88).

Cronkhite-Canada syndrome. This syndrome, first described in 1955 (89), consists of bowel polyposis and neuroectodermal abnormalities. It is seen primarily in middle age. The polyps occur throughout the gastrointestinal tract, but the stomach is consistently involved (90). The polyps are hamartomata, it is believed that there is no potential for malignant transformation, and the syndrome is not familial. The neuroectodermal abnormalities consist of alopecia, nail dystrophy and skin hyperpigmentation and can develop before the gastrointestinal lesions appear. A severe protein-losing enteropathy can be present (90–92). A scleroderma-like pattern develops in the skin (93). The specific abnormality is not known, although some patients have a hormone abnormality (94). The condition can be fatal.

References

1. Blatt LJ: Polyps of the colon and rectum; incidence and distribution. Dis Colon Rectum 4:277–282, 1961.
2. Welin S: Results of the Malmö technique of colon examination. JAMA 199:369–371, 1967.
3. Ekelund G: On cancer and polyps of colon and rectum. Acta Pathol Microbiol Scand 59:165–170, 1963.
4. Ott DJ, Gelfand DW: Colorectal tumors: pathology and detection. AJR 131:691–695, 1978.
5. Press HC Jr, Davis TW: Ingested foreign bodies simulating polyposis: report of six cases. AJR 127:1040–1042, 1976.
6. Youker JE, Welin S: Differentiation of true tumors of the colon from extraneous material: a new roentgen sign. Radiology 84:610–615, 1965.
7. Skucas J, Gluckman JB, Fowler EH, Turner MD, Narisawa T: Radiological evaluation of the growth characteristics of rat colonic tumors. Invest Radiol 13:34–39, 1978.
8. Delamarre J, Descombes P, Marti R, Remond A, Trinez G: Villous tumors of the colon and rectum: double-contrast study of 47 cases. Gastrointest Radiol 5:69–73, 1980.
9. Kaye JJ, Bragg DG: Unusual roentgenologic and clinicopathologic features of villous adenomas of the colon. Radiology 91:799–806, 1968.
10. Turek RE, Davis WC, Wilson WJ, Olson RO Jr: The roentgenographic diagnosis of villous tumors of the colon. AJR 113:349–351, 1971.
11. Wolf BS, Melamed M, Khilnani MT: Lipoma of the colon. J Mount Sinai Hosp 21:80–86, 1954.
12. O'Connell DJ, Shaw DG, Swain VAJ: Epiploic lipomatosis and lipomatous polyposis of the colon. Br J Radiol 49:969–971, 1976.
13. Danoff DM, Nisenbaum HL, Stewart WB, Moore RC, Clahassey EB: Segmental polypoid lipomatosis of the colon. AJR 128:858–860, 1977.
14. Swain VAJ, Young WF, Pringle EM: Hypertrophy of the appendices epiploicae and lipomatous polyposis of the colon. Gut 10:587–589, 1969.

15. Margulis AR, Jovanovich A: The roentgen diagnosis of submucous lipomas of the colon. AJR 84:1114–1120, 1960.
16. Morson BC, Dawson IMP: Gastrointestinal Pathology, p. 610. Blackwell Scientific, Oxford, 1979.
17. Estrada RG, Spjut HJ: Hyperplastic polyps of the large bowel. Am J Surg Pathol 4:127–133, 1980.
18. Sumner HW, Wasserman NF, McClain CJ: Giant hyperplastic polyposis of the colon. Dig Dis Sci 26:85–89, 1981.
19. Morson BC, Dawson IMP: Gastrointestinal Pathology, p. 81. Blackwell Scientific, Oxford, 1979.
20. Fenlon JW, Schackelford GD: Peutz-Jeghers syndrome: case report with angiographic evaluation. Radiology 103:595–596, 1972.
21. Korobkin M, Shapiro H, Lawson D, Golden D, Palubinskas AJ: Arteriographic diagnosis of a juvenile cecal polyp. Gastroenterology 63:1059–1061, 1972.
22. Langhans T: Über einen Drüsenpolyp im Ileum. Arch Path Anat. 38:559, 1867.
23. Lubarsch O: Über den primären Krebs des Ileum nebst Bemerkungen über das gleichzeitige Vorkommen von Krebs und Tuberculose. Arch Path Anat 111:280–317, 1888.
24. Godwin JD II: Carcinoid tumors. An analysis of 2837 cases. Cancer 36:560–569, 1975.
25. Greenwood SM, Huvos AG, Erlandson RA, Malt SH: Rectal carcinoid and rectal adenocarcinoma: a case report and review of the literature. Dis Colon Rectum 17:644–655, 1974.
26. Balthazar EJ: Carcinoid tumors of the alimentary tract. I. Radiographic diagnosis. Gastrointest Radiol 3:47–56, 1978.
27. Shulman H, Ginstra P: Invasive carcinoids of the colon. Radiology 98:139–143, 1971.
28. Kinkhabwala M, Balthazar EJ: Carcinoid tumors of the alimentary tract. II. Angiographic diagnosis of small intestinal and colonic lesions. Gastrointest Radiol 3:57–61, 1978.
29. Shauffer IA, Sequeira J: Suture granuloma simulating recurrent carcinoma. AJR 128:856–857, 1977.
30. Exner A: Über nichtmelanotische Sarcome des Mastdarmes. Med Klin (Berlin) 4:858–861, 1908.
31. Nemer FD, Stoeckinger JM, Evans OT: Smooth muscle rectal tumors: a therapeutic dilemma. Dis Colon Rectum 20:405–413, 1977.
32. Forde KA, Di Sant'Agnese P: Inflammatory tumor of the cecum simulating neoplasm. Am J Gastroenterol 74:366–367, 1981.
33. Lawson JP, Myerson PJ, Myerson DA: Colonic lymphangioma. Gastrointest Radiol 1:85–89, 1976.
34. Dodds WJ: Clinical and roentgen features of intestinal polyposis syndromes. Gastrointest Radiol 1:127–142, 1976.
35. Ranzi T, Castagnone D, Velio P, Bianchi P, Polli EE: Gastric and duodenal polyps in familial polyposis coli. Gut 22:363–367, 1981.
36. Editorial: Polyposis coli and the stomach. Br Med J 2 (6041):900, 1976.
37. Itai Y, Kogure T, Okuyama Y, Muto T: Radiographic features of gastric polyps in familial adenomatosis coli. AJR 128:73–76, 1977.
38. Schulman A: Gastric and small bowel polyps in Gardner's syndrome and familial polyposis coli. J Can Assoc Radiol 27:206–209, 1976.
39. Ushio K, Sasagawa M, Doi H, Yamada T, Ichikawa H, Hojo K, Koyama Y, Sano R: Lesions associated with familial polyposis coli. Studies of lesions of the stomach, duodenum, bones, and teeth. Gastrointest Radiol 1: 67–80, 1976.
40. Denzler TB, Harned RK, Pergam CJ: Gastric polyps in familial polyposis coli. Radiology 130:63–66, 1979.
41. Yao T, Iida M, Ohsato K, Watanabe H, Omae T: Duodenal lesions in familial polyposis of the colon. Gastroenterology 73:1086–1092, 1977.
42. Hamilton SR, Bussey HJR, Mendelsohn G, Diamond MP, Pavlides G, Hutcheon D, Harbison M, Shermeta D, Morson BC, Yardley JH: Ileal adenomas after colectomy in nine patients with adenomatous polyposis coli/Gardner's syndrome. Gastroenterology 77:1252–1257, 1979.
43. Utsunomiya J, Nakamura T: The occult osteomatous changes in the mandible in patients with familial polyposis coli. Br J Surg 62:45–51, 1975.
44. Anderson DE: An inherited form of large bowel cancer. Muir's syndrome. Cancer 45:1103–1107, 1980.
45. Qizilbash AH: Familial polyposis coli and periampullary carcinoma. Can J Surg 19:166–168, 1976.
46. Cripps WH: Two cases of disseminated polypus of the rectum. Trans Pathol Soc (Lond) 33:165–168, 1882.
47. Handford H: Disseminated polypi of the large intestine becoming malignant. Trans Path Soc (Lond) 41:133–137, 1890.
48. Bussey HJR, Veale AMO, Morson BC: Genetics of gastrointestinal polyposis. Gastroenterology 74:1325–1330, 1978.
49. Erbe RW: Inherited gastrointestinal-polyposis syndromes. N Engl J Med 294:1101–1104, 1976.
50. Shepherd JA: Familial polyposis of the colon with special reference to regression of rectal polyposis after subtotal colectomy. Br J Surg 58:85–91, 1971.
51. Moertel CG, Hill JR, Adson MA: Surgical management of multiple polyposis. The problem of cancer in the retained bowel segment. Arch Surg 100:521–526, 1970.
52. Bess MA, Adson MA, Elveback LR, Moertel CG: Rectal cancer following colectomy for polyposis. Arch Surg 115:460–467, 1980.
53. Lockhart-Mummery HE: Intestinal polyposis: the present position. Proc R Soc Med 60:381–388, 1967.
54. DeCosse JJ, Bussey HJR, Thomson JPS, Eyers AA, Ritchie SM, Morson BC: Ascorbic acid in polyposis coli. In: Winawer S, Schottenfeld D, Sherlock P (eds) Colorectal Cancer: Prevention, Epidemiology, and Screening, pp 59–64. Raven Press, New York, 1980.
55. Gardner EJ: A genetic and clinical study of intestinal polyposis, a predisposing factor for carcinoma of the colon and rectum. Am J Hum Genet 3:167–176, 1951.
56. Gardner EJ, Richards RC: Multiple cutaneous and subcutaneous lesions occurring simultaneously with hereditary polyposis and osteomatosis. Am J Hum Genet 5:139–147, 1953.
57. Gardner EJ: Follow-up study of a family group exhibiting dominant inheritance for a syndrome including intestinal polyps, osteomas, fibromas and epidermal cysts. Am J Hum Genet 14:376–390, 1962.
58. Devic M, Bussy M: Un cas de polypose adénomateuse généralisée à tout l'intestin. Arch Fr Mal App Dig 6:278–299, 1912.
59. Weston SD, Wiener M: Familial polyposis associated with a new type of soft-tissue lesion (skin pigmentation): report of three cases and a review of the literature. Dis Colon Rectum 10:311–321, 1967.
60. Coli RD, Moore JP, LaMarche PH, DeLuca FG, Thayer WR: Gardner's syndrome. A revisit to a previously described family. Dig Dis Sci 15:551–568, 1970.
61. Parks TG, Bussey HJR, Lockhart-Mummery HE: Familial

polyposis coli associated with extracolonic abnormalities. Gut 11:323–329, 1970.
62. Erbe RW: Case Records of the Massachusetts General Hospital. Clinicopathological exercises. N Engl J Med 299:1237–1245, 1978.
63. Ohsato K, Yao T, Watanabe H, Iida M, Itoh H: Small intestinal involvement in familial polyposis diagnosed by operative intestinal fiberoscopy. Dis Colon Rectum 20:414–420, 1977.
64. Bussey HJR: Extracolonic lesions associated with polyposis coli. Proc R Soc Med 65:294, 1972.
65. Mir-Madjlessi SH, Farmer RG, Hawk WA, Turnbull RB Jr: Adenocarcinoma of the ampulla of Vater associated with familial polyposis coli. Report of a case. Dis Colon Rectum 16:542–546, 1973.
66. Camiel MR, Mulé JE, Alexander LL, Benninghoff DL: Association of thyroid carcinoma with Gardner's syndrome in siblings. N Engl J Med 278:1056–1058, 1968.
67. Wennstrom J, Pierce ER, McKusick VA: Hereditary benign and malignant lesions of the large bowel. Cancer 34:850–857, 1974.
68. Pierce ER, Weisbord T, McKusick VA: Gardner's syndrome: formal genetics and statistical analysis of a large Canadian kindred. Clin Genet 1:65–80, 1970.
69. Naylor EW, Gardner EJ, Richards RC: Desmoid tumors and mesenteric fibromatosis in Gardner's syndrome. Arch Surg 114:1181–1185, 1979.
70. Turcot J, Després J-P, St. Pierre F: Malignant tumors of the central nervous system associated with familial polyposis of the colon: report of two cases. Dis Colon Rectum 2:465–468, 1959.
71. Baughman FA Jr, List CF, Williams JR, Muldoon JP, Segarra JM, Volkel JS: The glioma-polyposis syndrome. N Engl J Med 281:1345–1346, 1969.
72. Franca LCM, Sanvito WL: Tumor maligno do sistema nervoso central associado a polipose do colon com degeneracao maligna. Arq Neuro-Psiquiat (Sao Paulo) 27:67–72, 1969.
73. Sayed AK, Jafri SZH, Shenoy SS: Intestinal polyposis and brain tumor in a family. Dis Colon Rectum 22:486–491, 1979.
74. Peutz JLA: Over een zeer merkwaardige, gecombineerde familiaire polyposis van de slijmvliezen van den tractus intestinalis met die van de neuskeelholte en gepaard met eigenaardige pigmentaties van huid- en slijmvliezen. Nederl Maandschr Geneesk 10:134–146, 1921.
75. Jeghers H, McKusick VA, Katz KH: Generalized intestinal polyposis and melanin spots of the oral mucosa, lips and digits: a syndrome of diagnostic significance. N Eng J Med 241:993–1005, 1949.
76. Sommerhaug RG, Mason T: Peutz-Jeghers syndrome and ureteral polyposis. JAMA 211:120–122, 1970.
77. Jancu J: Peutz-Jeghers syndrome: involvement of the gastrointestinal and upper respiratory tracts. Am J Gastroenterol 56:545–549, 1971.
78. Utsunomiya J, Gocho H, Miyanaga T, Hamaguchi E, Kashimure A: Peutz-Jeghers syndrome: its natural course and management. Johns Hopkins Med J 136:71–82, 1975.
79. Hsu S-D, Zaharopoulos P, May JT, Costanzi JJ: Peutz-Jeghers syndrome with intestinal carcinoma. Cancer 44:1527–1532, 1979.
80. Veale AMO, McColl I, Bussey HJR, Morson BC: Juvenile polyposis coli. J Med Genet 3:5–16, 1966.
81. Reed K, Vose PC: Diffuse juvenile polyposis of the colon: a premalignant conditions? Dis Colon Rectum 24:205–210, 1981.
82. Šandler RS, Lipper S: Multiple adenomas in juvenile polyposis. Am J Gastroenterol 75:361–366, 1981.
83. Goodman ZD, Yardley JH, Milligan FD: Pathogenesis of colonic polyps in multiple juvenile polyposis. Cancer 43:1906–1913, 1979.
84. Marks MM, Atkinson KG: Heterotopic bone in a juvenile rectal polyp. Dis Colon Rectum 7:345–347, 1964.
85. Todd I: Juvenile polyps. Proc R Soc Med 56:969–970, 1963.
86. Stemper TJ, Kent TH, Summers RW: Juvenile polyposis and gastrointestinal carcinoma. A study of a kindred. Ann Intern Med 83:639–646, 1975.
87. Soyer RT, Kent TH: Fatal juvenile polyposis in infancy. Surgery 69:692–698, 1971.
88. Schwartz AM, McCauley RGK: Juvenile gastrointestinal polyposis. Radiology 121:441–444, 1976.
89. Cronkhite LW, Canada WJ: Generalized gastrointestinal polyposis: an unusual syndrome of polyposis, pigmentation, alopecia, and onychotropia. N Engl J Med 252:1011–1015, 1955.
90. Lipper S, Kahn LB: Superficial cystic gastritis with alopecia. Arch Pathol Lab Med 101:432–436, 1977.
91. Kindblom L-G, Angervall L, Santesson R, Selander S: Cronkhite-Canada syndrome: case report. Cancer 39:2651–2657, 1977.
92. Johnson GK, Soergel KH, Hensley GT, Dodds WJ, Hogan WJ: Cronkhite Canada syndrome: gastrointestinal pathophysiology and morphology. Gastroenterology 63:140–152, 1972.
93. Ali M, Weinstein J, Biempica L, Halpern A, Das KM: Cronkhite-Canada syndrome: report of a case with bacteriologic, immunologic, and electron microscopic studies. Gastroenterology 79:731–736, 1980.
94. Hidaka T, Miyoshi A: Cronkhite Canada syndrome. Nippon Rinsho 35:860–861, 1977.
95. Skucas J, Spataro R, Cannucciari D: The radiologic appearance of small colon carcinomas. Radiographics 1:66–72, 1981.

III.3.C. Malignant tumors

a. Introduction

Approximately 120,000 new cases of cancer of the colon and rectum are found in the United States each year. Approximately 55,000 will die of cancer of the colon and rectum. Because most studies show a high cure rate if the cancer is found early, emphasis should be placed on diagnosing the small and thus potentially curable lesions. In general, early lesions have approximately a 70% or greater survival rate compared to less than 15% for late lesions. Unfortunately, the age-adjusted colon cancer death rate has not changed much during the last several decades (1).

There is considerable variation in the incidence of colon cancer throughout the world (2). A direct relationship exists with the socioeconomic status;

with some exceptions, those populations having a high standard of living have a higher incidence of colon cancer (2). The incidence of colon cancer changes with a change in living conditions. Migration can change the bowel cancer risk in about two decades. Children within a family from a low risk country who emigrate to a high risk country acquire the high risk of the host country (3).

The incidence of colon cancer increases gradually with age, with the incidence beginning to rise from approximately the age of 35 years (4). Although colon cancer does appear in children and young adults, it is relatively uncommon; some of these young patients have an underlying predisposing factor. It is our impression that colon cancer in young patients tends to be considerably more malignant than in the older population, with few survivors (Fig. C.1). Some studies confirm this impression (5), while others have found no difference (6). Lesions in young patients tend to be more homogeneously distributed than in older patients (7).

The 1982 estimated cancer incidence in males and females in the United States was 14–15% of all cancers (8) and for both males and females cancer of the colon and rectum now has the second highest mortality. In males lung cancer has a higher mortality, while in females breast cancer leads the list. The incidence of colorectal carcinoma is about equal in men and women (9). In men, however, there is a greater incidence of carcinoma of the rectosigmoid, while in women the carcinomata tend to be more proximal. Overall, cancers involving the right side of the colon are increasing in frequency (10–12), while left-sided cancers are decreasing.

Prior radiation therapy leads to a somewhat increased incidence of cancer. These cancers are usually detected more than five years after the

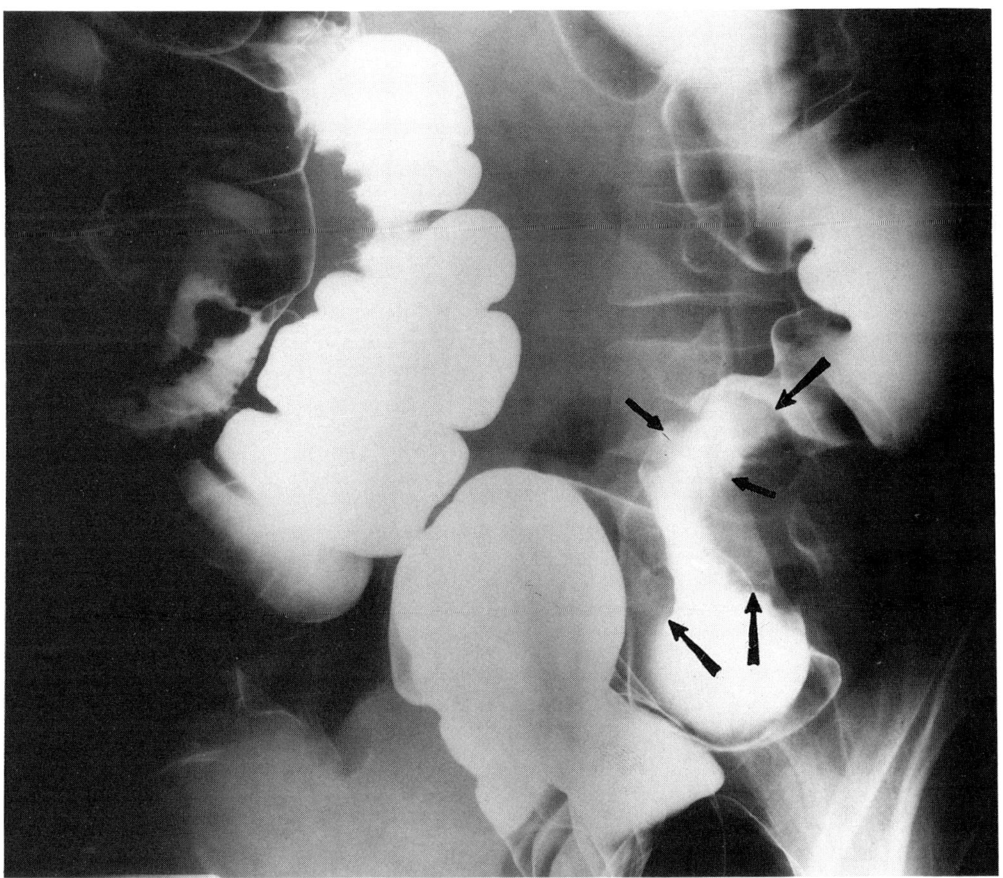

Fig. C.1. A 26-year-old male, investigated for unexplained anemia, who was asymptomatic. A long, ulcerated adenocarcinoma is present in the descending colon (arrows). Widespread metastases were found.

radiation therapy. Colon carcinoma develops more often after ureterosigmoidostomy (13, 14), although here also a latent period exists between the surgical procedure and subsequent development of cancer (15, 16). Colon cancer is more common in a setting of some of the colitides and polyposis syndromes (Table C.1). There is an increased incidence of colon cancer in patients with an earlier breast or genital cancer (17).

Table C.1. Increased risk of colorectal cancer (120).

Group of patients	Lifetime risk (%)
Average patient population	5
Prior breast or genital cancer	7–8
Colon cancer in relatives	15
Prior colon cancer (metachronous cancer)	15
Ulcerative colitis	50
Familial polyposis	100

A low residue diet has been associated with a high incidence of colon cancer (18). Populations on a high fiber diet tend to have a low incidence of colon cancer, although some investigators have questioned such an association (19, 20). In some populations there is a direct correlation between the amount of dietary fat and meat and the incidence of colon cancer (18, 21), yet some exceptions occur (20, 22). Populations increasing their consumption of meat experience an increased incidence of colon and rectal cancer (23).

The role of bacteria in the induction of cancer is still unsettled and results so far are controversial (24). The large bowel may also contain carcinogenic compounds. A person's diet can obviously affect the composition of colon content, although no specific carcinogen has been definitely implicated in the diet.

It has been proposed that excessive beer consumption is associated with an increased risk of developing rectal cancer (25). Here also not all studies support such a conclusion (22).

Several reports describe an association of *Streptococcus bovis* infection with colon neoplasms (26, 27). *S. bovis* bacteremia has also been associated with other carcinomata, lymphoma, and polyposis syndromes (28). Likewise, *Clostridium septicum* sepsis has been associated with underlying colon carcinoma (29). Whether such associations are fortuitous or real remains to be seen.

A relatively common indication for a barium enema prior to an inguinal or femoral hernia repair used to be exclusion of an associated cancer (30). Currently it is believed that there is no association between colon cancer and subsequent development of inguinal or femoral hernia (31).

The Dukes' classification (32) of staging colon cancer is based on pathological specimens and the radiographic appearance of a cancer cannot be used for Dukes' staging. Yet, radiologists should still be familiar with this almost universally used system for estimating a patient's prognosis. Dukes initially used his classification only for rectal cancers (32); however, his system has been extended to the entire colon. Dukes' 'A' means that the cancer is limited to the wall of the colon and thus has not spread beyond the muscle layers. The majority of patients with a Dukes' 'A' tumor are cured if the tumor is resected. Excision of a tumor that has invaded only the *submucosa* should result in cure (33). Dukes' 'B' means that the cancer has extended beyond the colon wall into the pericolic tissues but no regional lymph node metastases are present. Over one-half of these patients will be cured if the entire tumor is resected. Dukes' 'C' signifies that the regional lymph nodes are invaded. Even if the tumor is resected, only approximately one-third of these patients will be cured. Thus a very important prognostic sign is the presence or absence of lymph node metastases. Several confusing 'modified Dukes'' classifications have been proposed (34). Many investigators use Dukes' stage 'D' to mean distal tumor spread.

b. Clinical considerations

Colon cancers can have an insidious course. Small lesions are generally asymptomatic. They tend to grow slowly and metastasize late (Fig. C.2). It is not unusual for the radiologist to discover a large and infiltrating tumor which obviously has been present for a number of years, yet the patient admits having only mild symptoms (Fig. C.3). Likewise, most radiologists have encountered in their practice patients who first present with obstruction. Generally, on close questioning, the patient does admit to a previous change in bowel habits; minor changes in bowel habit are commonly overlooked by the patient and sometimes by the patient's physician.

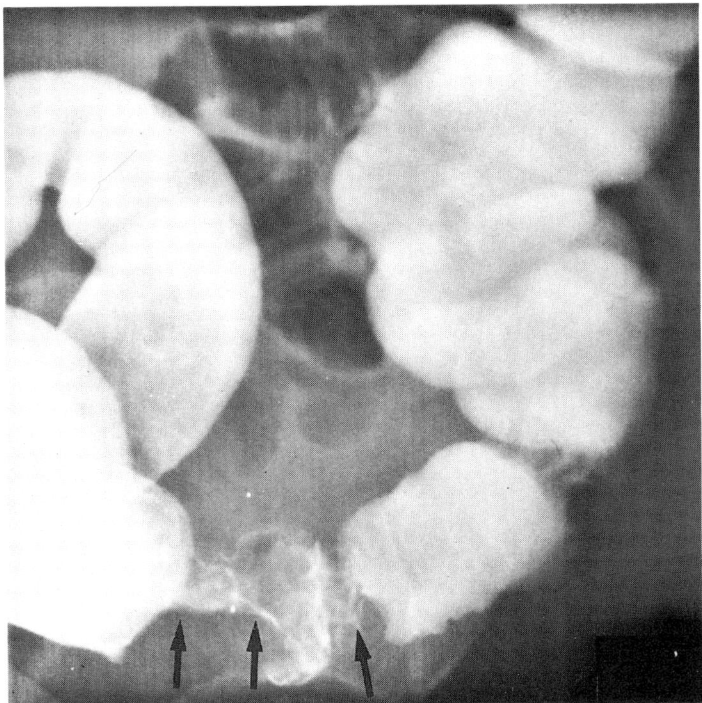

a

b

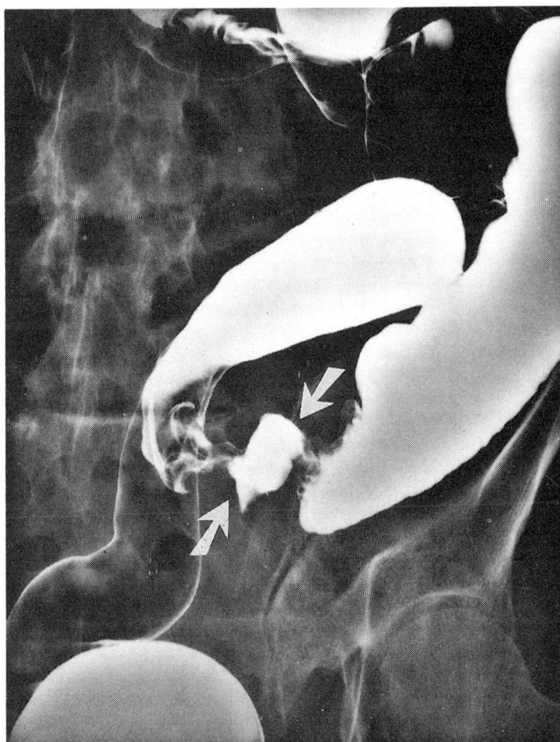

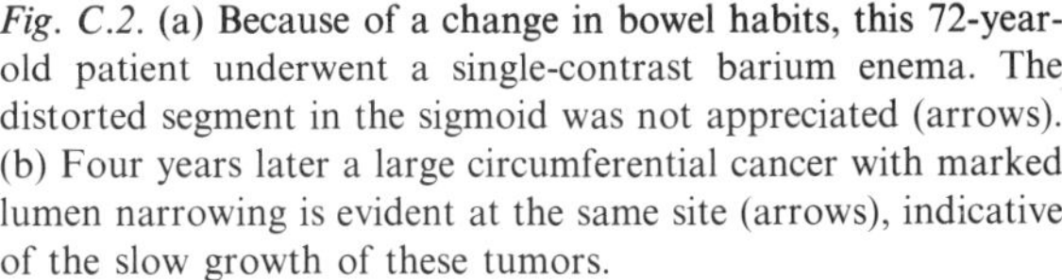

Fig. C.2. (a) Because of a change in bowel habits, this 72-year-old patient underwent a single-contrast barium enema. The distorted segment in the sigmoid was not appreciated (arrows). (b) Four years later a large circumferential cancer with marked lumen narrowing is evident at the same site (arrows), indicative of the slow growth of these tumors.

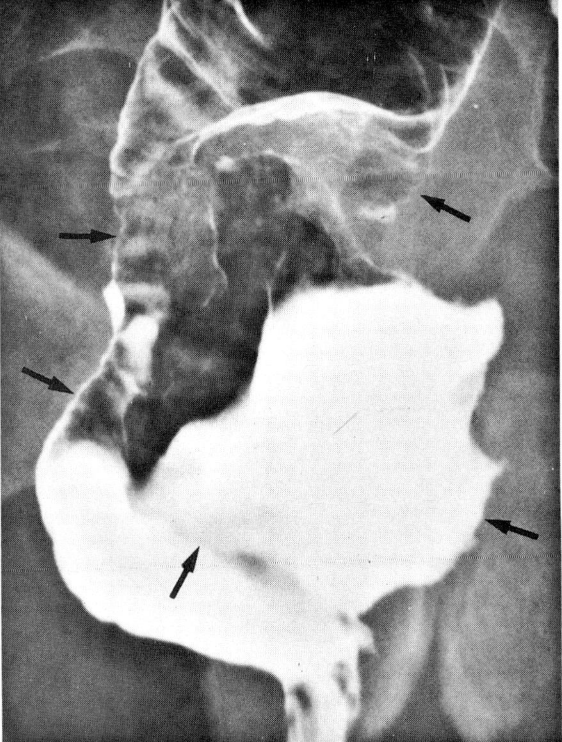

Fig. C.3. A large fungating, infiltrating carcinoma involves almost the entire rectum (arrows). The patient sought medical attention because of 'maroon stools'.

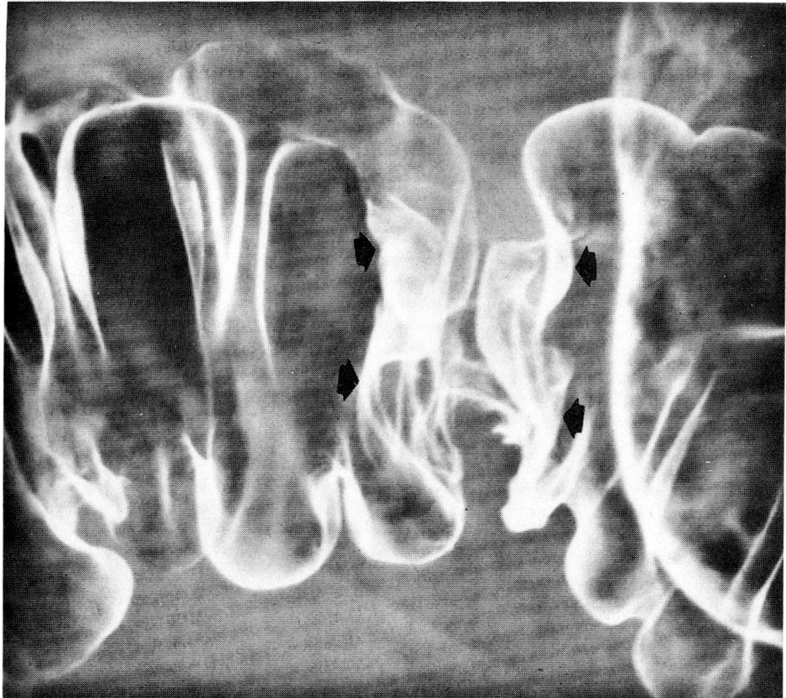

Fig. C.4. This 38-year-old patient had vague left lower quadrant pain and the referring physician requested the barium enema to check for possible diverticular disease. No diverticula were present but there is a far advanced circumferential carcinoma in the transverse colon (arrowheads). Surgery revealed extensive mesenteric node metastases.

Many patients with cancer have vague pain, diarrhea, or varying amounts of bleeding (Fig. C.4). Recognition of such subtle symptoms appears to be a good indicator of cancer (35). Unfortunately, some patients still seek medical help only when absolutely necessary.

The symptoms tend to be different between lesions in the right and left sides of the colon.

Because of the fluid nature of the right colon content, it is unusual for carcinoma of the right colon to obstruct. A cecal carcinoma can act as a lead point for intermittent intussusception, with the patient experiencing vague episodes of intermittent right lower quadrant pain (Figs. C.5 and C.6). A cecal carcinoma can also necrose, perforate, or obstruct the appendix, thus mimicking the clinical presentation of appendicitis (Fig. C.7). Occasionally a carcinoma will arise at the ileocecal valve and the initial presentation will be small bowel obstruction. These lesions thus tend to grow to a large size before a diagnosis is made (Fig. C.8). In particular, with cecal and ascending colon carcinomata it is not unusual for the patient to simply present with occult blood or melena.

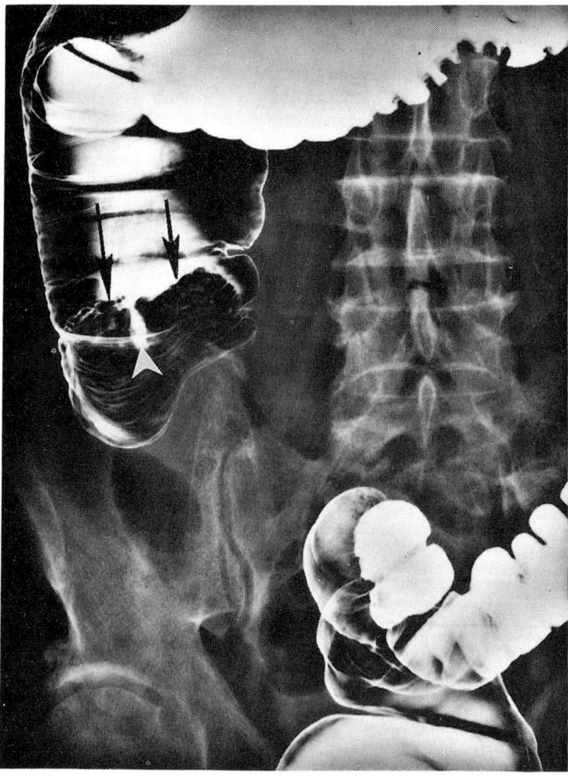

Fig. C.5. Cecal adenocarcinoma acting as a lead point for intussusception (arrows). There is an ulcer within the tumor (arrowheads).

Carcinoma of the left colon presents with rectal

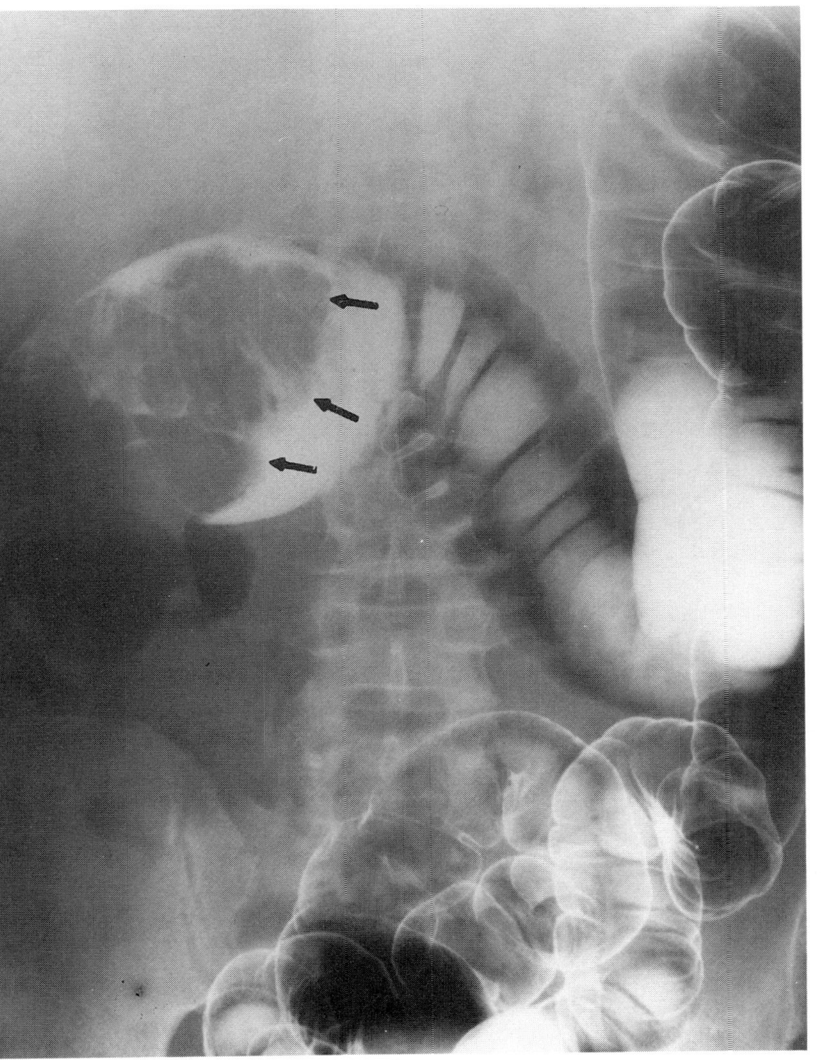

a

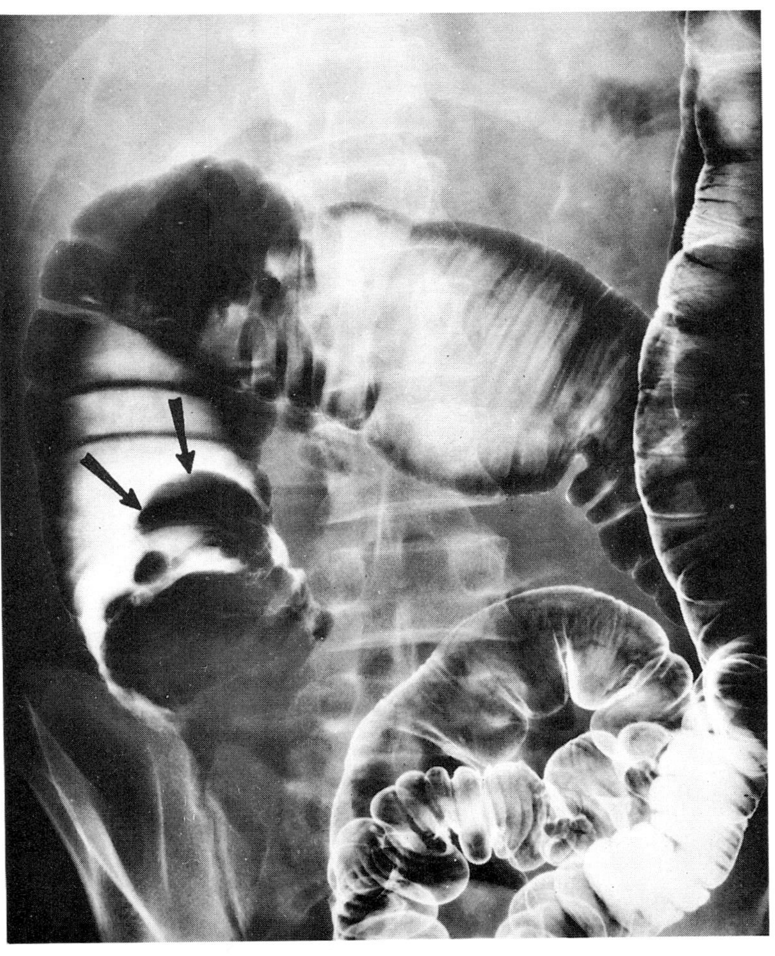

b

Fig. C.6 (a) An intussusception has extended into the transverse colon (arrows). (b) With gradual pressure the intussusception was reduced to the right colon. The intussusception lead point was a cecal adenocarcinoma (arrows).

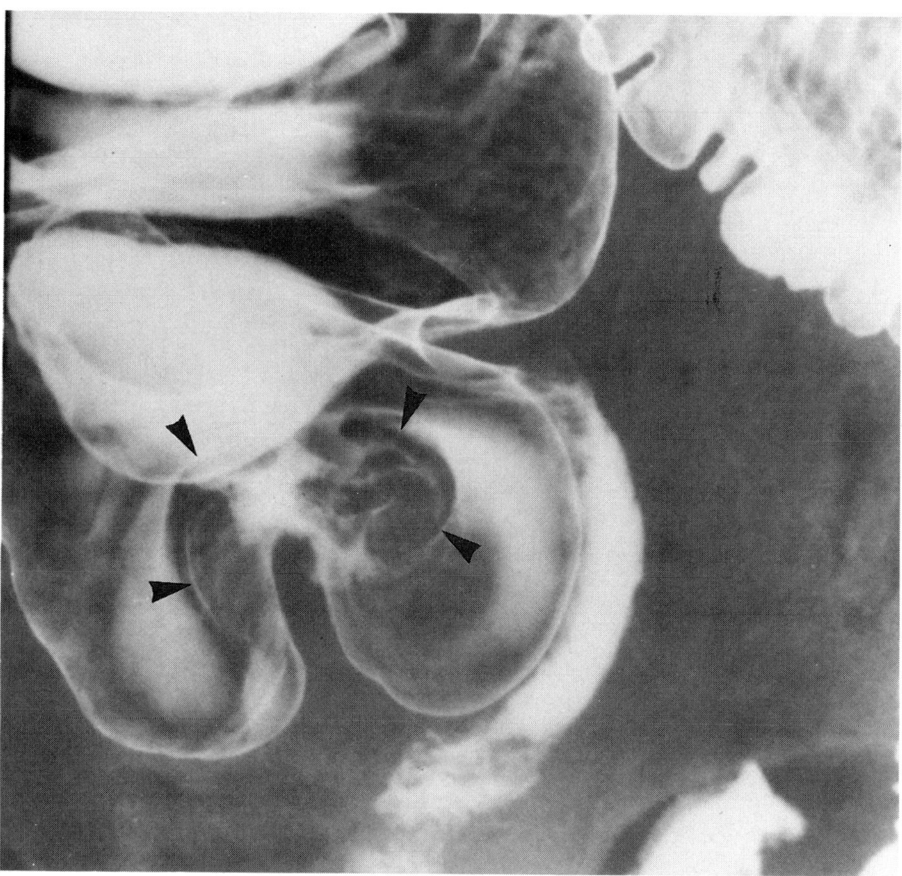

Fig. C.7. Small cecal adenocarcinoma (arrowheads) originating at the base of the appendix. The appendix was obstructed. Although clinical signs suggested appendicitis, a barium enema was requested because the patient was 76 years old.

bleeding or with varying degrees of bowel obstruction. Vague abdominal pain, especially on the left side, is common. Diarrhea may alternate with constipation. Excessive mucus in the stool is not uncommon. Because stool in the left colon is more solid than on the right, left colon cancers tend to obstruct earlier than right colon cancers and these patients generally tend not to be as anemic as patients with right colon lesions.

The large, bulky and well differentiated tumors tend to metastasize less than poorly differentiated smaller lesions. Patients with a polypoid cancer tend to have a better prognosis than those with an infiltrating tumor.

The earliest and most reliable clinical sign of an underlying colon neoplasm is occult blood in the stool. Numerous patient population groups have been screened for occult blood with varying results. Patient compliance with such screening is a major factor; both high compliance (36) and low compliance have been reported (37). It cannot be emphasized enough that all adult patients with occult blood in the stool and with no obvious source of bleeding, even if otherwise asymptomatic, should undergo a thorough investigation of the colon to exclude a colon carcinoma (38). The bleeding often is sufficiently slow enough that it is not noticed by the patient. Even when the patient has melena or bright red rectal bleeding it is not unusual to have the patient or the patient's physician ascribe this bleeding to hemorrhoids. Occasionally, the initial investigation is because of

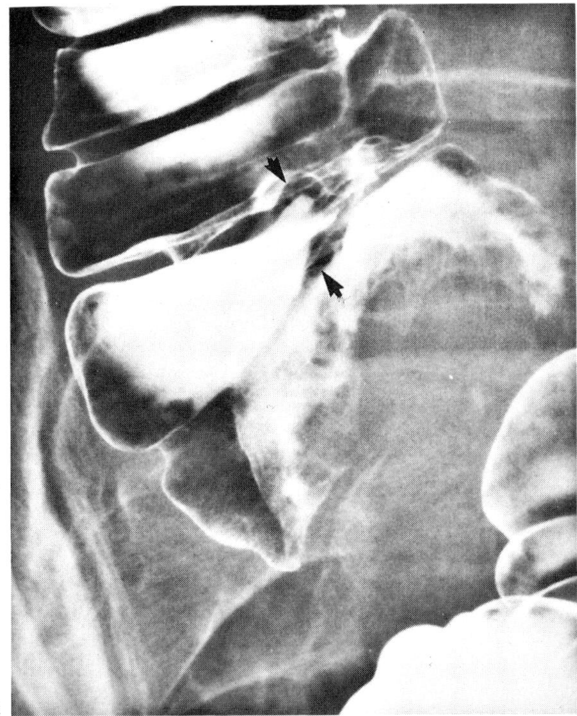

a

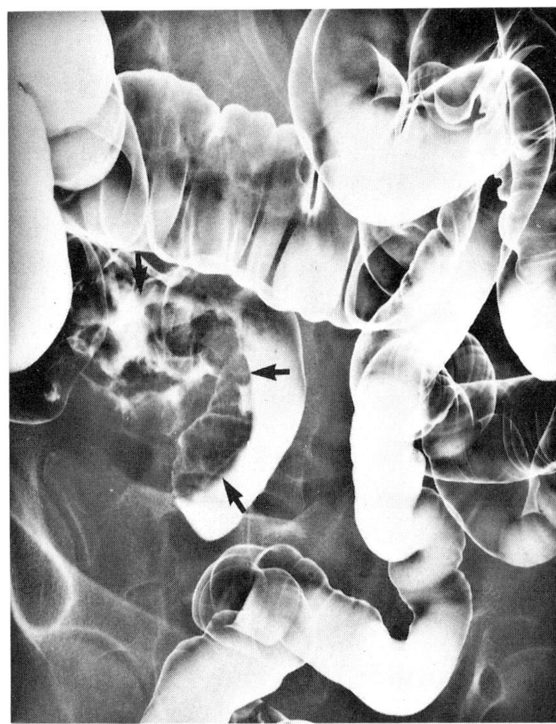

b

Fig. C.8. (a) An adenocarcinoma has destroyed most of the cecum. The ileocecal valve (arrowheads) is distal to the cancer and no obstruction is present. The patient was anemic. (b) An even larger carcinoma of the cecum (arrows). The irregular collections of barium represent ulcerations. The patient had rectal bleeding.

shortness of breath and a tired sensation because of underlying anemia. The anemia generally develops over a prolonged period of time and the patient may not be aware of any change.

We believe that colonoscopy should be performed *after* a double-contrast barium enema. Such an approach allows the clinician to evaluate the radiological findings and concentrate on any suspicious areas during colonoscopy.

In 1965, a substance present in fetal colon tissue was isolated from tumors of the digestive tract (39). Because of this association, the substance was named carcinoembryonic antigen (CEA). This antigen, having a molecular weight of approximately 2,000,000, appears to be associated with the tumor cell surface. Although it was hoped initially that this antigen would be specific for gastrointestinal tumors (40), it has not turned out to be either tumor specific or organ specific.

The CEA test should not be used as a screening test for colorectal cancer (41). Likewise, it is not a sensitive test for the detection of early local recurrence of tumor (42). Many patients with colon cancer, Dukes' C classification, have an elevated CEA level. Unfortunately, at this point an extensive tumor is generally present. The CEA level may still be useful as a prognostic tool, because patients with a low level have a longer survival (43). Serial readings are important and increased readings following cancer resection should raise the suspicion of metastases (44), especially to the liver.

The CEA levels in patients receiving chemotherapy can be confusing (45). Changes in CEA are not predictive of survival, although a persistent elevation of CEA is indicative of therapeutic failure. The CEA levels are comparable with serum alkaline phosphatase in assessing response of liver metastases to chemotherapy.

Elevated CEA levels have been reported in various benign liver and gastrointestinal diseases such as some of the polyposis syndromes and various colitides (46, 47). Patients with pulmonary emphysema may have elevated CEA titers. The CEA test is expensive and in actual practice only rarely changed the clinical management of a patient (48) or resulted in improved patient benefit (49). Maximum benefit appears to be in the follow-up of colon cancer patients after 'curative' treatment.

Other antigens, such as the zinc glycinate marker (ZGM), have been proposed as tumor markers (50). Undoubtedly, other tests will be available in the future, hopefully allowing earlier cancer detection.

c. Radiology of adenocarcinomata

The diagnostic yield of a double-contrast barium enema depends primarily upon the examiner. A competent examiner, using the best available double-contrast enema technique, can achieve reliable and reproducible results. A well performed double-contrast barium enema will detect most lesions measuring more than several millimeters in diameter (4, 51–53).

Approximately 75% of all missed carcinomata have been missed because the radiologist mistook the lesion for retained stool in a patient with poor colon preparation, or the radiologist simply described poor preparation but left a choice of repeating the examination to the clinician (54). The final radiological report should indicate whether the examination was normal, abnormal, or whether the examination must be repeated. All patients suspected of having an obstructive colon carcinoma should first be studied with an acute abdominal examination. With obstruction, the abdominal examination shows a distended colon and small bowel proximally, with the amount of distension depending upon the degree and chronicity of obstruction (Fig. C.9). Quite often one can locate the

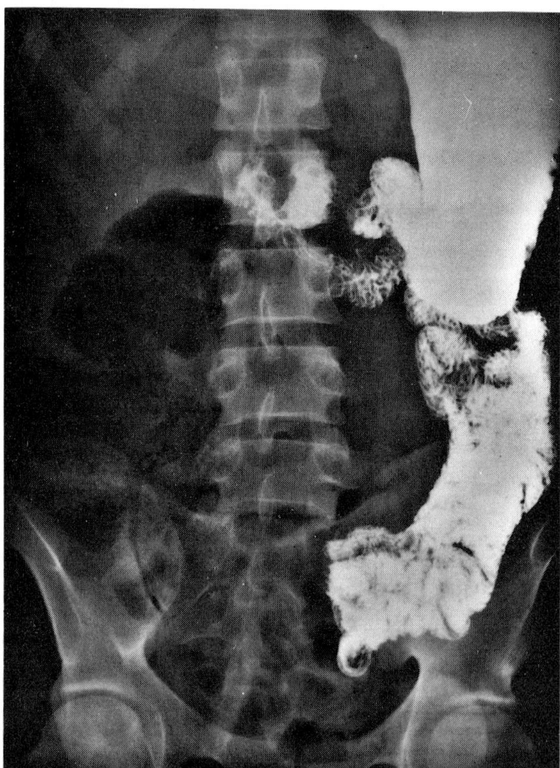

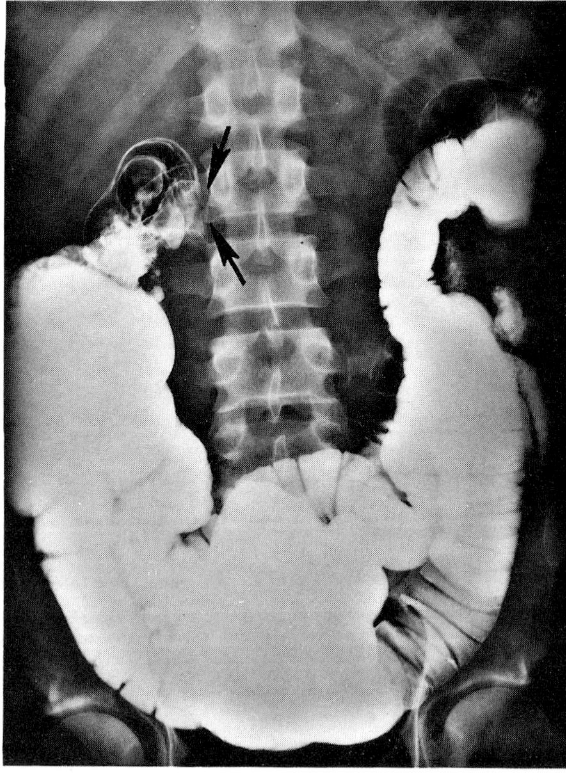

Fig. C.9. 31-year-old male with abdominal pain. An upper gastrointestinal and small bowel examination was requested. (a) The proximal small bowel is normal. Right colic dilatation is already apparent. (b) 24 hours later the barium column has reached the site of obstruction in the transverse colon (arrows). At this point not only is the right colic dilation obvious, but the obstruction has also resulted in distal small bowel dilatation. A mid-transverse colon adenocarcinoma was resected. In retrospect, the colic dilation should have been identified initially, a barium enema should have been performed to identify the site of obstruction, and the addition of barium sulfate proximal to the obstruction avoided.

approximate point of obstruction on these radiographs. Reliance on non-contrast radiographs alone, however, is dangerous because occasionally the obstruction will be in a different site than apparent on these radiographs. In addition, the colon can be dilated with no obstruction being present. Dilation of the transverse colon can be associated both with benign disease and with extracolic carcinoma invading from adjoining structures.

Occasionally, fine speckled calcifications are present in a colon cancer (55). High quality radiographs are necessary to appreciate such a finding. These calcifications generally imply that the tumor is relatively well differentiated and that considerable mucus is being produced (Fig. C.10). A metastatic focus may likewise calcify. These calcifications are readily apparent on CT scans (Fig. C.11).

Although gas in the bowel wall can represent benign pneumatosis cystoides intestinalis, the majority of such patients with obstruction will have bowel ischemia. The increased intraluminal pressure proximal to an obstruction tends to decrease the venous blood return (56). Because most of these patients are elderly, quite often there is superimposed arteriosclerotic cardiovascular disease. The overall result is decreased blood flow and bowel ischemia. We believe that, in general, a finding of gas within the bowel wall in a patient with suspected distal colon obstruction requires emergency surgical decompression. Radiological contrast studies in such a setting are rarely warranted and are usually contraindicated.

It is unusual for a colon carcinoma to perforate into the peritoneum at the site of the lesion. Most perforations occur proximal to the lesion and are the result of increased intraluminal pressure from obstruction. Occasionally encountered, however, is a carcinoma with an adjacent pericolic abscess (57). Most such abscesses presumably arise from a localized perforation through the tumor and subsequent infection. The radiological examination can be confusing if the primary appearance is that of inflammation. A colon carcinoma can result in portal venous gas (58).

A fistula can develop at the site of a tumor. The fistula can be to any of the adjacent intraabdominal organs or even extend cutaneously (57, 59). If it is known that the patient's symptoms have been present for some time and if the patient does not have acute abdominal signs or symptoms, barium sulfate is the contrast agent used for the barium enema. Obviously, if there are peritoneal signs an enema examination is contraindicated. In general, however, if it is desired to know the site of origin of a cutaneous fistula, a fistulogram is more productive and should be obtained first.

A contraindication to the performance of any barium enema is recent colonoscopy or sigmoidoscopy with biopsy. If there has been a biopsy, the barium enema should be postponed for approximately one week or longer after the biopsy.

Occasionally there is obstruction to the retrograde flow of barium yet clinically the patient is not obstructed. Such a check-valve mechanism can be seen with both tumors and inflammatory disease, although it is more common with a carcinoma. A barium enema can evaluate only the distal end of such a lesion and in most cases the full extent of the lesion cannot be appreciated (Fig. C.12). Even if minimal contrast flows proximal to the obstruction, the true nature of the lesion becomes apparent (Fig. C.13).

Although a pathologist generally describes a carcinoma by the degree of differentiation and extent of invasion, a radiologist describes it by its gross radiographic appearance. A carcinoma can thus be primarily intraluminal and appear like a typical polyp, it can infiltrate through the wall of the colon, it can be either long or short in length, it can contain ulcers, or it can encircle and narrow the colon lumen to varying degrees. All of these terms are descriptive and simply convey to the referring physician the general appearance of the lesion. Annular lesions have been referred to as 'napkin-ring' or 'apple-core', terms simply describing an annular and circumferential lesion with varying degrees of lumen narrowing.

A colon carcinoma can thus have one of several appearances. It should be emphasized that a small carcinoma is generally smooth (60) (Fig. C.14). It is only after some growth that an irregular outline appears.

One typical radiographic appearance is that of a polypoid or fungating mass and an almost completely intraluminal extension (Fig. C.15). These fungating carcinomata are prone to ulcerate and bleed. When large, they are relatively easy to diagnose (Fig. C.16). When small, they appear like any intraluminal polyp.

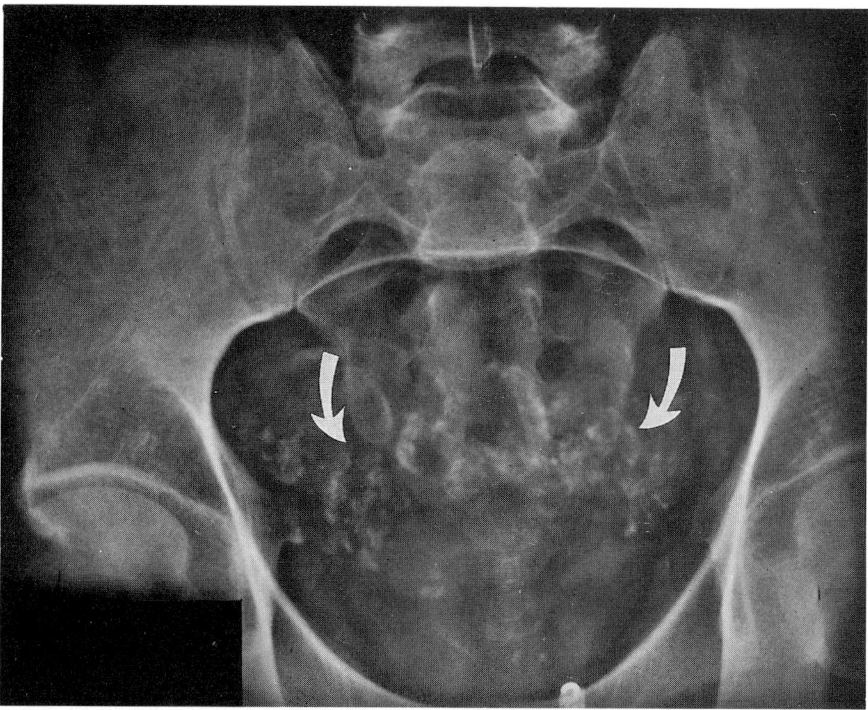

Fig. C.10. A mucin-producing adenocarcinoma results in diffuse speckled calcifications throughout the pelvis (arrows).

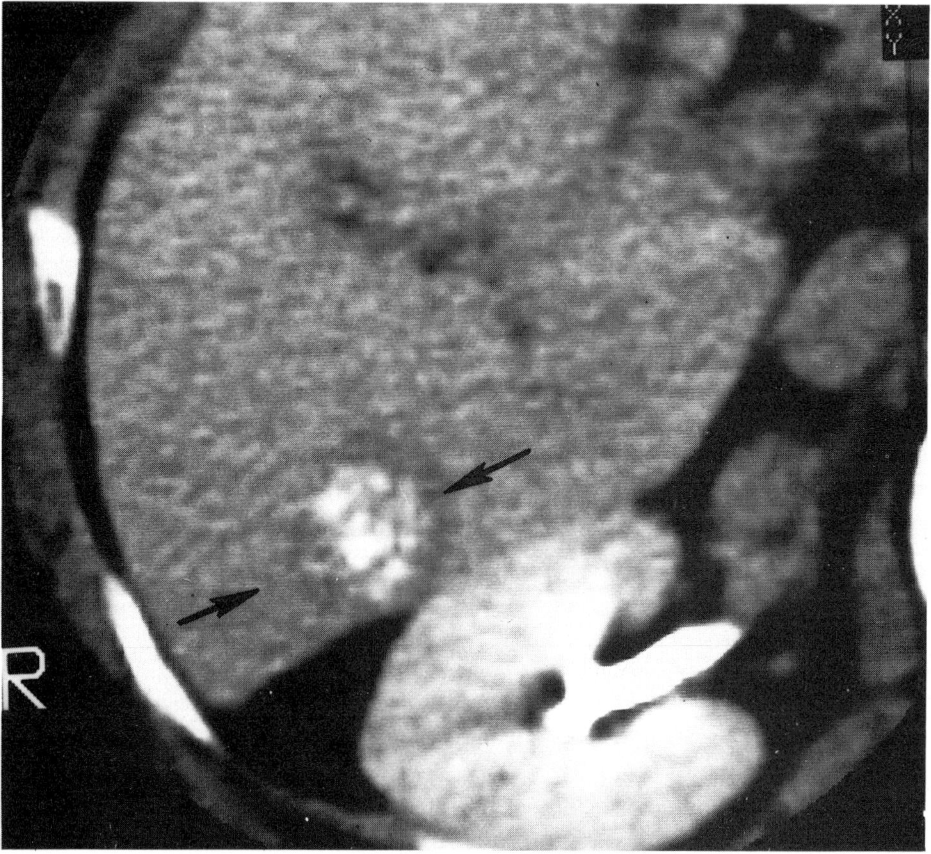

Fig. C.11. Calcified liver metastasis (arrows). The calcifications were poorly seen on conventional radiographs.

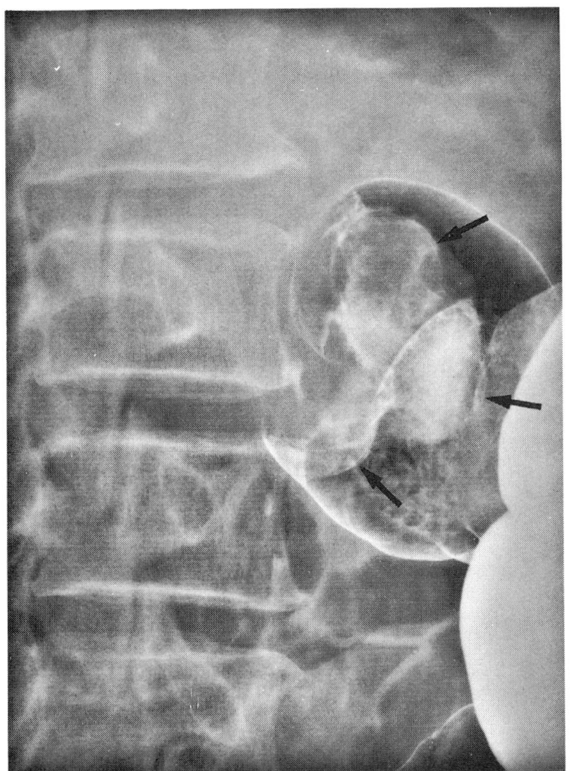

Fig. C.12. Retrograde obstruction by an adenocarcinoma (arrows). The tumor was acting as a lead point for an intussusception. Clinically, the patient did not have bowel obstruction.

When an infiltrating tumor is still small, it has a plaque-like appearance (Fig. C.17). With growth, the tumor envelops a portion of the colon wall (Fig. C.18); some radiologists use the term 'saddle cancer' to describe these lesions (61). These infiltrating carcinomata tend to be aggressive. If undetected early, or if the patient refuses treatment, these tumors continue infiltrating the bowel wall and eventually result in an annular carcinoma (Figs. C.19 and 20).

A carcinoma can infiltrate circumferentially early in its growth and thus barely narrow the lumen (Fig. C.21). Or, the circumferential infiltration can eventually be so extensive that the lumen is almost completely obliterated (Fig. C.22). They can infiltrate extensively and result in considerable wall rigidity. The proximal and distal tumor margins tend to be sharply demarcated with an overhanging edge usually being present. Within the tumor, the normal colon folds are destroyed and barium tends to be trapped in irregular and haphazard crevices, often the result of multiple ulcerations (Fig. C.23). The circumferential involvement can be asymmetrical (Fig. C.24). At times a circumferential neoplasm is associated with an additional eccentric com-

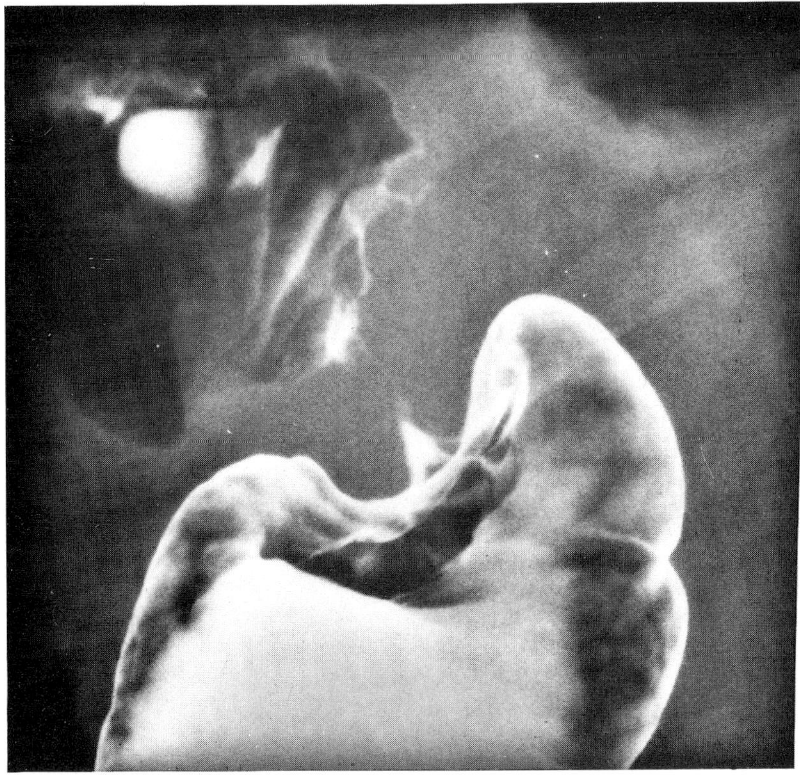

Fig. C.13. Almost complete retrograde obstruction at the splenic flexure. The colon proximal to the lesion is not dilated and clinically no obstruction was evident. The small amount of barium and air introduced proximal to the lesion allows identification of the lesion as most likely a carcinoma. Surgical resection revealed an adenocarcinoma.

ponent (Fig. C.25). The absence of normal folds helps differentiate a tumor from diverticulitis. Although annular carcinomata occur anywhere in the colon, they are more common on the left side.

Some carcinomata tend to form large ulcers. Even when a large tumor component is present the lumen is wide in the central portion of the tumor because of the ulceration. If obstruction does occur, it is usually at the leading edges of the cancer (Fig. C.26).

A carcinoma originating close to the ileocecal valve usually invades locally (Fig. C.27). Once the tumor has spread outside the serosa, invasion of adjacent structures, including the terminal ileum, occurs. It is unusual to see a carcinoma spread through the ileocecal valve because there are no direct lymphatic communications between the colon and terminal ileum (62). If a tumor does involve both the terminal ileum and the colon, a lymphoma should be suspected. The exception is a cecal

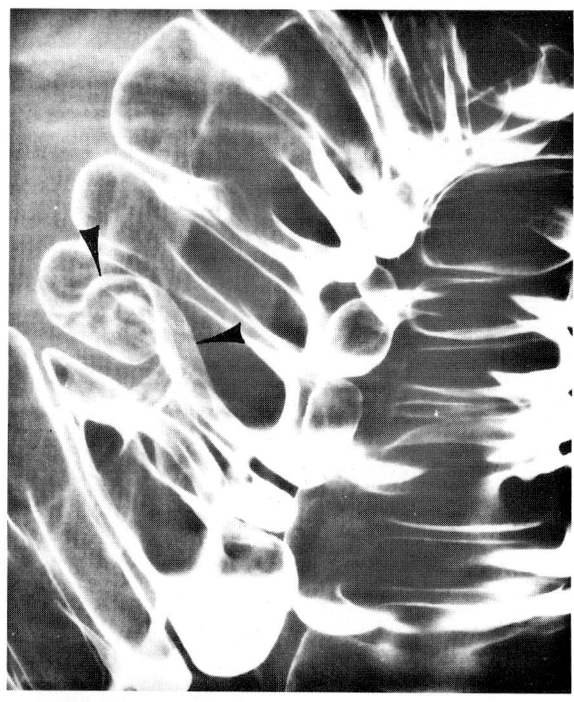

a

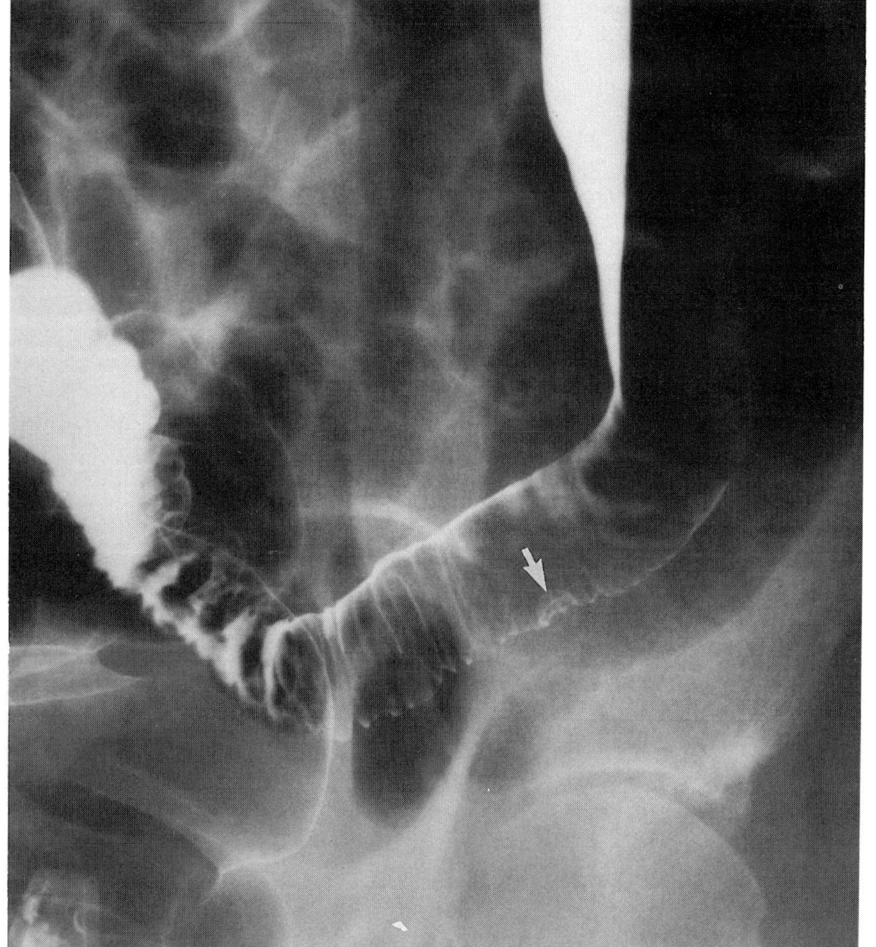

b

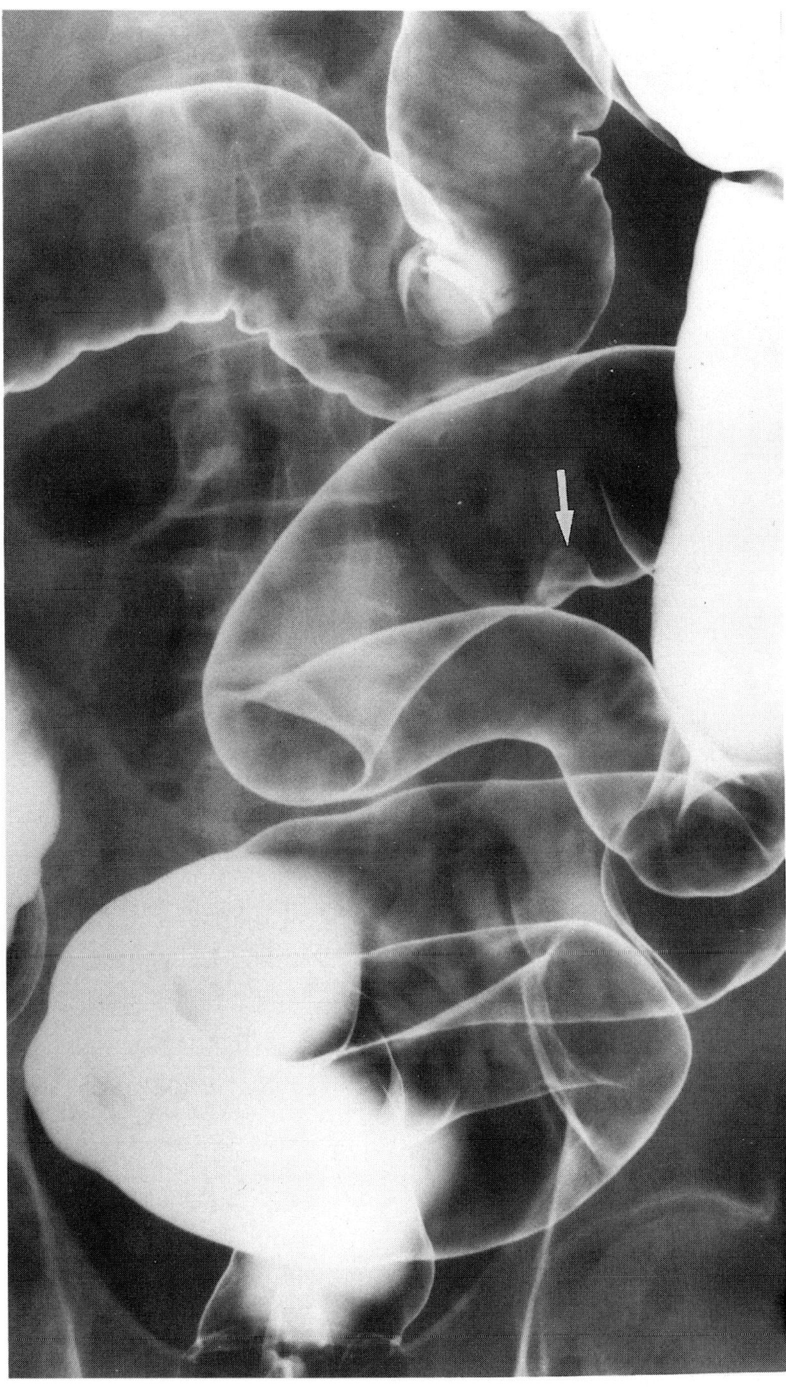

Fig. C.14. (a) Moderately differentiated adenocarcinoma (arrowheads). The lesion is smooth in outline although resection 10 days later showed extension to the serosa. (b) Small, smooth polyp (arrow). It was an adenocarcinoma. (c) Smooth polyp approximately 1.0 cm in diameter (arrow). Initial colonoscopy could not locate the polyp, probably because of the marked redundancy. Repeat colonoscopy and biopsy revealed an adenocarcinoma. (From Skucas et al. (60); copyright, RSNA, 1982.)

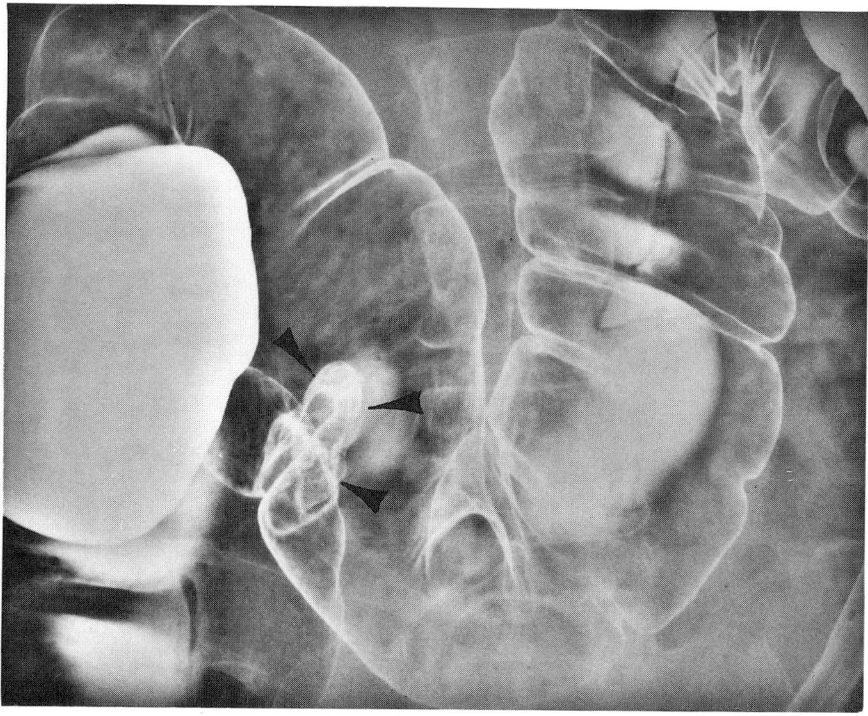

Fig. C.15. A lobulated intraluminal polyp in the transverse colon (arrowheads). Colonoscopic biopsy two days after the barium enema revealed 'adenomatous polyp with marked epithelial atypia'. Surgical resection five days later showed a 'well differentiated adenocarcinoma arising in an adenomatous polyp with invasion of the stalk'.

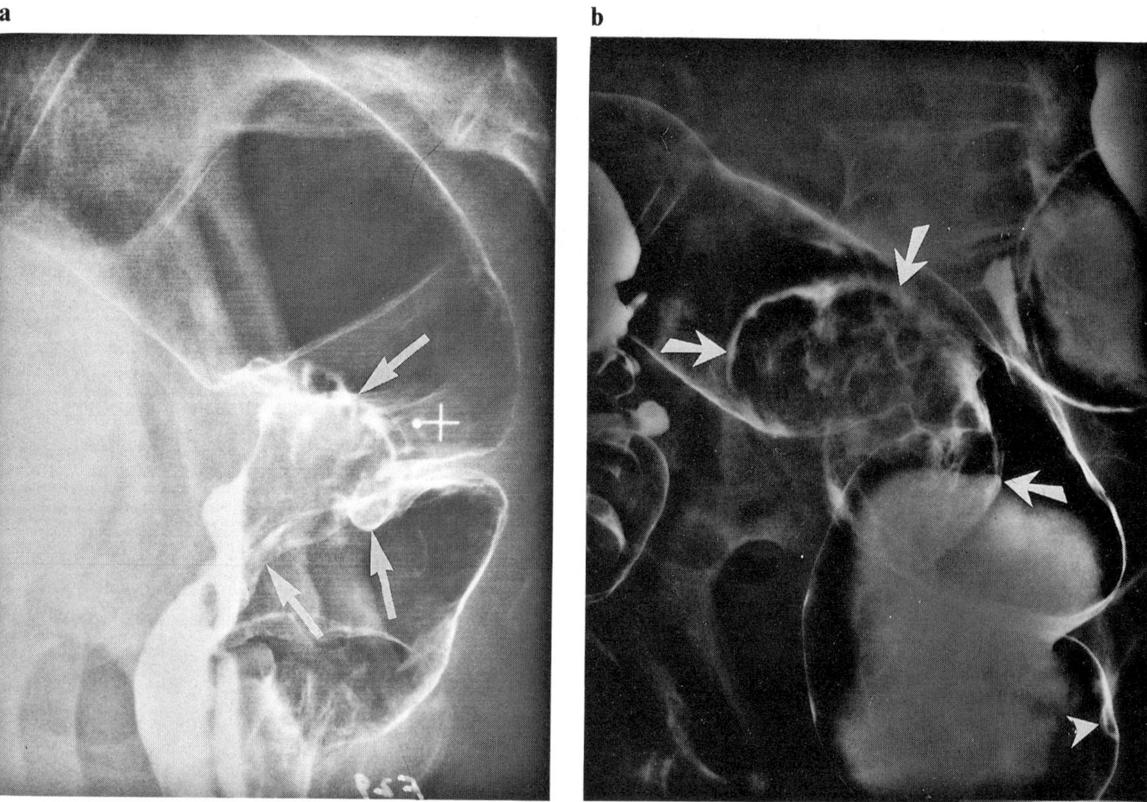

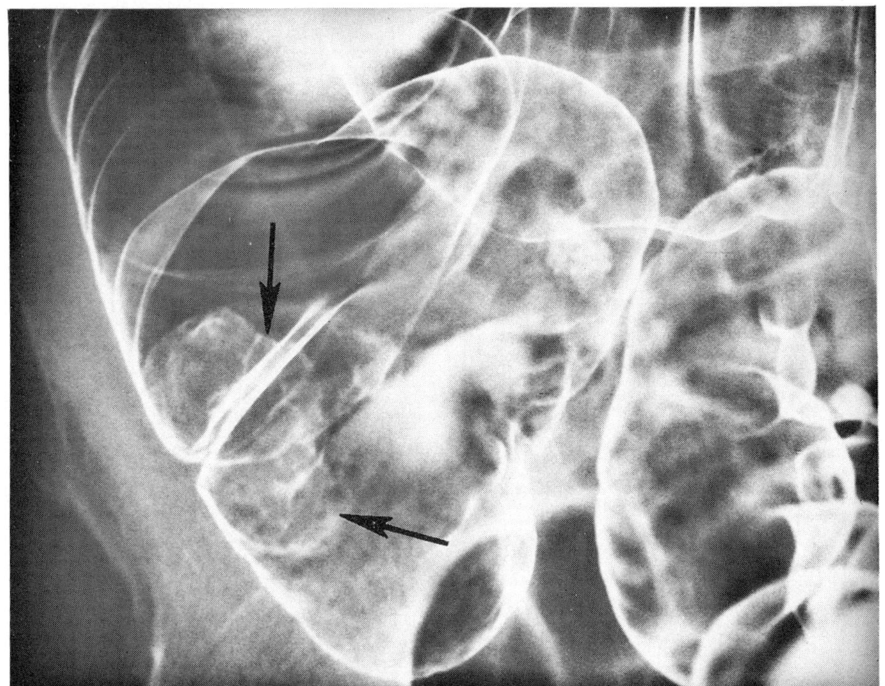

c

d

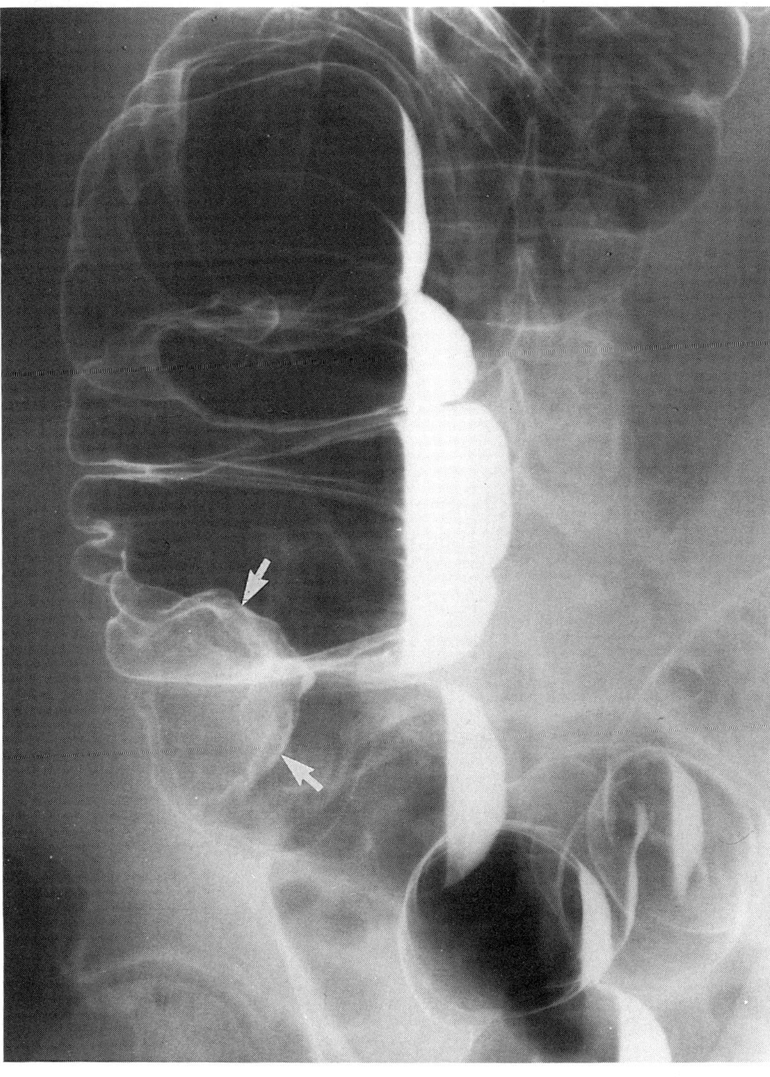

Fig. C.16. (a) Large polypoid rectal adenocarcinoma (arrows). The shaggy, ulcerated outline strongly supports the diagnosis of a malignancy. (b) An even larger polypoid adenocarcinoma of the rectosigmoid (arrows). A small adenoma is present in the rectum (arrowhead). (c) Intraluminal adenocarcinoma of the cecum (arrows). The tumor is irregular in outline, a typical finding in carcinomata this size. (d) Large intraluminal adenocarcinoma (arrows). The appearance is very similar to the previous figure although this polyp is considerably larger.

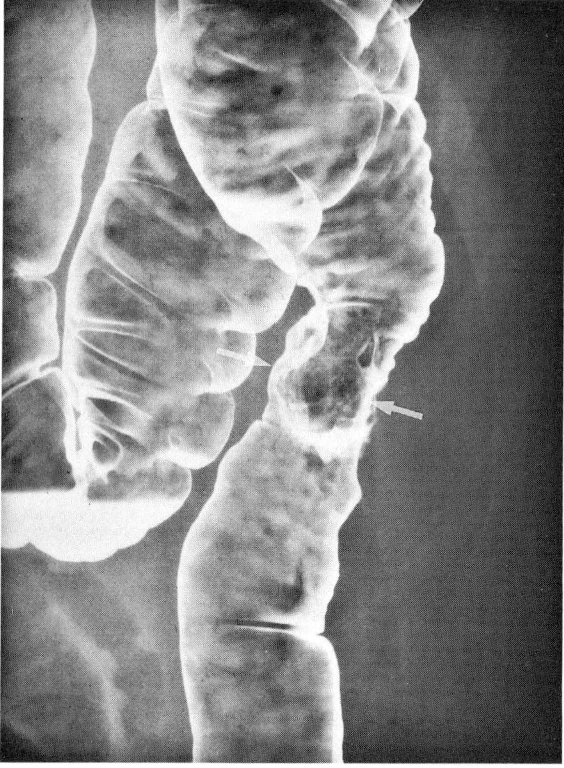

a

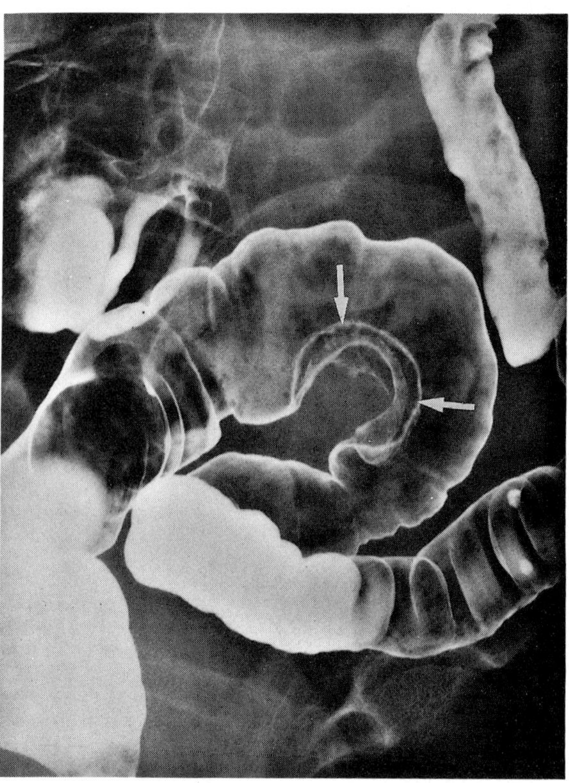

b

Fig. C.17. (a) A plaque-like adenocarcinoma extends primarily in the intramural tissues, with little intraluminal extension (arrows). (b) A more advanced plaque-like infiltrating adenocarcinoma of the sigmoid (arrows).

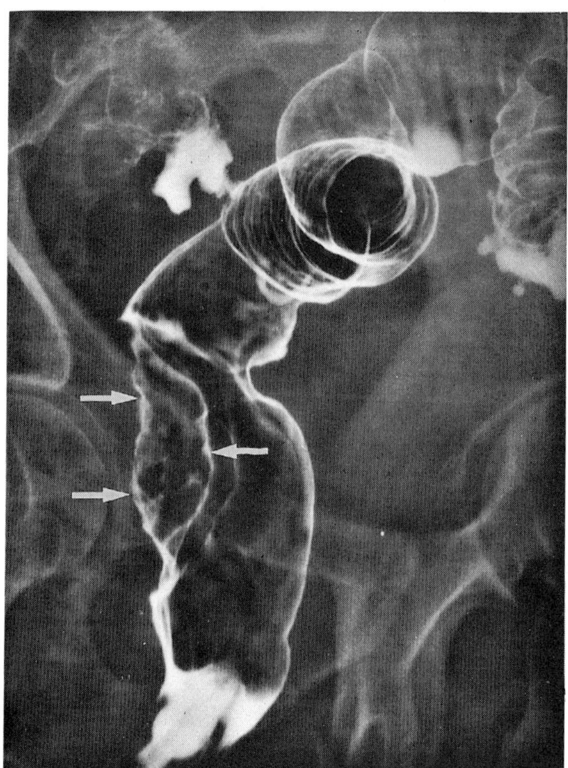

Fig. C.18. Large rectal 'saddle carcinoma' (arrows).

carcinoma with extensive lymphatic metastasis, lymphatic obstruction, and retrograde lymphatic embolization to the ileum (63).

A carcinoma can be associated with considerable spasm. During a barium enema the radiologist can thus be initially confronted with a smooth obstruction to the retrograde flow of barium. If this area is in the sigmoid, differentiation from diverticulitis may initially be impossible. A hypotonic agent generally helps relieve the spasm and allows the radiologist to outline the true nature of the lesion. With persistent spasm, the radiologist can apply gradual pressure and the spasm should clear, at least intermittently. Occasionally both a carcinoma and diverticulitis occur in the same segment and differentiation is not possible.

Only rarely does an infiltrating carcinoma involve a long segment of the colon (Fig. C.28). The proximal and distal margins of the cancer are either sharply marginated or smooth and poorly defined. If eccentric in location, the uninvolved wall can distend normally. The lumen can be smooth or irregular. The overall picture is similar to that seen

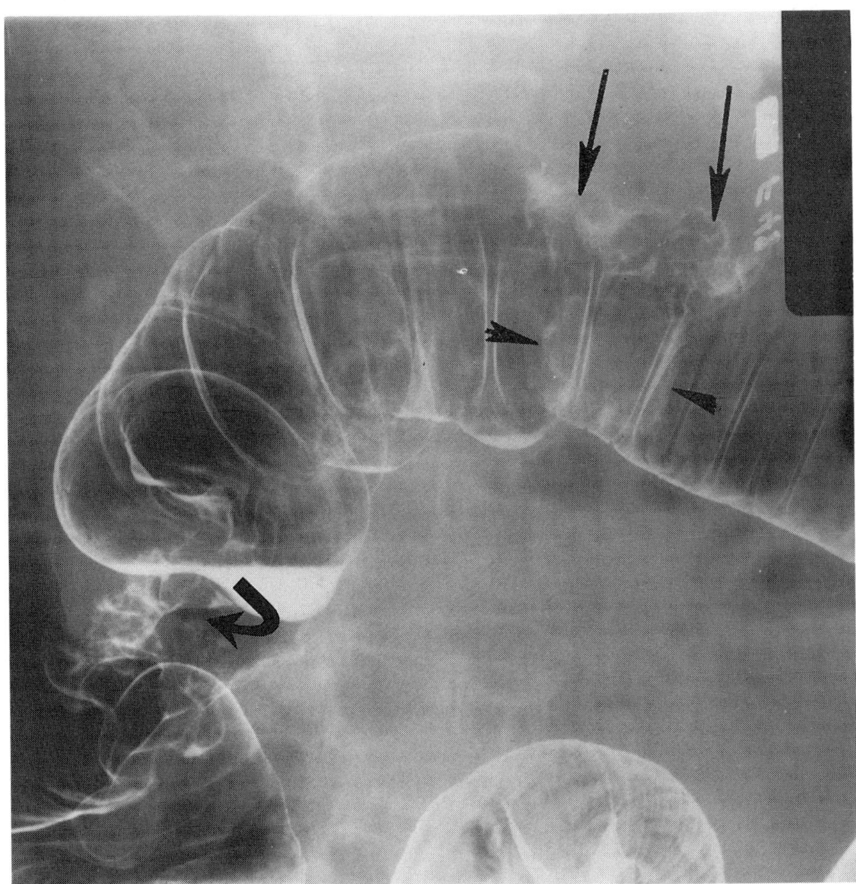

Fig. C.19. An infiltrating adenocarcinoma at the hepatic flexure. The tumor is primarily along one side of the colon (arrows), although circumferential invasion has started (arrowheads). Another synchronous adenocarcinoma is present in the ascending colon (curved arrow).

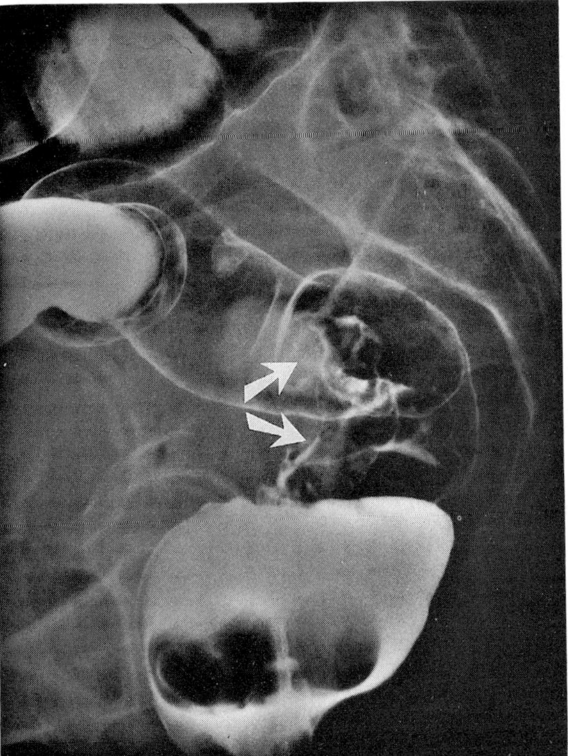

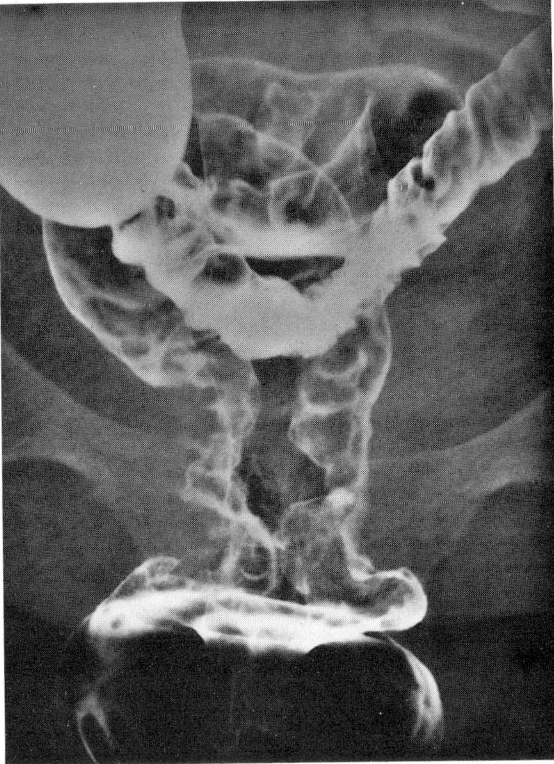

Fig. C.20. Infiltrating rectal adenocarcinoma. (a) The tumor appears primarily along the anterior wall of the rectum (arrows) in the lateral view. (b) A frontal view reveals that the tumor is extending along both side walls and that only a portion of the posterior wall is not involved.

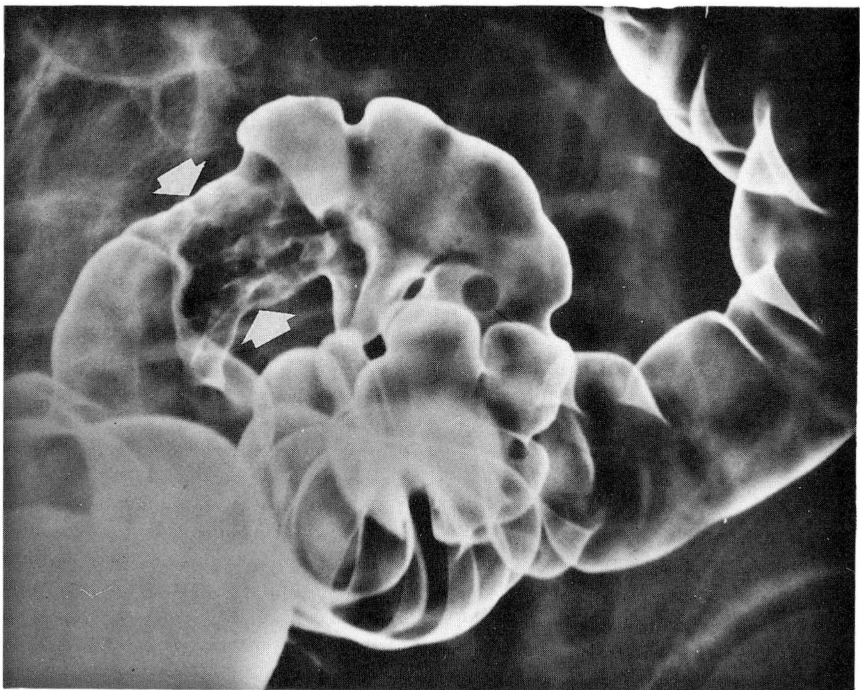

a

b

Fig. C.21. (a) Circumferential adenocarcinoma of the sigmoid. There is minimal narrowing of the lumen (arrowheads). (b) Another patient with circumferential adenocarcinoma of the sigmoid. Although the lumen is only slightly narrowed, there already is full-thickness invasion of the bowel wall. Both the proximal and distal tumor edges are sharply defined (arrows), a characteristic finding of carcinomata.

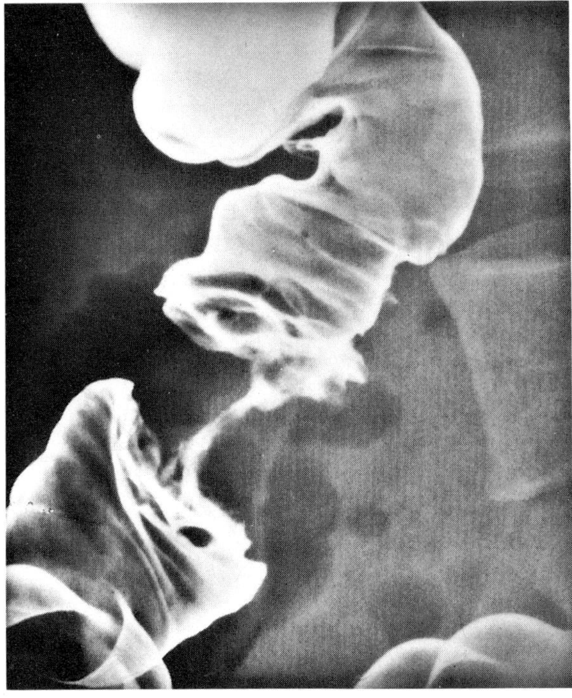

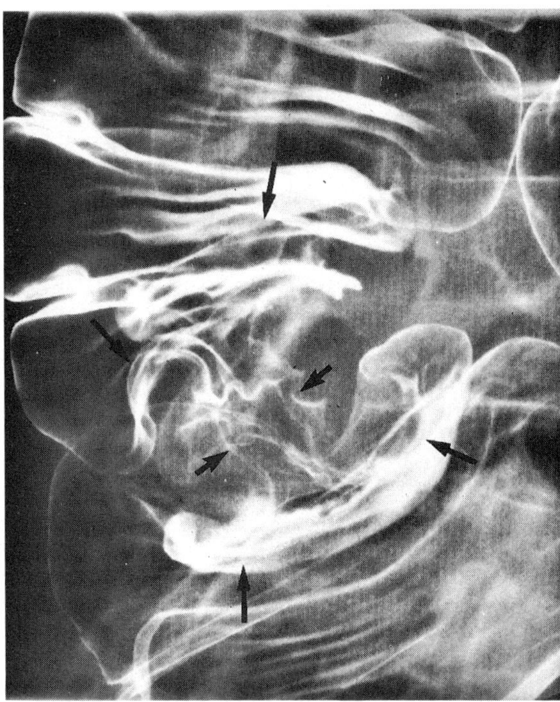

Fig. C.22. (a) Adenocarcinoma of descending colon in a 26-year-old male. Almost complete obstruction is present and both the proximal and distal tumor margins are sharply defined. Metastasis to regional lymph nodes was present. (b) Annular adenocarcinoma of the ascending colon in a 47-year-old male. A narrow channel is present and both tumor edges are sharply defined (arrows). (c) Only a very narrow channel is present through the tumor (arrows), yet there was no evidence of obstruction.

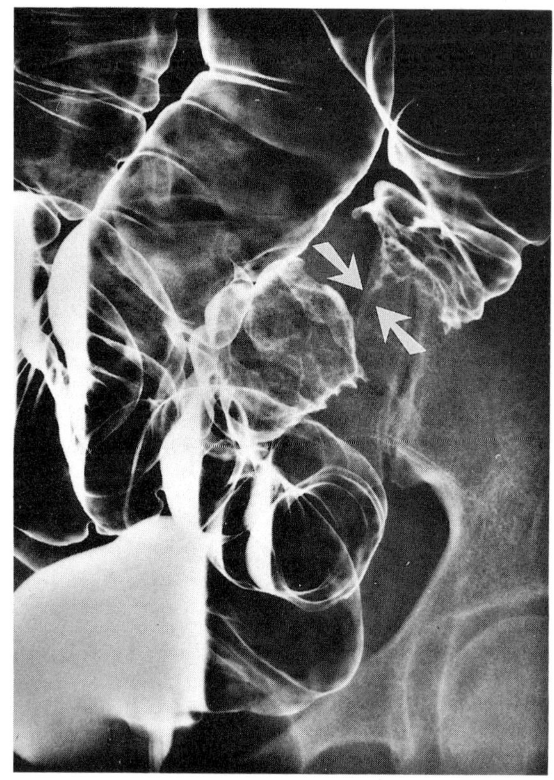

with extensive infiltrating gastric carcinomata (64). These scirrhous lesions have been called linitis plastica of the colon, generally have a considerable desmoplastic reaction, and often are seen in a setting of one of the colitides. Histologically, these tumors are anaplastic mucinous adenocarcinomata. Because infiltration is primarily submucosal, a portion of the overlying mucosa can be intact. Colonoscopic biopsy may not reveal any tumor, which leads to possible confusion with inflammatory disease. The hallmark of these lesions is the lack of pliability of the involved segment and the fixed appearance of at least a portion of the wall. These are usually extremely malignant tumors and extracolic invasion and metastasis to the regional lymph nodes is common, although distal metastasis appears to be unusual (65).

Such primary scirrhous carcinomata of the colon are unusual, with most occuring in the rectosigmoid region (65, 66). These tumors appear to be more common in patients with ulcerative colitis who subsequently develop a carcinoma, although some investigators believe the association is simply coin-

a

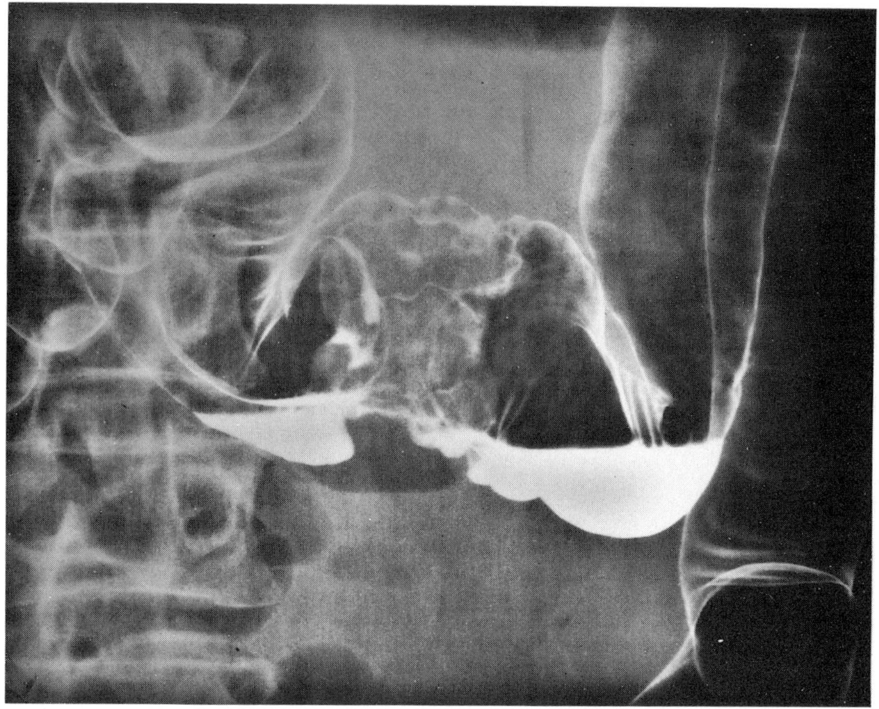

Fig. C.23. (a) A circumferentially infiltrating adenocarcinoma in a 48-year-old physician. He had a previous single-contrast barium enema and the lesion was missed. The tumor is irregular in outline but sharply defined, and barium is trapped in irregular crevices. Ten years later, he is alive and well. (From RE Miller MD (122); copyright, Year Book Medical Publishers, 1975.) (b) Long sigmoid adenocarcinoma. The proximal and distal tumor margins are sharply defined, the lumen is narrowed considerably, and tumor nodules are scattered throughout the involved segment.

b

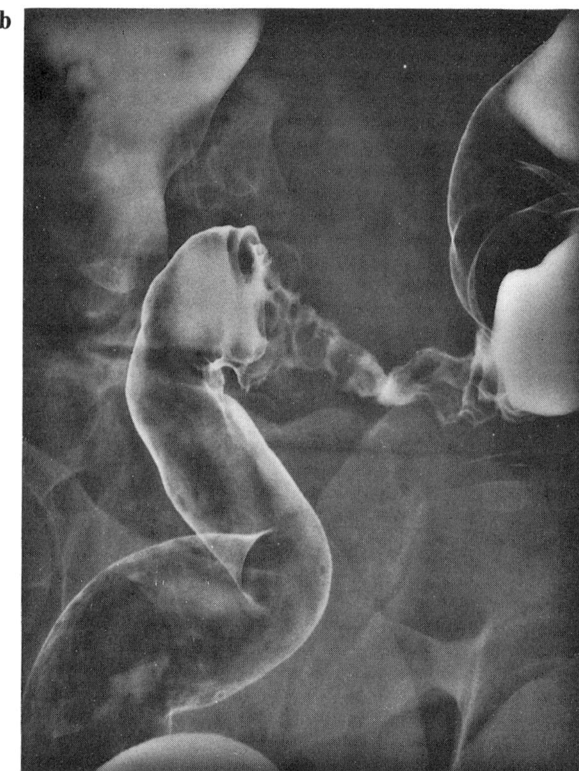

*Fig. C.23.***b**

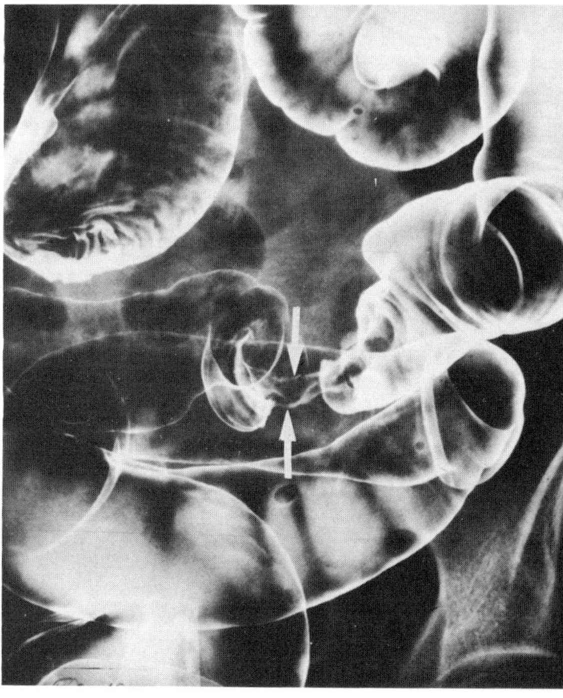

Fig. C.24. An annular adenocarcinoma (arrows) is markedly asymmetrical in its appearance. Only a narrow channel through the tumor remains.

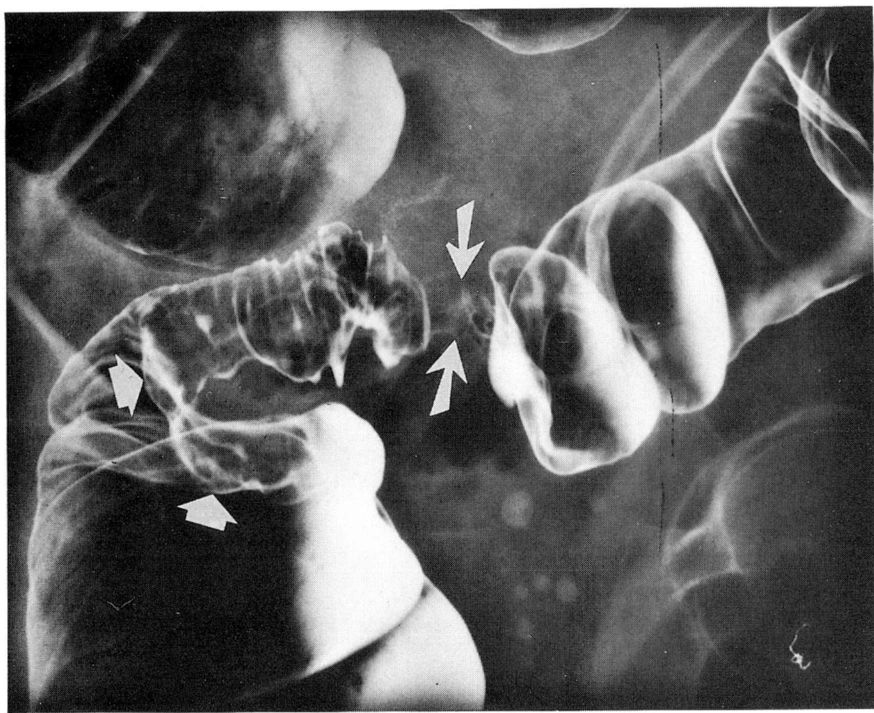

Fig. C.25. This cancer has a circumferential component (arrows) resulting in a stricture, and an eccentric component (arrowheads) invading the colon distally.

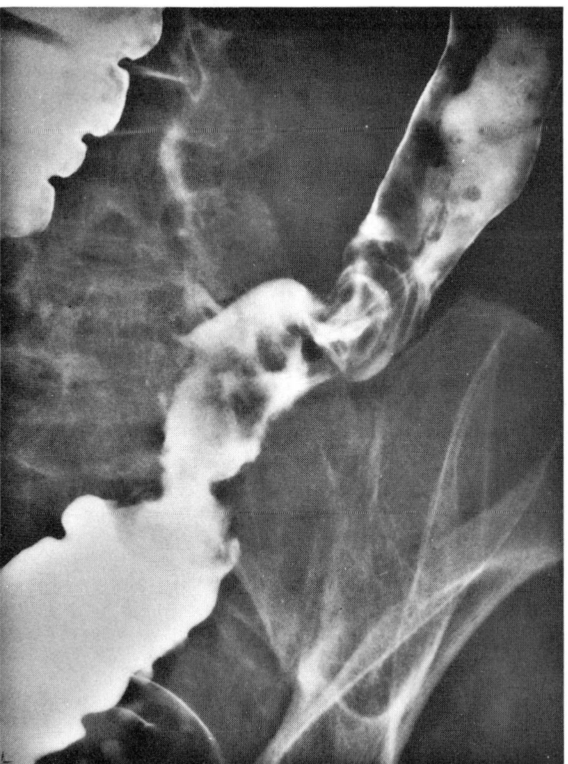

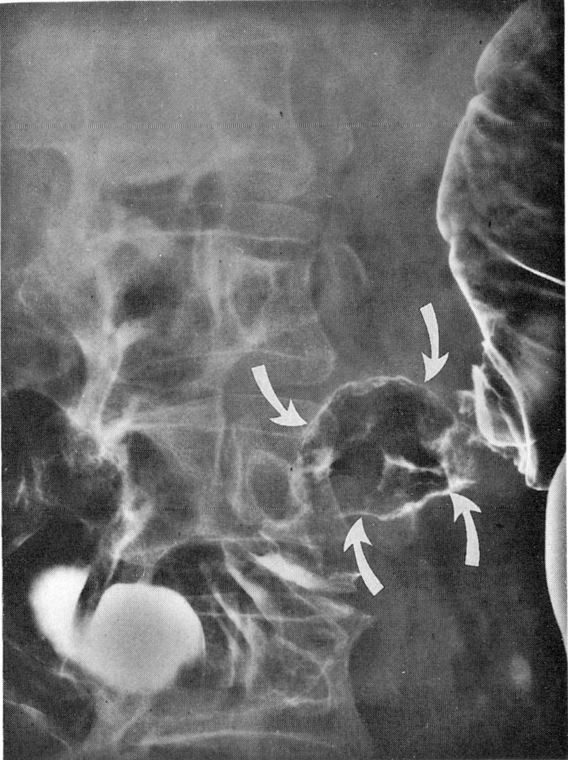

b

Fig. C.26. (a) Large descending colon adenocarcinoma. The bowel lumen within the tumor is irregular in appearance, indicative of ulceration. No obstruction was present. Tumor was present in regional lymph nodes. (b) Mid-transverse colon adenocarcinoma. The central dilatation (arrows) represented tumor necrosis. Serosal tumor nodules and nodal metastases were present.

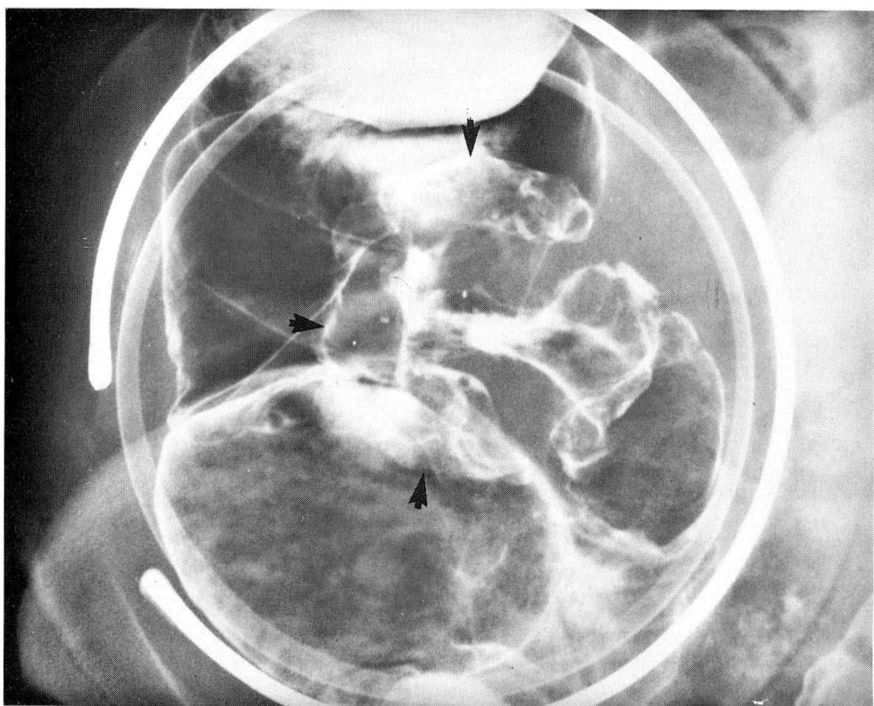

Fig. C.27. Adenocarcinoma arising at the ileocecal valve (arrowheads). Although a large, irregular tumor is present, there was no obstruction.

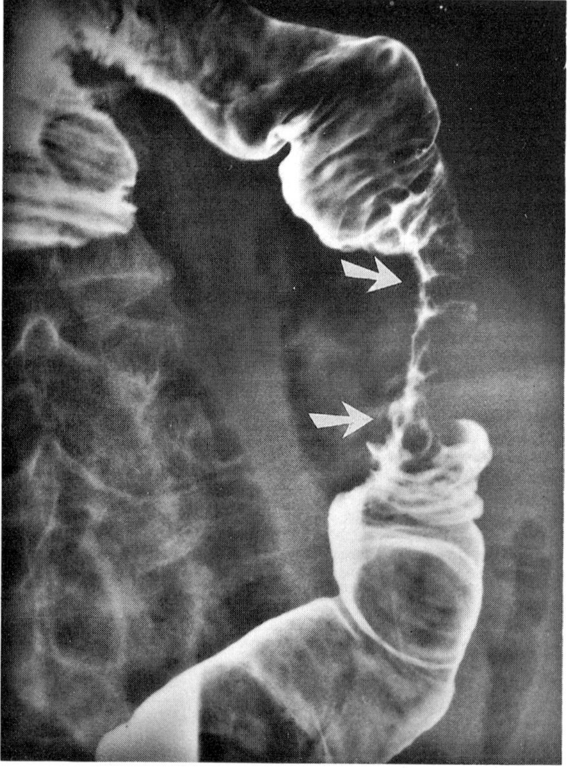

Fig. C.28. A moderately differentiated adenocarcinoma involves a long segment of the colon (arrows). The tumor had penetrated through the serosa. In spite of the long length of involvement, no obstruction was present.

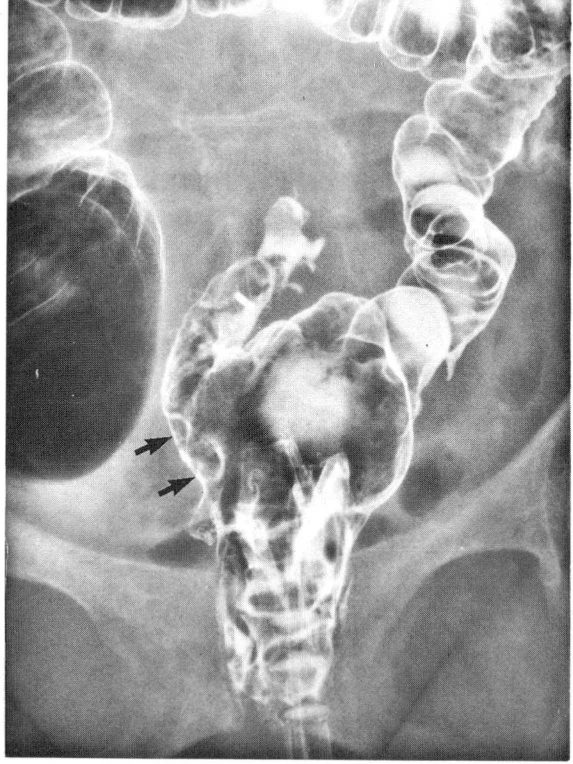

Fig. C.29. Post sigmoid resection and end-to-side anastomosis. Numerous nodules are present in the rectum (arrows), representing recurrent carcinoma.

cidental (64). In patients with longstanding ulcerative colitis such a carcinoma can be mistaken for a benign stricture (67). In general, these lesions mimic diverticulitis, serosal metastasis, and regional enteritis. Metastases to the colon from the stomach and breast, in particular, can be indistinguishable from a primary scirrhous carcinoma.

Primary squamous carcinomata of the colon are rare. Some are adenosquamous rather than purely squamous. Some of these squamous carcinomata have an association with an underlying condition, such as ulcerative colitis (68) or colon duplication (69).

d. Recurrent carcinoma

Recurrence of tumor depends considerably on the Dukes' stage of the initial tumor. When there is recurrence, approximately 60% will be local only, 15% will be local together with distal metastases, and approximately 25% will have distal metastases only (70). Rectosigmoid tumors tend to recur locally (Fig. C.29) while tumors from the remainder of the colon tend to recur at distal sites (71).

We have been impressed with the few patients seen with recurrent tumor at the anastomotic site, with involvement of other sites being more common. When there is recurrence at the anastomosis, it is difficult to differentiate surgical deformity from recurrence or inflammatory changes in the area (Fig. C.30). This is one reason why, we believe, a postoperative baseline barium enema should be obtained after partial colon resection. A baseline study helps evaluate any deformity or mass that subsequently develops (72). CT likewise is very useful in evaluating postoperative recurrence (73–75). However, because of the distortion produced by surgery and subsequent fibrosis, it is imperative to obtain baseline CT in order to aid subsequent evaluation (76). After an abdominoperoneal resection, not only tumor recurrence but also other complications, such as an abscess, are ideally suited for CT evaluation (77) (Fig. C.31).

Patients with one colon cancer are at a higher risk for developing other metachronous cancers. Thus, after cancer resection, these patients require sequential colon follow-up examinations (44).

Because the primary venous drainage from the colon is into the liver, it is not surprising that the liver is most frequently involved in distal metastases. The lungs place second in the incidence of metastases. The radiologist should realize, however, that any organ in the body can be involved (Fig. C.32).

Numerous palliative procedures have been performed on patients with recurrent or metastatic disease. Systemic chemotherapy offers little hope at present. Liver infusion chemotherapy, hepatic artery ligation, or partial hepatic resection may palliate selected patients (78). Intraoperative electron beam radiation therapy is being tried by some (79).

e. Sarcoma

Characteristically, these lesions are associated with few symptoms and are large when initially diagnosed. A mass may be palpable through the abdominal wall. When small or moderate in size, a sarcoma can be indistinguishable from a carcinoma radiographically. However, usually when seen, the tumor's large size and the few symptoms voiced by the patient should raise suspicion of the true diagnosis.

A sarcoma can either grow into the lumen and present as a polyp, or grow intramurally. Sometimes a primarily extrinsic component is present. Occasionally a sarcoma bleeds or acts as a lead point for an intussusception.

Usually it is not possible to distinguish with a barium enema between a fibrosarcoma, angiosarcoma, leiomyoma or a leiomyosarcoma. It is not unusual for a smooth muscle tumor to have a very large central ulcerated cavity and relatively small tumor mass (Fig. C.33). If multiple lesions are present, lymphoma should be considered in the differential diagnosis. If a tumor grows primarily on the serosa, no intraluminal changes may be visible. Leiomyosarcomata are very vascular tumors and angiography reveals a dense tumor stain, a well defined margin and quite often enlargement of the feeding vessels. Unfortunately, some leiomyosarcomata are hypovascular and no draining vein is identified. Angiographically, malignant lesions cannot be differentiated from benign tumors unless arterial invasion is present (80).

f. Lymphoma and leukemia

The gastrointestinal tract is the most common site of primary extranodal lymphoma. It can also be involved as part of generalized disease (81). The

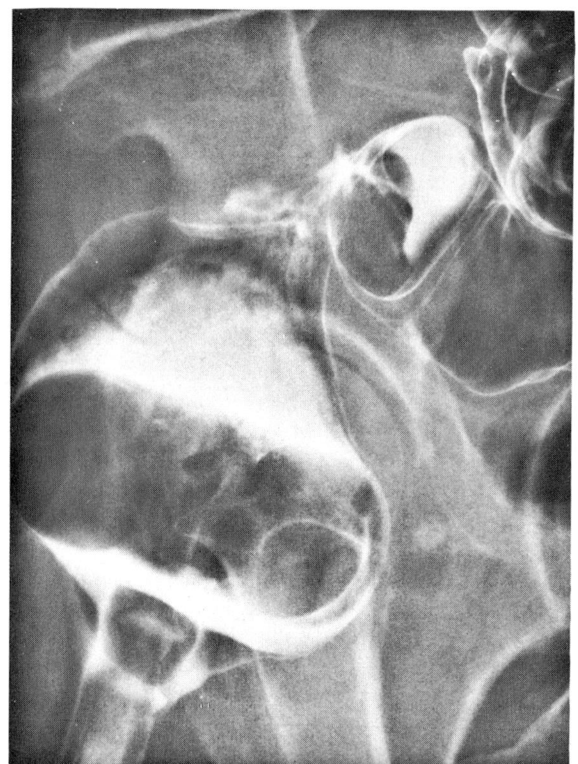

a

most common site of primary gastrointestinal lymphoma is in the stomach. The next common site is in the small bowel and least common involvement is in the colon (82). Within the colon the cecum is most frequently involved; rectal involvement comes second (83). Both adults and children are affected. Males predominate in children while the sex incidence is about equal in adults (84).

A lymphoma can grow to an exceedingly large size before significant symptoms are present (Fig. C.34). A lymphomatous mass can act as the lead point for colocolic or ileocolic intussusception.

There is poor correlation between the radiographic appearance and the histological diagnosis. The extent of lymphoma is of prognostic significance, with disseminated disease having the worst

Fig. C.30. (a) Recurrent rectal carcinoma one year after initial resection. The presacral space is wide and there is marked stenosis at the anastomotic site. (b) Recurrent carcinoma at the site of resection (arrows). The tumor is primarily intramural in location. (c) Multiple tumor nodules surround the anastomotic site (arrows). A base-line examination is very useful to exclude deformity secondary to previous surgery. (From RE Miller MD (122); copyright, Year Book Medical Publishers, 1975.)

b

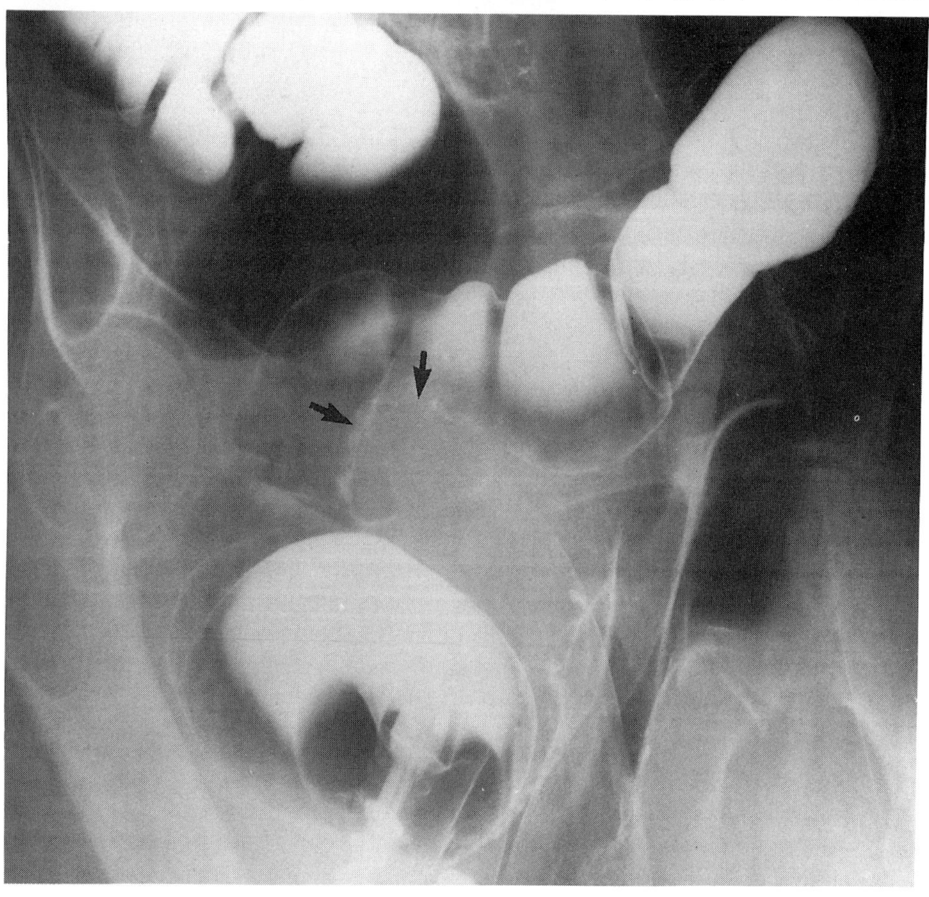

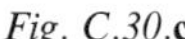

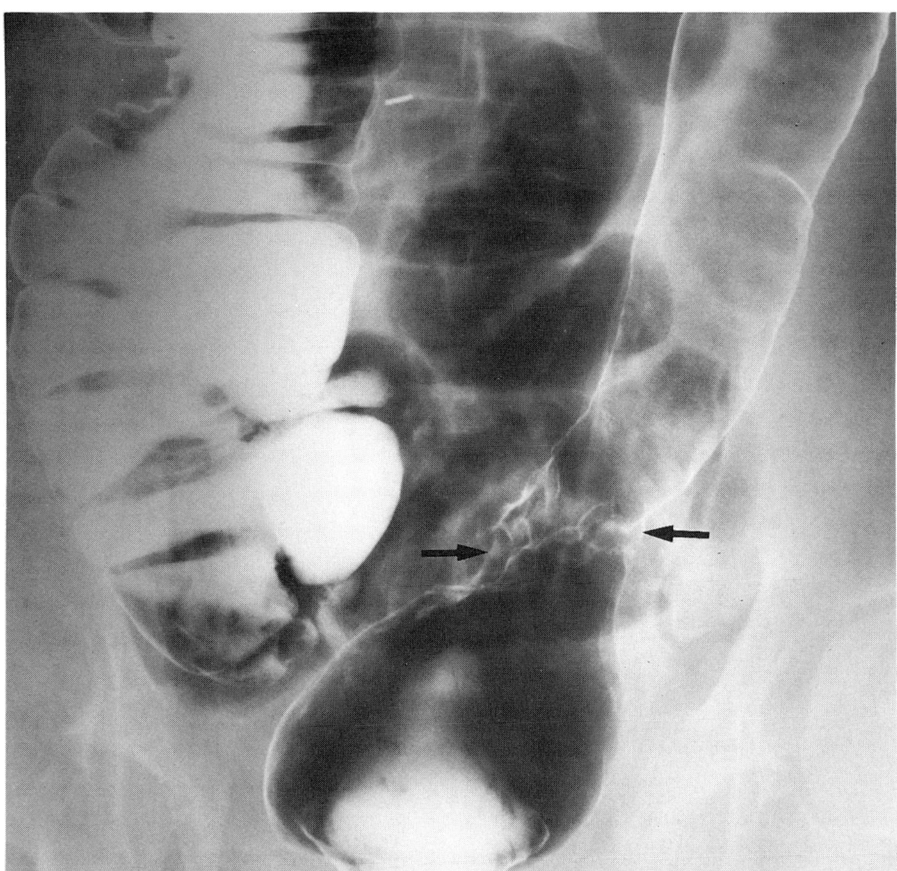

Fig. C.30.c

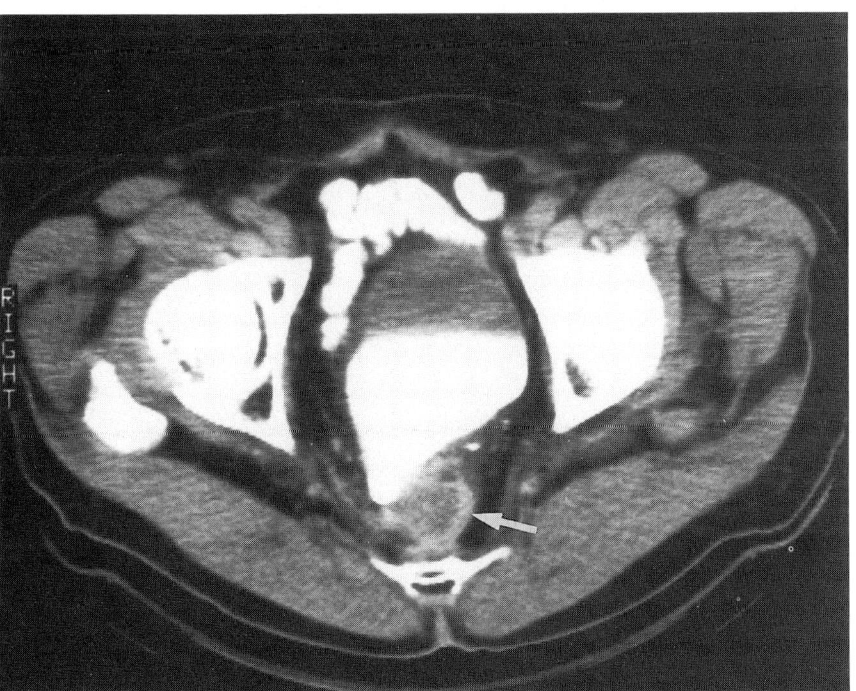

Fig. C.31. Recurrent tumor (arrow) after abdominoperoneal resection. Contrast in the bladder aids in outlining the anterior extent of the tumor.

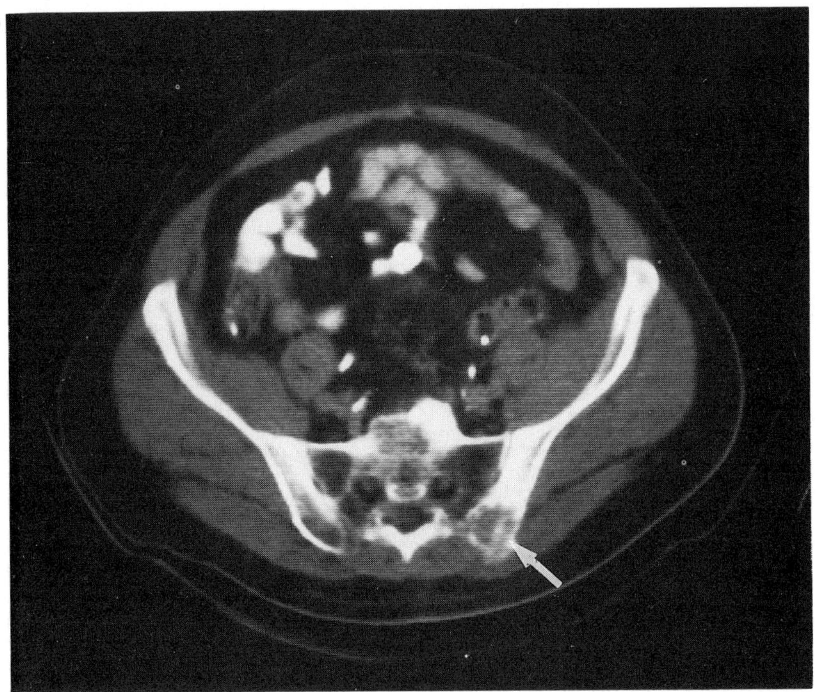

Fig. C.32. The patient had had a colon carcinoma resected one year previously and was being evaluated for recurrent symptoms. A metastasis is present in the sacrum (arrow).

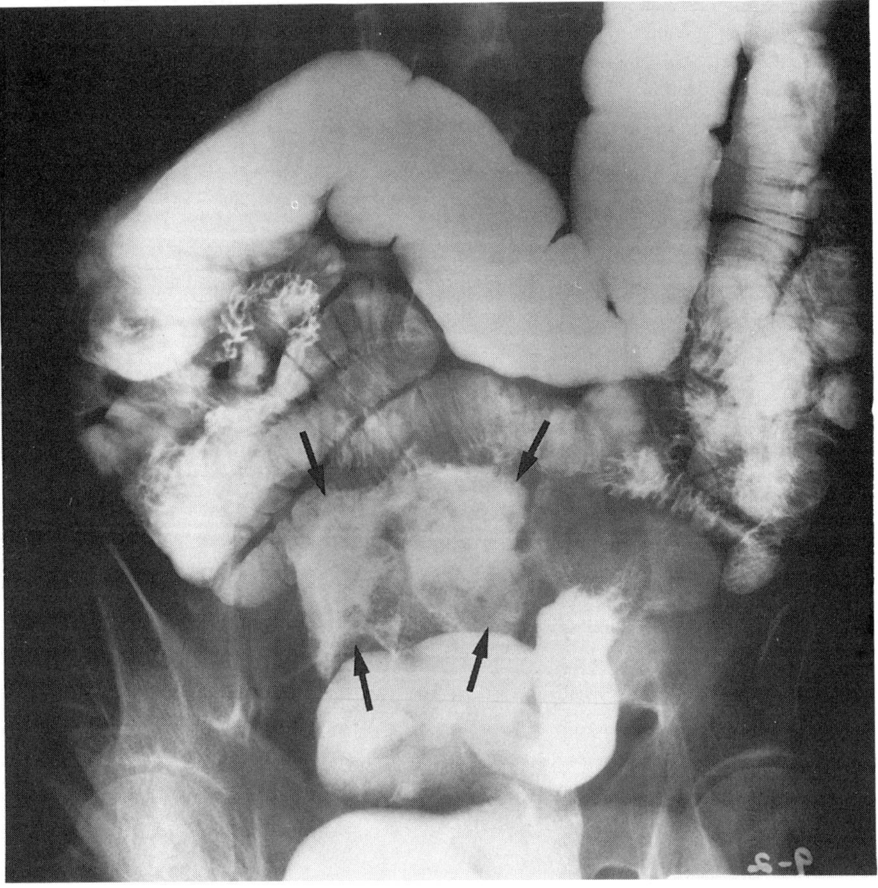

Fig. C.33. Ileal leiomyoblastoma (arrows). A reflux small bowel examination reveals a large irregular cavity in the distal ileum with little surrounding mass.

prognosis (85). The staging listed in Table C.2 is often employed in lymphoma classification.

Radiographically, colon lymphoma can show several patterns.

Table C.2. Staging of gastrointestinal lymphomas (Adapted from (121).).

Stage Ie	Gastrointestinal involvement only
Stage IIe	Gastrointestinal and regional lymph nodes only are involved
Stage III	Involvement above and below diaphragm
Stage IV	Widespread dissemination

Lymphoma occasionally mimics lymphoid hyperplasia. A common appearance is that of diffuse smooth and sessile nodules (86). These nodules can range from small polyps (Fig. C.35), to large, irregular palpable masses with extensive in-

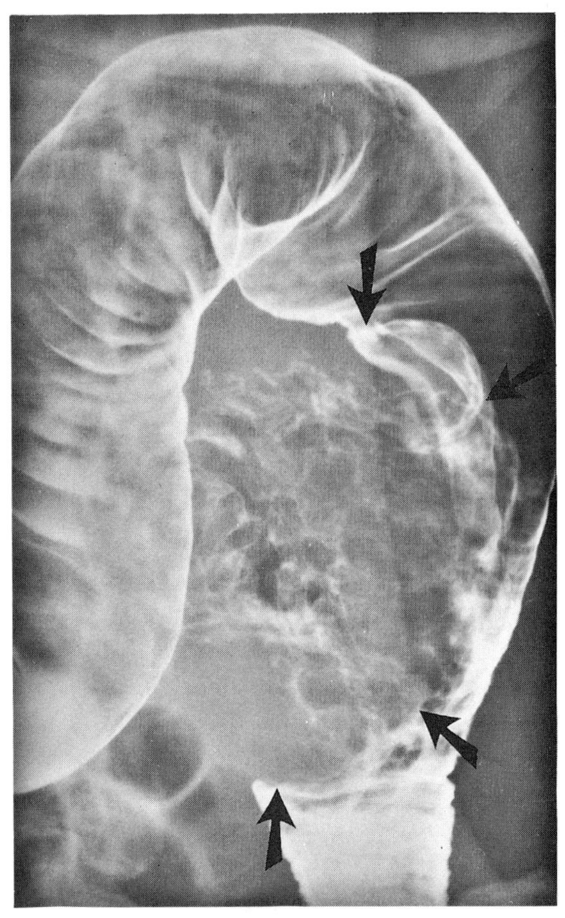

Fig. C.34. Lymphosarcoma involving the proximal descending colon. A large ulcerated mass is present (arrows). The overall appearance is similar to a leiomyosarcoma.

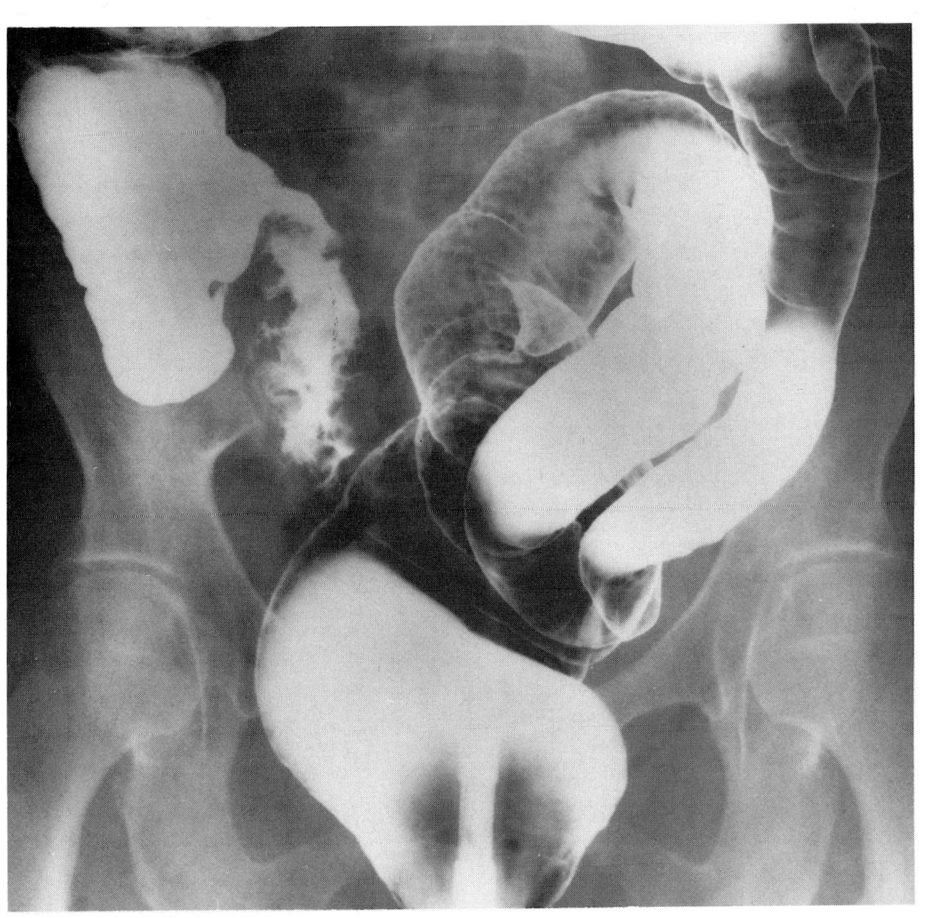

Fig. C.35. Lymphoma appearing as small polyps scattered throughout. The pattern resembled that seen with familial polyposis.

tramural infiltration (Fig. C.36). Occasionally, only a single lesion is present (Fig. C.37). Ulceration is unusual with small polyps. If there is extensive infiltration, however, ulcers or fistula can be present (Fig. C.38). An extracolic component can be apparent from associated colon or small bowel displacement (Fig. C.39). Rarely, lymphoma is completely extrinsic and located in such structures as the mesentery; it then presents simply as a soft-tissue mass displacing bowel.

Lymphoma can mimic a carcinoma or present with 'thumb-printing' suggestive of ischemia (87, 88). Pneumatosis coli can be present (83, 89). Splenomegaly is not unusual (Fig. C.40). Two children have been reported with massive ileocecal valves secondary to lymphoid infiltration (90).

While carcinoma involving an extended segment of the colon generally narrows the lumen, a diffuse lymphoma tends to widen the lumen. The exception is Hodgkin's lymphoma which can narrow the lumen.

Hodgkin's lymphoma most often involves the rectum. The tumor can present simply as rectal ulcers (91) or it can mimic adenocarcinoma (Fig. C.41). The generally known systemic disease aids in suggesting the true diagnosis.

It is not uncommon to confuse diffuse lymphoma with regional enteritis (Fig. C.42). When a long segment is involved ulcerative colitis is also in the differential diagnosis. Complicating the picture further is the increased incidence of lymphoma in long-standing ulcerative colitis (92, 93).

There are few radiological descriptions of colon plasmacytoma. These lesions can obstruct, infiltrate, ulcerate varying lengths of colon, or appear as polyps (94). They can mimic colon carcinoma or ulcerative colitis. There can be rapid progression in severity and extent of involvement, thus raising suspicion that one is not dealing with a typical carcinoma.

Most patients with leukemic infiltration of the gastrointestinal tract are relatively asymptomatic; some patient's present with massive gastrointestinal bleeding (95, 96). The colon infiltration can have a radiographic appearance of multiple polyps (97), typical carcinoma (98), or the infiltration can be diffuse. In some patients cecal distortion, or typhlitis may be present. The involvement may be

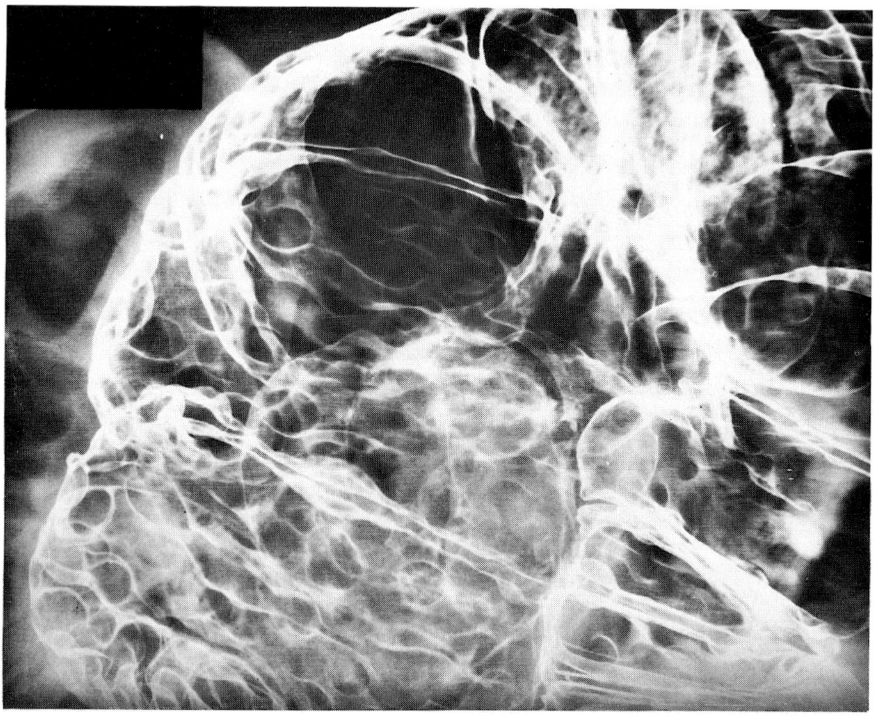

Fig. C.36. Multiple polyps of different size are scattered throughout the right colon. The polyps represented Hodgkin's lymphoma although superficially the appearance was that of familial polyposis.

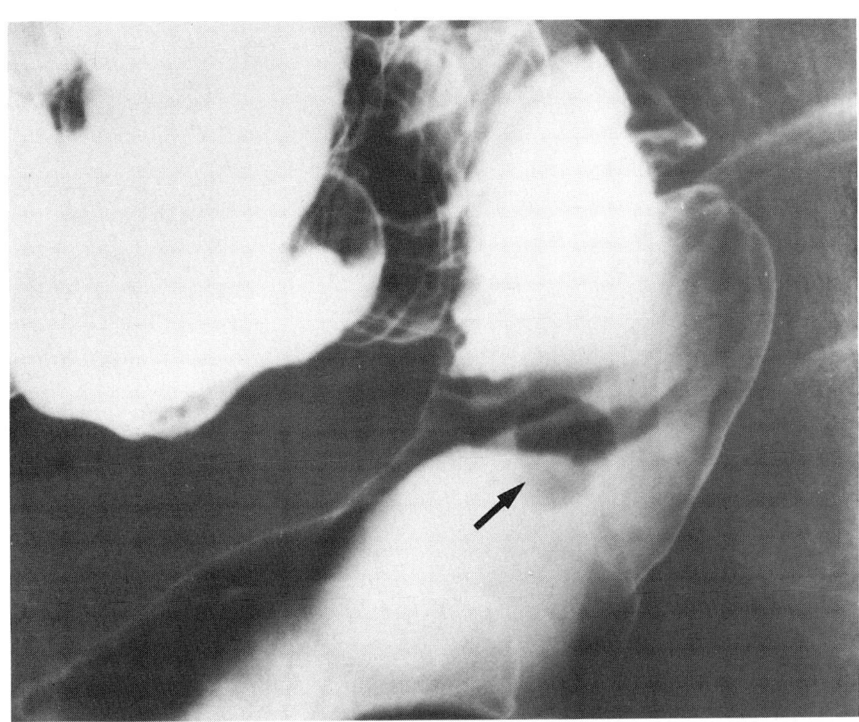

Fig. C.37. Histiocytic lymphoma involving a pedunculated polyp (arrow). The polyp was primarily adenomatous in nature.

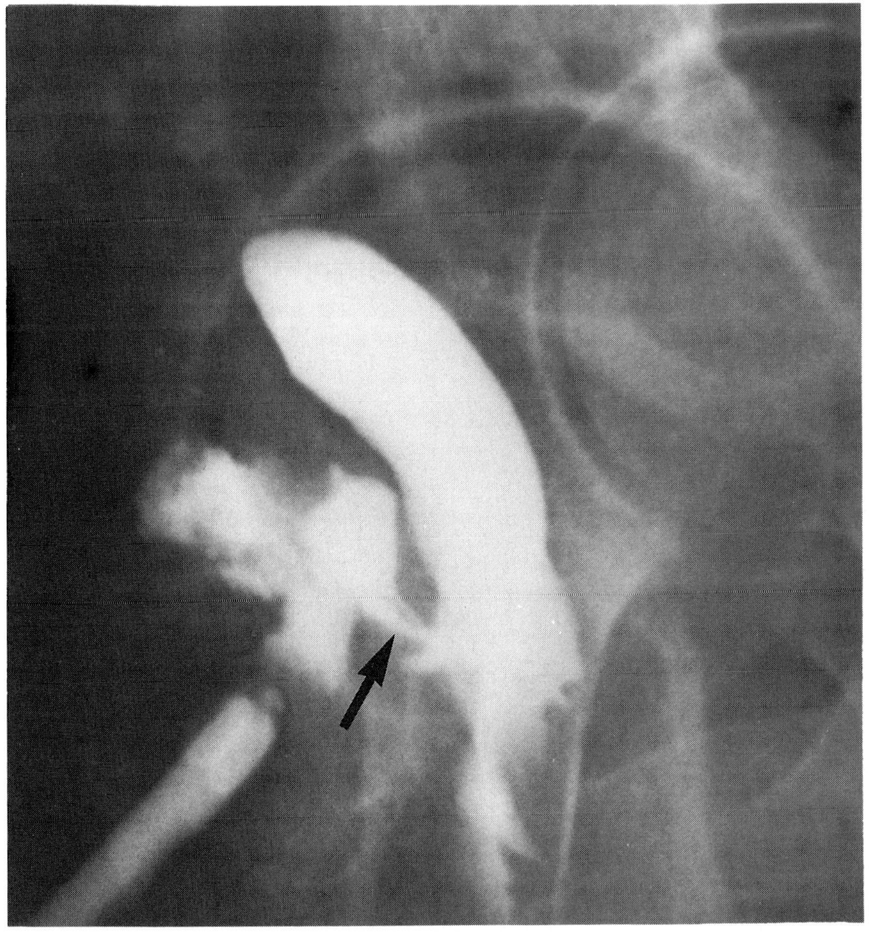

Fig. C.38. Spontaneous rectovaginal fistula (arrow). The rectum was considerably deformed and was infiltrated by a histiocytic lymphoma.

related to therapy (99), with no leukemic infiltration being identified on pathological studies and the cecum simply showing an inflammation. Such inflammatory infiltrates have been seen both in patients who are immunosuppressed and in those receiving chemotherapy (100, 101). In some patients the cecal inflammatory reaction is related to infection (99) and has been described as necrotizing enterocolitis (102). In others the cecum is involved by the leukemia or lymphoma and necrosis is secondary to ischemic changes (103). Oral vancomycin has been used to treat some of the patients with necrotizing enterocolitis (104).

The radiographic appearance of typhlitis varies. Some patients have no bowel gas in the cecum and bowel wall edema is demonstrated on a barium enema. An occasional patient will have cecal ulcers.

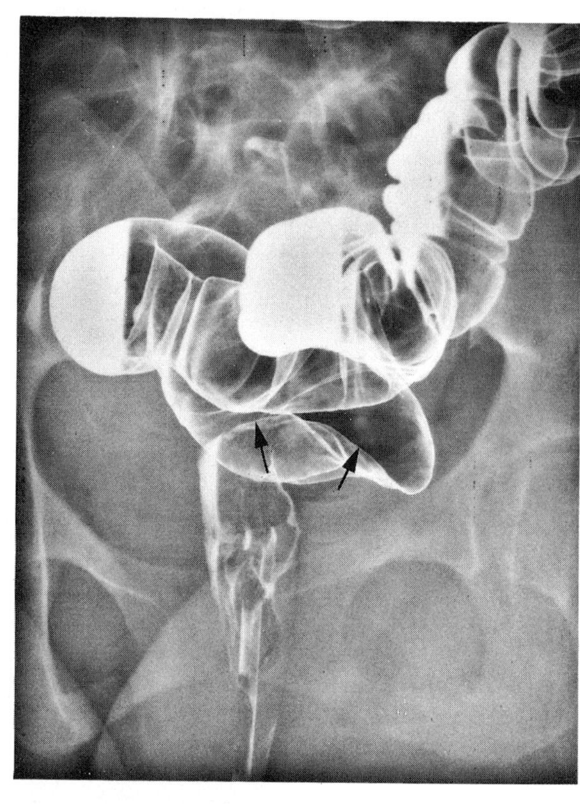

Fig. C.39. Rectal lymphoma. The extrinsic mass (arrows) has invaded and narrowed the rectum. Multiple small ulcers are present.

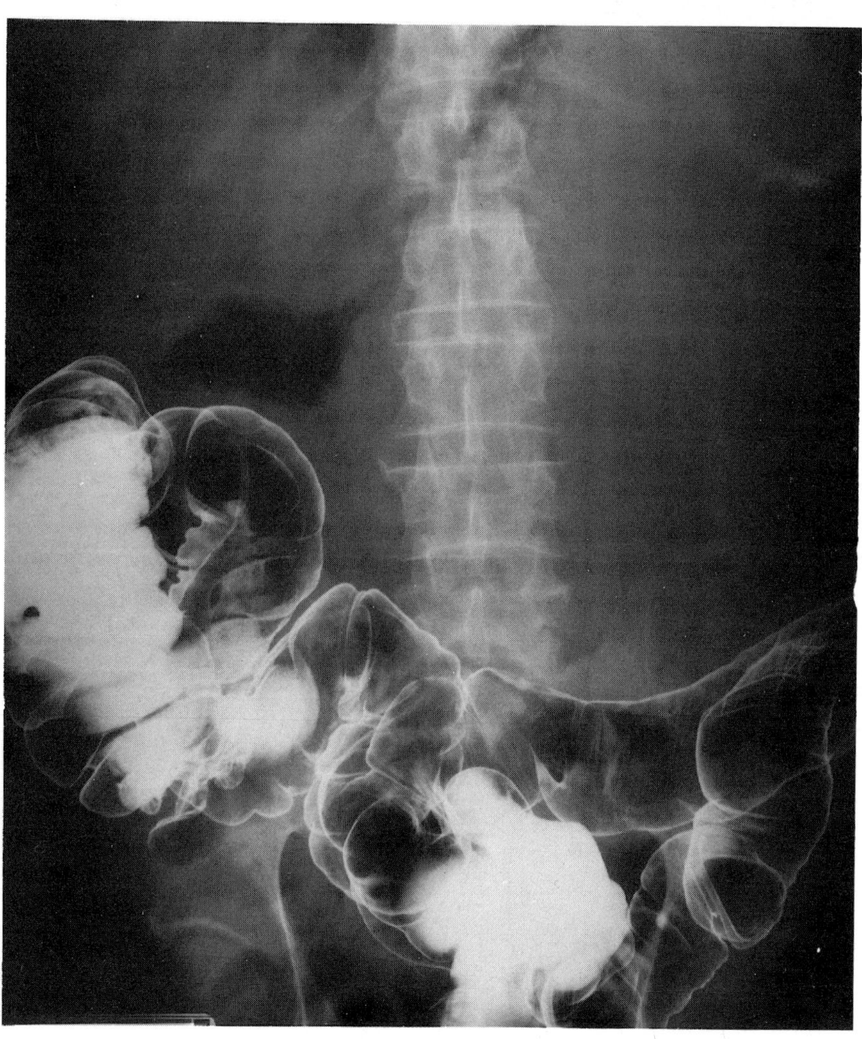

Fig. C.40. Marked splenomegaly secondary to lymphomatous involvement. The colon is displaced inferiorly.

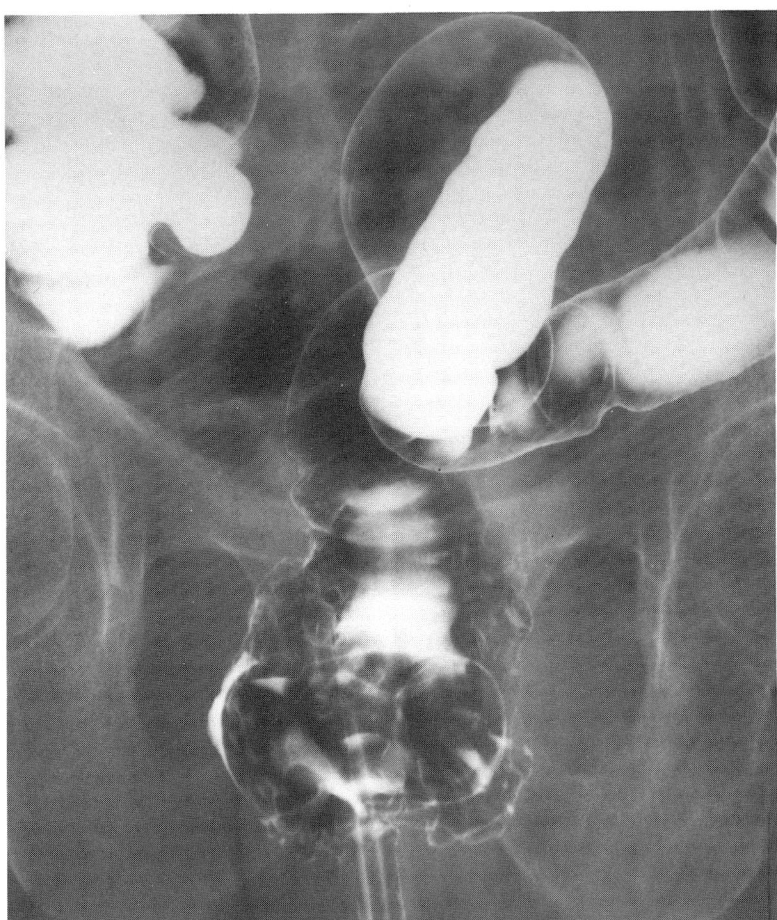

a

Fig. C.41. (a) Rectal Hodgkin's lymphoma. An ulcerated, irregular outline is present in the rectum. (b) Hodgkin's lymphoma involving the right colon (arrow). The size and irregular outline closely resembles a carcinoma or villous adenoma. (c) Cecal Hodgkin's lymphoma appearing as a large, irregular, intraluminal polyp (arrows). The appearance mimics a carcinoma.

b

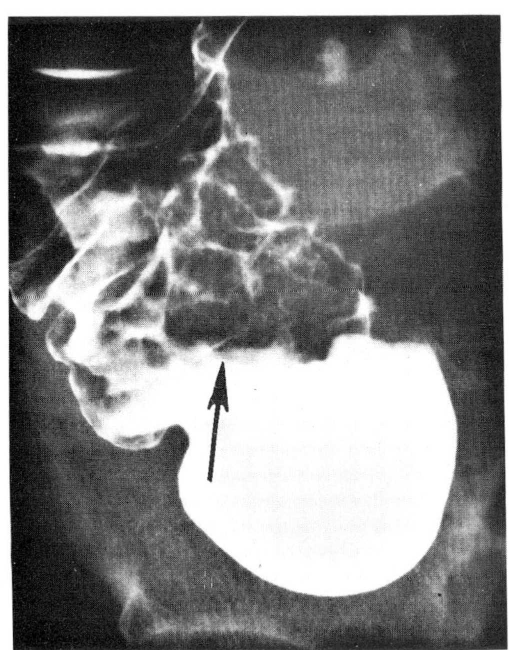

c

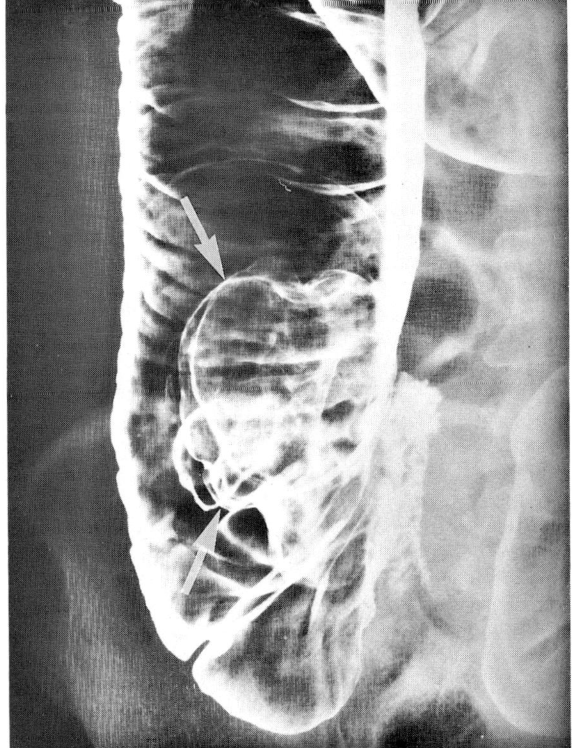

With severe involvement, the cecum becomes dilated and appears as 'toxic cecitis'. Subsequent perforation is usually fatal (105).

In childhood, the differential diagnosis includes appendicitis. Although cecal inflammation with leukemia in adults is unusual (101), the radiographic appearance is similar to that seen in cecal diverticulitis.

g. Secondary neoplasms

The colon can be involved by neoplasms in other organs by hematogenous metastases, lymphatic spread, direct invasion, or through intraperitopeal spread. Direct invasion is not necessarily from adjacent organs, because a tumor can spread along the mesentery and involve noncontiguous segments of the bowel.

Hematological tumor spread results in tumor deposition in the wall of the colon with eventual intramural growth (Fig. C.43). These nodules can be essentially the same size or can vary in size. The antimesenteric border of the colon is a common site for these deposits (106).

A common hematological metastasis to the colon is from the breast. The patients can present with symptoms suggesting one of the colitides (107, 108). If long segments of the colon are involved, it can mimic regional enteritis (109) or diffuse infiltration of the colon wall mimics linitis plastica.

Whether the tumor is initially deposited directly on the colon serosa or deposited intramurally by hematogenous spread, the tumor grows and invades adjacent layers. When the muscle is infiltrated it is usual for the colon to foreshorten, resulting in a 'corrugated' or 'accordion-like' appearance, described by some as a 'striped' colon (110) (Fig. C.44). With further growth the tumor invades all layers of the colon wall, the colon folds become

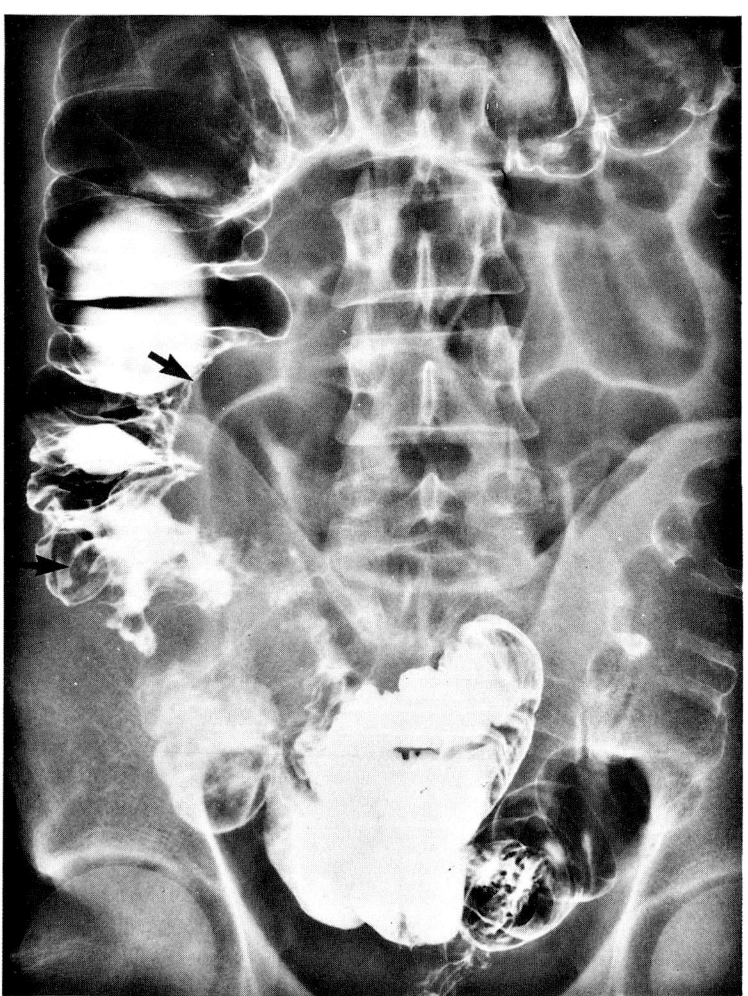

Fig. C.42. Ileocolic lymphoma. The colic involvement is asymmetrical and multiple small ulcers are scattered throughout the involved segment (arrows). The radiographic appearance is similar to that of regional enteritis.

destroyed, and irregular ulcers appear.

A metastasis can obstruct. If the fluoroscopist is not able to pass barium proximal to the lesion, the true etiology of the obstruction may not be apparent because the distal end of the obstruction can have a smooth and relatively benign appearance. Several obstructive sites can be present.

Although a single metastasis is occasionally seen, it is more common for multiple metastatic foci to be scattered throughout the small bowel and colon. The metastases can be poorly defined or sharply marginated. In particular, metastatic malignant melanoma can present as multiple colon polyps (111). Mucosal metastasis is rare. When it does occur, distinction from a primary colon cancer may not be possible unless biopsy reveals a cell type not normally found in the colon (112).

The role of lymphatics in the spread of tumor to the colon is poorly understood. Occasionally encountered is lymphatic blockage and altered pathways of lymph flow, with metastases to unusual sites.

The transverse colon is in continuity with the stomach through the gastrocolic ligament. Posteriorly, the transverse colon is attached to the pancreas through the transverse mesocolon. Thus, neoplasms from the stomach and pancreas can spread directly to the transverse colon. A gastric carcinoma spreads along the gastrocolic ligament, with these tumors typically involving that segment of the colon located between the mesocolic taenia and the omental taenia (113, 114). The colon folds throughout the involved segment become distorted yet they usually remain intact because the mucosa and submucosa are initially preserved. With extension of the tumor, the entire colon circumference becomes involved (Fig. C.45).

Pancreatic carcinoma invades the transverse colon through the transverse mesocolon and involves the mesocolic and free taenia. Typically one sees

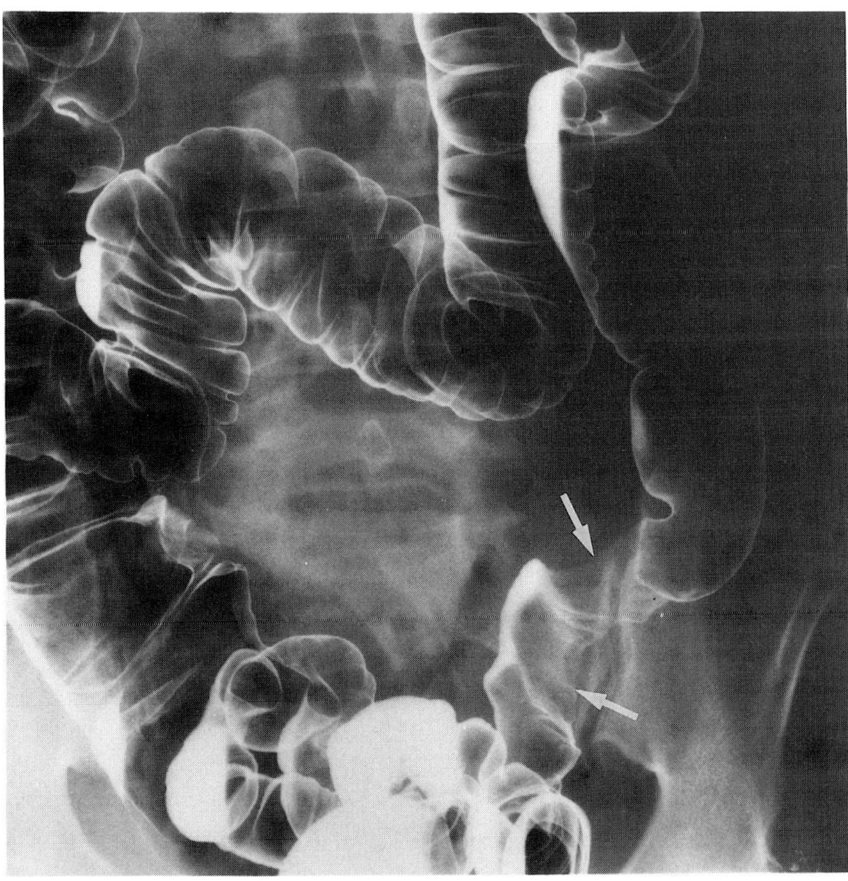

Fig. C.43. Metastatic carcinoma to the colon. Relatively long segments of the cecum and sigmoid are infiltrated (arrows). The extrinsic origin of the metastasis is readily apparent.

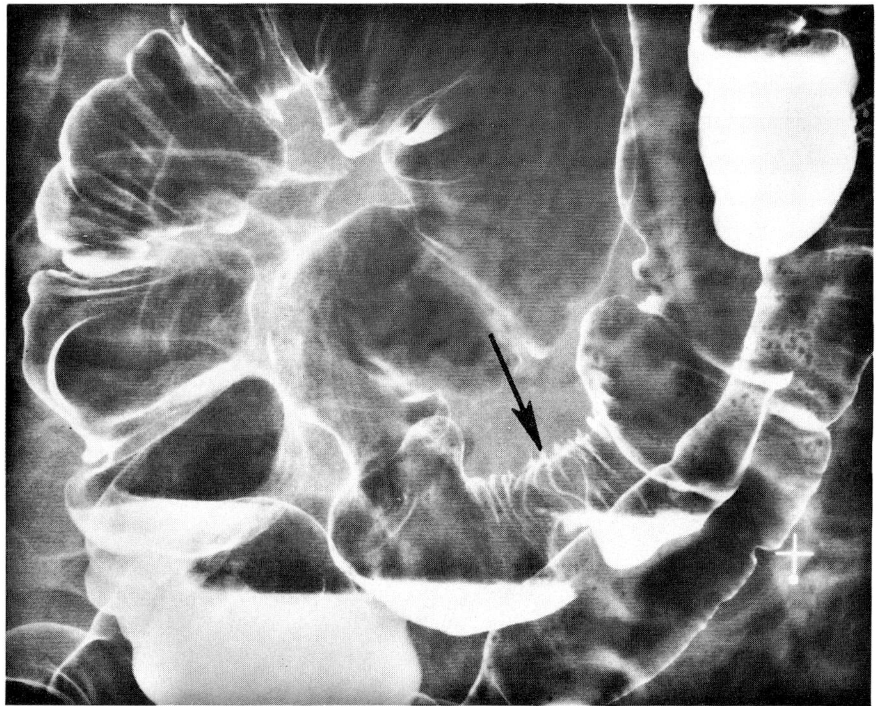

a

b

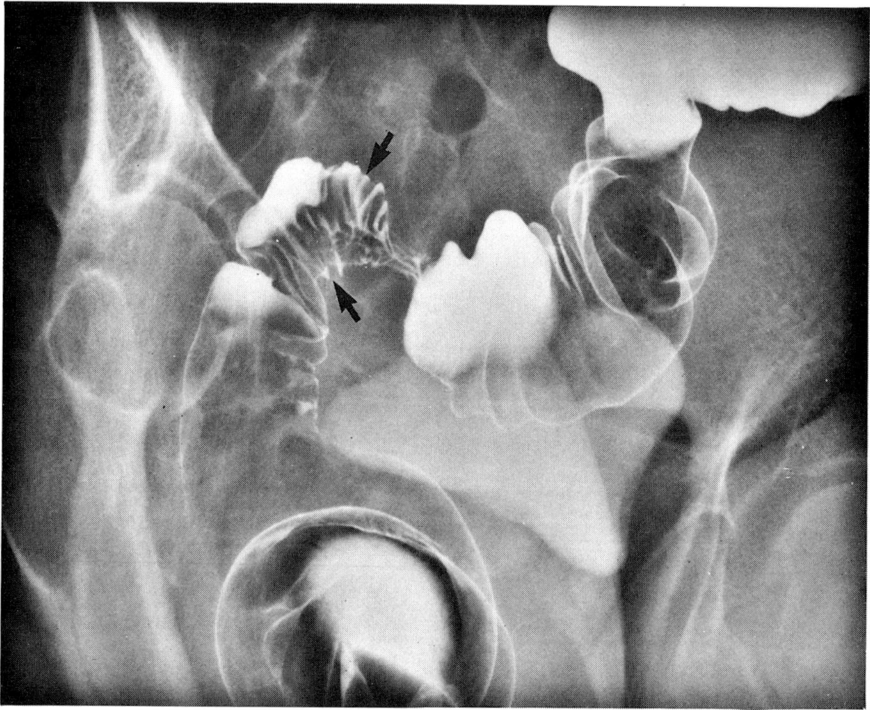

Fig. C.44. (a) Serosal metastasis resulting in a corrugated appearance (arrow). The primary source of the carcinoma was not known. (b) Metastasis to sigmoid. The corrugated appearance is more extensive (arrows) and a stricture is developing.

major involvement along the posterior and inferior aspects of the colon. As with a gastric carcinoma, with extensive pancreatic tumor invasion the entire colon circumference becomes infiltrated, even to the point of obstruction (Fig. C.46).

A tumor originating in the superior pole of the right kidney displaces the hepatic flexure both inferiorly and anteriorly. A tumor in the lower pole of the right kidney displaces the hepatic flexure superiorly. Likewise, a tumor in the upper pole of the left kidney displaces the adjacent segment of colon. Because the anatomic flexure is fixed in position by its ligamentous attachment, it is usually not displaced unless there has been gross distortion of the involved anatomy. A recurrent hypernephroma on either side can first be detected as a recurrence in the colon (106) (Fig. C.47).

It is not unusual to find a large palpable pelvic tumor when a patient first presents for examination. Malignant pelvic neoplasms can either displace the colon or invade. If the tumor only displaces the colon, the colon folds are simply distorted and fixed in their new position. With invasion, the appearance is similar to that seen with metastases; the colon becomes foreshortened and assumes a corrugated appearance (Fig. C.48). Ulcers result if the mucosa is invaded. Because invasion is generally into adjacent bowel, most pelvic malignancies invade the sigmoid and rectum. Prostatic carcinoma spreads extraperitoneally and can involve the rectum. Invasion can be limited to the anterior wall of the rectum (Fig. C.49) or it can extend circumferentially, thus widening the presacral space (Fig. C.50).

Spreading intraperitoneal tumors first involve colon serosa. Tumors in the peritoneal cavity flow with ascitic fluid (115) and tend to gravitate to the most inferior portions of the peritoneal cavity, one of which is the pouch of Douglas. The tumor presents as a shelf-like mass located just anterior to

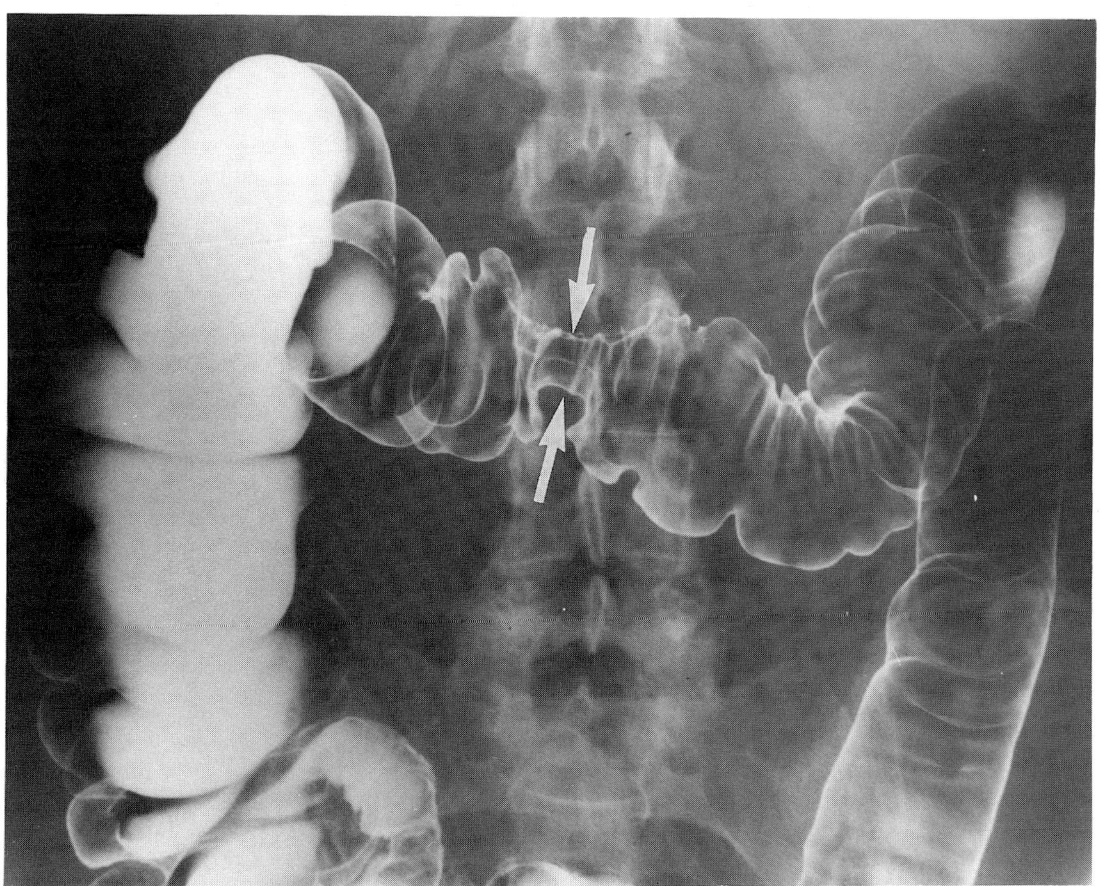

Fig. C.45. Gastric carcinoma invading the transverse colon through the gastrocolic ligament. The entire bowel circumference is involved although the lesion is eccentric (arrows).

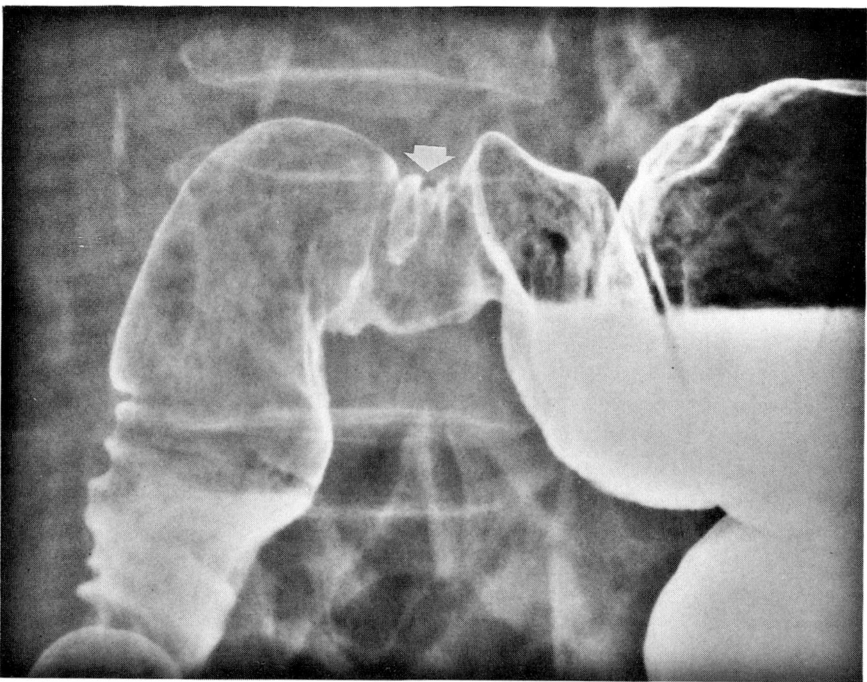

Fig. C.46. Mucin-secreting pancreatic adenocarcinoma with spread to the transverse colon. The entire circumference of the colon is involved, with a portion of the wall having an 'accordion-like' appearance (arrow).

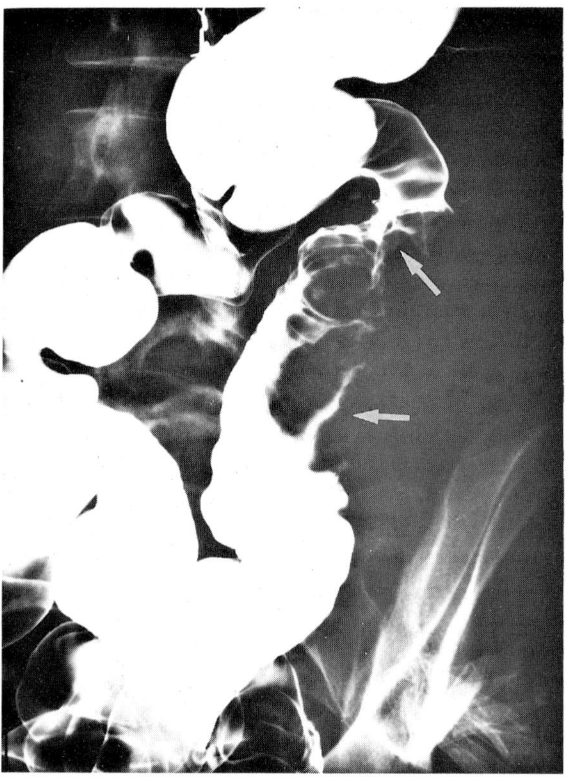

Fig. C.47. Recurrent hypernephroma invading the descending colon (arrows). A left renal hypernephroma had been resected three years previously.

the rectum. Although there were occasional case reports in the nineteenth century of tumors in the pouch of Douglas, George Blumer, in 1909, was first to publicize this finding in the English language (116, 117). He correctly emphasized that although in the vast majority of patients a rectal shelf is due to intraperitoneal tumor, occasionally peritonitis secondary to tuberculosis or other infection can result in a similar finding. Endometriosis in this location likewise will have a similar appearance. Ascites, with the patient upright, can also present with a mass in the pouch of Douglas (118). This shelf has a characteristic radiographic appearance on a lateral view of the rectum. The rectum is narrowed in caliber, with fixed distortion throughout the area of involvement (Fig. C.51).

Intraperitoneal seeding to the right lower quadrant can present with an extrinsic mass indenting the cecum. Quite often the adjacent small bowel is also involved. It may not be possible to distinguish between tumor and an inflammatory process such as appendicitis or regional enteritis. Often the patient's clinical presentation will allow one to make a definitive diagnosis.

Occasionally an ovarian dermoid tumor involves the colon. If the dermoid perforates into the peri-

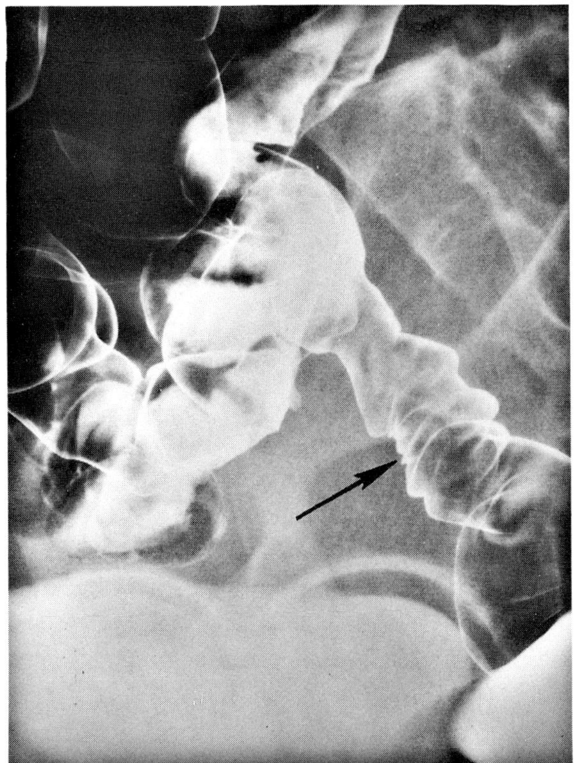

a

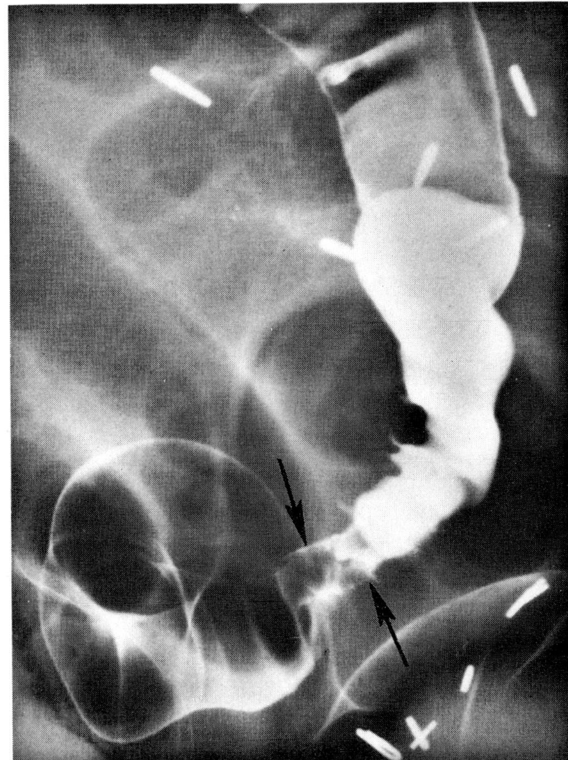

b

c

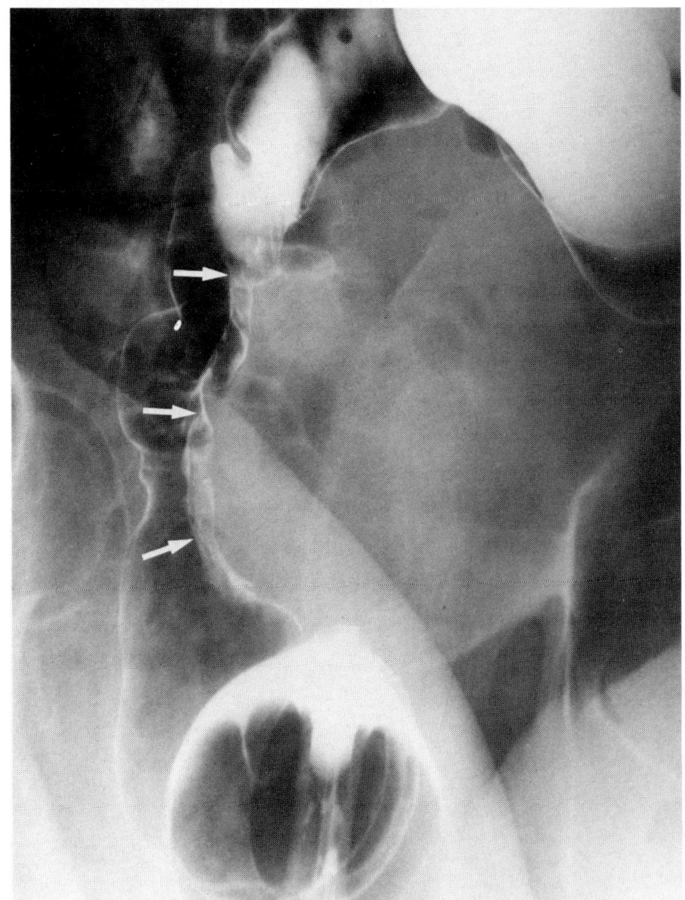

Fig. C.48. (a) Ovarian papillary cystadenocarcinoma with invasion of the anterior wall of the rectum (arrow). The corrugated appearance is typical for serosal involvement. (b) Ovarian adenocarcinoma invading the sigmoid colon (arrows). The lumen is narrowed, there is circumferential involvement and the distal tumor margin is sharply defined. (c) Ovarian papillary adenocarcinoma invading the recto-sigmoid primarily from the left side (arrows). A long segment of bowel is invaded by clearly an extrinsically originating tumor.

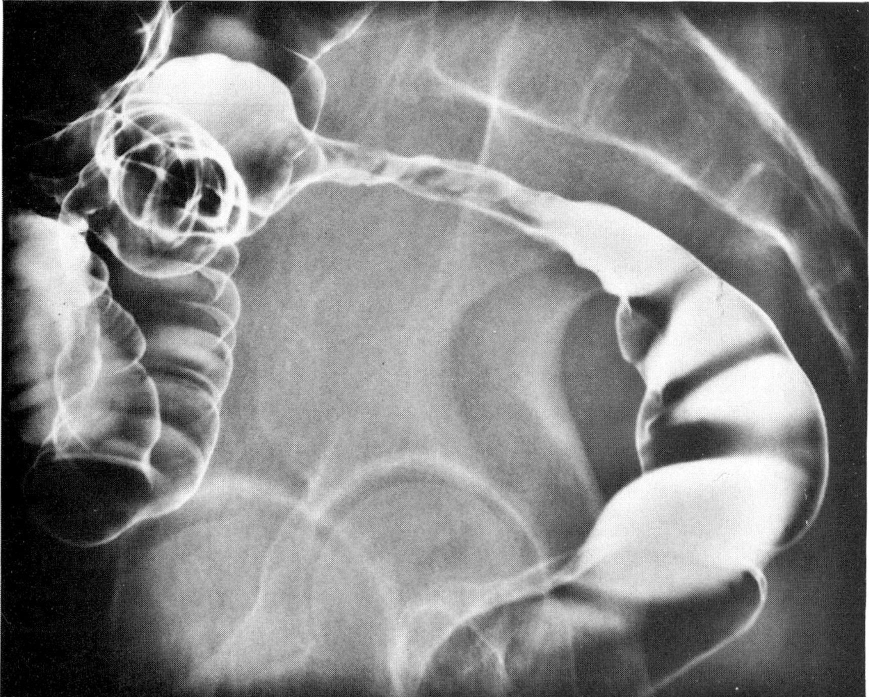

a

b

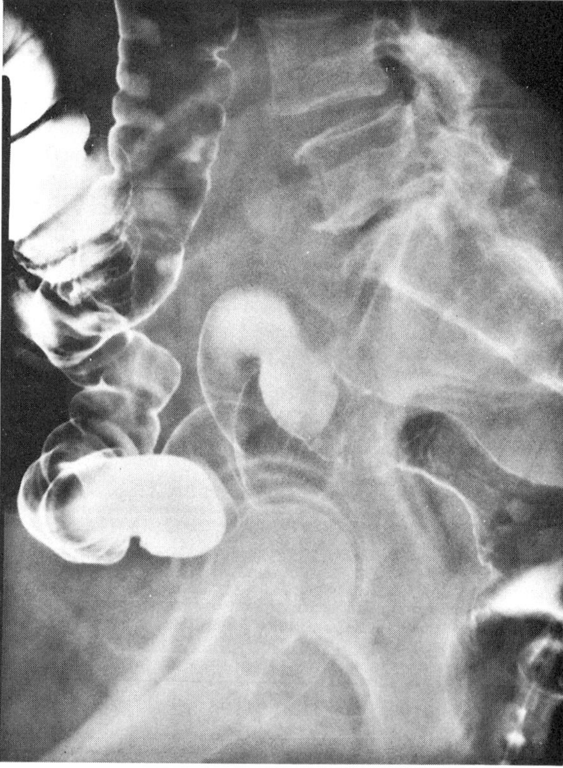

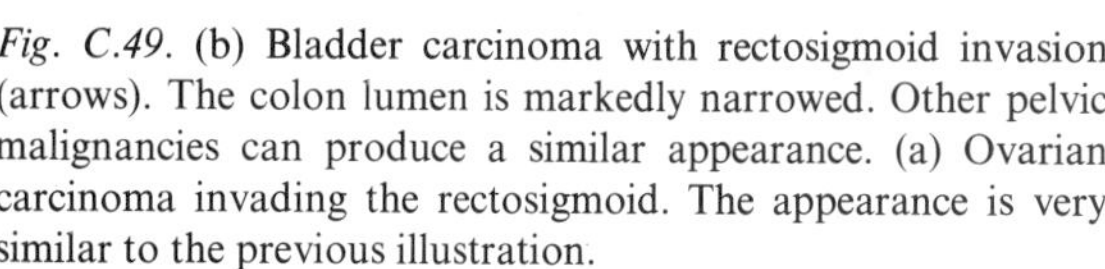

Fig. C.49. (b) Bladder carcinoma with rectosigmoid invasion (arrows). The colon lumen is markedly narrowed. Other pelvic malignancies can produce a similar appearance. (a) Ovarian carcinoma invading the rectosigmoid. The appearance is very similar to the previous illustration.

Fig. C.50. Diffuse involvement of the rectum by an infiltrating poorly-differentiated carcinoma. The rectal lumen is narrowed, numerous shallow ulcers are present, and the presacral space is widened. The origin of the primary tumor was not known.

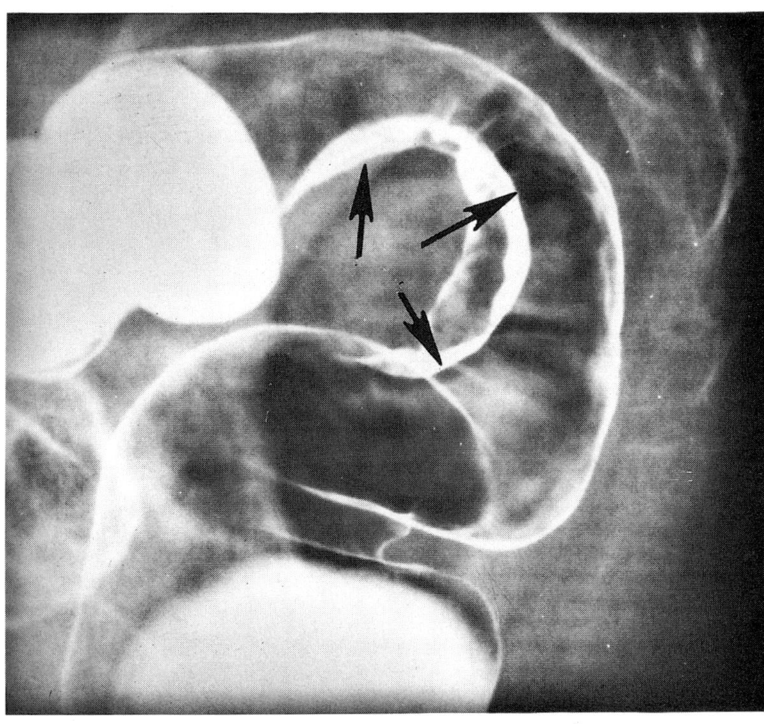

Fig. C.51. Blumer's shelf in the pouch of Douglas (arrows). The primary site for this adenocarcinoma was never determined.

toneal cavity, peritonitis can result. If the dermoid perforates into the colon, the dermoid contents extrude into the lumen (119).

References

1. Doll R: General epidemiologic considerations in etiology of colorectal cancer. In: Winawer S, Schottenfeld D, Sherlock P (eds) Colorectal Cancer: Prevention, Epidemiology, and Screening, p. 9. Raven Press, New York, 1980.
2. Kassira E, Parent L, Vahouny G: Colon cancer. An epidemiological survey. Am J Dig Dis 21:205–214, 1976.
3. Haenszel W, Berg JW, Segi M, Kurihara M, Locke FB: Large-bowel cancer in Hawaiian Japanese. J Natl Cancer Inst 51:1765–1779, 1973.
4. Ott DJ, Gelfand DW: Colorectal tumors: Pathology and detection. AJR 131:691–695, 1978.
5. Simstein NL, Kovalcik PJ, Cross GH: Colorectal carcinoma in patients less than 40 years old. Dis Colon Rectum 21:169–171, 1978.
6. Bülow S: Colorectal cancer in patients less than 40 years of age in Denmark, 1943–1967. Dis Colon Rectum 23:327–336, 1980.
7. Martin EW Jr, Joyce S, Lucas J, Clausen K, Eperman M: Colorectal carcinoma in patients less than 40 years of age: Pathology and prognosis. Dis Colon Rectum 24:25–28, 1981.
8. Silverberg E: Cancer Statistics, 1982. Ca — Cancer J Clin 32:15–31, 1982.
9. Wynder EL, Shigematsu T: Environmental factors of cancer of the colon and rectum. Cancer 20:1520–1561, 1967.
10. Rhodes JB, Holmes FF, Clark GM: Changing distribution of primary cancers in the large bowel. JAMA 238:1641–1643, 1977.
11. Snyder DN, Heston JF, Meigs JW, Flannery JT: Changes in site distribution of colorectal carcinoma in Connecticut, 1940–1973. Am J Dig Dis 22:791–797, 1977.
12. Abrams JS, Reines HD: Increasing incidence of right-sided lesions in colorectal cancer. Am J Surg 137:522–526, 1979.
13. Sooriyaarachchi GS, Johnson RO, Carbone PP: Neoplasms of the large bowel following ureterosigmoidostomy. Arch Surg 112:1174–1177, 1977.
14. Preissig RS, Barry WF Jr, Lester RG: The increased incidence of carcinoma of the colon following ureterosigmoidostomy. AJR 121:806–810, 1974.
15. Schipper H, Decter A: Carcinoma of the colon arising at ureteral implant sites despite early external diversion: pathogenetic and clinical implications. Cancer 47:2062–2065, 1981.
16. Recht KA, Belis JA, Kandzari SJ, Milam DF: Ureterosigmoidostomy followed by carcinoma of the colon. Cancer 44:1538–1542, 1979.
17. Schoenberg BS, Greenberg RA, Eisenberg H: Occurrence of certain multiple primary cancers in females. J Natl Cancer Inst 43:15–32, 1969.
18. Armstrong B, Doll R: Environmental factors and cancer incidence and mortality in different countries, with special reference to dietary practices. Int J Cancer 15:617–631, 1975.
19. Hill MJ: Colon cancer: a disease of fiber depletion or of dietary excess? Digestion 11:289–306, 1974.
20. Reddy BS: Dietary fibre and colon cancer: epidemiologic and experimental evidence. Can Med Assoc J 123:850–856, 1980.
21. Wynder EL: The epidemiology of large bowel cancer. Cancer Res 35:3388–3394, 1975.
22. Lyon JL, Klauber MR, Gardner JW, Smart CR: Cancer

incidence in Mormons and non-Mormons in Utah, 1966–1970. N Engl J Med 294:129–133, 1976.
23. Lee JAH: Recent trends of large bowel cancer in Japan compared to United States and England and Wales. Int J Epidemiol 5:187–194, 1976.
24. International Agency for Research on Cancer, Intestinal Microecology Group. Dietary fibre, transit-time, faecal bacteria, steroids, and colon cancer in two Scandinavian populations. Lancet ii:207–211, 1977.
25. Dean G, MacLennan R, McLoughlin H, Shelley E: Causes of death of blue-collar workers at a Dublin brewery, 1954–73. Br J Cancer 40:581–589, 1979.
26. Smith TR, Friedman SN, Adler H: *Streptococcus bovis* Septicemia as a clue to colon neoplasms in two cases. AJR 131:887–888, 1978.
27. Klein RS, Recco RA, Catalano MT, Edberg SC, Casey JI, Steigbigel NH: Association of *Streptococcus bovis* with carcinoma of the colon. N Engl J Med 297:800–802, 1977.
28. Marshall JB, Gerhardt DC: Polyposis coli presenting with *Streptococcus bovis* endocarditis. Am J Gastroenterol 75:314–316, 1981.
29. Schaaf RE, Jacobs N, Kelvin FM, Gallis HA, Akwari O, Thompson WM: *Clostridium septicum* infection associated with colonic carcinoma and hematologic abnormality. Radiology 137:625–627, 1980.
30. Davis WC, Jackson FC: Inguinal hernia and colon carcinoma. CA — Cancer J Clin 18:143–145, 1968.
31. Juler GL, Stemmer EA, Fullerman RW: Inguinal hernia and colorectal carcinoma. Arch Surg 104:778–780, 1972.
32. Dukes CE: The classification of cancer of the rectum. J Pathol Bacteriol 35:323–332, 1932.
33. Morson BC, Bussey HJR, Samoorian S: Policy of local excision for early cancer of the colorectum. Gut 18:1045–1050, 1977.
34. Roseman DL, Straus AK: Staging of carcinoma of the colon and rectum. Surg Gynecol Obstet 151:93–95, 1980.
35. Kurnick JE, Walley LB, Jacob HH, Nakayama L: Colorectal cancer detection in a community hospital screening program. JAMA 243:2056–2057, 1980.
36. Winawer SJ, Andrews M, Flehinger B, Sherlock P, Schottenfeld D, Miller DG: Progress report on controlled trial of fecal occult blood testing for the detection of colorectal neoplasia. Cancer 45:2959–2964, 1980.
37. Winchester DP, Shull JH, Scanlon EF, Murrell JV, Smeltzer C, Vrba P, Iden M, Streelman DH, Magpayo R, Dow JW, Sylvester J: A mass screening program for colorectal cancer using chemical testing for occult blood in the stool. Cancer 45:2955–2958, 1980.
38. Winawer SJ, Sherlock P, Schottenfeld D, Miller DG: Screening for colon cancer. Gastroenterology 70:783–789, 1976.
39. Gold P, Freedman SO: Specific carcinoembryonic antigens of the human digestive system. J Exp Med 122:467–481, 1965.
40. Thomson DMP, Krupey J, Freedman SO, Gold P: The radioimmunoassay of circulating carcinoembryonic antigen of the human digestive system. Proc Nat Acad Sci 64:161–167, 1969.
41. Green JB III, Trowbridge AA: The use of carcinoembroyonic antigen in the clinical management of colorectal cancer. Surg Clin North Am 59:831–839, 1979.
42. Moertel CG, Schutt AJ, Go VLW: Carcinoembryonic antigen test for recurrent colorectal carcinoma. Inadequacy for early detection. JAMA 239:1065–1066, 1978.
43. Wanebo HJ, Rao B, Pinsky CM, Hoffman RG, Stearns M, Schwartz MK, Oettgen HF: Preoperative carcinoembryonic antigen level as a prognostic indicator in colorectal cancer. N Engl J Med 299:448–451, 1978.
44. Bloch R, Warm K, Rosemeyer D, Weithofer G: Bedeutung der Nachsorgeuntersuchung beim Dickdarmkarzinom. Dtsch Med Wochenschr 104:1555–1559, 1979.
45. Shani A, O'Connell MJ, Moertel CG, Schutt AJ, Silvers A, Go VIW: Serial plasma carcinoembryonic antigen measurements in the management of metastatic colorectal carcinoma. Ann Intern Med 88:627–630, 1978.
46. Loewenstein MS, Zamcheck N: Carcinoembryonic antigen (CEA) levels in benign gastrointestinal disease states. Cancer 42:1412–1418, 1978.
47. Ali M, Weinstein J, Biempica L, Halpern A, Das KM: Cronkhite-Canada syndrome: report of a case with bacteriologic, immunologic, and electron microscopic studies. Gastroenterology 79:731–736, 1980.
48. Meeker WR Jr.: The use and abuse of CEA test in clinical practice. Cancer 41:854–862, 1978.
49. Gray BN, Walker C, Barnard R: Value of serial carcinoembryonic antigen determinations for early detection of recurrent cancer. Med J Aust 1:177–178, 1981.
50. Saravis CA, Oh SK, Pusztaszeri G, Doos W, Zamcheck N: Present status of the zinc glycinate marker (ZGM). Cancer 42:1621–1625, 1978.
51. Andren L, Frieberg S, Welin S: Roentgen diagnosis of small polyps in the colon and rectum. Acta Radiol 43:201–208, 1955.
52. Miller RE: Detection of colon carcinoma and the barium enema. JAMA 230:1195–1198, 1974.
53. Welin S: Modern trends in diagnostic roentgenology of the colon. Br J Radiol 31:453–464, 1958.
54. Eyler W: In: Detection of Colon Lesions, p 108. 1st Standardization Conference, 1969. American College of Radiology, Chicago, 1973.
55. Ghahremani GG, Meyers MA, Port RB: Calcified primary tumors of the gastrointestinal tract. Gastrointest Radiol 2:331–339, 1978.
56. Schwartz SS, Boley SJ: Ischemic origin of ulcerative colitis associated with potentially obstructing lesions of the colon. Radiology 102:249–252, 1972.
57. Freeman HP, Oluwole SF, Ganepola GAP: Unusual presentations of carcinoma of the right colon. Cancer 44:1533–1537, 1979.
58. Gold RP, Seaman WB: Splenic flexure carcinoma as a source of hepatic portal venous gas. Radiology 122:329–330, 1977.
59. Schabel SI, Rogers CI, Rittenberg GM: Duodeno-duodenal fistula — A manifestation of carcinoma of the colon. Gastrointest Radiol 3:15–17, 1978.
60. Skucas J, Spataro RF, Cannucciari DP: The radiographic features of small colon cancers. Radiology 143:335–340, 1982.
61. Dreyfuss JR, Benacerraf B: Saddle cancers of the colon and their progression to annular carcinomas. Radiology 129:289–293, 1978.
62. Bargen JA, Wesson HR, Jackman RJ: Studies on the ileocecal junction (ileocecus). Surg Gynecol Obstet 71:33–38, 1940.
63. Moffat RE, Gourley WK: Ileal lymphatic metastases from cecal carcinoma. Radiology 135:55–58, 1980.
64. Raskin MM: Some specific radiological findings and consideration of linitis plastica of the gastrointestinal tract. Crit Rev Clin Radiol 8:87–106, 1976-77.
65. Bonello JC, Quan SHQ, Sternberg SS: Primary linitis

plastica. of the rectum. Dis Colon Rectum 23:337–342, 1980.
66. Balthazar EJ, Rosenberg HD, Davidian MM: Primary and metastatic scirrhous carcinoma of the rectum. AJR 132:711–715, 1979.
67. Fennessey JJ, Sparberg MB, Kirsner JB: Radiological findings in carcinoma of the colon complicating chronic ulcerative colitis. Gut 9:388–397, 1968.
68. Crissman JD: Adenosquamous and squamous cell carcinoma of the colon. Am J Surg Pathol 2:47–54, 1978.
69. Hickey WF, Corson JM: Squamous cell carcinoma arising in a duplication of the colon: case report and literature review of squamous cell carcinoma of the colon and of malignancy complicating colonic duplication. Cancer 47:602–609, 1981.
70. Cass AW, Million RR, Pfaff WW: Patterns of recurrence following surgery alone for adenocarcinoma of the colon and rectum. Cancer 37:2861–2865, 1976.
71. Malcolm AW, Perencevich NP, Olson RM, Hanley JA, Chaffey JT, Wilson RE: Analysis of recurrence patterns following curative resection for carcinoma of the colon and rectum. Surg Gynecol Obstet 152:131–136, 1981.
72. Hippeli R, Schindler G, Hans U: Gestörte Heilungsvorgänge an Kolonanastomosen nach Tumorresektion. ROEFO 131:581–587, 1979.
73. Zaunbauer W, Haertel M, Fuchs WA: Computed tomography in carcinoma of the rectum. Gastrointest Radiol 6:79–84, 1981.
74. Steinbrich W, Mödder U, Rosenberger J, Friedmann G: Computertomographische Diagnostik lokaler Rezidive nach Operationen von Rektumkarzinomen. ROEFO 131:499–503, 1979.
75. Husband JE, Hodson NJ, Parsons CA: The use of computed tomography in recurrent rectal tumors. Radiology 134:677–682, 1980.
76. Grabbe E, Buurman R, Winkler R, Bücheler E, Schreiber H-W: Computertomographische Befunde nach Rektumamputation. ROEFO 131:135–139, 1979.
77. Grabbe E, Winkler R: Radiologische Diagnostik nach abdomino-perinealer Rektumamputation. ROEFO 131:127–135, 1979.
78. Williams JAR: Salvage and palliation of patiens with metastatic colorectal cancer. Med J Aust 2:143–146, 1980.
79. Cohen AM, Gunderson LL, Wood WG: Intraoperative electron beam radiation therapy boost in the treatment of recurrent rectal cancer. Dis Colon Rectum 23:453–455, 1980.
80. Uflacker R, Amaral NM, Lima S, Wholey M, Pereira EC, Nobrega M, Tavares T: Angiography in primary myomas of the alimentary tract. Radiology 139:361–369, 1981.
81. Herrmann R, Panahon AM, Barcos MP, Walsh D, Stutzman L: Gastrointestinal involvement in non-Hodgkin's Lymphoma. Cancer 46:215–222, 1980.
82. Contreary K, Nance FC, Becker WF: Primary lymphoma of the gastrointestinal tract. Ann Surg 191:593–598, 1980.
83. O'Connell DJ, Thompson AJ: Lymphoma of the colon: the spectrum of radiologic changes. Gastrointest Radiol 2:377–385, 1978.
84. Bush RS: Primary lymphoma of the gastrointestinal tract. JAMA 228:1291–1295, 1974.
85. Lewin KJ, Ranchod M, Dorfman RF: Lymphomas of the gastrointestinal tract. Cancer 42:693–707, 1978.
86. Weyman PJ, Koehler RE: Diffuse colonic modularity and splenomegaly. Invest Radiol 15:2–5, 1980.
87. Harned RK, Sorrell MF: Hodgkin's disease of the rectum. Radiology 120:319–320, 1976.
88. Perry PM, Cross RM, Morson BC: Primary malignant lymphoma of the rectum (22 cases). Proc Roy Soc Med 65:72, 1972.
89. O'Connell DJ, Thompson AJ: Pneumatosis coli in non-Hodgkins lymphoma. Br J Radiol 51:203–205, 1978.
90. Selke AC Jr, Jona JZ, Belin RP: Massive enlargement of the ileocecal valve due to lymphoid hyperplasia. AJR 127:518–520, 1976.
91. Shapiro HA: Primary Hodgkin's disease of the rectum. Arch Intern Med 107:270–273, 1961.
92. Renton P, Blackshaw AJ: Colonic lymphoma complicating ulcerative colitis. Br J Surg 63:542–545, 1976.
93. Wagonfeld JB, Platz CE, Fishman FL, Sibley RK, Kirsner JB: Multicentric colonic lymphoma complicating ulcerative colitis. Am J Dig Dis 22:502–508, 1977.
94. Rao KG, Yaghmai I: Plasmacytoma of the large bowel: A review of the literature and a case report of multiple myeloma involving the rectosigmoid. Gastrointest Radiol 3:225–228, 1978.
95. Wolma FJ, Lynch JB: Leukemic infiltration of colon. An unusual cause for massive melena. Arch Surg 78:71–74, 1959.
96. Prolla JC, Kirsner JB: The gastrointestinal lesions and complications of the leukemias. Ann Intern Med 61:1084–1103, 1964.
97. Rabin MS, Bledin AG, Lewis D: Polypoid leukemic infiltration of the large bowel. AJR 131:723–724, 1978.
98. Javett SL, Tefft M, Drummond CP, Levitan R: Leukemic infiltration of the sigmoid colon. Report of a case simulating carcinoma with obstruction. Am J Dig Dis 8: 299–304, 1963.
99. Wagner ML, Rosenberg HS, Fernbach DJ, Singleton EB: Typhlitis: a complication of leukemia in childhood. AJR 109:341–350, 1970.
100. Cronin TG, Calandra JD, Del Fava RL: Typhlitis presenting as toxic cecitis. Radiology 138:29–30, 1981.
101. Del Fava RL, Cronin TG Jr: Typhlitis complicating leukemia in an adult: barium enema findings. AJR 129:347–348, 1977.
102. Archibald RB, Nelson JA: Necrotizing enterocolitis in acute leukemia: radiographic findings. Gastrointest Radiol 3:63–65, 1978.
103. O'Connell TX, Kadell B, Tompkins RK: Ischemia of the colon. Surg Gynecol Obstet 142:337–342, 1976.
104. Freeman HJ, Rabeneck L, Owen D: Survival after necrotizing enterocolitis of leukemia treated with oral vancomycin. Gastroenterology 81:791–794, 1981.
105. Varki AP, Armitage JO, Feagler JR: Typhlitis in acute leukemia: succesful treatment by early surgical intervention. Cancer 43:695–697, 1979.
106. Meyers MA, McSweeney J: Secondary neoplasms of the bowel. Radiology 105:1–11, 1972.
107. Meyers MA, Oliphant M, Teixidor H, Weiser P: Metastatic carcinoma simulating inflammatory colitis. AJR 123:74–83, 1975.
108. Chang SF, Burrell MI, Brand MH, Garsten JJ: The protean gastrointestinal manifestations of metastatic breast carcinoma. Radiology 126:611–617, 1978.
109. Lammer J, Dirschmid K, Hugel H: Carcinomatous metastases to the colon simulating Crohn's disease. Gastrointest Radiol 6:89–91, 1981.
110. Ginaldi S, Lindell MM Jr, Zornoza J: The striped colon: a new radiographic observation in metastatic serosal implants. AJR 134:453–455, 1980.

111. Sacks BA, Joffe N, Antonioli DA: Metastatic melanoma presenting clinically as multiple colonic polyps. AJR 129:511–513, 1977.
112. Khan AQ, Griffin JW, Tedesco FJ: Squamous cell carcinoma of the ascending colon. Am J Gastroenterol 72:565–567, 1979.
113. Meyers MA, Volberg F, Katzen B, Abbott G: Haustral anatomy and pathology: a new look. I. Roentgen identification of normal pattern and relationships. Radiology 108:497–504, 1973.
114. Meyers MA, Volberg F, Katzen B, Abbott G: Haustal anatomy and pathology: a new look. II. Roentgen interpretation of pathologic alterations. Radiology 108:505–512, 1973.
115. Meyers MA: Distribution of intra-abdominal malignant seeding: Dependency on dynamics of flow of ascitic fluid. AJR 119:198–206, 1973.
116. Blumer G: The rectal shelf: a neglected rectal sign of value in the diagnosis and prognosis of obscure malignant and inflammatory disease within the abdomen. Albany Med Ann 30:361–366, 1909.
117. Corman ML: Classic articles in colonic and rectal surgery. Dis Colon Rectum 23:445–448, 1980.
118. Schulman A, Fataar S: Extrinsic stretching, narrowing and anterior indentation of the rectosigmoid junction. Clin Radiol 30:463–469, 1979.
119. Goldenberg NJ: Dermoid perforation of the colon. Gastrointest Radiol 3:221–222, 1978.
120. Fraumeni JF Jr, Mulvihill JJ: Who is at risk of colorectal cancer? In: Schottenfeld D (ed) Cancer Epidemiology and Prevention, p 404. CC Thomas, Springfield, IL, 1975.
121. Brady LW: Malignant lymphoma of the gastrointestinal tract. Radiology 137:291–298, 1980.
122. Miller RE: Examination of the colon. Curr Probl Radiol 5:2–40, 1975.

III.4. MISCELLANEOUS LESIONS

III.4.A. Appendiceal lesions

a. Introduction

In herbivorous animals the appendix helps in the digestion of fibrous substances such as cellulose. In humans, however, the vermiform appendix is a structure without any significant function, yet considerable morbidity and mortality is associated with this essentially useless structure. Especially in the pediatric age group, inflammation and resultant appendicitis are by far of greatest importance in diseases involving the appendix. In the adult population, appendicitis tends to present in an atypical fashion and mimics other intraabdominal inflammatory diseases and in these patients the radiologist plays a vital role in the differential diagnosis.

The appendix can be the site of such essentially incidental findings as diverticulae. Most of these are acquired, although a congenital diverticulum is occasionally encountered (1). Or, the appendix can harbor life-threatening neoplasms. The appendix can also be the site of a curious entity known as a mucocele, a condition which is also found in some gynecological organs. Rarely, unusual diseases can involve the appendix. As an example, Whipple's disease has been reported in the appendix (2).

Agenesis of the appendix is rare (1, 3, 4). Even rarer are duplications (1, 5) and abnormal insertions of the appendix (6).

b. Appendicitis

Although earlier appendectomies probably had been performed, the first described successful appendectomy, performed inadvertently during a scrotal hernia repair, was in 1735 (7). There was considerable discussion over the subsequent years as to whether right lower quadrant inflammation is due primarily to disease in the appendix or disease in the cecum. It was not until 1886 that Dr. Reginald Fitz finally showed convincingly that the inflammation originates in the appendix and not in the cecum (8).

Appendicitis is a relatively common disease, with the peak incidence being in the second decade. Some believe that the overall incidence of appendicitis is decreasing (9). It is rare in the very young; unfortunately, it is not rare and is quite often misdiagnosed in the elderly. Elderly patients, in particular, may first present with generalized peritonitis and secondary paralytic ileus.

The typical young patient has an appropriate history and physical findings, making clinical diagnosis relatively simple. Most of these patients do not require radiological examination. The overall preoperative diagnostic accuracy rate, however, is only approximately 70% (10).

Obstruction with subsequent infection and inflammation is a major factor in the pathogenesis of appendicitis. A calculus commonly serves as the nidus of obstruction. Rarely, a swallowed foreign body acts as the nidus (1, 11) (Fig. A.1). The incidence of appendicitis is independent of the length and position of the appendix (12). Occasionally an unusual organism may produce appendicitis; as an example, in some endemic areas amebic appendicitis is seen (13).

Although over the years there have been intermittent reports that retained barium in the appendix can be associated with appendicitis (14–17), we have personally not encountered this condition. The few reports of barium appendicitis suggest that this entity is rare if it exists at all. Little, if any, relationship exists between prolonged barium retention in an appendix and future acute appendicitis (18). A normal appendix can expel barium over a variable period of time. Occasionally barium can coat an appendiceal calculus making it more readily seen on radiographs. If the patient subsequently develops appendicitis, it is tempting to ascribe the pathogenesis of appendicitis to the retained barium.

Considerable controversy exists as to whether recurrent appendicitis is a real entity or not. An occasional patient with recurrent right lower quadrant pain will subsequently be shown to have a chronically inflamed appendix. After appendectomy, some of these patients continue to have pain and thus some other disease must be implicated. Others are free of symptoms after the appendectomy. In some of the latter patients, the appendix had filled readily during a barium enema (19), and thus appendicitis without appendiceal obstruction must be postulated.

If radiographic examination is necessary, the initial study should be an acute abdominal examination. The radiographic findings vary considerably, depending upon the stage of the disease. Many patients, especially children seen early in the course of the disease, have normal radiographic examinations.

The most important radiographic finding of appendicitis is a calculus within the appendix (Fig. A.2). In patients with appendicitis the reported incidence of appendiceal calculi has ranged from a few percent to almost one-third, with 22% seen in children being typical (20). These calculi generally contain fat derivatives, inorganic material such as calcium phosphate, and organic residue. The calculus can be small or large, or there can be multiple calculi (Fig. A.3). Lamination of the calculus is not unusual. The ability to see a calculus radiographically will obviously depend upon the amount of calcium present and the quality of the radiographic technique used. Radiographs of resected specimens reveal some calcium in approximately one-third of these patients.

Of interest is the asymptomatic patient with an incidentally seen appendiceal calculus. Some believe that a calculus in the appendix will eventually result in acute appendicitis in most patients (21). An appendiceal calculus is also associated with a higher incidence of complications during an acute attack of appendicitis. Because patients with calculi are at a relatively large risk for the subsequent development of acute appendicitis, together with increased

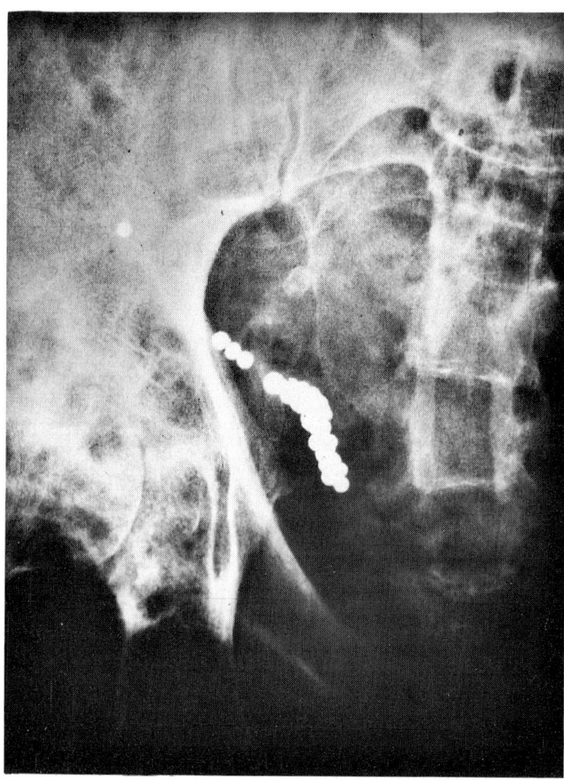

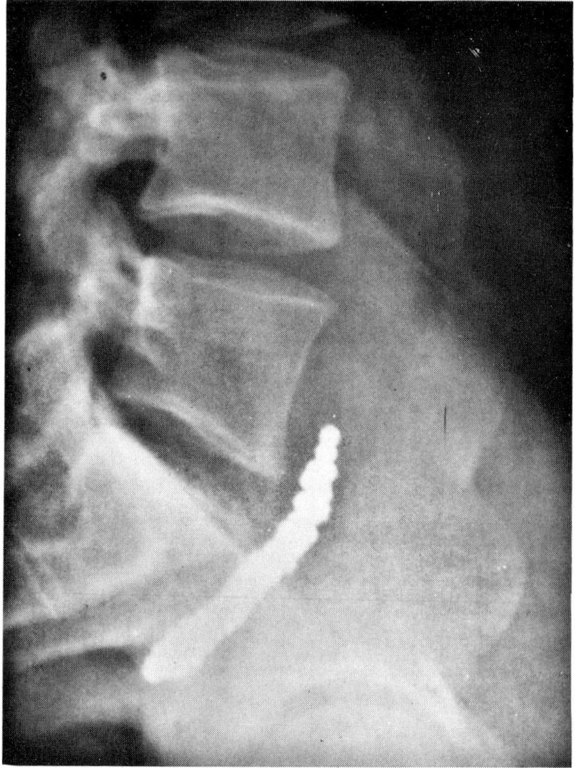

b

Fig. A.1. Lead shot appendicitis. (a) Frontal and (b) lateral radiographs reveal numerous round lead shot aligned in the patient's appendix. (Courtesy of Dr. Klas Mare, Gothenburg.)

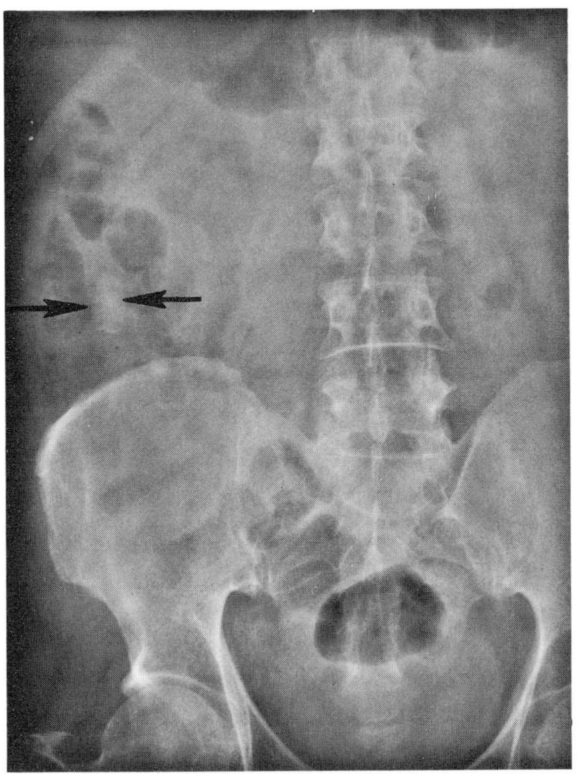

Fig. A.2. Large calculus (arrows) in a retrocecal appendix. The right psoas outline is poorly defined. No lumbar scoliosis is present. The patient presented with clinical signs of appendicitis. Surgery revealed a periappendiceal abscess.

complications during the acute attack, some have argued for a prophylactic appendectomy. Such an approach, however, remains controversial and many physicians advocate watchful waiting.

A recently described sign of appendicitis with perforation is dilation of the transverse colon and collapse of the cecum and ascending colon (22). It is postulated that the transverse colon dilation is because of adynamic ileus and collapse of the right side of the colon results from spasm. Presumably dilation of the right colon occurs later in the disease.

Less than one-half of all patients with acute appendicitis have an air-fluid level in the cecum. Also, somewhat less than one-half have an air-fluid level in a dilated distal ileum. Although it is more common to see either one or the other sign, some patients will have both. Unfortunately, both signs are nonspecific and can be seen not only with other diseases, but occasionally also in normal individuals (20). With appendicitis these signs usually represent localized adynamic ileus. The small bowel can also be dilated because of obstruction by a periappendiceal abscess. A not unusual picture is dilation of the cecum because of adynamic ileus and dilation of the ileum because of both adynamic ileus

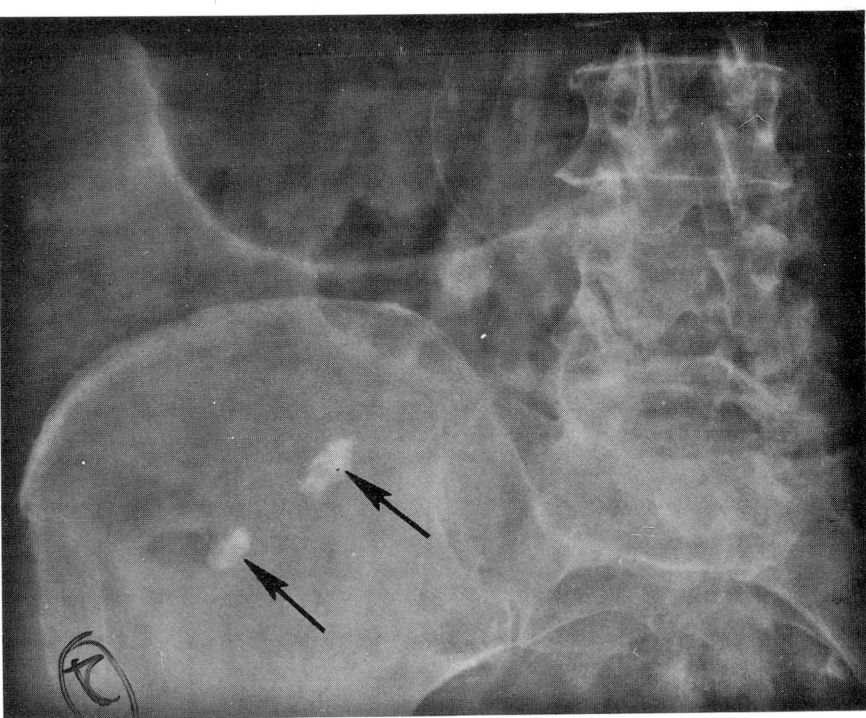

Fig. A.3. 78-year-old female with two calculi in the appendix (arrows). She presented with appendicitis.

and superimposed mechanical ileus.

Approximately one-third of patients with appendicitis have a lumbar scoliosis, with the convexity to the left. There is obliteration of the inferior aspect of the right psoas outline, loss of the right obturator muscle outline, or obliteration of the right peritoneal fat stripe. Considerable variation in the amount of extraperitoneal fat can be seen in different individuals and occasionally there is obliteration of these outlines in normal patients. Usually, however, both sides tend to be symmetrical and asymmetrical loss of a portion of the right flank stripe should be viewed with suspicion.

Pneumoperitoneum is rare in acute appendicitis (23), because the perforation is usually in the obstructed segment of the appendix, which contains little gas. Also, the inflammatory reaction together with adhesions tend to limit and localize the perforation to the right lower quadrant. Such localized perforations appear more frequent in young children. A perforation can progress to an abscess, followed by secondary peritoneal irritation and generalized paralytic ileus. A mottled appearance or a mass displacing bowel should be viewed with suspicion for an abscess. The abscess is usually in the right lower quadrant but it can be anywhere in the abdomen because of the considerable variability in the location of the appendix. The cecum can be displaced medially by a soft tissue mass lying between the peritoneal fat stripe and the lateral wall of the cecum (24). This sign is probably seen only with advanced disease. A perforated retrocecal appendix can lead to a subhepatic abscess (25). Rarely, a right subphrenic abscess develops and associated changes are present in the right lung base. An abscess can occasionally persist even after appendectomy; eventual drainage into an adjacent organ can lead to spontaneous resolution.

Gas in the appendix has been reported as a sign of appendicitis (26). Unfortunately, gas can be seen in the appendix even in normal and asymptomatic individuals (27). If one sees, however, a gas-filled appendix with a meniscus at the base caused by the obstructing calculus, whether calcified or not, then one has presumptive evidence for appendicitis (28).

Of all of the above signs, a calculus has by far the greatest significance (Table A.1). Although approximately 50% of patients with subsequently proven acute appendicitis do have some type of abnormality on noncontrast radiographs, aside from a calculus the other findings are relatively nonspecific and can only suggest the diagnosis. The findings will obviously vary considerably with the severity of the disease. It should also be realized that approximately 50% of all patients with acute appendicitis will have normal radiographic findings.

Table A.1. Radiographic signs in appendicitis.

Radiographic signs
Non-contrast study
1. Calculus
2. Air-fluid level in cecum
3. Air-fluid level in distal ileum
4. Soft-tissue mass
5. Lumbar scoliosis
6. Obliterated psoas outline
7. Obliterated peritoneal fat stripe
8. Adynamic ileus
9. Small bowel obstruction
10. Dilated transverse colon
11. Pneumoperitoneum
12. Gas in the appendix
Barium enema
1. Soft-tissue mass at base of cecum
2. Barium spill into abscess
3. Partial filling of appendix with irregular cut-off

A barium enema should be limited to those patients where the preoperative diagnosis of appendicitis is being questioned. In the absence of significant peritoneal irritation, a barium enema is a relatively safe examination. Orally administered barium has only a minor role in the diagnosis, because even a normal appendix may not fill with barium and the cecum tends to stay collapsed. An oral study also tends to delay diagnosis. In most of these patients there generally is only one question to be answered: is appendicitis present? We perform a single contrast rather than a double-contrast examination. Likewise, these patients should be studied when they first present to the hospital and no colon preparation should be attempted prior to the examination; in most patients with appendicitis the colon tends to be relatively empty because of spasm. If there is an adjacent inflammatory mass, either the cecum, terminal ileum, or the sigmoid colon (29) is deformed, indented, or displaced by the mass (Fig. A.4). At times a large pelvic abscess (Fig. A.5) or abdominal abscess (Fig. A.6) is present. With extensive inflammation and deformity it may not be possible to pinpoint the origin of an abscess.

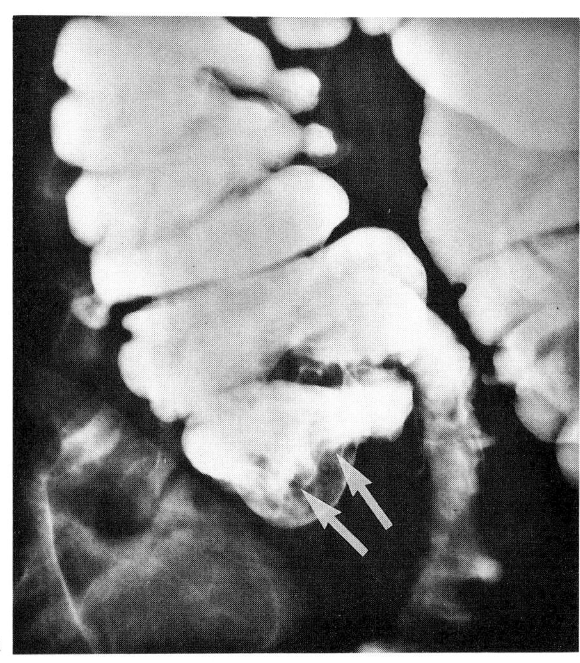

a

Fig. A.4. (a) Appendicitis was suspected in this 54-year-old male. A single-contrast barium enema performed on an unprepared colon reveals nonfilling of the appendix and a mass indenting the base of the cecum (arrows). The mass also displaces the terminal ileum medially. A periappendiceal abscess was drained at surgery. (b) An inflammatory mass indents the base of the cecum in this 25-year-old female with appendicitis. (c) 39-year-old male with appendicitis. The appendix did not fill with barium and there is a prominent mass at the base of the cecum (arrows). A single-contrast barium enema was adequate for diagnosis.

b

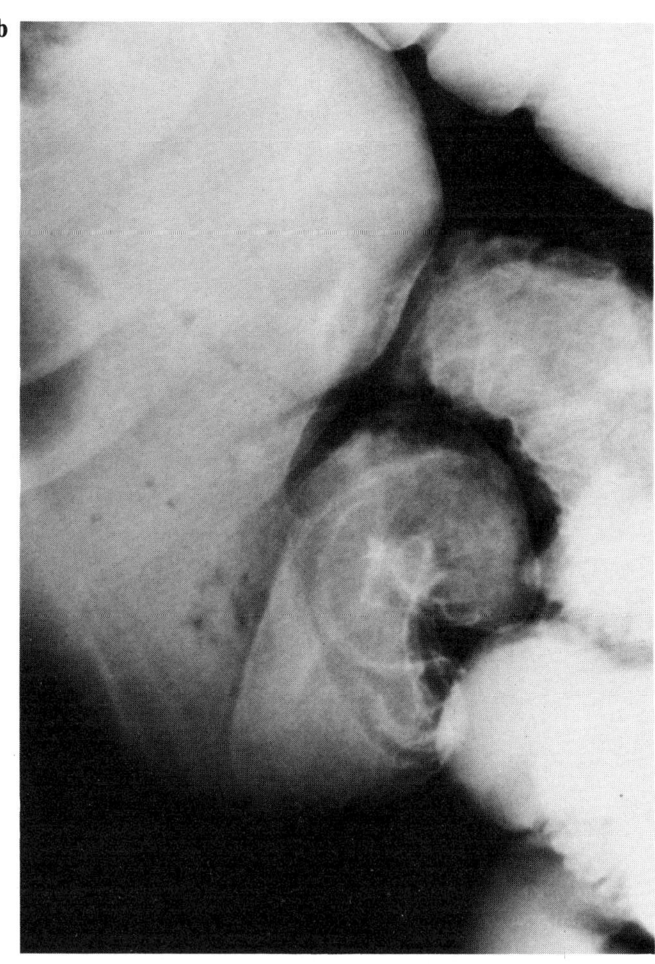

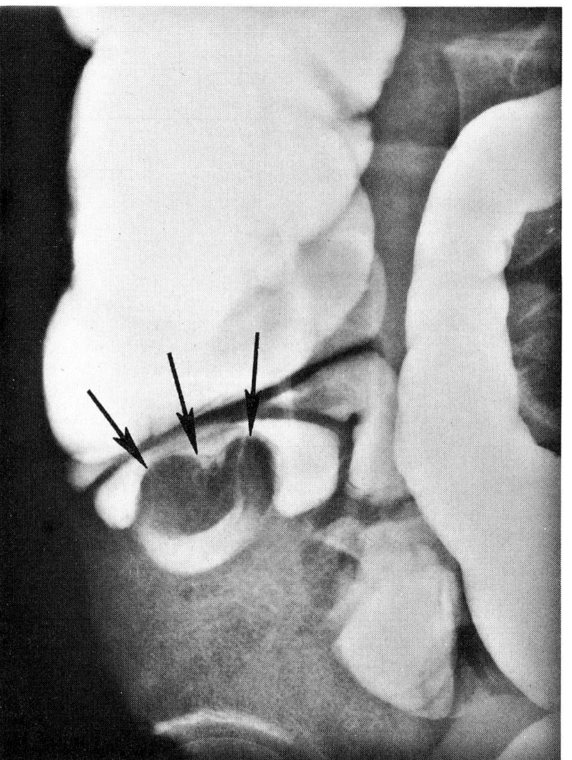

*Fig. A.4.*c

If the appendix fills completely during the examination one can conclude with reasonable certainty that the patient does not have appendicitis. Unfortunately, even in individuals with no prior appendectomy, the appendix may not fill during a barium enema in approximately 10 to 20% of patients (30). In children the incidence of nonfilling of the appendix is less (31). With initial nonfilling of the appendix, postevacuation radiographs should be obtained because occasionally the appendix will fill only at this time.

Occasionally barium will trickle into a periappendiceal abscess; whenever such a communication is seen, the colon should be drained immediately and postevacuation radiographs obtained. The main purpose in draining the colon is to avoid possible spill of a walled-off abscess into the peritoneal cavity.

Often in patients with cystic fibrosis the appendiceal lumen is plugged by mucus and does not fill during a barium enena (32). A mass can be present in the cecum, representing the tenacious intraluminal content seen in these patients.

Obstruction of only a part of the appendix can result in appendicitis (33). Such partial filling of the appendix, shown by an irregular outline, is more reliable than complete nonfilling (Fig. A.7). When the entire appendix fills there is a normal convex appearance to the tip of the barium column; with obstruction in the mid-appendix such a convex appearance is lacking.

An appendiceal fistula is rare, both preoperatively and postoperatively (1). Preoperative fistulas have been reported between the appendix and most of the adjacent structures and, rarely, to relatively distal structures. Most preoperative fistulas are seen in relatively advanced stages of appendicitis. A fistula should raise the possibility of regional enteritis. If a persistent appendiceal-cutaneous fistula is seen postoperatively, a retained appendiceal calculus should be suspected, because without an obstructing calculus most fistulas heal readily. Also, with a chronic postoperative fistula, infection with *Actinomyces israeli* should be considered.

Acute appendicitis can generally be excluded from the differential diagnosis if there is a history of a previous appendectomy and a scar is present in the right lower quadrant. On rare occasions, however, a residual appendiceal stump may become inflamed and the patient can present with appendicitis (34).

Angiography in the few reported examples of periappendiceal abscess has shown an avascular mass surrounded by a hypervascular stain (35). Computerized tomography shows a similar mass.

The differential diagnosis of a mass indenting the tip of the appendix includes other lesions of the appendix and tumors originating in adjacent structures (Fig. A.8). It is unusual for appendicitis to involve the wall of the terminal ileum, while both regional enteritis and infection by *Yersinia enterocolitica* characteristically involve the distal ileum. Correlation with the patient's clinical history will generally allow the radiologist to provide a meaningful differential diagnosis.

c. Tumors

Appendiceal tumors can be divided into benign and malignant (Table A.2). By far the most common epithelial neoplasm of the appendix is a carcinoid. Approximately 99% of appendiceal carcinoids behave as a benign tumor, with only an occasional one having malignant characteristics (36). The typi-

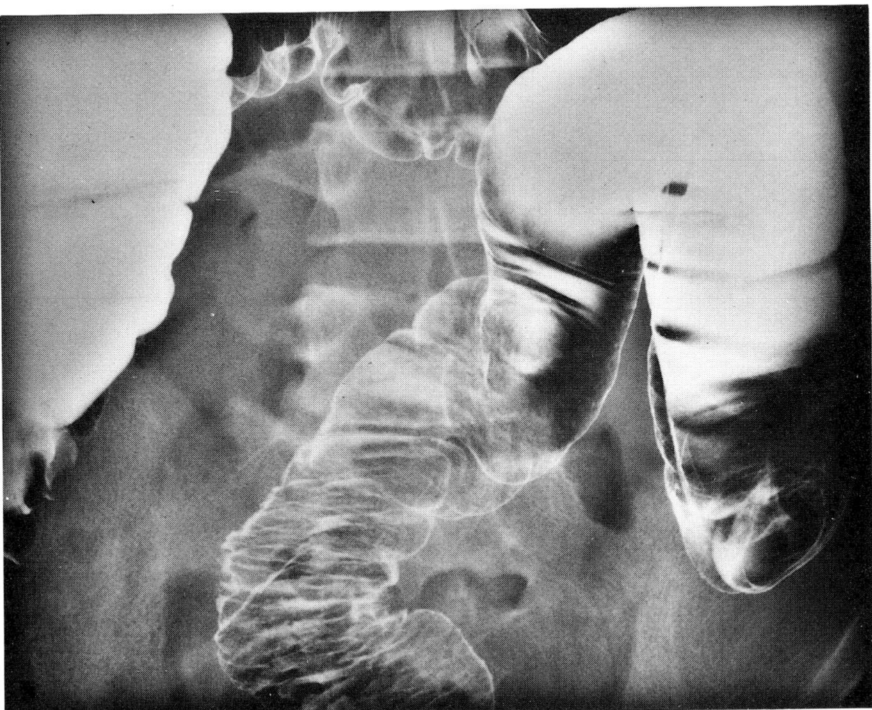

a

b

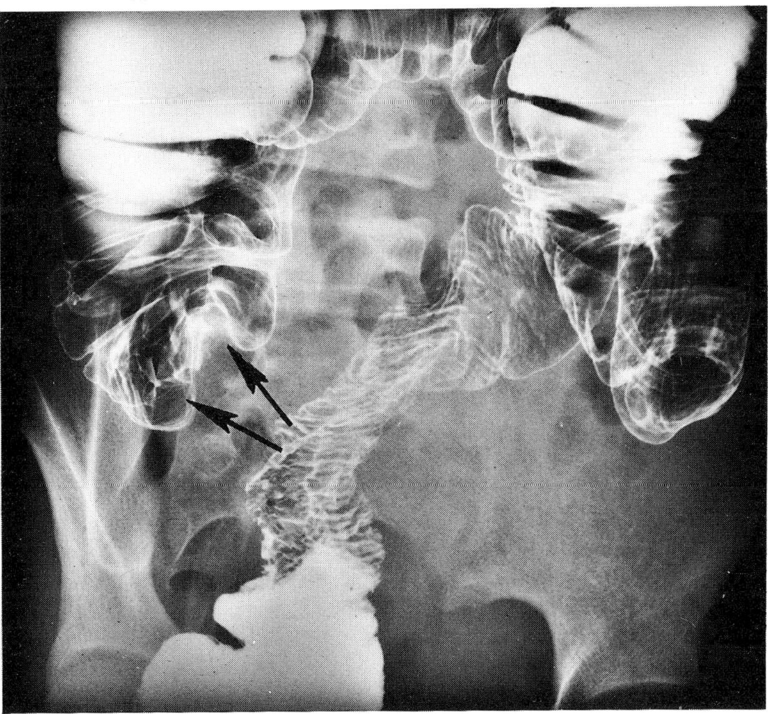

Fig. A.5. (a) Frontal and (b) oblique radiographs reveal a mass at the base of the cecum (arrows) and extensive infiltration and deformity of the rectosigmoid. A large abscess originating from the appendix has extended into the pelvis and lower abdomen. (Courtesy of Drs. A. Schulman and S. Fataar, Groote Schuur Hospital, Capetown).

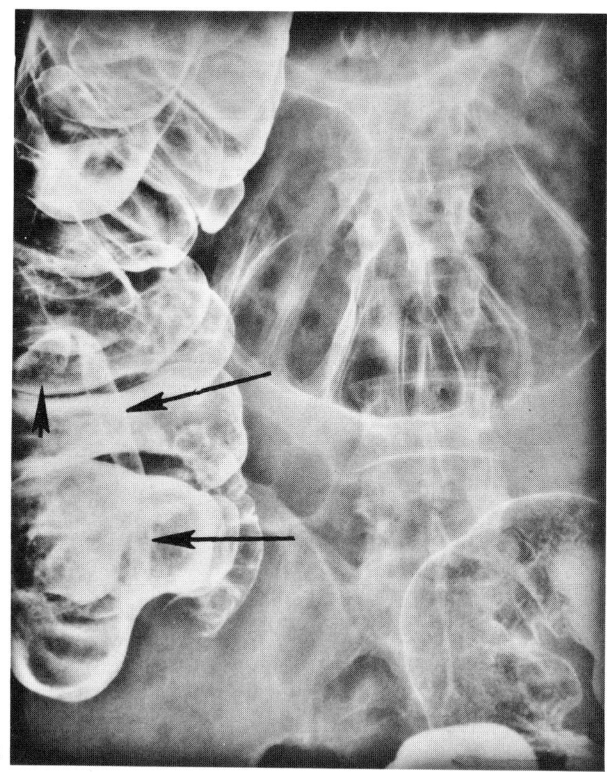

a

Fig. A.6. (a) A barium enema in a 63-year-old male reveals a retrocecal appendix (arrows) and a calculus at the tip of the appendix (arrowhead). The right colon distends normally. (b) 10 months later the patient presented with right mid-abdominal pain. A 'napkin-ring' lesion is present in the ascending colon (arrows), the appendix does not fill with barium, and an air–fluid level is present alongside the colon (arrowheads). All of these factors pointed towards appendicitis rather than a neoplasm as the source of this patient's symptoms.

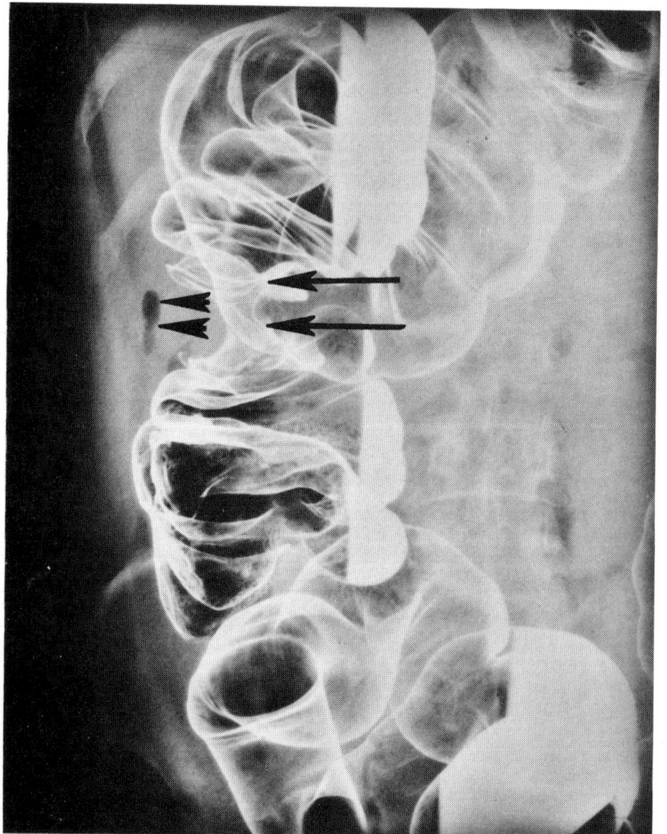

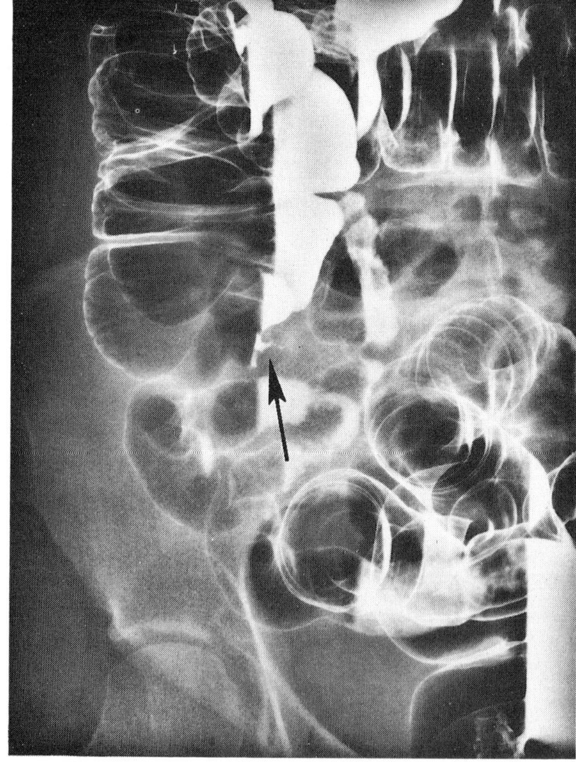

Fig. A.7. Partial filling of the appendix (arrow) in a 48-year-old female with right lower quadrant pain. The irregular tapering of the appendiceal lumen is characteristic of appendicitis with obstruction in the mid-appendix.

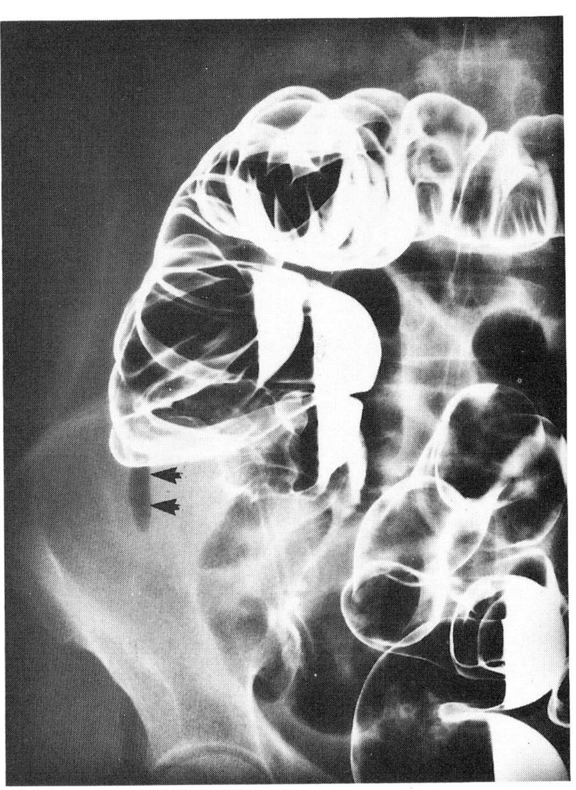

cal carcinoid syndrome is only rarely seen with appendiceal carcinoids (37). Liver metastases are also rare if the primary tumor is in the appendix, with most metastases originating from ileal carcinoids.

Most appendiceal carcinoids are not seen on radiographic examination. Most are incidental findings after appendectomy for appendicitis, with some being the cause of appendicitis (38).

Rectal and appendiceal carcinoids tend to be most benign while carcinoids originating in the remainder of the colon tend to grow more rapidly and are more aggressive. Nonappendiceal carcinoids arising directly from the colon generally are large, sessile and fungating masses or they mimic a circumferential carcinoma (37).

Fig. A.8. Cecal carcinoma and adjacent abscess. Clinically this 68-year-old female was suspected to have acute appendicitis. The barium enema reveals an air–fluid level in the abscess (arrowheads) and an intraluminal mass (arrows), representing the cancer. Because the ileocecal valve was not involved, no obstruction was present. At surgery the appendix could not be identified because of the surrounding abscess.

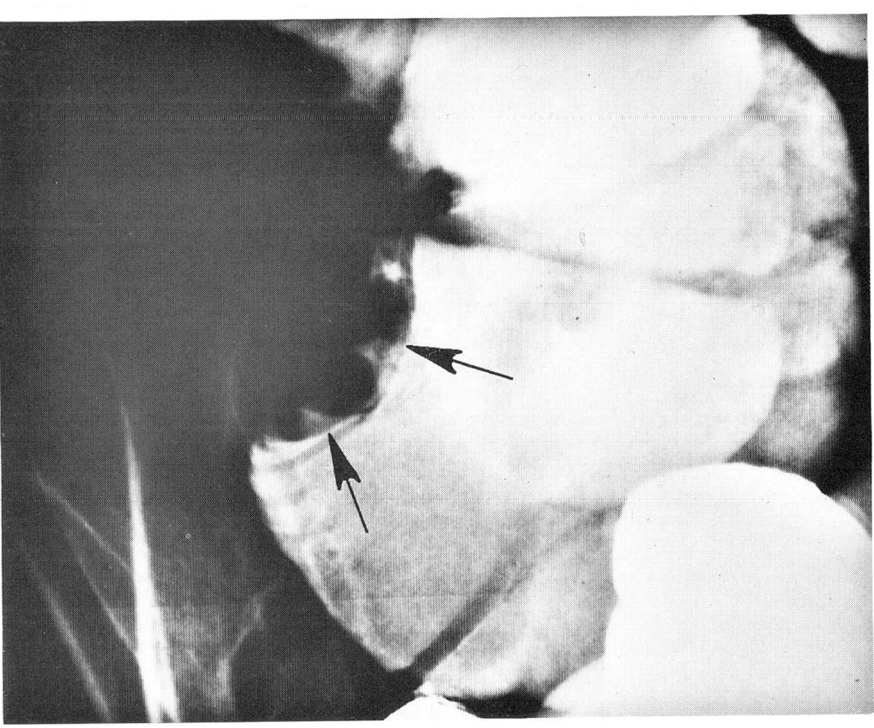

Fig. A.9. Appendiceal adenocarcinoma. This 69-year-old patient was suspected of having appendicitis and a single contrast barium enema was performed to confirm the diagnosis. A periappendiceal abscess surrounding a retrocecal appendix has a similar appearance.

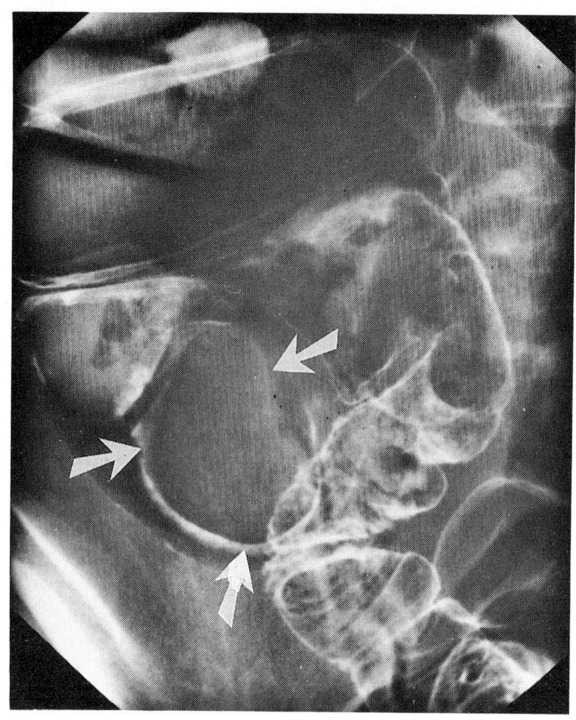

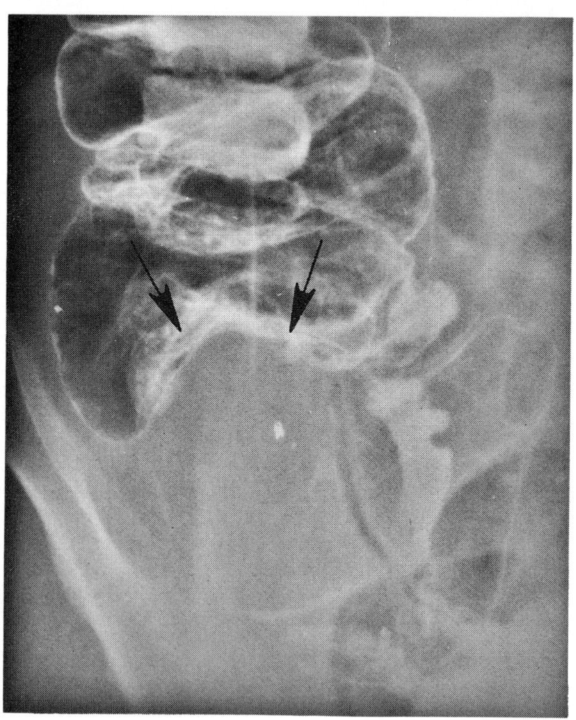

Fig. A.10. (a) Appendiceal mucocele in a 34-year-old female (arrows). The appendix did not fill during the barium enema. The mucocele presents as a smooth extraluminal mass. A large lipoma can have a similar appearance. (b) Another patient with an appendiceal mucocele. A large, smooth mass indents the base of the cecum (arrows).

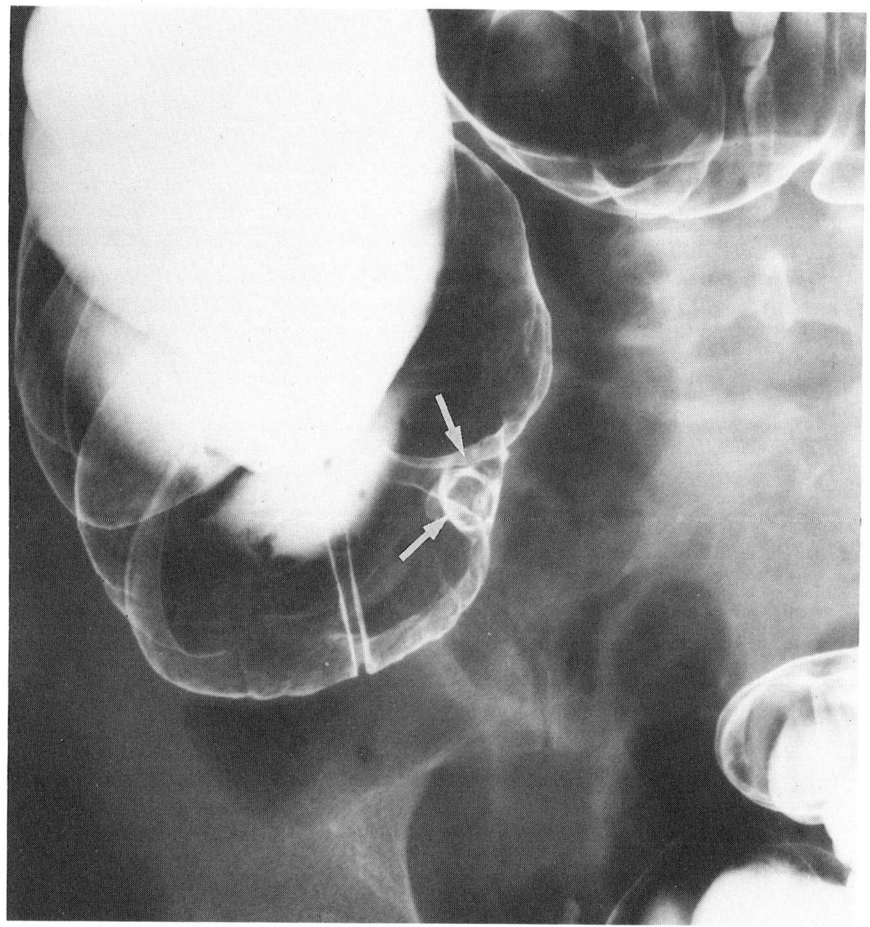

Fig. A.11. Prominent appendiceal stump (arrows) after an appendectomy. The patient's clinical presentation and knowledge of a prior appendectomy generally allow ready differentiation from other conditions.

Table A.2. Classification of appendiceal epithelial tumors (44).

Benign
1. Mucinous cystadenoma
2. Papillary adenoma

Malignant
1. Mucinous cystadenocarcinoma
2. Nonmucin producing adenocarcinoma
3. Carcinoid (52)
4. Adenoacanthoma

Nonneoplastic
1. Mucosal hyperplasia

A nonmucin producing adenocarcinoma of the appendix is generally identified only by the pathologist, with most of these patients presenting with acute appendicitis because of obstruction of the lumen (Fig. A.9). Only approximately one-third of these cancers can be correctly diagnosed intraoperatively (39).

There is an increased incidence of synchronous or metachronous colon neoplasms in patients with an appendiceal adenoma (40). It has been suggested that if a surgically removed appendix reveals the presence of a neoplasm, the colon should be studied to exclude any associated malignant neoplasm (40, 41). Metastatic carcinoma to the appendix is rare (42).

The term appendiceal 'mucocele' refers to an appendix where the lumen is dilated and filled with mucus (43). Unfortunately, some consider a mucocele simply as dilation of the lumen because of obstruction, others believe that all mucoceles are a single entity, while still others try to divide mucoceles into benign and malignant entities (44). A dilated lumen filled with mucus can be caused by mucosal hyperplasia, a mucinous cystadenoma, or a mucinous cystadenocarcinoma. Thus, the term 'mucocele' is simply descriptive of the gross appearance without specifying the pathogenesis of a lesion.

These patients can be either asymptomatic or they have right lower quadrant pain. Preceding episodes of appendicitis can occur. Depending upon the size of the mucocele, a mass may be palpable.

Radiographic examination can show curvilinear calcifications within the wall of the mass. During a barium enema the greatly distended appendix appears as an extraluminal mass indenting the cecum (Fig. A.10). There is nonfilling of the appendix. Rarely the mass may intussuscept (45). A mucocele can become infected, leading to an abscess.

Occasionally a mucocele ruptures either spontaneously or during surgery. The resultant spread throughout the peritoneal cavity produces 'pseudomyxoma peritonei', a descriptive term for numerous mucinous deposits scattered throughout the peritoneal cavity (46). Multiple curvilinear calcifications are uncommon but characteristic finding of pseudomyxoma peritonei (47).

Myxoglobulosis is an unusual form of mucocele, consisting of numerous white globules of mucus scattered throughout the appendix. Myxoglobulosis is generally associated with a high content of calcium and calcifications can be seen scattered throughout the right lower quadrant. A barium enema reveals the extraluminal mass, generally smooth in outline, indenting the cecum and sometimes displacing the ileum medially.

An inverted appendiceal stump in considerably smaller than a mucocele (Fig. A.11). Although radiographically a periappendiceal abscess can appear similar to a mucocele, the patient's clinical presentation generally allows ready differentiation. If there has been intussusception, differentiating whether the lead point is a cecal carcinoma or a mucocele may not be possible.

d. Intussusception

Rarely the appendix may intussuscept into the cecum (48, 49). There can also be varying degrees of colocolic intussusception with the appendix acting as a lead point for the intussusception. These patients can be relatively asymptomatic, have vague cramp-like right lower quadrant pain, or can present with acute colon obstruction. The intussusception may be intermittent in occurrence.

A barium enema reveals the intussusception as a soft tissue mass within the cecum. If the appendix is completely invaginated into the cecum, a barium enema reveals a fingerlike intraluminal mass arising from where the base of the appendix should be. Occasionally the enema will reduce an intussusception (48, 50); a postevacuation radiograph should be obtained, because following evacuation intussusception can again occur.

It should be emphasized that most colon intussusceptions in the adult are caused by a tumor, most likely a malignant neoplasm. In young children, most colon intussusceptions are idiopathic, and if the radiologist is able to reduce the intussusception and it does not recur, little other therapy is necessary. The exception is in neonates, where a mass, such as a congenital cyst, Meckel's diverticulum, a neoplasm. or necrotizing enterocolitis, appears to be a common predisposing cause (51). In children, Meckel's diverticulum or a polyp can be encountered. In older children lymphoma can result in ileocecal intussusception.

References

1. Collins DC: 71,000 human appendix specimens. A final report, summarizing forty years' study. Am J Proctol Gastroenterol Colon Rectal Surg 14:365–381, 1963.
2. Misra PS, Lebwohl P, Laufer H: Hepatic and appendiceal Whipple's disease with negative jejunal biopsies. Am J Gastroenterol 75:302–306, 1981.
3. Tilson MD, Touloukian MD: Agenesis of the vermiform appendix. J Pediatr Surg 7:74, 1972.
4. Pester GH: congenital absence of the vermiform appendix. Arch Surg 91:461–462, 1965.
5. Wallbridge PH: Double appendix. Br J Surg 50:346–347, 1962.
6. Gayen S: Anomalous origin of the vermiform appendix. Br Med J 2:549, 1973.
7. Amyand C: Of an inguinal rupture, with a pin in the appendix caeci, encrusted with stone; and some observations on wounds in the guts. Philos Trans R Soc Lond 39:329–342, 1736.
8. Fitz RH: Perforating inflammation of the vermiform appendix; with special reference to its early diagnosis and treatment. Trans Assoc Am Physicians 1:107–144, 1886.
9. Noer T: Decreasing incidence of acute appendicitis. Acta Chem Scand 141:431–432, 1975.
10. Jess P, Bjerregaard B, Brynitz S, Holst-Christensen J, Kalaja E, Lund-Kristensen J: Acute appendicitis. Prospective trial concerning diagnostic accuracy and complications. Am J Surg 141:232–234, 1981.
11. Carey LS: Lead shot appendicitis in northern native people. J Can Assoc Radiol 28:171–174, 1977.
12. Buschard K, Kjaeldgaard A: Investigation and analysis of the position, fixation, length, and embryology of the vermiform appendix. Acta Chir Scand 139:293–298, 1973.
13. Cardoso JM, Kimura K, Stoopen M, Cervantes LF, Elizondo L, Churchill R, Moncada R: Radiology of invasive amebiasis of the colon. AJR 128:935–941, 1977.
14. Vukmer GJ, Trummer MJ: Barium appendicitis. Arch Surg 91:630–632, 1965.
15. Merten DF, Lebowitz ME: Acute appendicitis in a child associated with prolonged appendiceal retention of barium (barium appendicitis). South Med J 71:81–82, 1978.
16. Totty WG, Koehler RE, Cheung LY: Significance of retained barium in the appendix. AJR 135:753–756, 1980.
17. Bergman JJ, Rosen GD, Moeller DA: Appendicitis associated with recent barium study. J Fam Pract 8:931–935, 1979.
18. Maglinte DDT, Bush ML, Aruta EV, Bullington GE: Retained barium in the appendix: diagnostic and clinical significance. AJR 137:529–533, 1981.
19. Homer MJ, Braver JM: Recurrent appendicitis: reexamination of a controversial disease. Gastrointest Radiol 4:295–301, 1979.
20. Bakhda RK, McNair MM: Useful radiological signs in acute appendicitis in children. Clin Radiol 28:193–196, 1977.
21. Beneventano TC, Schein CJ, Jacobson HG: The roentgen aspects of some appendiceal abnormalities. AJR 96:344–360, 1966.
22. Swischuk LE, Hayden CK: Appendicitis with perforation: the dilated transverse colon sign. AJR 135:687–689, 1980.
23. Farman J, Kassner EG, Dallemand S, Stein HD: Pneumoperitoneum and appendicitis. Gastrointest Radiol 1:277–279, 1976.
24. Casper RB: Fluid in the right flank as a roentgenographic sign of acute appendicitis. AJR 110:352–354, 1970.
25. Harned RK: Retrocecal appendicitis presenting with air in the subhepatic space. AJR 126:416–418, 1976.
26. Joffe N: Radiology of acute appendicitis and its complications. CRC Crit Rev Diagn Imaging 7:97–160, 1975.
27. Lim MS: Gas-filled appendix: lack of diagnostic specificity. AJR 128:209–210, 1977.
28. Bigongiari LR, Wicks JD: Gas-filled appendix with meniscus: outline of the appendicolith. Gastrointest Radiol 3:229–231, 1978.
29. Halls JM, Meyers HI: Acute appendicitis with abscess simulating carcinoma of the sigmoid. AJR 129:1057–1059, 1977.
30. Sakover RP, Del Fava RL: Frequency of visualization of the normal appendix with the barium enema examination. AJR 121:312–317, 1974.
31. Schey WL: Use of barium in the diagnosis of appendicitis in children. AJR 118:95–103, 1973.
32. Fletcher BD, Abramowsky CR: Contrast enemas in cystic fibrosis: implications of appendiceal nonfilling. AJR 137:323–326, 1981.
33. Ekberg O: Ileocecal abnormalities in appendiceal abscess. Acta Radiol (Diagn) 19:343–347, 1978.
34. Soter CS: The contribution of the radiologist to the diagnosis of acute appendicitis. Semin Roentgenol 8:375–388, 1973.
35. Winograd J, Palubinskas AJ: Arteriographic diagnosis of appendiceal abscess. Br J Radiol 50:229–230, 1977.
36. Godwin DJ II: Carcinoid tumors. An analysis of 2837 cases. Cancer 36:560–569, 1975.
37. Balthazar EJ: Carcinoid tumors of the alimentary tract. I. Radiographic diagnosis. Gastrointest Radiol 3:47–56, 1978.
38. Ryden SE, Drake RM, Franciosi RA: Carcinoid tumors of the appendix in children. Cancer 36:1538–1542, 1975.
39. Chang P, Attiyeh FF: Adenocarcinoma of the appendix. Dis Colon Rectum 24:176–180, 1981.
40. Wolff M, Ahmed N: Epithelial neoplasms of the vermiform appendix (exclusive of carcinoid). II. Cancer 37:2511–2522, 1976.
41. Morson BC, Dawson IMP: Gastrointestinal Pathology, p 473. Blackwell Scientific, Oxford, 1979.
42. Dieter RA Jr: Carcinoma metastatic to the vermiform appendix: report of three cases. Dis Colon Rectum 13:336–340, 1970.
43. Qizilbash AH: Mucoceles of the appendix: their relationship to hyperplastic polyps, mucinous cystadenomas and cystadenocarcinomas. Arch Pathol Lab Med 99:548–555, 1975.
44. Aranha GV, Reyes CV: Primary epithelial tumors of the

appendix and a reappraisal of the appendiceal 'mucocele' Dis Colon Rectum 22:472–476, 1979.
45. Douglas NJ, Cameron DC, Nixon SJ, Rensberg MV, Samuel E: Intussusception of a mucocele of the appendix. Gastrointest Radiol 3:97–100, 1978.
46. Limber GK, King RE, Silverberg SG: Pseudomyxoma peritonaei: a report of ten cases. Ann Surg 178:587–593, 1973.
47. Douds HN, Pitt MJ: Calcified rims: characteristic but uncommon radiologic finding in pseudomyxoma peritonei. Gastrointest Radiol 5:263–266, 1980.
48. Bachman AL, Clemett AR: Roentgen aspects of primary appendiceal intussusception. Radiology 101:531–538, 1971.
49. Atkinson GO, Gay BB Jr, Naffis D: Intussusception of the appendix in children AJR 126:1164–1168, 1976.
50. Kleinman PK: Intussusception of the appendix: hydrostatic reduction. AJR 134:1268–1270, 1980.
51. Patriquin HB, Afshani E, Effman E, Griscom NT, Johnson F, Kramer SS, Rapp K, Reilly BJ: Neonatal intussusception. Report of twelve cases. Radiology 125:463–466, 1977.
52. Morson BC, Dawson IMP: Gastrointestinal Pathology, p 470. Blackwell Scientific, Oxford, 1979.

III.4.B. Endometriosis

Endometriosis is an unusual lesion first put in its proper perspective by Sampson in 1921 (1). Since then endometrial-like tissue has been described most commonly in the pelvis and abdomen although it can also occasionally be found in other locations. Common sites of endometrial implantation are the uterosacral ligaments and the rectovaginal septum. Endometriosis in the latter location can lead to rectosigmoid infiltation and symptoms referrable to this region. Involvement of the remainder of the colon and appendix is unusual but can occur (2).

No single theory explains adequately the wide diversity of location for this entity. There probably are several causes for endometriosis, with implantation of aberrant tissue simply being one of them. Endometrial tissue is not neoplastic in nature. The changes occurring in this tissue are hormone dependent and the periodic proliferation and subsequent necrosis eventually results in fibrosis and constriction. The resultant bowel damage can appear radiographically similar to other intrinsic diseases, including a carcinoma.

Most patients with endometriosis are between the ages of 25 and 45. Many of the patients are nulliparous. Symptoms of colon involvement tend to be in the older age group, with some patients being past menopause. Regression of symptoms can occur with pregnancy. The patients have various disturbances of menstruation, with some patients exhibiting relatively few symptoms, although pain is generally most prominent during menstruation. Most patients with rectosigmoid involvement have endometriosis either on the serosa or in the intramural portion of the bowel wall and have an intact mucosa. These patients thus do not present with rectal bleeding. Mucosal involvement is associated with cyclic bleeding. A mass in the rectosigmoid, together with rectal bleeding during the menstrual period, is strong presumptive evidence for bowel involvement by endometriosis.

If an endometrioma is located adjacent to the colon, a barium enema may simply show colon displacement. If the colon is directly involved, the characteristic radiographic appearance is an eccentric and infiltrating tumor. These lesions usually are single, have well-defined discreet edges, and the colon folds tend to be intact although they are splayed (3). If the colon wall is foreshortened because of fibrosis, the folds have a spiculated appearance. Circumferential involvement is less common, and can be asymmetrical, but the superficial folds still are only distorted and not destroyed. An intraluminal irregular polyp mimicking a neoplasm is occasionally seen. Least common is diffuse pelvic involvement with multiple colon lesions

With chronic involvement eventual fibrosis of the involved segment ensues and the colon lumen narrows. At this stage endometriosis can mimic peritoneal carcinomatosis, with the lesions in these patients simply being due to serosal fibrosis and resultant foreshortening of the involved area. The younger age group and association of symptoms with menstruation should suggest endometriosis in the differential diagnosis.

Most of the lesions we have seen have been along the anterior wall of the rectosigmoid, where endometriosis mimics metastatic deposits in the pouch of Douglas (Figs. B.1 and B.2). Endometriosis can appear similar to diverticulitis (4). Generally there is little confusion with a primary colon carcinoma because endometriosis tends to distort, but the folds remain intact. Intraluminal masses are unusual in endometriosis.

Rarely encountered is endometriosis involving the appendix; here it can mimic an intramural cecal mass or a periappendiceal abscess. The appendix may not fill with barium.

The development of a malignancy in an area of endometriosis is extremely rare (2, 5).

Often the endometrial inplants can be removed surgically. With extensive bowel involvement an oophorectomy generally results in regression of the endometriosis.

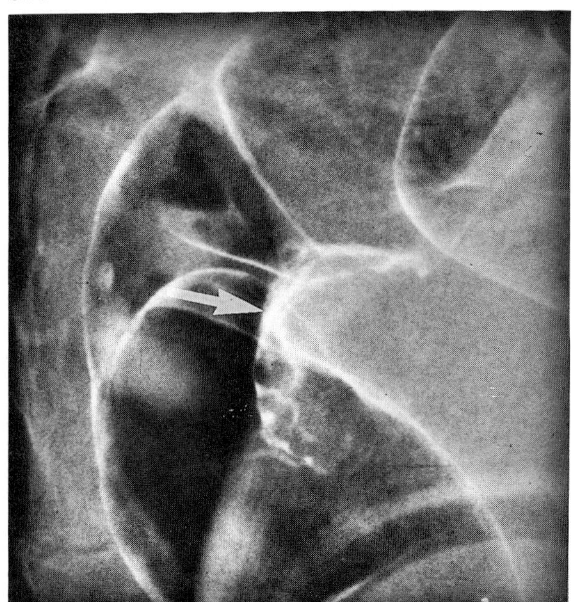

a

b

Fig. B.1. Two examples of endometriosis involving the anterior rectal wall. Their similarity to metastases in the pouch of Douglas is obvious. (a) There is a single, ulcerated and sharply defined lesion (arrow) in this patient. (b) The lesion in this patient is similar to the previous one; in addition, a smaller focus of endometriosis is present proximally (arrow).

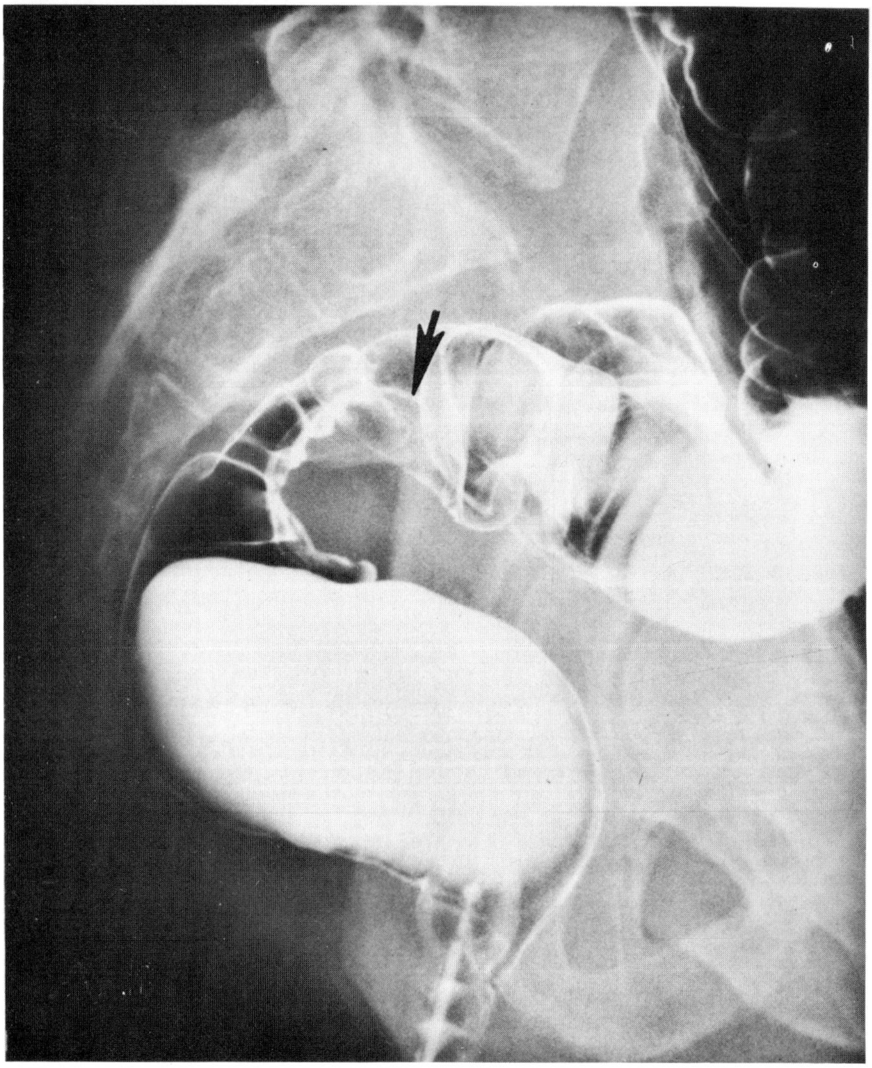

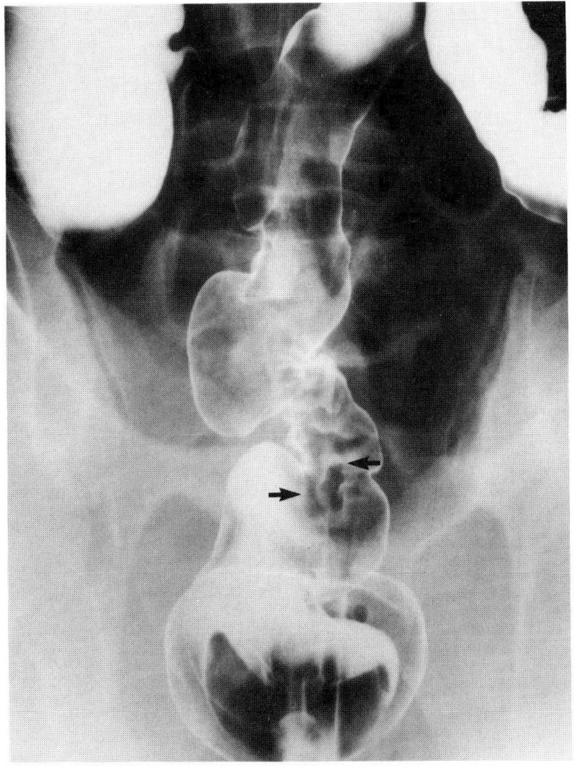

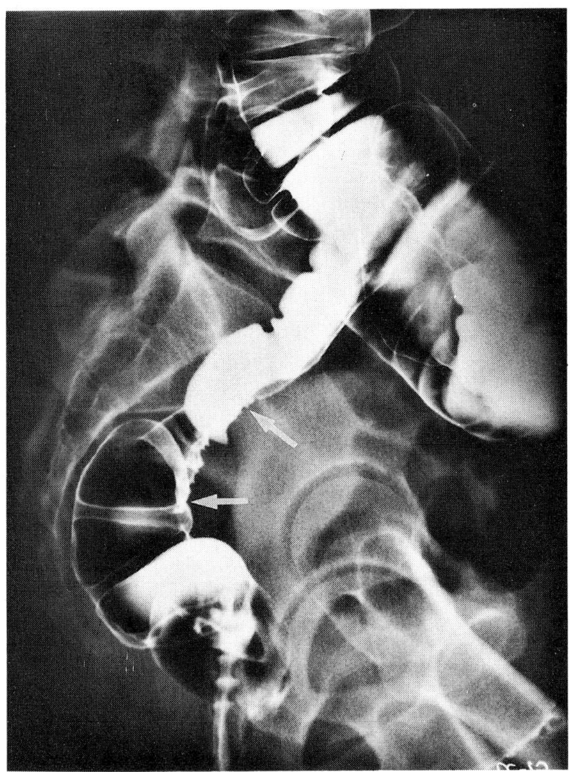

Fig. B.2. 28-year-old patient with pain and bleeding. The rectosigmoid involvement is more extensive (arrows) than in the previous patients. (a) Frontal and (b) lateral views. Because of the lesion's anterior location the lateral view shows the infiltration better.

References

1. Sampson JA: Perforating hemorrhagic (chocolate) cysts of the ovary. Arch Surg 3:245–323, 1921.
2. MaCafee CHG, Hardy Greer HL: Intestinal endometriosis. Report of 29 cases and survey of literature. J Obstet Gynecol Br Emp 67:539–555, 1960.
3. Tavernier C, Jourde L, Dhamlencourt A-M, Delafolie A: L'endométriose colique: diagnostic radiologique. J Radiol 61:437–445, 1980.
4. Fagan CJ: Endometriosis: clinical and roentgenographic manifestations. Radiol Clin North Am 12:109–125, 1974.
5. Labay GR, Feiner F: Malignant pleural endometriosis. Am J Obstet Gynecol 110:478–480, 1971.

III.4.C. Amyloidosis

Amyloidosis is an uncommon entity consisting of deposits of an abnormal protein in divers organs. A wide radiographic spectrum is found in the various organs of the human body. Over two-thirds of patients with amyloidosis have involvement of the gastrointestinal tract. A common diagnostic test involves rectal biopsy for amyloid.

Although a separation into primary and secondary amyloidosis is simplistic, from a patient management standpoint this division is useful. Primary amyloidosis occurs without any precedent or underlying disease; secondary amyloidosis consists of depositions of amyloid in the presence of a chronic disease, such as infection, inflammation, tumor and possibly steroid therapy.

The amyloid is generally deposited around blood vessels. With sufficient such deposition there is narrowing of the lumen and secondary ischemic changes in the organ involved. Amyloid can also be deposited in the mucosa. With severe involvement the mucosal glands are deformed and eventually destroyed. Infiltration of the muscle layers leads to loss of tonicity and peristalsis.

Generally there are no radiographic findings unless sufficient amyloid infiltration has resulted in significant ischemia. Thus, with mild colon infiltration a rectal biopsy can be positive but even a technically excellent double-contrast barium enema will not reveal any abnormality. Endoscopy has revealed mucosal petechiae (1). With significant colon involvement one finds decreased colon tonicity and loss of haustrations (2). Occasionally adynamic ileus involving both the small bowel and the colon is present.

The differential diagnosis of amyloidosis includes chronic ulcerative colitis (3), regional enteritis, ischemic colitis, and infectious colitis. Foreshortening of the colon, as found in ulcerative colitis, generally is not seen in amyloidosis. Because amyloidosis results in ischemia, there is overlap with ischemic colitis both radiographically and clinically. Amyloidosis can develop in a setting of regional enteritis. The invariable involvement of the kidneys by amyloidosis in these patients suggests the true nature of the condition (4).

References

1. Schmidt H, Fruehmorgen P, Riemann JF, Becker V: Mucosal suggillation in the colon in secondary amyloidosis. Endoscopy 13:181–183, 1981.
2. Seliger G, Krassner RL, Beranbaum ER, Miller F: The spectrum of roentgen appearance in amyloidosis of the small and large bowel: radiologic-pathologic correlation. Radiology 100:63–70, 1971.
3. Cassad DE, Bocian JJ: Primary systemic amyloidosis simulating acute ideopathic ulcerative colitis: report of a case. Dig Dis Sci 10:63–74, 1965.
4. Greenstein AJ, Janowitz HD, Sachar DB: The extra-intestinal complications of Crohn's disease and ulcerative colitis: a study of 700 patients. Medicine 55:401–412, 1976.

III.4.D. Volvulus

a. Introduction

Volvulus, from the Latin verb 'volvere' (to twist), results in partial or complete bowel obstruction. Although volvulus can occur in both the stomach and the small bowel, by far the most common sites are in the colon. A twist of a loop of colon produces blockage at two points, with a closed loop obstruction in between. With sufficient twist there is interruption of the blood supply to that loop of bowel. Intraluminal distension of the colon and the resultant increased pressure help interrupt colon blood circulation and can result in ischemia.

A common prerequisite to colon volvulus is the presence of a long and mobile mesentery to that loop of bowel (Fig. D.1). Because the two segments of the colon that have a relatively long mesentery are the cecum and the sigmoid, it is here that most colon volvulus is seen. The ascending colon, descending colon, and rectum, usually in a fixed extraperitoneal location, are prevented from twisting unless there is an associated congenital anomaly and these segments of the colon are on lax mesenteries.

The onset of volvulus can be either insidious or sudden. With acute onset abdominal pain is usually present and abdominal distension develops. It is not uncommon to have multiple episodes of intermittent colon torsion prior to the actual episode of volvulus. Such intermittent obstruction makes possible the enormous distension occasionally encountered (Fig. D.2).

Sigmoid volvulus is considerably more common in patients from mental institutions and those prone to chronic constipation. Throughout the world, volvulus is more common in those populations subsisting on a high roughage diet. Sigmoid volvulus is likewise more common in males and in the elderly. Cecal volvulus is more common in females and is usually seen in adults, although it can occur in children (1). Volvulus has been associated with sprue (2), muscular dystrophy (3, 4), occurs more frequently than normal in pregnancy, in association with distal colon obstruction (5), and may confuse the clinical picture in a setting of adynamic ileus. A differentiation between colon ileus, discussed elsewhere, and cecal volvulus can be difficult.

One of the radiographic hallmarks of colon volvulus is the enormous distension seen on abdominal radiographs (Fig. D.3). In fact, quite often the dramatic distension is out of proportion to the symptoms present. Radiographs of the abdomen are generally diagnostic for both cecal and sigmoid volvulus. Angiography on patients with volvulus reveals ischemia (6); there is a whirlpool and 'bundled' appearance to the arteries, intense bowel-wall opacification, and poor or nonfilling of the draining veins.

b. Cecal volvulus

Volvulus of the cecum often also involves portions of the ascending colon and ileum. The classic radiographic appearance of cecal volvulus is that of a greatly distended loop of bowel extending from the right lower quadrant to the left upper quadrant, with the axis of the cecum diagonally across the abdomen. However, depending upon the degree of

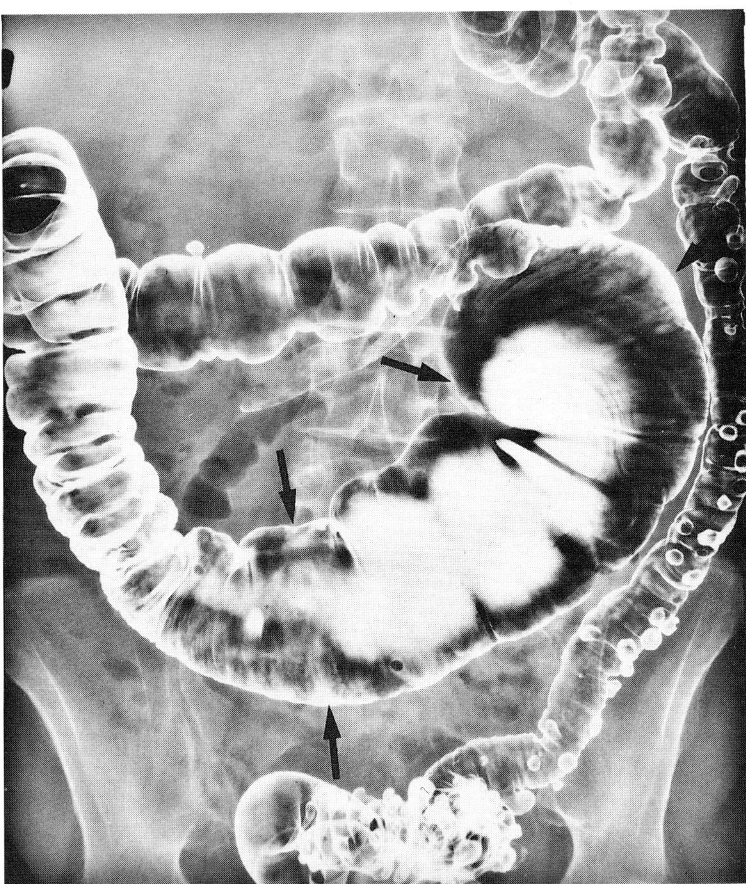

Fig. D.1. The cecum and a portion of the ascending colon (arrows) are very mobile in this patient. A portion of the ascending colon is intraperitoneal in location and on a mesentery, conditions predisposing to volvulus.

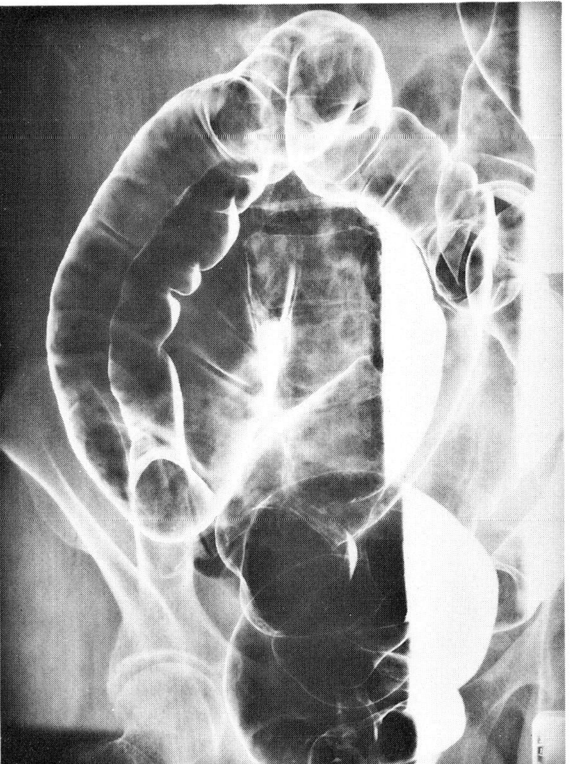

a

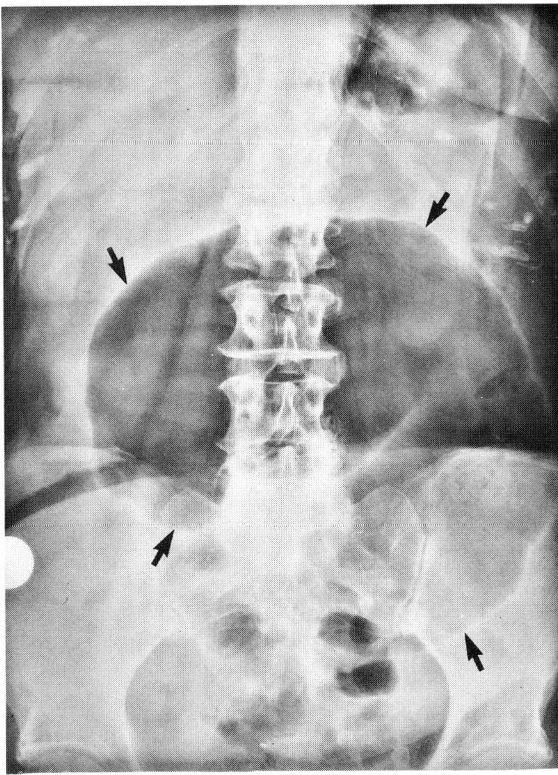

b

Fig. D.2. (a) The patient underwent a barium enema for abdominal pain. The cecum and portion of the ascending colon are rotated around their axis. No obstruction was present. (b) Four years later the patient presented with acute cecal volvulus. The cecum is greatly dilated (arrows). The patient had had intermittent symptoms over the intervening years.

twist, or volvulus, and the original location of the cecum, the cecum can be located almost anywhere in the abdomen. The appearance resembles that of a large lucent kidney (Fig. D.4). The haustra are preserved unless there already is significant ischemia and bowel wall edema. There generally is a decrease in caliber of the remaining colon distal to the volvulus. With uncomplicated cecal volvulus the small bowel is also considerably dilated. The small bowel, however, can be filled with fluid with little or no gas being present and, as a result, the small bowel obstruction can be missed on noncontrast radiographs. At times the appendix fills with gas; if it is in an unusual location and is attached to a dilated viscus the diagnosis is readily apparent (7). Chronic cecal volvulus is unusual (Fig. D.3).

At times, noncontrast radiographs of the abdomen are adequate and no other radiographic study is necessary for diagnosis. Usually, however, a barium enema is required for confirmation. We perform a single contrast barium enema. The reasons why a double-contrast barium enema is not performed is that no great accuracy of detail is necessary to make the diagnosis and for the double-contrast examination the patient would have to lie prone for at least a portion of the examination. Because these patients generally have abdominal pain and distension, the prone position can be intolerable.

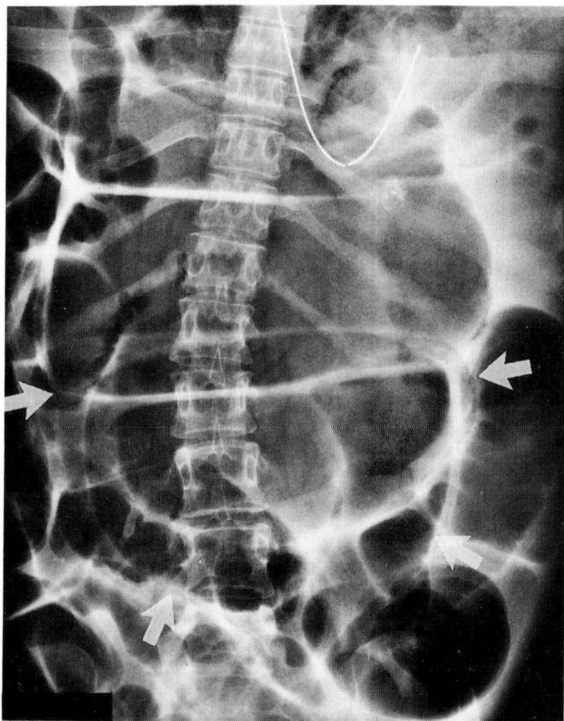

Fig. D.3. Chronic cecal volvulus. The greatly dilated cecum fills most of the abdomen (arrows). Such enormous dilation of the cecum could occur only on a chronic basis.

One purpose in performing a barium enema is to try to reduce the volvulus. We maintain the enema bag at 1 m above the table top and depend on the resultant increased intraluminal pressure to help reduce the volvulus. The barium sulfate suspension used for double-contrast examinations is considerably more viscous than that for single contrast. No pressure should be applied to the enema bag. During the double-contrast examination one usually adds air into the colon and it is then difficult to estimate the resultant intraluminal pressure. With a single contrast examination, on the other hand, the intraluminal pressure can be maintained at 1 m of water, assuming colon spasm can be abolished. Thus, prior to the barium enema, we premedicate these patients with glucagon. Without glucagon, it is not unusual to see spasm and difficulty in retention of the enema. In addition, with spasm distal to the obstruction it is impossible to control or even estimate the resultant intraluminal pressure. Glucagon tends to abolish or at least diminish this unknown factor although it is not known whether glucagon actually aids in the reduction of a volvulus.

The contraindications for performing a barium enema are clinical signs of peritonitis, rectal bleeding, or the radiographic finding of gas in the bowel wall. Likewise, the presence of pneumoperitoneum on abdominal radiographs is a contraindication to the performance of a barium enema.

A barium enema demonstrates a nondilated colon up to the point of torsion.

There are two radiographic appearances of cecal volvulus. A twist along the longitudinal axis of the ascending colon is called axial torsion. The appearance of the twisted segment during a barium enema is similiar to that seen with sigmoid volvulus; barium trapped in the twisted and narrowed folds has a spiral or 'bird-beak' appearance (Fig. D.5). If the retrograde obstruction is not complete and barium does reflux into the volvulized segment, the full extent of the twist will readily become apparent.

If the cecum twists along its transverse axis there

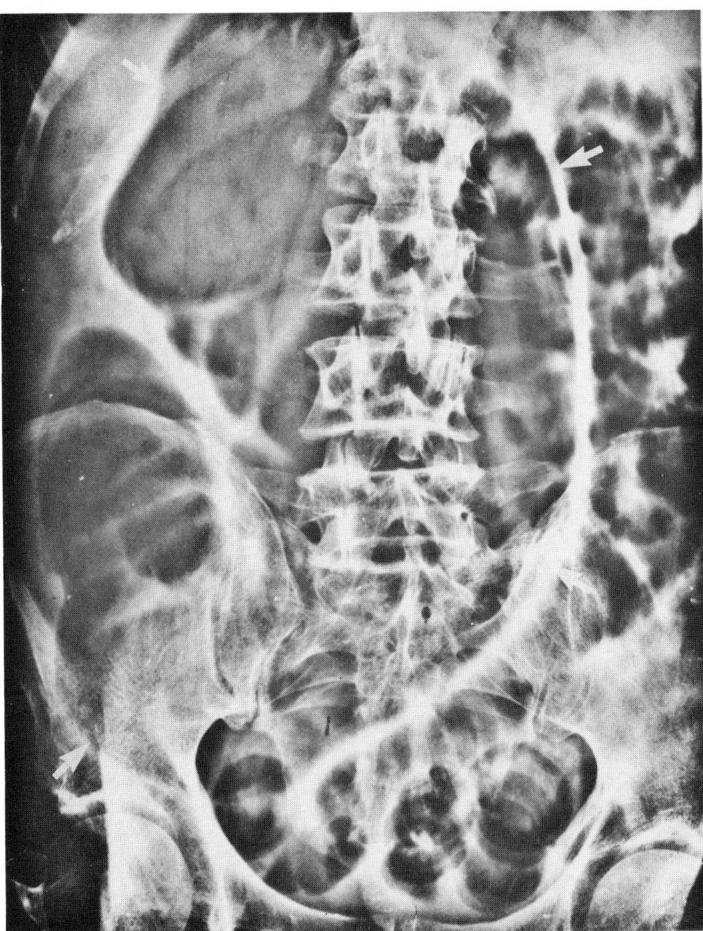

a

b

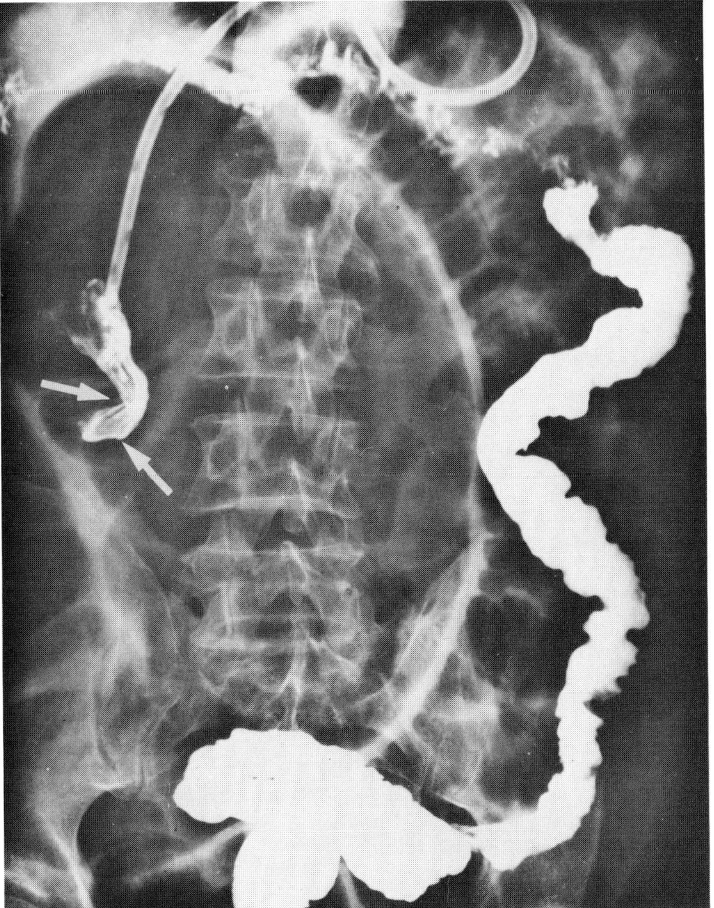

Fig. D.4. Cecal volvulus. (a) A large gas-filled structure resembling a kidney fills most of the right side of the abdomen (arrows). (b) The post-evacuation radiograph obtained after an unsuccessful attempt at reduction of the volvulus reveals the twisted segment (arrows).

may not be a spiral twist. Such volvulus, commonly called cecal bascule, can lead to a smooth-appearing obstructed segment. Depending upon the degree of twist and resultant obstruction with both types of volvulus, barium may pass into the cecum or it may stop at the twist. The cecal bascule is associated either with fibrous bands or adhesions, with the cecum simply twisting around these fixed points.

Occasionally the dilated cecum will not change its appearance during the barium enema, but will be reduced during evacuation. We thus obtain a post-evacuation radiograph to check for this possibility. The reverse may also occur: a barium enema can be normal but the postevacuation radiograph will reveal a volvulus (8) (Fig. D.6). An unusual association is between cecal volvulus and urticaria involving the cecum (9) (see Fig. K.1, page 353). Biopsy of the involved segment revealed submucosal edema and cellular infiltration. Whether these changes are secondary to ischemia is not known.

c. Transverse colon volvulus

Transverse colon volvulus is rare (10). Splenic flexure volvulus is even less common (11–13). These conditions are seen primarily in adults with only a few case reports in children (14, 15). Although the transverse colon is on a mesentery, the hepatic and splenic flexures are relatively fixed in position and as a result the transverse colon can volvulize only under unusual conditions. Such factors as absent or redundant colic ligaments, mid-gut malrotation with loss of fixation of the flexures or close proximity of the flexures, together with a long mesocolon, predispose the transverse colon to volvulize (16, 17). Distal obstruction, even sigmoid volvulus, likewise appears to predispose to transverse colon volvulus (16). It has been described after a hemicolectomy (18).

Clues to the correct diagnosis are the distended loop involved in the volvulus and, on a barium enema, the spiraling colon folds at the twist. A 'bird-beak' deformity can be present. The overall picture mimics obstruction due to a fibrous band, another rare cause of transverse colon obstruction (Fig. D.7).

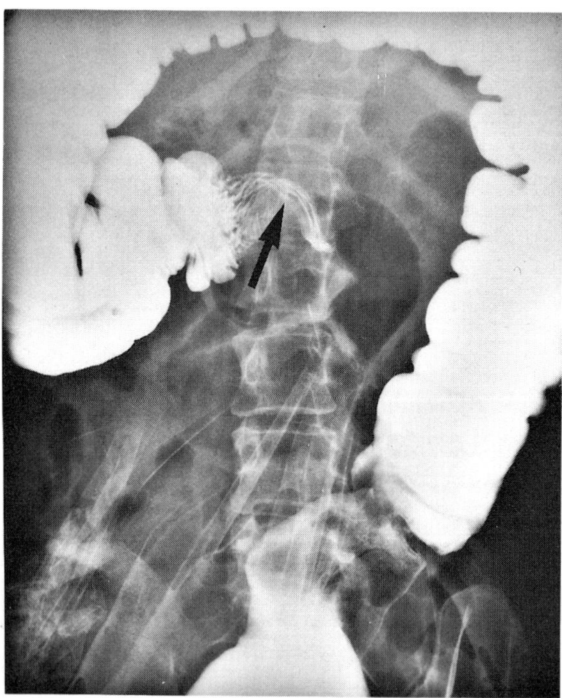

Fig. D.5. Cecal volvulus. The twisted colon folds, just distal to the volvulus, have a typical spiral appearance (arrow). The patient has had sigmoid resection for prior sigmoid volvulus.

d. Ileosigmoid knot

A rare cause of volvulus is a loop of small bowel wrapped around the sigmoid (19, 20). These patients have an abrupt onset of pain and in untreated cases the course is fulminant. When first examined the patient may already be in shock and exhibit rebound tenderness, probably secondary to infarction of the twisted ileal loops. The radiographic appearance is that of a dilated sigmoid, normal caliber or slightly dilated proximal colon, and a dilated small bowel. In effect, this entity consists of distal small bowel obstruction and a volvulus-like sigmoid obstruction.

e. Sigmoid volvulus

In any population the incidence of sigmoid volvulus appears to be inversely related to the incidence of diverticular disease. Most of the involved patients have a redundant sigmoid colon on a long and mobile mesentery. The sigmoid colon can be far superior to its usual location even when the patient is not obstructed.

Noncontrast abdominal radiographs show a greatly dilated sigmoid. The appearance is that of several parallel and vertical loops of greatly distended bowel extending from the pelvis to the upper abdomen. Haustra are generally obliterated be-

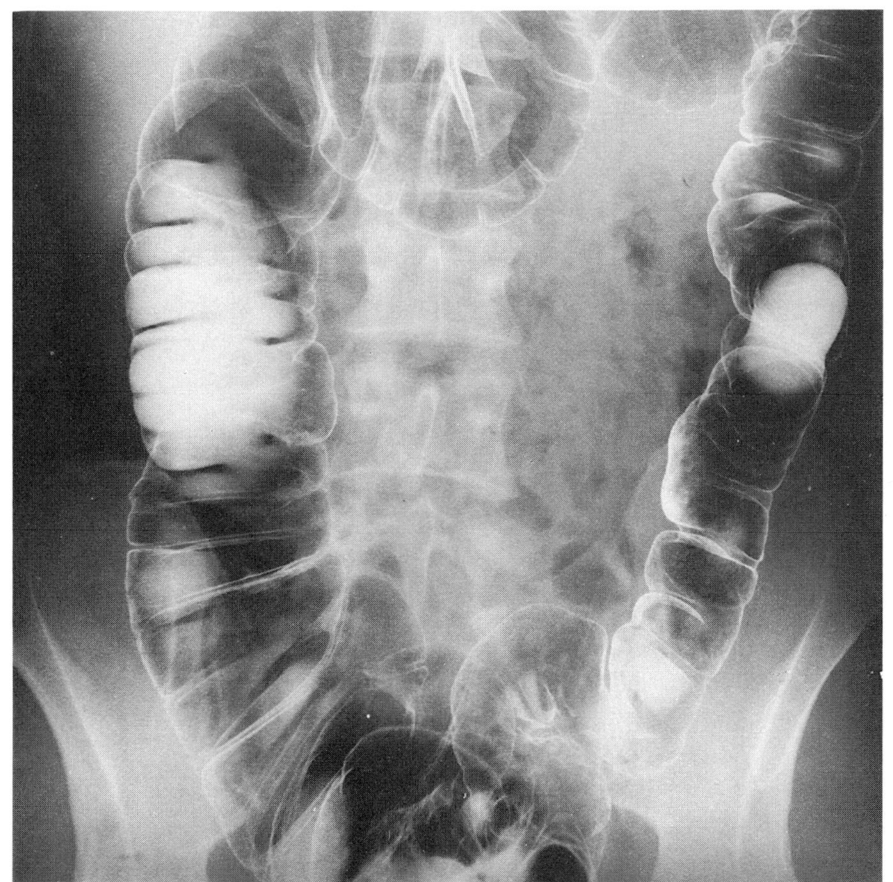

a

b

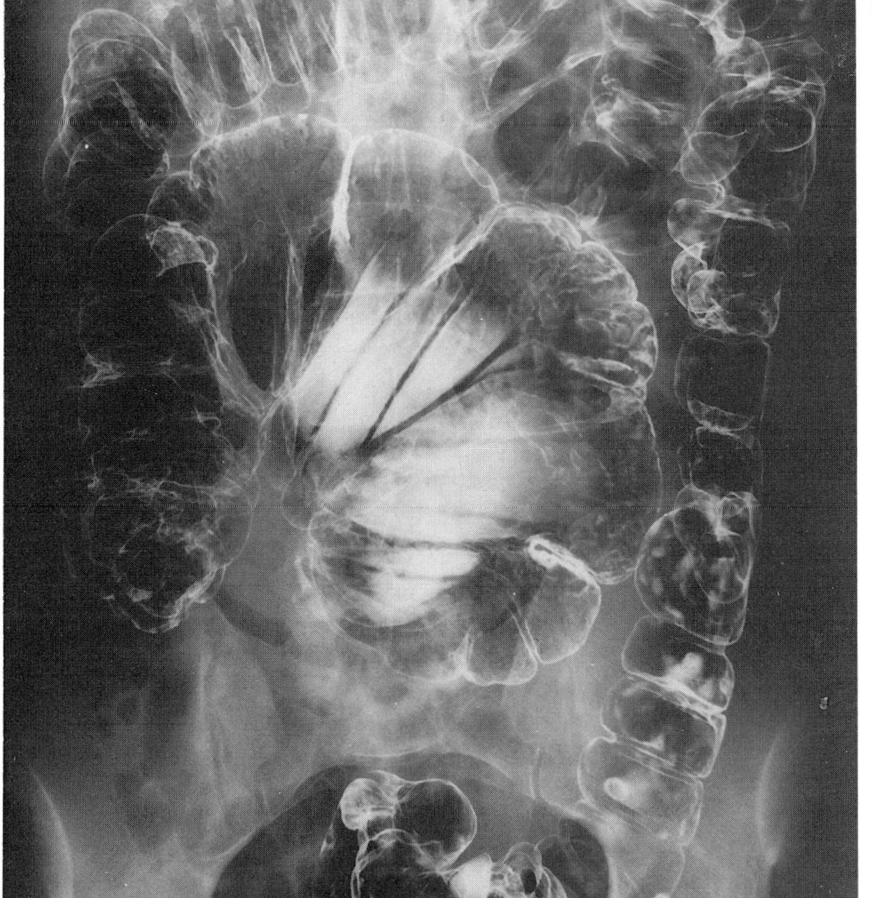

Fig. D.6. (a) The barium enema reveals a normally placed cecum. (b) Following evacuation the patient experienced severe pain, tenderness was present, and the post-evacuation radiograph showed a cecal volvulus. (Courtesy Dr. A. Hemingway (8); copyright, British Institute of Radiology, 1980)

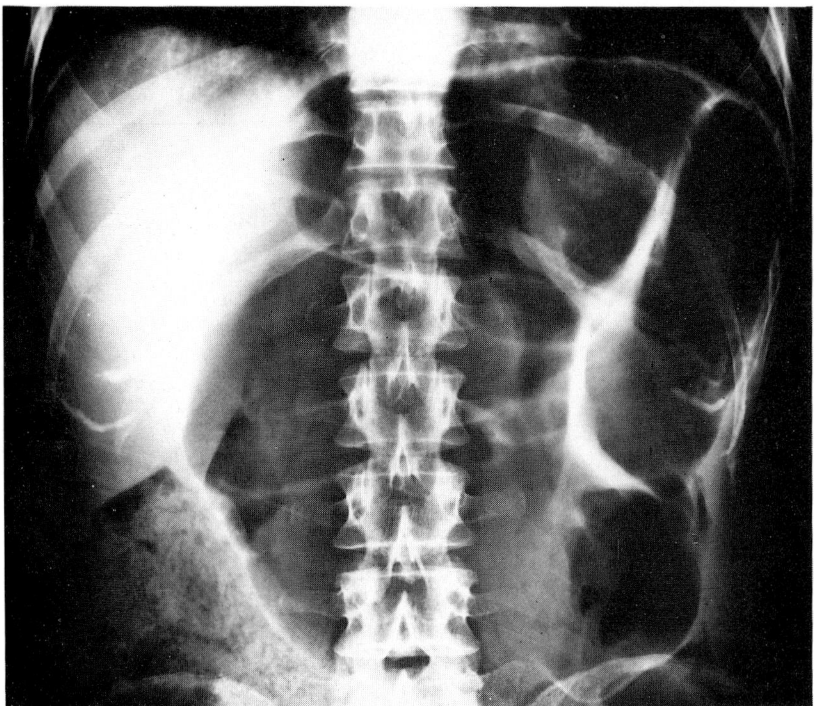

a

b

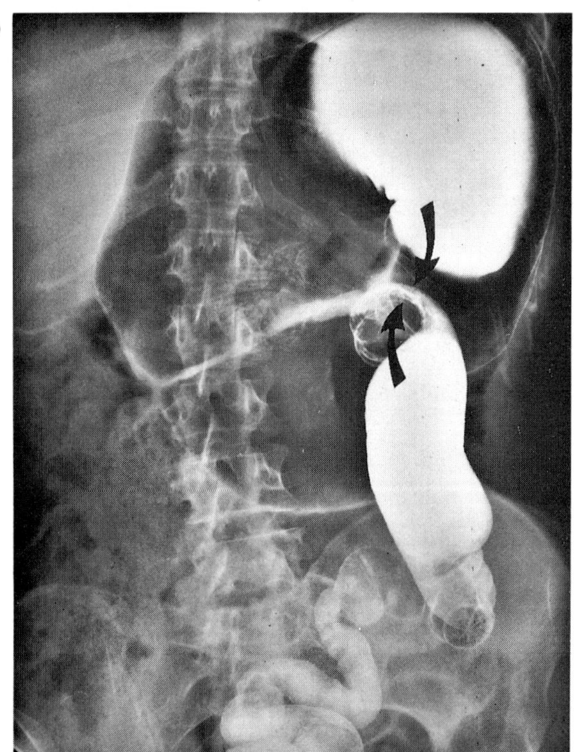

Fig. D.7. Splenic flexure volvulus. (a) There is a greatly dilated loop of colon in the left upper quadrant. Sigmoid volvulus can have a similar appearance. (b) A barium enema reveals an intact sigmoid and a twisted segment in the descending colon (arrows).

cause of the marked distension (21). It is not unusual for the obstructed loop to extend to just beneath the diaphragm. Because the obstructed twist involves both a proximal and a distal segment, not only is there a closed loop obstruction of the sigmoid, but the colon proximal to the sigmoid is also obstructed. It is usual, therefore, to see the greatly distended loop of sigmoid lying vertically in the mid-abdomen or somewhat diagonally to the right, the dilated descending colon lying on the left side lateral to the sigmoid and a dilated ascending colon lying lateral to the sigmoid on the right side. The two sigmoid colon walls, lying side-by-side in the middle, have an appearance of a dense vertical line running from the upper abdomen inferiorly to the pelvis. This distended loop with a mid-line stripe has been called the 'coffee bean' sign (Fig. D.8). If the proximal obstruction is not complete, there is little dilation proximal to the volvulus. Small bowel distension is unusual (21).

With sigmoid volvulus we likewise perform a single-contrast barium enema. The patient is premedicated with glucagon, with glucagon being used simply to decrease spasm and allow better filling of the colon.

A barium enema fills the rectum, with the barium

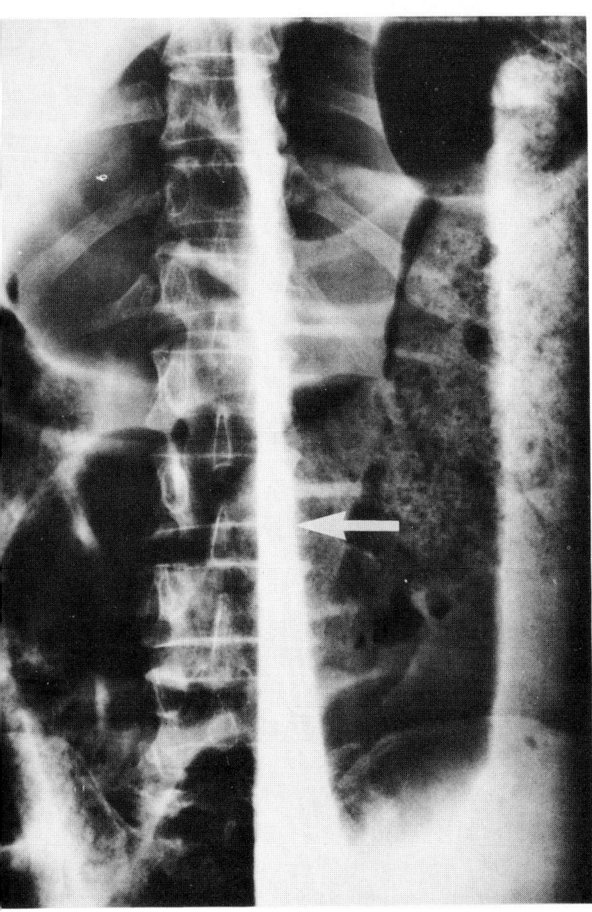

column stopping abruptly at the distal point of obstruction (Fig. D.9). The colon folds here merge together and twist in a characteristic spiral 'bird-beak' configuration. If the retrograde obstruction is not complete, the full extent of the distal obstruction can be identified.

The contraindications to a barium enema are similar to those in patients with cecal volvulus; patients suspected of sigmoid volvulus having signs of peritonitis or radiographic evidence of gas within the bowel wall should not undergo any enema. Likewise, the introduction of a rectal tube or even sigmoidoscopy should be viewed with suspicion if peritonitis is suspected.

Fig. D.8. Sigmoid volvulus. (a) Decubitus and (b) upright radiographs reveal two large loops of colon parallel to each other in the mid-abdomen. A dense vertical stripe (arrow) corresponding to the twisted mesentery and adjacent bowel walls separates the two loops. The ascending and descending portions of the colon, lying laterally, are also considerably dilated.

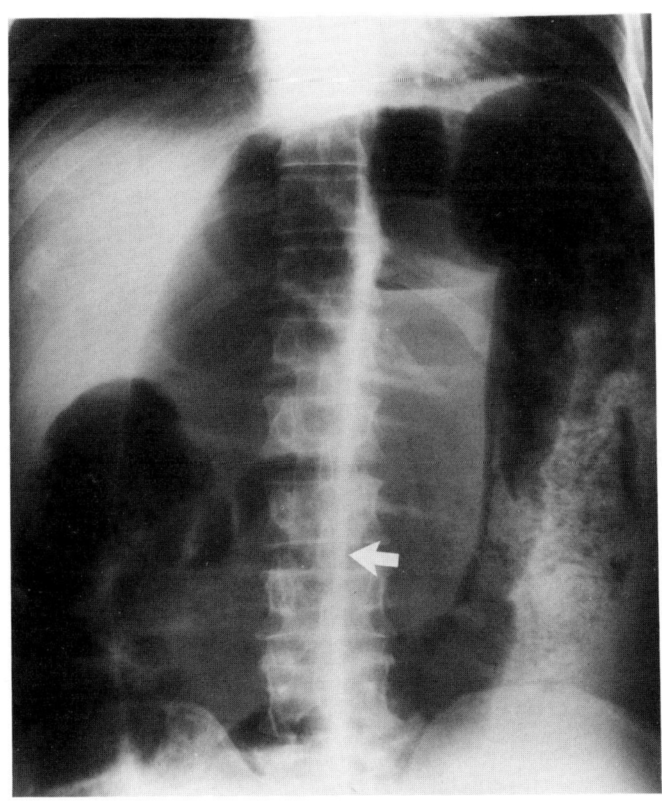

A barium enema can reduce the volvulus. If not successful, sigmoidoscopy and placement of a rectal tube can reduce the volvulus. Unfortunately, after any reduction there is a high recurrence rate and many of these patients eventually undergo surgical resection. Caution is necessary during the attempted reduction to prevent bowel perforation.

If surgery is required, the type of operation will be influenced by the presence or absence of gangrene. Most surgeons tend to resect a generous portion of the sigmoid, because otherwise there can be recurrence of the volvulus (22).

Chronic volvulus involving the sigmoid can reduce spontaneously, with intermittent obstruction or obstipation being the only clue to the underlying disease process. Chronic sigmoid volvulus results in a moderately dilated sigmoid colon with incomplete obstruction, or, with an acute exacerbation, the colon twists around its axis resulting in a tight and complete obstruction that cannot be reduced by a barium enema or sigmoidoscopy.

Some patients, especially those in chronic care institutions, experience multiple bouts of chronic sigmoid volvulus. These patients are obstructed only intermittently. Generally during an acute attack they have signs of complete colon obstruction. Quite often, however, the attack resolves spontaneously and the patient reverts to chronic sigmoid volvulus. A barium enema in these patients with chronic volvulus reveals a redundant sigmoid colon. The colon proximal to the sigmoid can also be considerably dilated depending upon the degree of obstruction. A postevacuation radiograph generally shows considerable retained barium in a hypotonic and dilated colon. Although medical or radiologic decompression can relieve the acute obstruction at any one time, the eventual outcome is resection of the involved colon segment. Whenever these intermittent bouts of volvulus are sufficiently severe or frequent to interfere with the patients well being or life style, surgical therapy should be considered.

In most patients with sigmoid volvulus the diagnosis is readily apparent. Gastric outlet obstruction can result in a very large stomach extending to the right side of the abdomen but the vertical loops of bowel present with sigmoid volvulus are not seen. With small bowel obstruction, regardless of etiology, there generally is marked small bowel distension proximally, with little, if any, gas in the colon. With cecal volvulus the distal colon is collapsed and small bowel distension can be seen. Distal sigmoid

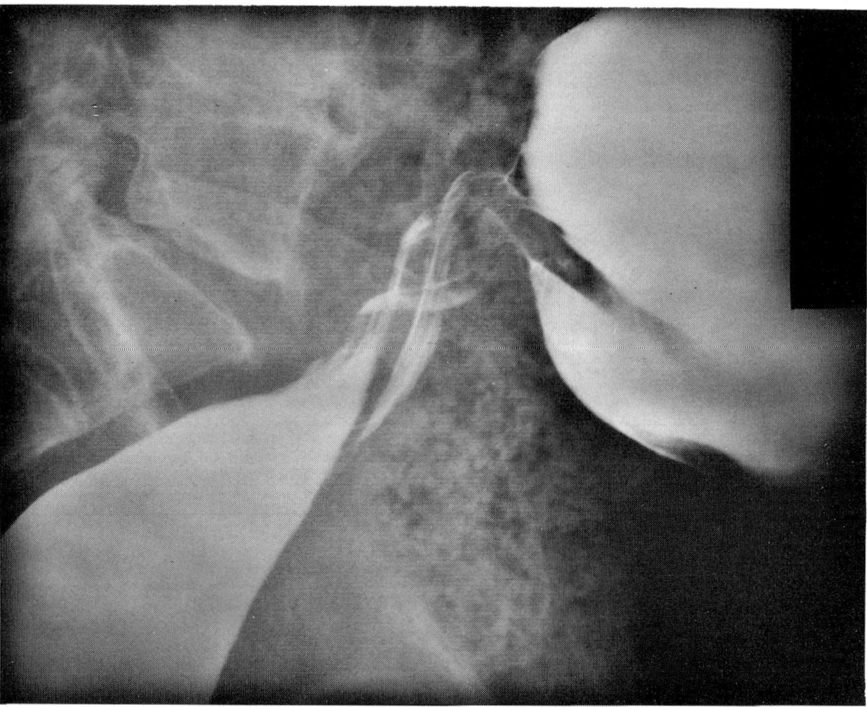

Fig. D.9. Barium enema findings in sigmoid volvulus. A spiral appearance is present at the twist.

obstruction, such as with a carcinoma, may mimic sigmoid volvulus although generally there is less sigmoid distension and more cecal distension. If there is any doubt about the diagnosis, a barium enema provides ready differentiation.

References

1. Kirks DR, Swischuk LE, Merten DF, Filston HC: Cecal volvulus in children. AJR 136:419–422, 1981.
2. Glazer I, Adlersberg D: Volvulus of the colon: a complication of sprue. Gastroenterology 24:159–172, 1953.
3. Simpson AJ, Khilnani MT: Gastrointestinal manifestations of the muscular dystrophies; a review of roentgen findings. AJR 125:948–955, 1975.
4. Greenstein AJ, Kark AE: Sigmoid volvulus in muscular dystrophy. Am J Gastroenterol 57:571–577, 1972.
5. Wecksell A, Gordon LA: Simultaneous double obstruction of the proximal colon: a case report. Gastrointest Radiol 4:303–305, 1979.
6. Kadir S, Athanasoulis CA, Greenfield AJ: Intestinal volvulus: angiographic findings. Radiology 128:595–599, 1978.
7. Young WS: Further radiological observations in cecal volvulus. Clin Radiol 31:479–483, 1980.
8. Hemingway AP: Caecal volvulus — a new twist to the barium enema. Br J Radiol 53:806–807, 1980.
9. Yousefzadeh DK, Teplick JG: Urticaria of the colon. Radiology 132:315–316, 1979.
10. Anderson JR, Lee D, Taylor TV, McLean Ross AH: Volvulus of the transverse colon. Br J Surg 68:179–181, 1981.
11. Lantieri R, Teplick SK, Labell MJ: Splenic flexure volvulus. AJR 132:463–464, 1979.
12. Sachidananthan CK, Soehner B: Volvulus of the splenic flexure of the colon: report of a case and review of the literature. Dis Colon Rectum 15:466–469, 1972.
13. Ghahremani GG, Bowie JD: Volvulus of the splenic flexure: report of a case. Dis Colon Rectum 17:100–102, 1974.
14. Dadoo RC, Keswani RK: Volvulus of the transverse colon in a child: a case report of a rare disorder. Clin Pediatr 16:751–752, 1977.
15. Howell HS, Freeark RJ, Bartizal JF: Transverse colon volvulus in pediatric patients. Arch Surg 111:90, 1976.
16. Zinkin LD, Katz LD, Rosin JD: Volvulus of the transverse colon. Dis Colon Rectum 22:492–496, 1979.
17. Newton NA, Reines HD: Transverse colon volvulus: case reports and review. AJR 128:69–72, 1977.
18. Smith MF, Dalling R: Volvulus of the transverse colon, a long-term complication of hemicolectomy. Dis Colon Rectum 19:684–685, 1976.
19. North LB, Weens HS: The intestinal knot syndrome. AJR 92:1042–1047, 1964.
20. Young WS, White A, Grave GF: The radiology of ileosigmoid knot. Clin Radiol 29:211–216, 1978.
21. Young WS, Engelbrecht HE, Stoker A: Plain film analysis in sigmoid volvulus. Clin Radiol 29:553–560, 1978.
22. Harbrecht PJ, Fry DE: Recurrence of volvulus after sigmoidectomy. Dis Colon Rectum 22:420–424, 1979.

III.4.E. Progressive systemic sclerosis (Scleroderma)

Scleroderma is a systemic disorder of unknown etiology which can involve the gastrointestinal tract. It is seen in adults. In this disease there is excessive deposition of connective tissue in various organs. Collagen tends to predominate. It is postulated that the connective tissue defect is a derangement in collagen degradation (1). It is believed that the functional abnormalities seen are due primarily to atrophy of the muscularis propria and the extensive infiltration by collagen tissue.

Within the gastrointestinal tract, the esophagus is involved in the vast majority of patients; the stomach is least often involved (2). The colon, when involved, presents primarily with dilation and scleroderma is one of the conditions responsible for colon 'pseudo-obstruction' (Ogilvie's syndrome). These patients can have few gastrointestinal symptoms, or, with sufficient involvement there is pain and bloating. Malabsorption can develop. The intestinal lesions often are associated with skin involvement. Likewise, dysphagia secondary to esophageal involvement can occur. The physician must bear in mind that the initial symptoms for some of these patients refer only to the gastrointestinal tract.

Scleroderma is a progressive and relentless disease, although the course is variable. Some patients have a fulminant course while others have episodic periods of exacerbation between times of quiescence. Women are afflicted more often than men, although men have a worse prognosis.

With significant bowel involvement abdominal radiographs show marked dilation of the small bowel and colon. It is not unusual to suspect obstruction on the initial examinations. Occasionally pneumatosis cystoides intestinalis is present.

A barium enema shows an atonic colon with no site of obstruction. The ileocecal valve tends to be wide open. There are relatively large saccular out-pouchings, suggestive of prominent haustra, usually situated on the antimesenteric border of the colon. These out-pouchings probably are caused by atrophy of the underlying muscles. The haustra can be effaced (3) and the colon dilated and elongated. Asymmetrical involvement is common, with part of the colon lacking haustra and another part having accentuation of sacculations. Inconstant contractures are not unusual.

An antegrade small bowel study generally reveals prolonged small bowel transit through considerably dilated bowel. It is not unusual to see barium reach the colon only 24 hours later. Such prolonged stasis in the small bowel can result in bacterial overgrowth and subsequent malabsorption.

Scleroderma is one of the causes of bowel ischemia, subsequent stricture, and perforation (4). The ischemia is secondary to intimal proliferation in the feeding vessels, with subsequent narrowing of the vessel's lumen.

Although barium impaction has been reported in patients with scleroderma (5), presumably similar findings would occur with severe obstipation regardless of etiology. The gastrocolic reflex is absent in patients with scleroderma (6), leading to colon stasis.

Patients with severe scleroderma have been managed with total parenteral nutrition. These patients generally require two to three liters of nutrient solution every 24 hours. The complications encountered include catheter infection, venous thrombosis, and catheter migration. Unfortunately, the annual cost of such total parenteral nutrition averages over $ 24,000 or more (7).

There is no specific treatment for scleroderma.

The loss of haustra is not associated with foreshortening. Thus, scleroderma is readily differentiated from those colitides that lead to inflammation, ulceration, and foreshortening, such as ulcerative colitis. The differential diagnosis includes cathartic colitis and amyloidosis. The history of laxative abuse, if obtainable, should lead to the correct diagnosis. Amyloidosis mimics scleroderma radiographically; however, biopsy of the involved segment should allow a differentiation. If the small bowel is dilated, sprue is in the differential diagnosis. If the peroral jejunal biopsy is normal in clinically and radiologically suspected sprue, scleroderma should be considered in the differential.

References

1. Jiminez SA, Yankowski RI, Frontino PM: Biosynthetic heterogeneity of sclerodermatous skin in organ cultures. J Mol Med 2:423–430, 1977.
2. Olmsted WW, Madewell JE: The esophageal and small bowel manifestations of progressive systemic sclerosis. Gastrointest Radiol 1:33–36, 1976.
3. Martel W, Chang SF, Abell UR: Loss of colonic haustration in progressive systemic sclerosis. AJR 126:704–713, 1976.
4. Battle WM, McLean GK, Brooks JJ, Herlinger H, Trotman BW: Spontaneous perforation of the small intestine due to scleroderma. Dig Dis Sci 24:80–84, 1979.
5. Thompson MA, Summers R: Barium impaction as a complication of gastrointestinal scleroderma. JAMA 235:1715–1717, 1976.
6. Battle WM, Snape WJ, Cohen S, Myers A: Disordered colonic motility in scleroderma. Clin Res 27:577A, 1979.
7. Cohen S, Laufer I, Snape WJ Jr, Shiau Y-F, Levine GM, Jiminez S: The gastrointestinal manifestations of scleroderma: pathogenesis and management. Gastroenterology 79:155–166, 1980.

II.4.F. Pneumatosis intestinalis

Pneumatosis intestinalis is characterized by accumulation of gas in the bowel wall and surrounding structures. It is not necessarily associated with gastrointestinal disease and can be idiopathic in origin. Even if there is underlying gastrointestinal disease, pneumatosis can have little significance or it can be a grave prognostic sign. Pneumatosis intestinalis is not a disease entity but rather a finding usually first seen on radiographs.

Pneumatosis intestinalis consists of multiple gas filled cysts in the wall of the bowel. The cysts may be small or up to several centimeters in diameter. They can increase in size or clear spontaneously (1). An associated pneumoperitoneum is sometimes seen, although the patient's clinical condition is benign. The gas can dissect into the extraperitoneum and extend into the thorax. The pneumoperitoneum presumably is caused by rupture of subserosal cysts. Sigmoidoscopy has revealed these cysts as soft masses protruding into the lumen. If the mass in punctured during sigmoidoscopy the cyst collapses.

In general, patients exhibiting pneumatosis intestinalis and having underlying disease can be divided into two broad groups: 1) those patients with disrupted mucosa and increased intraluminal pressure, and 2) those patients who have an intrinsic abnormality of the bowel wall itself. Disorders of the first group include intestinal obstruction (2, 3), instrumentation (4) and pelvic or abdominal surgery even when the bowel is not resected (5). When obstruction is present, the increased intraluminal pressure causes gas to accumulate in the bowel wall and dissect within the wall.

Disorders in the second group, consisting of an intrinsic abnormality of the bowel wall itself, include bowel ischemia, infiltration, and inflamation. Leukemia (6, 7), lymphoma (8), the various vasculitides (9), and therapy with chemotherapeutic (10) and immunosuppressive (11) drugs have been associated with pneumatosis. Likewise, infection by gas forming organisms (12), inflammation secondary to regional enteritis (4, 13), or appendicitis (14) have resulted in pneumatosis intestinalis. Pneumatosis can be related to underlying malignant disease, secondary ischemic necrosis, or can reflect acute necrotizing enterocolitis because of superimposed infection (15). In particular, in premature infants the presence of pneumatosis should raise the possibility of necrotizing enterocolitis, a relatively lethal disease (3).

An unlikely but real association exists between pneumatosis intestinalis and jejunoileal bypass for obesity (16–20). Either the unbypassed or the bypassed bowel segment can be involved (20). Some associations are poorly understood. Pneumatosis intestinalis has been found in a setting of milk intolerance (21) and in various collagen diseases such as scleroderma (22), systemic lupus erythematosus (23), and dermatomyositis (22, 24). There is a higher than expected incidence of pneumatosis in patients with pyloric stenosis (4). Hepatodia phragmatic interposition of the colon, or Chilaiditi's syndrome (25), is likewise associated with pneumatosis (4).

No single etiology of pneumatosis intestinalis is known. There probably are several etiologies for the formation of these cysts. Pneumatosis in some patients with the vasculitides is probably caused by localized ischemia and resultant necrotizing enterocolitis (9). If *Clostridium perfringens* is injected into the bowel wall of germ-free rats, eventually an appearance similar to pneumatosis intestinalis develops (26). Similarly, after mucosal injury and bowel distension, a pneumatosis may be produced.

These patients can be asymptomatic or have nonspecific bowel complaints ranging from pain to diarrhea and occasional bleeding. The pneumatosis by itself seldom requires treatment. When the pneumatosis is produced by an underlying disease, treatment of that disease generally results in clearing of the pneumatosis.

In most patients no therapy is necessary and the pneumatosis clears spontaneously. Some investigators advocate a high concentration of oxygen and claim relatively successful results (27, 28), although oxygen therapy can be justified only for symptomatic patients because of possible pulmonary damage with prolonged oxygen exposure (29).

The early authors noted a preponderance of small bowel involvement; most recent reports stress colon involvement, with left colic involvement being not unusual. The cysts may be either in the submucosa or subserosa in location. Although some investigators try to differentiate between the submucosal and subserosal locations and try to associate each with a particular etiology, there is sufficient overlap that such a differentiation is not practical.

In the vast majority of patients an acute abdominal examination readily discloses the pneumatosis (27, 30). There is a mottled appearance around the colon circumference. These oval or linear lucencies alongside the colon lumen vary considerably in appearance (Fig. F.1). Occasionally

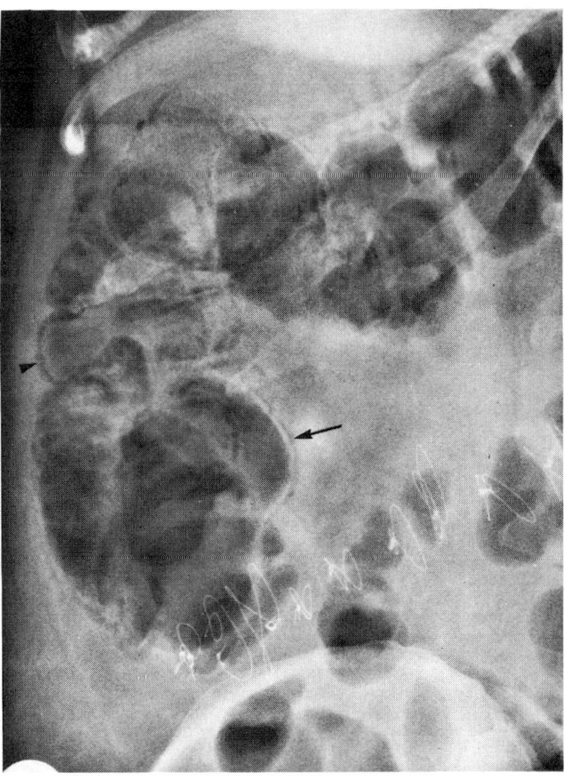

Fig. F.1. Pneumatosis intestinalis of the right colon. Linear collections of gas are present in the wall of the colon (arrows). The patient was 4 weeks after surgery for jejunoileal bypass. (Courtesy of Drs. J. Wandtke et al. (20); copyright 1977, ARRS.)

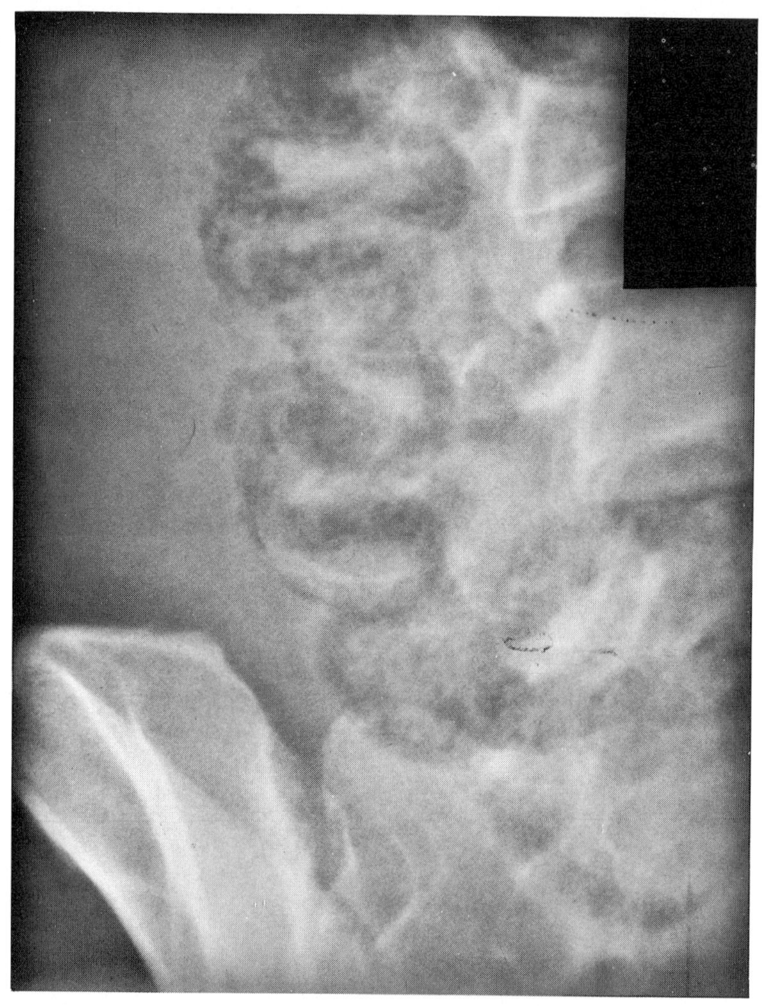

a

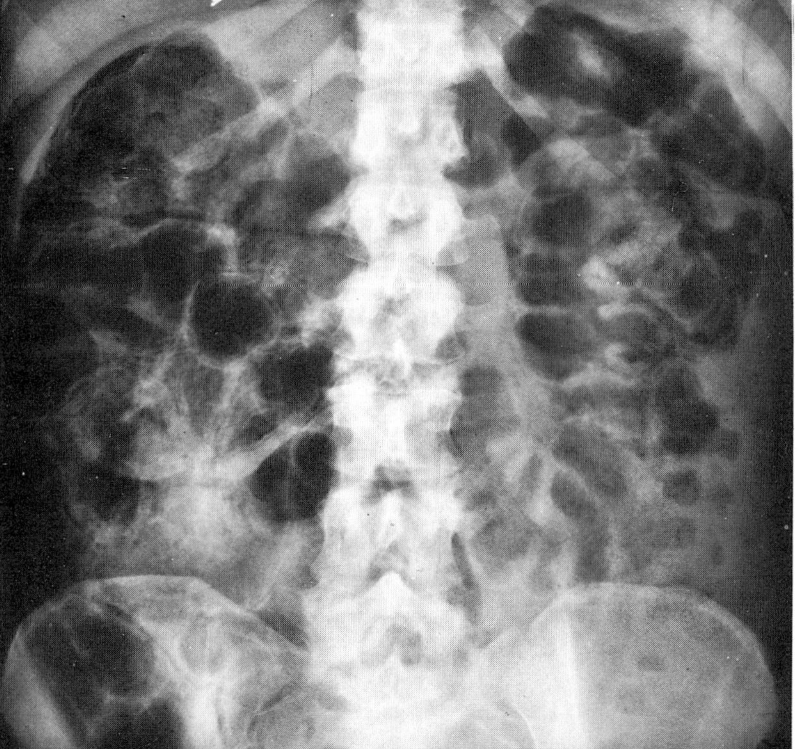

b

Fig. F.2. (a) Extensive pneumatosis is present in the right colon. The mottled appearance is similar to that seen with retained stool. (b) Another patient with pneumatosis intestinalis throughout the small bowel and colon and superimposed pneumoperitoneum. Such a prominent mottled appearance strongly suggests pneumatosis. (Courtesy of Drs. J. Wandtke et al. (20); copyright 1977, ARRS.)

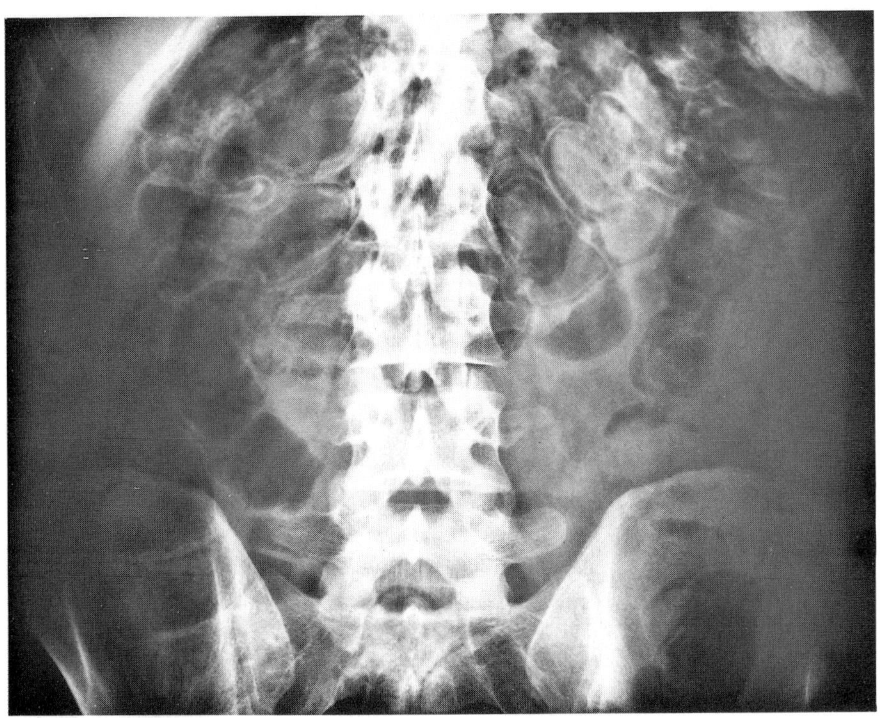

Fig. F.3. Nineteen-year-old male with leukemia developed fever, nausea, and vomiting after marrow transplantation. (a) A supine radiograph shows extensive pneumatosis surrounding the transverse colon. Both the inner and outer bowel margins are clearly seen. (b) Left lateral decubitus radiograph reveals extensive extra-peritoneal gas (arrows). The gas was not free in the peritoneal cavity because it did not rise to the uppermost part of the abdomen.

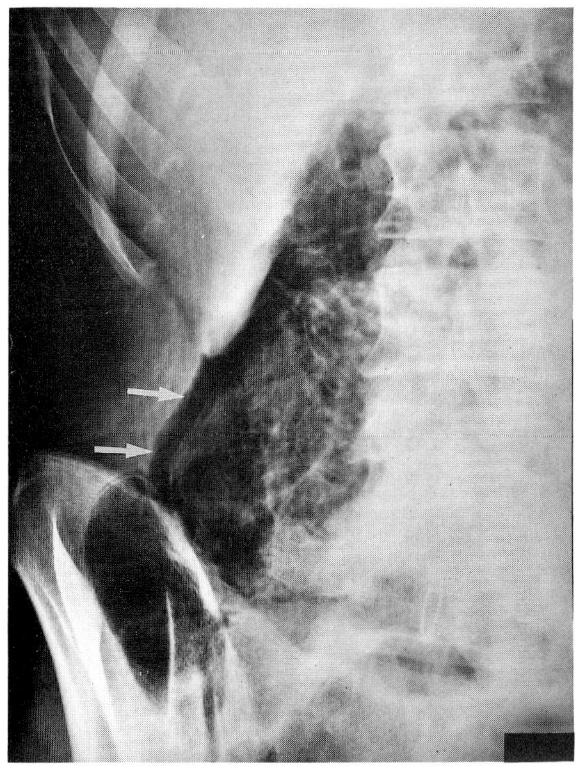

their shape makes differentiation from bowel content difficult (Fig. F.2). Usually only one segment of the colon is involved. Chest radiographs and decubitus radiographs of the abdomen will reveal if there has been extension of the pneumatosis to the peritoneal cavity, extraperitoneal structures, or spread into the thorax (Fig. F.3).

Occasionally, when there is a question whether these cysts are present, a barium enema will identify the gas outside of the bowel lumen. A barium enema will outline the gas-filled cysts by barium intraluminally and by the soft-tissue content of the abdomen outside of the colon wall (Fig. F.4). If the actual cyst wall can be identified, it is seen as a thin soft-tissue density adjacent to the colon lumen.

The diagnosis is usually relatively clear. If the gas content of the cysts cannot be identified, confusion exists with a lymphosarcoma (31); gas-filled cysts are not seen with lymphosarcoma (32). Thus, technically excellent radiographs are necessary for the early identification of these cysts. In colitis cystica profunda the rectum is usually involved, while in

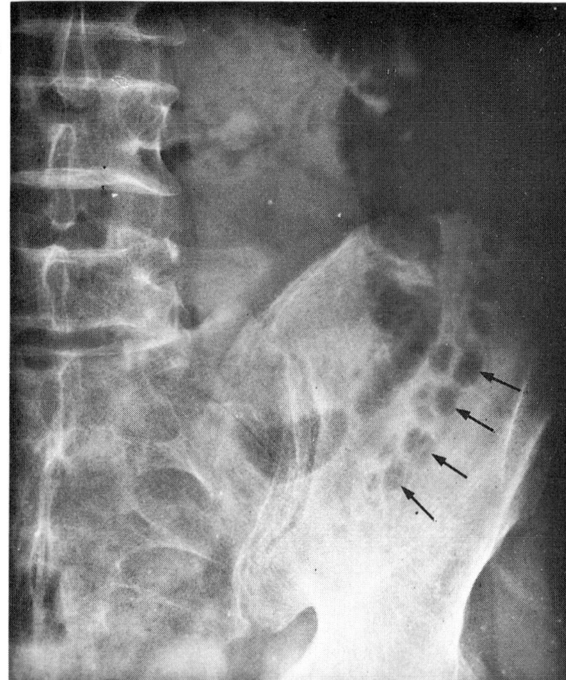

a

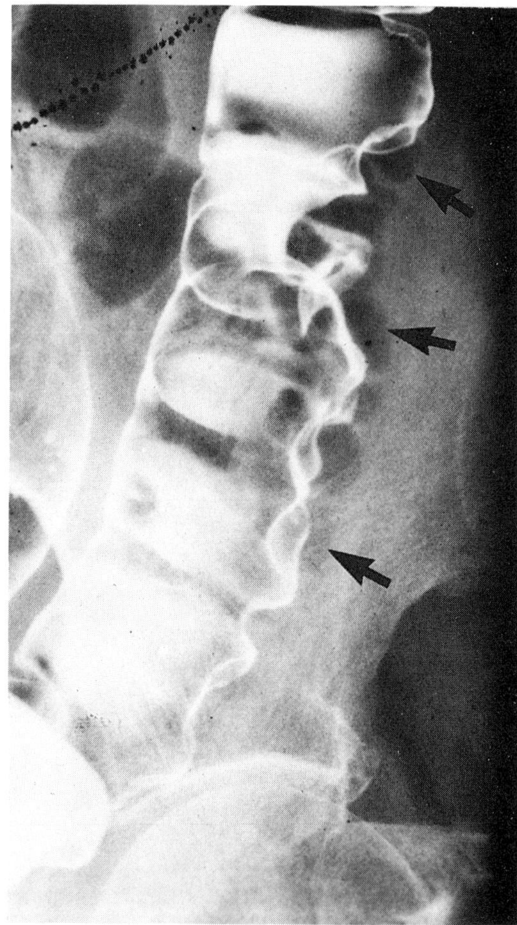

b

Fig. F.4. An asymptomatic 38-year-old male is followed for prior peptic ulcer disease. (a) Initial radiograph reveals unusual gas pockets in the left lower quadrant (arrows). (b) A barium enema shows that the gas is intramural in location. The colon lumen is markedly irregular in the involved segment (arrows).

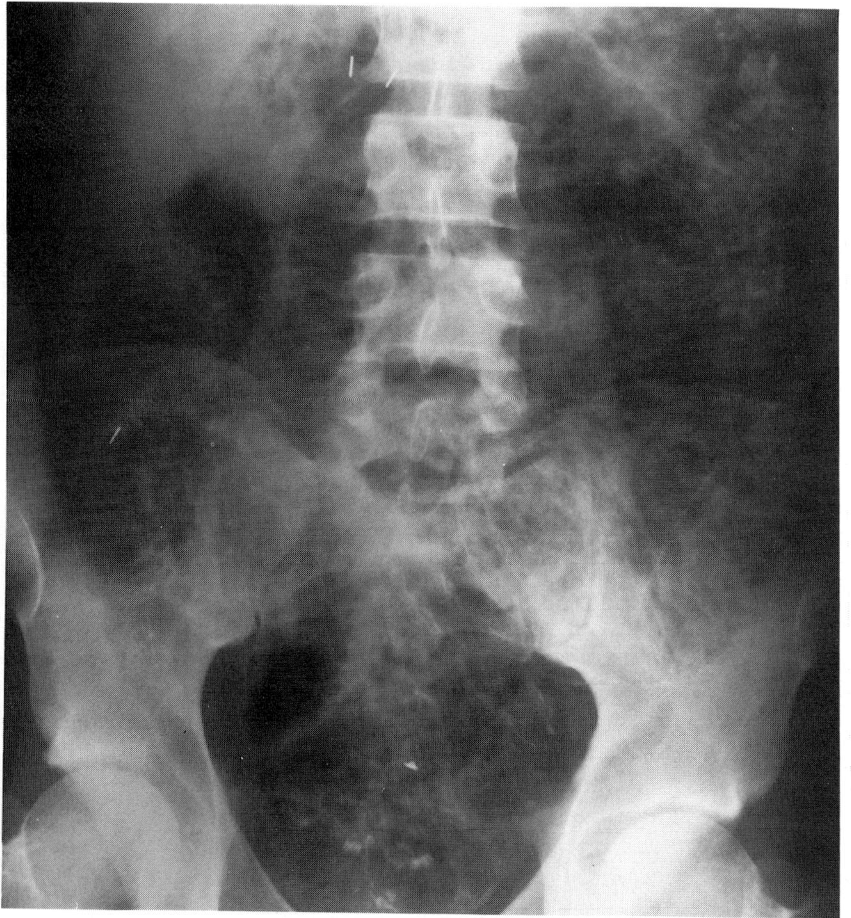

Fig. F.5. A 31-year-old male underwent resection of a transverse colon carcinoma. Surgery included dissection at the base of the mesentery. One week later the patient developed abdominal pain and an acute abdominal examination revealed a mottled pattern throughout the abdomen. The possibility of a major vascular accident was raised, but the patient's relatively benign condition pointed towards pneumatosis intestinalis. The intramural gas cleared gradually over the next several weeks.

pneumatosis intestinalis the rectum usually is spared. With rectal involvement the possibility of ischemia rather than benign pneumatosis should be considered. In general, ischemia and subsequent gas production can mimic benign pneumatosis (Fig. F.5). Yet even here the patient's clinical condition and the presence of any underlying disease aid in the differentiation.

Gas in the portal vein tributaries, in adults, should alert one to bowel ischemia and necrosis. Benign pneumatosis does not result in portal vein gas.

References

1. Bloch C: The natural history of pneumatosis coli. Radiology 123:311–314, 1977.
2. Shallal JA, Van Heerden JA, Bartholomew LG, Cain JC: Pneumatosis cystoides intestinalis. Mayo Clin Proc 49:180–184, 1974.
3. Robinson AE, Glossman H, Brumley GW: Pneumatosis intestinalis in the neonate. AJR 120:333–341, 1974.
4. Meyers MA, Ghahremani GG, Clements JL Jr, Goodman K: Pneumatosis intestinalis. Gastrointest Radiol 2:91–105, 1977.
5. Wenz W, Stremmel W: Seltene Ursache einer 'intramuralen' Gasansammlung im rechten Colon. Radiologe 15:442–445, 1975.
6. Jaffe N, Carlson DH, Vawtes GF: Pneumatosis cystoides intestinalis in acute leukemia. Cancer 30:239–243, 1972.
7. Keats TE, Smith TH: Benign pneumatosis intestinalis in childhood leukemia. AJR 122:150–152, 1974.
8. O'Connell DJ, Thompson AJ: Pneumatosis coli in non-Hodgkins lymphoma. Br J Radiol 51:203–205, 1978.
9. Kleinman P, Meyens MA, Abbott G, Kazam E: Necrotizing enterocolitis with pneumatosis intestinalis in systemic lupus erythematosus and polyarteritis. Radiology 121:595–598, 1976.
10. Shindelman LE, Geller SA, Wisch N, Bauer JJ: Pneumatosis cystoides intestinalis. A complication of systemic chemotherapy. Am J Gastroenterol 75:270–274, 1981.
11. Borns PF, Johnston TA: Indolent pneumatosis of the bowel wall associated with immune suppressive therapy. Ann Radiol 16:163–166, 1973.
12. Reyna R, Soper RT, Condon RE: Pneumatosis intestinalis. Am J Surg 125:667–671, 1973.
13. Ghahremani GG, Port RB, Beachley MC: Pneumatosis coli in Crohn's disease. Am J Dig Dis 19:315–323, 1974.
14. DiDonato LR: Pneumatosis coli secondary to acute appendicitis. Radiology 120:90, 1976.
15. Smith EEJ, Saunders JH, Bowley N: Pneumatosis intestinalis in the small bowel of an adult — a radiological sign of a serious post-operative complication. Br J Radiol 54:266–267, 1981.
16. Passaro E Jr, Drenick E, Wilson SE: Bypass enteritis. Am J Surg 131:169–173, 1976.
17. Martyak SN, Curtis LE: Pneumatosis intestinalis: a complication of jejunoileal bypass. JAMA 235:1038–1039, 1976.
18. Sicard GA, Vaughan R, Wise L: Pneumatosis cystoides intestinalis: an unusual complication of jejunoileal bypass. Surgery 79:480–484, 1976.
19. Menguy R: Pneumatosis intestinalis after jejunoileal bypass. Etiological mechanism in one case. JAMA 236:1721–1723, 1976.
20. Wandtke J, Skucas J, Spataro R, Bruneau RJ: Pneumatosis intestinalis as a complication of jejunoileal bypass. AJR 129:601–604, 1977.
21. Aziz EM: Neonatal pneumatosis intestinalis associated with milk intolerance. Am J Dis Child 125:560–562, 1973.
22. Mueller CF, Morehead R, Alter AJ, Michener W: Pneumatosis intestinalis in collagen disorders. AJR 115:300–305, 1972.
23. Freiman D, Chon HK, Bilaniuk L: Pneumatosis intestinalis in systemic lupus erythematosus. Radiology 116:563–564, 1975.
24. Oliveros MA, Herbst JJ, Lester PD, Ziter FA: Pneumatosis intestinalis in childhood dermatomyositis. Pediatrics 52:711–712, 1973.
25. Chilaiditi D: Zur Frage der Hepatoptose und Ptose im Allgemeinen im Anschluss und drei Fälle von temporärer, partieller Leberverlagerung. Fortschr Geb Roentgenstr 16:173–208, 1910-11.
26. Yale CE, Balish E, Wu JP: The bacterial etiology of pneumatosis cystoides intestinalis. Arch Surg 109:89–94, 1974.
27. O'Connell DJ, Dewbury KC, Green B, Wyatt AP: The plain abdominal radiograph in pneumatosis coli. Clin Radiol 27:563–568, 1976.
28. Gruenberg JC, Batra SK, Priest RJ: Treatment of pneumatosis cystoides intestinalis with oxygen. Arch Surg 112:62–64, 1977.
29. Simon NM, Nyman KE, Divertie MB, Rovelstad RA, King JE: Pneumatosis cystoides intestinalis: treatment with oxygen via close fitting mask. JAMA 231:1354–1356, 1975.
30. Olmsted WW, Madewell JE: Pneumatosis cystoides intestinalis: a pathophysiologic explanation of the roentgenographic signs. Gastrointest Radiol 1:177–181, 1976.
31. Marshak RH, Lindner AE, Milano AM: Pneumatosis coli. Am J Gastroenterol 56:68–73, 1971.
32. Marshak RH, Lindner AE, Maklansky D: Pneumatosis cystoides coli. Gastrointest Radiol 2:85–89, 1977.

III.4.G. Developmental abnormalities

Developmental abnormalities are of major importance in pediatric radiology, although some are also significant in adults. These abnormalities are covered here only superficially, and provide only an introduction to the field. Fuller discussions are available in pediatric radiology texts.

Some of the conditions encountered in adults, such as volvulus or internal herniation, cannot occur readily without an associated development abnormality. Because the clinical presentation depends upon an acquired condition superimposed upon a developmental anomaly, these entitites are discussed separately.

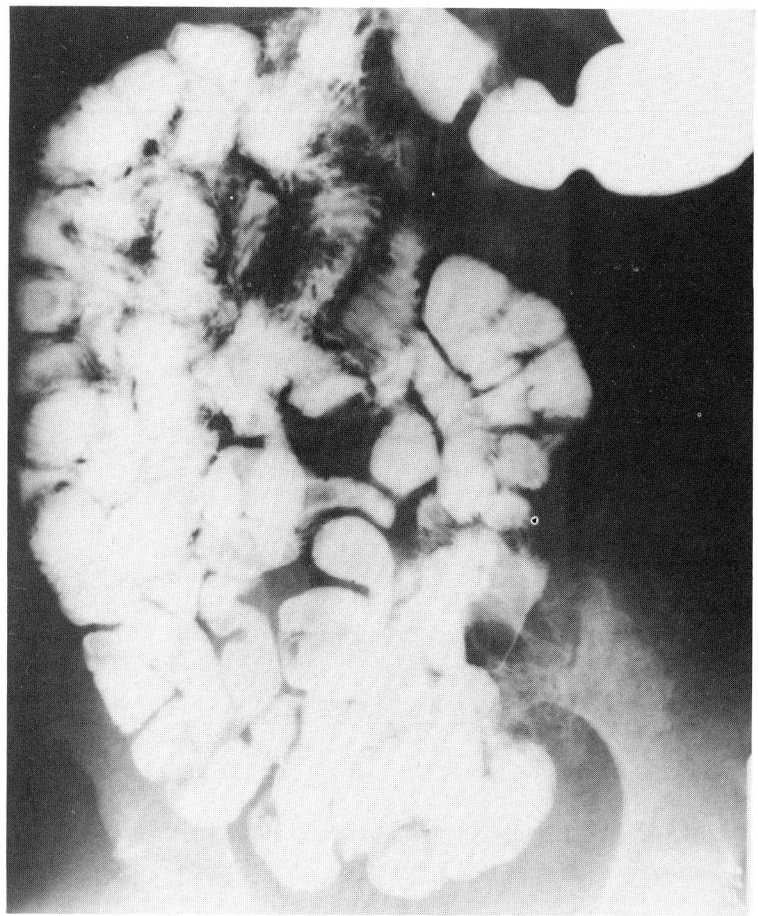

a

b

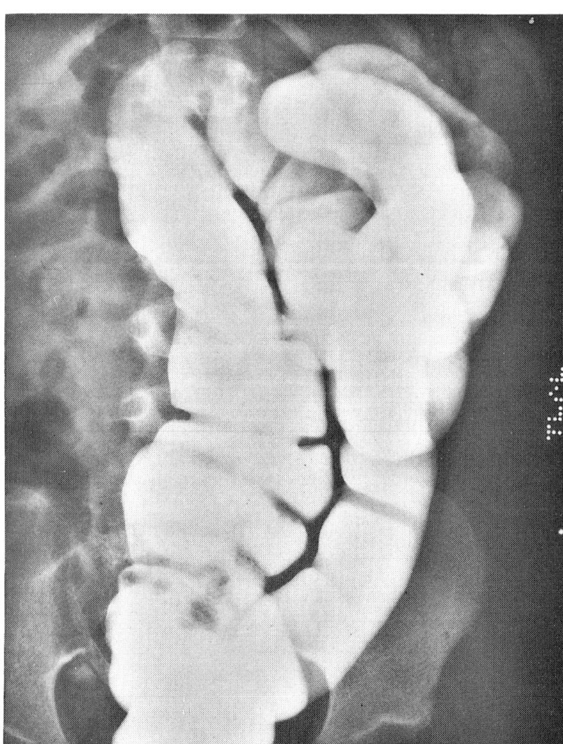

Fig. G.1. (a) Mid-gut nonrotation. The entire small bowel lies on the right side of the abdomen. The patient had had multiple bouts of obstruction. (b) Another patient with nonrotation. The ascending and descending portions of the colon lie parallel to each other on the left side of the abdomen.

a. Malrotation

Malrotation of the colon is generally but not always associated with small bowel malrotation. An arrest in rotation can occur at any time during the embryonic mid-gut development. It is not unusual to see minor degrees of malrotation in adults. With partial rotation of the proximal portion of the mid-gut, the colon can be in normal position, and vice versa (1, 2). By themselves these changes are usually not associated with any clinical problems and some radiologists look upon them simply as variations of normal.

With reversed rotation of the bowel, the cecum lies essentially in its usual position, but the transverse colon is more posterior in location and the small bowel lies anteriorly. With failure of full rotation, the small bowel lies on the right side of the abdomen and the cecum is either on the left or in the midline. Generally the ascending colon still has a mesentery. Thus the radiographic picture is of small bowel filling the right side of the abdomen and the ascending and descending colon being on the left side (Fig. G.1). Because the entire bowel is supported by a single mesentery, such bowel is prone to volvulus. However, if the patient reaches adulthood without any such complication, the malrotation is then usually regarded as a curiosity. In symptomatic patients, an associated volvulus should be considered.

With abnormal fixation of the cecum, the cecum is located either superior to its usual position and lies close to the normal hepatic flexure, with a long mesentery lies inferiorly in the pelvis, or extends across the midline to the left (Fig. G.2).

Hepatodiaphragmatic colon interposition, known as Chilaiditi's syndrome, is due to acquired factors and not to malrotation or abnormal fixation (3).

b. Situs inversus

If situs inversus is complete, it involves reversal of both the intrathoracic and the intraabdominal organs. If incomplete, only the intraabdominal organs may be involved. Incomplete situs inversus in adults generally represents a curiosity. Complete situs inversus, in association with bronchiectasis and nasal sinus abnormalities is known as Kartagener's syndrome.

c. Atresia

Atresia of the rectum is not an uncommon entity in pediatric radiology. This condition can be divided into low, intermediate, and high atresia or stenosis. Colon atresia outside of the rectum is rare. The atresia is probably a result of intrauterine bowel ischemia.

Although some radiologists use a head-down position to evaluate the atresia (Fig. G.3), it can sometimes be difficult to estimate the length of the atretic segment. A radiopaque marker at the anus or the distal point of obstruction may not adequately outline the atretic segment; colon gas may not be present to the level of obstruction. Whether the obstruction is high or low in the rectum can be gauged by any associated genitourinary abnormalities. A high obstruction should reveal a fistula to the genitourinary tract. Thus a cystogram may define the colorectal abnormality in these patients. The high atresias can also be associated with sacral abnormalities. An international classification has been proposed to describe these abnormalities (4).

A barium enema reveals a small caliber distal colon up to the point of obstruction and dilated, gas-filled bowel proximally. In general, the more distal the stricture or atresia, the smaller will be the colon lumen distal to the obstruction. Similar changes are seen in acquired microcolon in adults where a proximal colostomy had been performed years previously (5).

Atresia must be differentiated from meconium obstruction. Generally, a contrast enema allows differentiation of these entities and pinpoints the site of obstruction. Obstruction by meconium can be subdivided further; if a contrast study is performed, meconium ileus reveals an unused small colon distal to the obstruction, while the inspissated meconium syndrome has a normal distal colon (6).

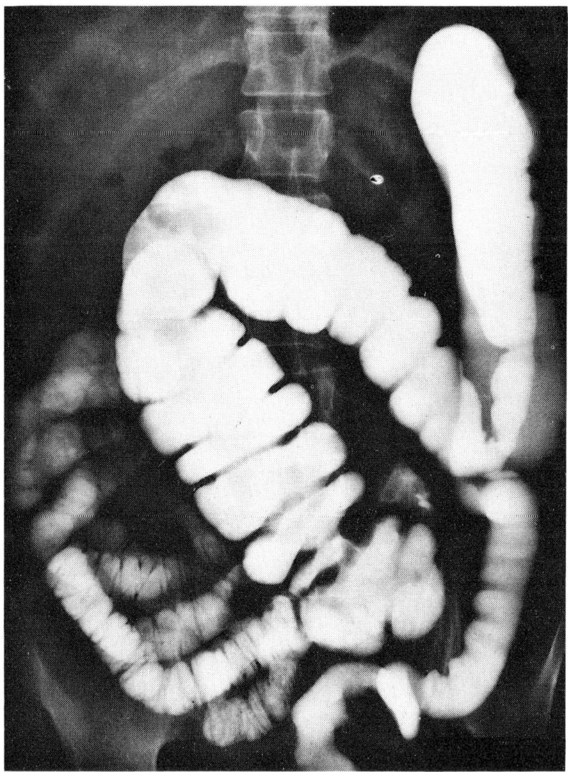

Fig. G.2. Mobile cecum and ascending colon. The entire right colon is on a mesentery and the cecum extends to the left lower quadrant (See also Fig. D.1., page 313).

An absent or partial rectovaginal septum is occasionally encountered (Fig. G.4). Although some of these are congenital in origin, many are acquired.

d. Bands

Fibrous bands may occasionally obstruct the colon, with the most common site being in the cecum. In adults it may not be possible to differentiate between obstruction caused by congenital bands and bands secondary to inflammation and adhesions (Fig. G.5).

Ladd's bands (7) are attached to a nonrotated or partly rotated cecum and generally result in duodenal obstruction. The majority of these patients are in the pediatric age group. Most adults are either asymptomatic or present with intermittent partial obstruction.

Peritoneal bands passing over the ascending colon (Jackson's membrane) can occasionally narrow the colon lumen sufficiently enough to result in obstruction. Similar bands can occasionally be encountered in the ileum.

e. Duplication

The more complex colon duplications are generally

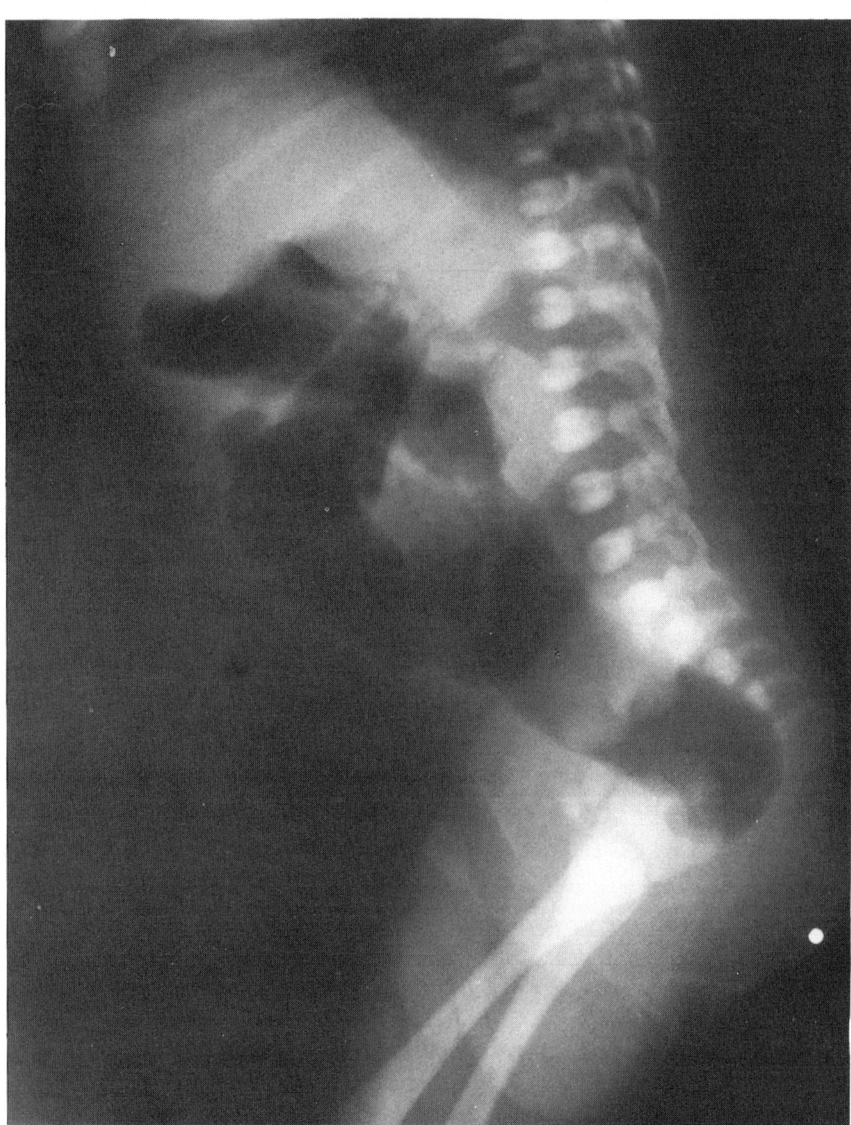

Fig. G.3. Imperforate anus, low type. A lead marker has been placed at the anus and the infant held in a head down position. Gas outlines the colon and part of the rectum.

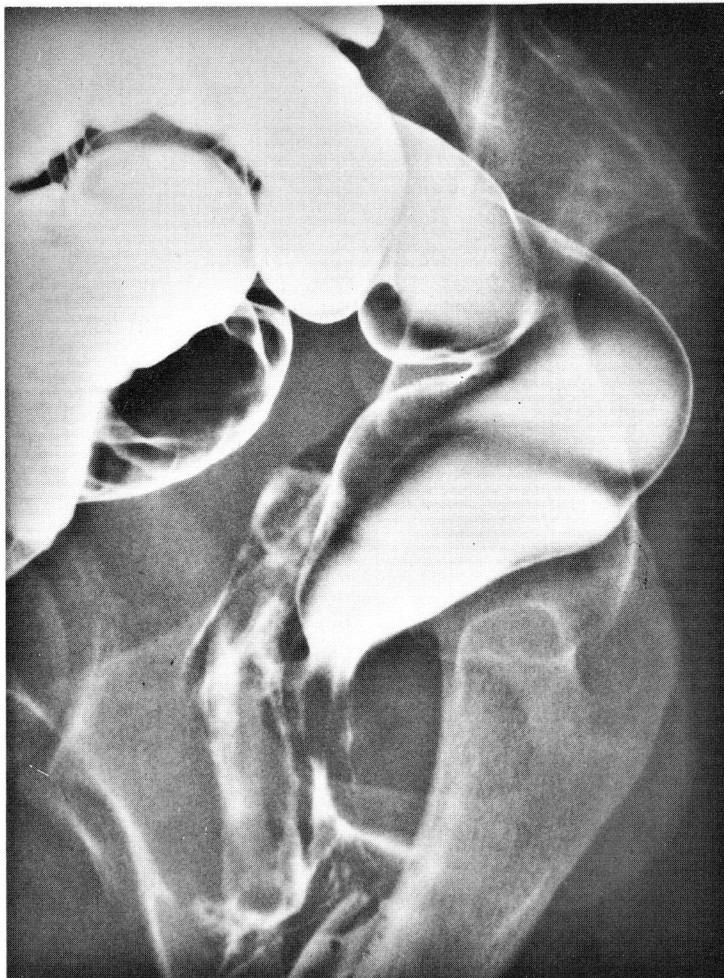

Fig. G.4. The inferior part of the recto-vaginal septum is absent in this 22-year-old patient. She has had two normal deliveries; trauma during delivery could result in identical findings.

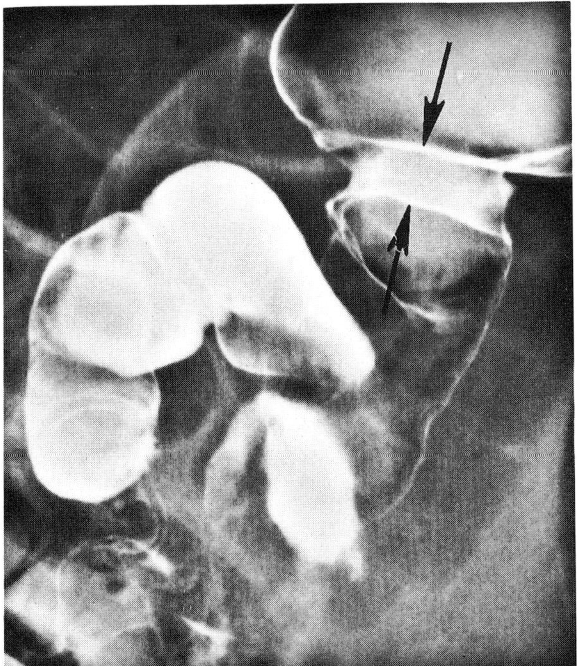

a

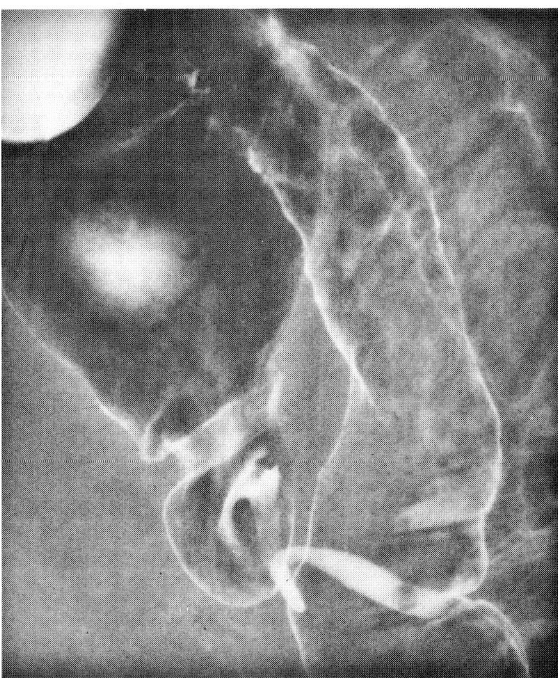

b

Fig. G.5. (a) A 62-year-old patient with right lower quadrant pain was found to have a small cecum and a circumferential 'band' (arrows) in the ascending colon. Numerous adhesions were lysed during surgery and presumably the patient's symptoms were secondary to partial obstruction. The resected cecum showed extensive fibrosis and ulcerations. (b) Another 62-year-old patient with right lower quadrant pain. The cecum is small and a 'band' surrounds the proximal portion of the cecum.

seen in the pediatric age group. There may be associated small bowel duplication. Most duplications occur in the ileum; only occasional ones are described in the colon (8). They are located on the mesenteric border of the colon. Associated genitourinary or bone abnormalities are not uncommon (9, 10) and an excretory urogram should be considered when a duplication is found. The duplication occasionally communicates with the colon although the majority do not. When the duplication does not communicate with the colon it is filled with fluid and can thus mimic an enteric cyst. A colon duplication usually has a muscle lining and a mucosa. Some of the colon duplications are lined by gastric mucosa (8).

A noncommunicating colon duplication can present as an abdominal mass. Because of secretion, the duplication can grow and result in obstruction of the adjoining colon. It can also act as the lead point for an intussusception. Both the communicating and noncommunicating duplications can ulcerate and bleed.

If the duplication is sufficiently large, radiographs reveal a round or tube-like configuration with possible displacement of adjacent organs. A communicating duplication can fill with gas and occasionally abdominal radiographs show two parallel collections of gas. A barium enema reveals colon compression by the extrinsic mass or a communicating duplication fills with contrast. Occasionally the duplication will fill only on the postevacuation radiographs (11). Rarely a duplication drains externally through the perineum and as a result it has a narrow caliber and a spiral appearance (12).

Both adenocarcinoma (13) and squamous cell carcinoma (14) have been reported in a duplication. If the duplication communicates with the colon, a mass in the duplication seen on a barium enema should raise suspicion for neoplasm.

f. Hirschsprung's disease

A greatly dilated colon with a narrowed distal segment was first described by Hirschsprung in 1888 (15). This disease is more common in males and there is some evidence for a familial inheritance. It is unusual in premature infants, but has been reported (16). There appears to be an increased incidence in mongolism.

This condition is most commonly found in infancy, although with mild involvement, the disease can manifest itself later in life (17). These children present with varying degrees of distal colon obstruction, and biopsy reveals absent ganglion cells from a narrowed segment in the distal colon and rectum. Why the aganglionotic segment does not dilate is not known. The aganglionotic segment ends at the anus. Skip areas are only rarely found (18).

Most of these patients have an abnormal barium enema and abnormal rectal manometry (19, 20). Occasionally either one or the other test is normal in a patient with subsequently proven Hirschsprung's disease. The radiographic changes tend to become more apparent sometime after birth; it may take time and use for the proximal portion of the colon to become sufficiently dilated (Fig. G.6).

These patients should not have any cleansing procedures prior to the barium enema, because the aganglionic segment may be dilated by the cleansing enemas and the transition zone not seen (19, 20). A barium enema shows a narrowed distal segment that can vary in length (Fig. G.7). Occasionally, a long narrowed segment is seen, with the disease extending far proximally.

The rectosigmoid index is obtained by dividing the widest diameter of the rectum by the widest diameter of the sigmoid (21). The dimensions are taken from a fully distended colon during a barium enema. If the index is less than 0.8, aganglionosis of the rectosigmoid should be suspected (22). Unfortunately the index is of little value if aganglionosis involves longer segments. Some radiologists rely extensively on retention of barium for 24 or even 48 hours to make the diagnosis of Hirschsprung's disease. While suggestive, other conditions can likewise lead to prolonged barium retention. It should be realized that Hirschsprung's disease cannot be *absolutely* excluded from a barium enema examination.

Rarely encountered is aganglionosis of the entire colon and even of the distal small bowel (23). A barium enema reveals a relatively narrow colon, small bowel dilatation proximally and no obvious obstructive lesion. Rapid reflux occurs into the ileum. There is considerable retention of barium in the colon, sometimes for days, and the colon tends to be foreshortened.

The diagnosis of Hirschsprung's disease can be established by an appropriate biopsy. Unfortunately, occasionally normal ganglion cells are present yet the patient's clinical and radiological findings still suggest Hirschsprung's disease. This condition has been called the adynamic bowel syndrome (24). Although ganglion cells are present, it is postulated that there is an abnormality in innervation. Study of the ganglion cells in these patients shows immaturity and a decreased number of ganglion cells (25) and an absent nerve network linking the ganglion cells (24).

A dilated colon can be seen in other conditions, such as partial distal colon obstruction and adynamic ileus. A dilated colon is associated with various neurological disorders, including spinal cord deformities. An association between total aganglionosis of the colon and congenital failure of automatic control of ventilation may exist (25). In the neonate, other diseases resulting in a dilated proximal colon include meconium plug syndrome, colon atresia and stricture. The meconium plug

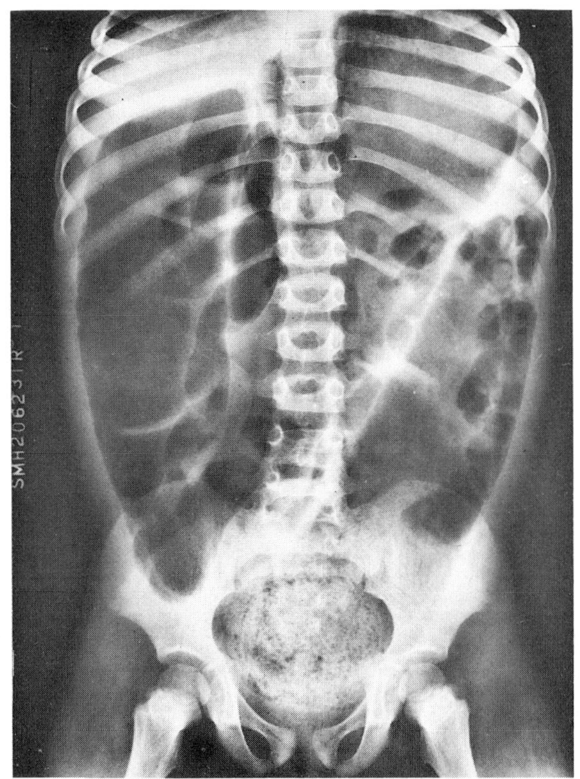

a

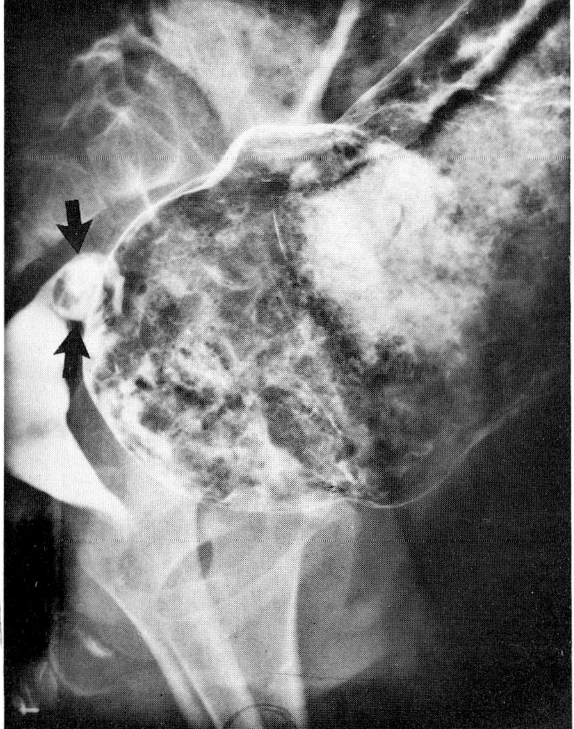

b

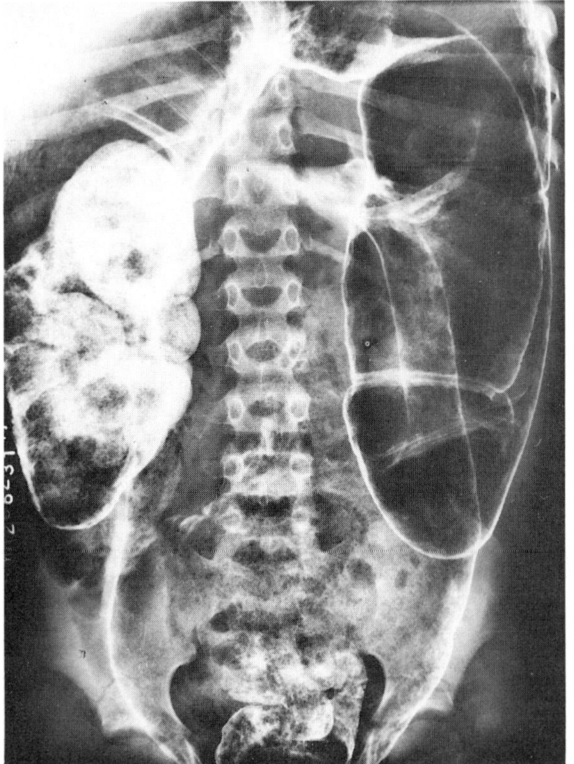

c

Fig. G.6. Five year old boy with constipation since birth. (a) A supine radiograph reveals colon dilatation. (b) The lateral rectal radiograph from a barium enema several years later shows the narrowed transition zone (arrows). (c) A postevacuation radiograph reveals the massive colon dilatation that had occurred in this patient. The resected portion of the colon showed absent myenteric ganglia.

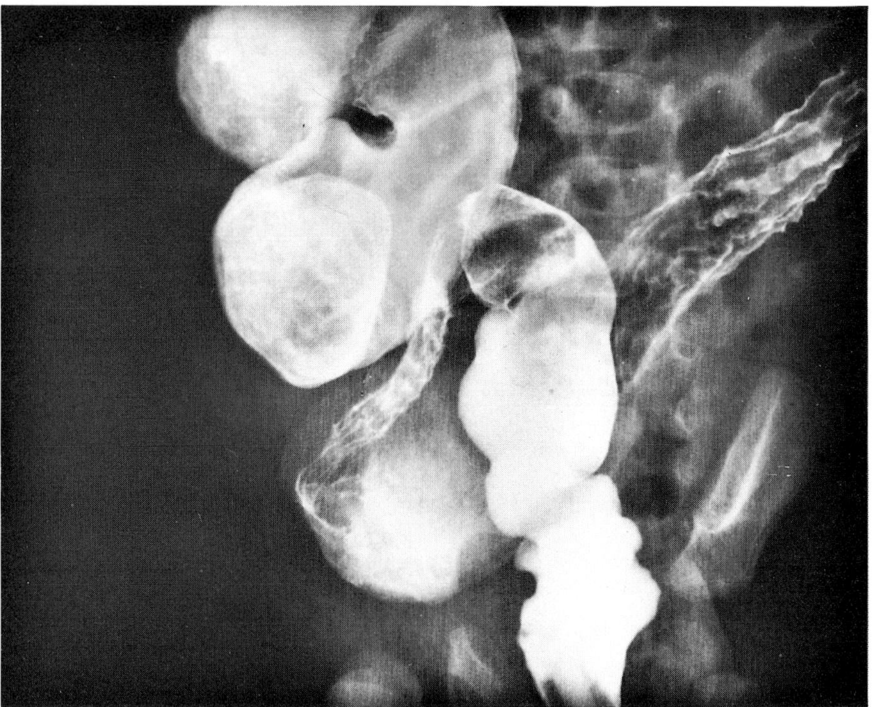

Fig. G.7. 8-week-old boy with Hirschsprung's disease. A relatively long segment of aganglionosis was present.

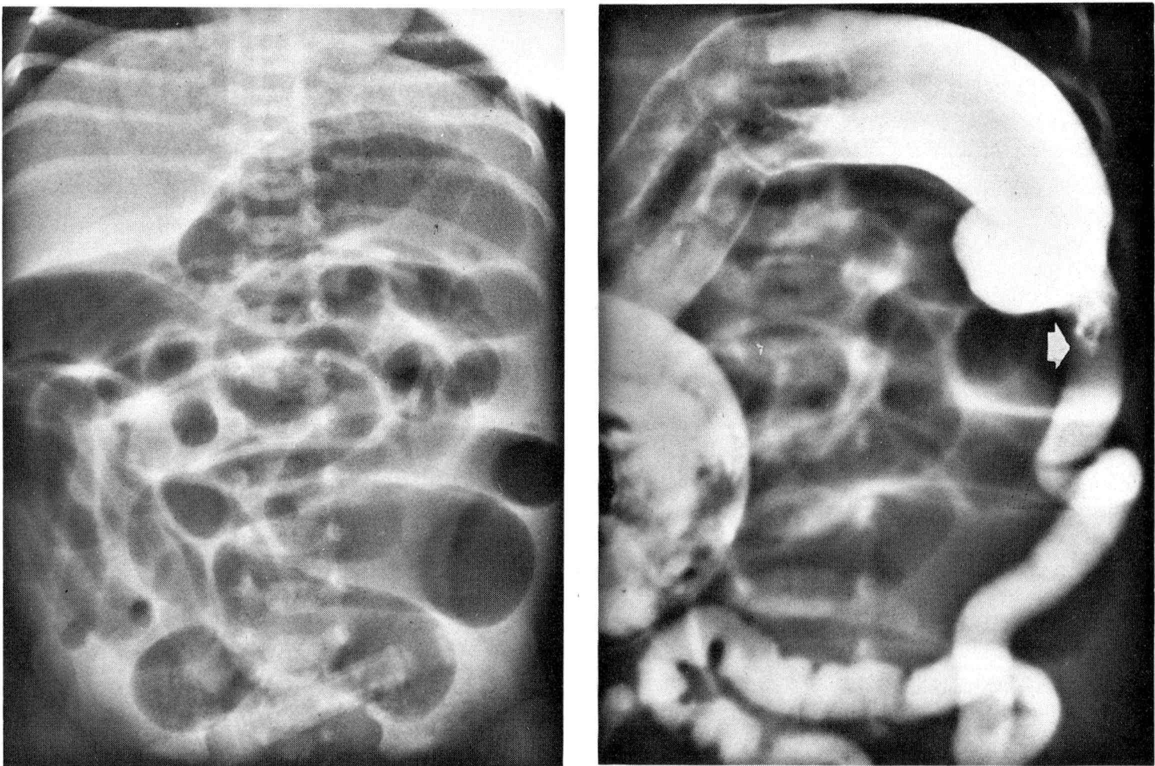

Fig. G.8. Probable neonatal small left colon syndrome. (a) Initial study reveals markedly dilated bowel. (b) A barium enema shows a transition between dilated and narrow bowel lumen in the descending colon (arrow).

syndrome and Hirschsprung's disease can have an identical radiographic appearance. A similar picture is also seen in the neonatal small left colon syndrome (26, 27), where varying lengths of descending colon are narrowed together with proximal dilation (Fig. G.8). A barium enema can be therapeutic to these infants, many of whom are born to diabetic mothers.

The differential diagnosis of a dilated proximal colon in the adult is more extensive and is covered in the section on colon ileus.

References

1. Balthazar EJ: Congenital positional anomalies of the colon: Radiographic diagnosis and clinical implication. I. Abnormalities of rotation. Gastrointest Radiol 2:41–47, 1977.
2. Balthazar EJ: Intestinal malrotation in adults. Roentgenographic assessment with emphasis on isolated complete and partial nonrotations. AJR 126:358–367, 1976.
3. Vessal K, Borhanmanesh F: Hepatodiaphragmatic interposition of the intestine (Chilaiditi's syndrome). Clin Radiol 27:113–116, 1976.
4. Santulli TV, Kiesewetter WB, Bill AH Jr: Anorectal anomalies: a suggested international classification. J Pediatr Surg 5:281–287, 1970.
5. Bryk D: Unused colon in the adult—Roentgen findings. Gastrointest Radiol 4:177–178, 1979.
6. Siegel MJ, Shackelford GD, McAlister WH: Neonatal meconium blockage in the ileum and proximal colon. Radiology 132:79–82, 1979.
7. Ladd WE: Congenital obstruction of the duodenum in children. N Engl J Med 206:277–283, 1932.
8. Toja K, Geissinger WT, Shaw A: Duplication of the transverse colon: report of a case. Dis Colon Rectum 18:430–434, 1975.
9. Bass EM: Duplication of the colon. Clin Radiol 29:205–209, 1978.
10. Hunter TB, Tonkin ILD: Complete duplication of the colon in association with urethral duplication. Gastrointest Radiol 4:93–95, 1979.
11. Bouliane R, Slonic A, Archambault H: La duplication colique. Ann Radiol 24:285–288, 1981.
12. Beyer D, Neuhaus H: Doppeltes Kolon—ein seltener Fall einer Darmduplikatur. ROEFO 131:47–49, 1979.
13. Arkema KK, Calenoff L: Adenocarcinoma in tubular duplication of the sigmoid colon. Gastrointest Radiol 2:137–139, 1977.
14. Hickey WF, Corson JM: Squamous cell carcinoma arising in a duplication of the colon: case report and literature review of squamous cell carcinoma of the colon and of malignancy complicating colonic duplication. Cancer 47:602–609, 1981.
15. Hirschsprung H: Stuhlträgheit Neugeborener in Folge von Dilatation und Hypertrophie des Colons. Jahrb Kinderheil 27:1–7, 1888.
16. Touloukian RJ, Duncan R: Acquired aganglionic megacolon in a premature infant: report of a case. Pediatrics 56:459–462, 1975.
17. Ponka JL, Grodsinsky C, Bush BE: Megacolon in teen-aged and adult patients. Dis Colon Rectum 15:14–22, 1972.
18. Kadair RG, Sims JE, Critchfield CF: Zonal colonic hypoganglionosis. JAMA 238:1838–1840, 1977.
19. Mahboubi S, Schnaufer L: The barium-enema examination and rectal manometry in Hirschsprung Disease. Radiology 130:643–647, 1979.
20. Mahboubi S, Schnaufer L: Manometry and barium enema in the diagnosis of Hirschsprung disease. Ann Radiol 24:117–120, 1981.
21. Pochaczevski R, Leonidas JC: The 'recto-sigmoid index'. A measurement for the early diagnosis of Hirschsprung's disease. AJR 123:770–777, 1975.
22. Siegel MJ, Shackelford GD, McAlister WH: The rectosigmoid index. Radiology 139:497–499, 1981.
23. Cremin BJ, Golding RL: Congenital aganglionosis of the entire colon in neonates. Br J Radiol 49:27–33, 1976.
24. Puri P, Lake BD, Nixon HH: Adynamic bowel syndrome. Report of a case with disturbance of the cholinergic innervation. Gut 18:754–759, 1977.
25. Munakata K, Okabe I, Morita K: Histologic studies of rectocolic aganglionosis and allied diseases. J Pediatr Surg 13:67–75, 1978.
26. Berdon WE, Slovis TL, Campbell JB, Baker DH, Haller JO: Neonatal small left colon syndrome: its relationship to aganglionosis and meconium plug syndrome. Radiology 125:457–462, 1977.
27. Davis WS, Allen RP, Favara BE, Slovis TL: Neonatal small left colon syndrome. AJR 120:322–329, 1974.

III.4.H. Extrinsic lesions

Because of its unique position and length, the colon is located adjacent to a number of other intra-abdominal structures. Thus, it is not surprising that both inflammatory and neoplastic disease of the extraperitoneal and intraperitoneal organs can secondarily involve the colon. Secondary neoplasms, originating in organs adjacent to the colon, are discussed more fully in the chapter on malignant tumors.

a. Gallbladder disease

The proximal portion of the transverse colon is closely related to the right lobe of the liver and the gallbladder; in the majority of individuals the body and fundus of the gallbladder are in close contract with the colon (1). An enlarged gallbladder can be seen as an impression upon the transverse colon. Acute cholecystitis, if associated with pericholecystic inflammation, can involve a localized segment of the transverse colon and result in an appearance similar to that seen with an adjacent abscess. With chronic cholecystitis adhesions can form between the gallbladder and colon and result in distortion. If the entire circumference of the colon is involved, the resultant radiographic picture appears similar to that of a colon carcinoma. When there is extensive inflammatory infiltration, the differentiation even at surgery can be difficult.

Because of the close anatomic relationship between the liver, gallbladder and the colon, a hepatoma or gallbladder carcinoma can spread to the contiguous colon segment. With sufficient colon invasion and subsequent mucosal ulceration these patients may present with rectal bleeding (2).

Cholecystitis occasionally results in a cholecystocolic fistula (1) together with gallstone ileus, although many individuals who develop a cholecystoenteric fistula do not develop obstruction (2) (Fig. H.1). A cholecystoduodenocolic fistula is rare and most reports consist of single examples (3, 4). The characteristic radiographic appearance with these fistula is gas in the gallbladder and in the bile ducts. A barium enema should demonstrate the fistula if it is still patent.

b. Renal disease

The distal segment of the ascending colon and the proximal segment of the transverse colon are adjacent to the right kidney. A similar relationship exists between the splenic flexure and the left kidney.

A barium enema examination in a patient with right renal agenesis or ectopia shows that the hepatic flexure is located more posteriorly than usual and occupies the renal fossa (5, 6). Similar changes are seen with left renal agenesis or ectopia as the anatomic splenic flexture occupies the renal fossa (7). Because the left kidney lies medially to the splenic flexure, with agenesis the flexure is more medial and posterior in position than usual. These changes should be interpreted with caution because a mobile splenic flexure can result in a medially displaced descending colon even when the kidney is normal.

Perinephric inflammation spreads along the adjacent fascial planes and can involve adjacent segments of the colon. The radiographic changes are characteristic for a serosal colon lesion and consist of infiltration, spiculation (palisading) and an asymmetrical fixed appearance of the involved segment (8) (Fig. H.2). A perinephrocolic fistula may occur secondary to chronic renal infection (9). Unfortunately, the serosal inflammatory involvement is very similar in appearance to a serosal metastasis.

c. Pancreatic disease

The pancreas is in continuity with the transverse colon through the transverse mesocolon. Also, the

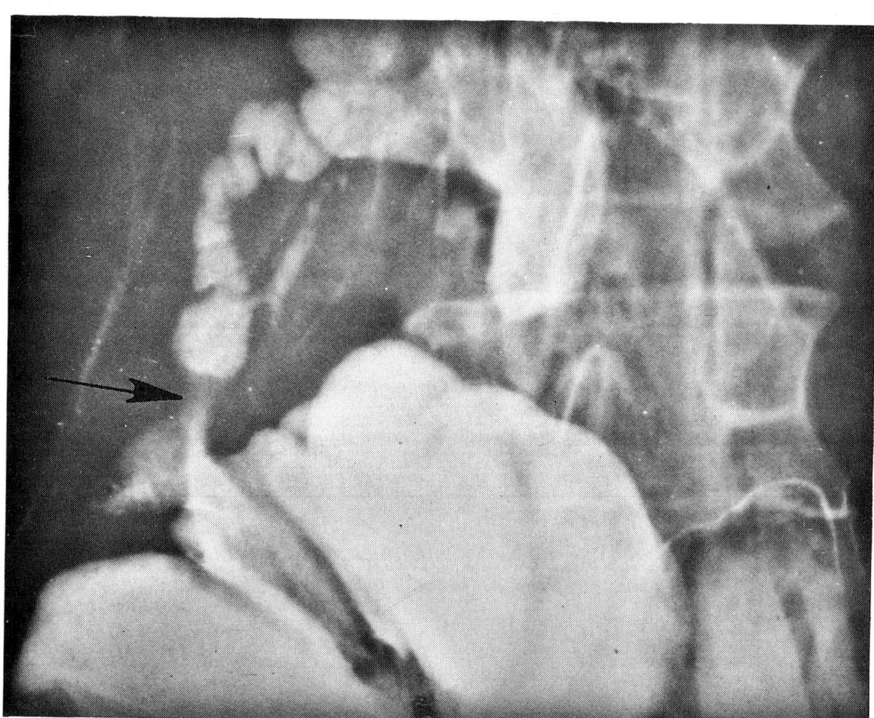

Fig. H.1. Cholecystocolic fistula in a patient who recently had acute cholecystitis. A barium enema shows the fistula (arrow), with partial filling of the common bile duct. Oral cholecystography usually is unrewarding in these patients.

tail of the pancreas extends to the splenic hilum and lies close to the splenic flexure. Thus, it is not unusual to see pancreatic inflammatory disease involve the colon (10), with either the transverse colon or the splenic flexure being affected. Because pancreatic enzymes can dissect along both paracolic gutters and along the small bowel mesentery, either the cecum, ascending, or descending colon may be involved (11).

Initially, the 'colon cut-off' sign was described as a radiographic sign indicative of acute pancreatitis (12, 13). This sign consists of distension of the right colon and narrowing of the transverse colon just distal of the hepatic flexure. Since then it has been shown that the 'colon cut-off' sign can be seen throughout the transverse colon or even in the proximal descending colon. Currently, this sign is applied rather loosely to any area of narrowing in the colon with proximal dilation, and not necessarily due to pancreatitis (Fig. H.3). Unfortunately, the 'colon cut-off' sign is an inconstant finding even in patients with pancreatitis (14).

The narrowed segment of the 'colon cut-off' as seen on abdominal radiographs often distends during a barium enema. A barium enema reveals bowel wall edema, narrowing, diffuse infiltration, necrosis or a colon perforation with a fistula to a pancreatic abscess (13, 15–17). The colon findings are asymmetrical and involve primarily the lower contour of the transverse colon (10). The constrictions can mimic a carcinoma (14, 18). A follow-up barium enema after the pancreatitis has cleared can reveal a normal colon (11) or a stenosis (19). The stenosis is probably secondary to ischemia, because pancreatitis can result in occlusion of the involved arteries and veins (20).

Most pseudocysts are located adjacent to the body or tail of the pancreas and, if large enough, indent the adjacent segment of colon. Occasionally a pseudocyst forms far away from the pancreas and

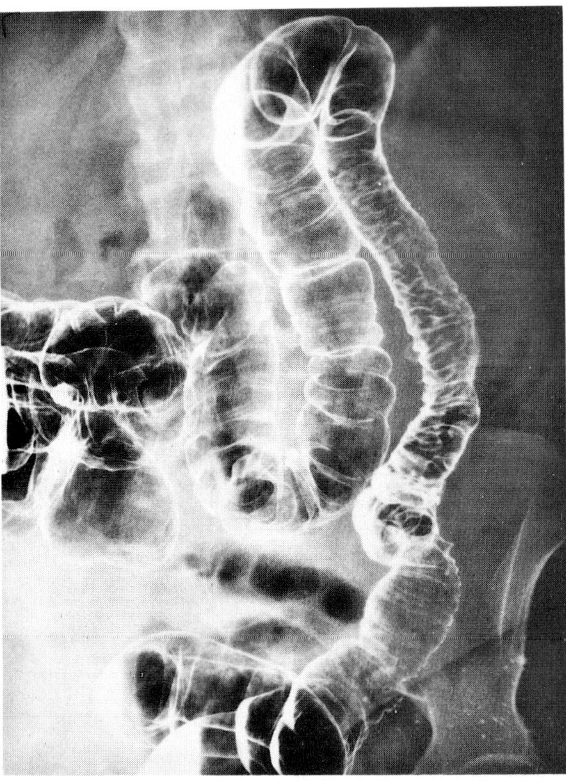

Fig. H.2. Left perinephric abscess with secondary involvement of the descending colon. The folds throughout the involved segment are fixed and have a spiculated appearance. Although serosal invasion by a tumor can result in a similar appearance in any one area, such a long segment of involvement by tumor is unusual. The clinical story also was consistent with infection.

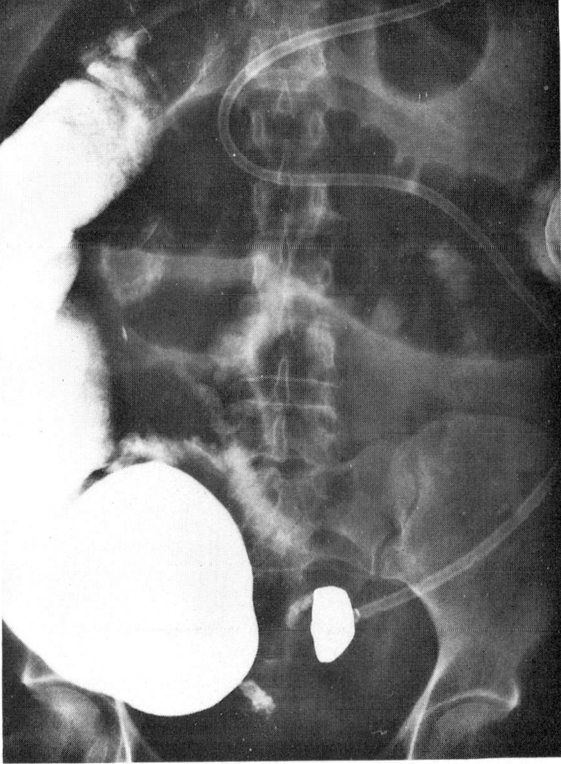

Fig. H.3. 'Colon cut-off' sign secondary to pancreatitis. The patient underwent an upper gastrointestinal examination several days previously and residual barium is present in a dilated right colon. The transverse colon is also dilated, with no gas seen distally. In fact, clinically the patient was suspected of being obstructed and a barium enema was required to show that no anatomic obstruction was present.

then it can involve the cecum, sigmoid, or even the rectum (21). The pseudocyst can rupture into the colon (22). If a pseudocyst is suspected, ultrasonography or computerized tomography is invaluable in determining the true nature of the cyst.

Pancreatic cancer can spread along the transverse mesocolon with the resultant changes in the colon being similar to those seen with pancreatitis. Intraperitoneal spread by a pancreatic cancer can involve the rectosigmoid colon, with the tumor seeding in the pouch of Douglas.

d. Pelvic lipomatosis

In pelvic lipomatosis there is extensive fatty infiltration and fibrosis throughout the pelvis. The condition is generally found as an incidental finding during a barium enema; few, if any, bowel complaints are related to pelvic lipomatosis. It usually affects the bladder but the rectum can also be involved. A barium enema may show the lipomatosis simply as a pelvic mass (23). In suspected cases CT is definitive.

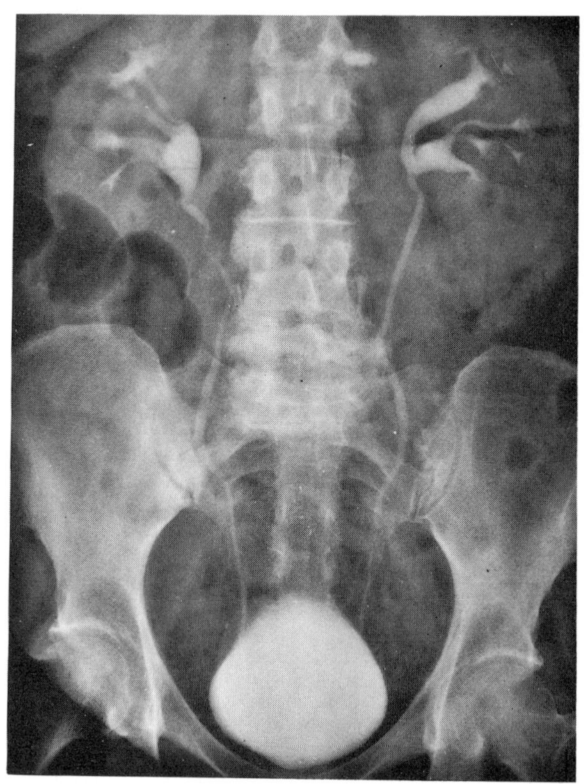

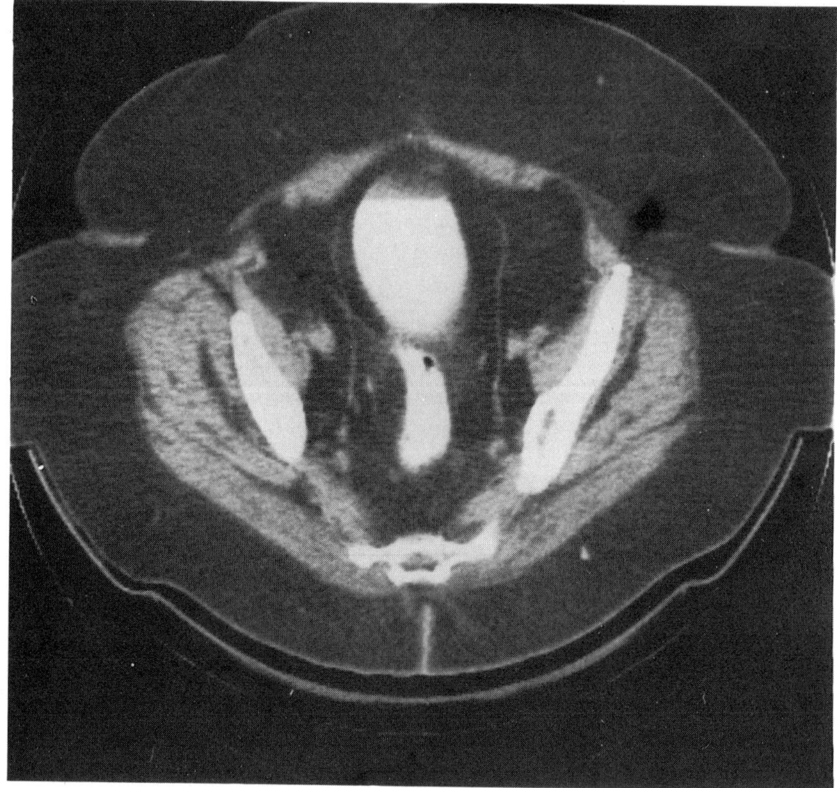

b

Fig. H.4. Pelvic lipomatosis. (a) Excretory urogram shows medial deviation of both ureters. (b) Extensive fat is present throughout the pelvis, with the bladder and rectum surrounded by fat.

Abdominal radiographs reveal a diffuse lucency throughout the involved area. A barium enema shows the rectum narrowed in symmetrical fashion and the sigmoid elevated above the pelvis. Even on post-evacuation radiographs the sigmoid remains elevated. The presacral space can be widened considerably. The fatty infiltration, however, is not limited to the presacral space but obviously also involves most of the pelvic structures (Fig. H.4).

The characteristic shape, the lack of bowel and bladder wall infiltration, and absence of significant bowel symptoms usually make the diagnosis readily apparent. If a question exists about the composition of the pelvic infiltration, computerized tomography readily diagnoses the excessive amounts of fat present.

e. Gastroduodenal disease

Although rare, occasionally either gastric or duodenal bulbar ulcers involve the colon. The ulcers are usually located along the greater curvature and as the ulcer penetrates through the wall the resultant inflammation spreads along the gastrocolic ligament to the transverse colon. A recurring ulcer after a subtotal gastrectomy and gastrojejunostomy can also involve the transverse colon. Radiographically, the colon changes appear similar to those seen with any extrinsic inflammation involving the colon serosa. These changes are secondary to the resultant edema, inflammatory infiltration and bowel wall thickening and should alert the radiologist to the extracolic nature of the disorder. Occasionally such a patient will be explored for suspected colon carcinoma (24).

The majority of gastrocolic fistulas are secondary to malignancies involving either the stomach, the colon or from post-surgical abscesses. Occasionally a benign gastric ulcer results in a fistula to the colon (25). Duodenocolic fistulas are even rarer. Most of these are secondary to peptic ulcer disease or regional enteritis, primary in either the duodenum or colon (Fig. H.5). There are occasional reports of a fistula extending from a duodenal diverticulum (26). The course of a fistula is usually easier to identify on a retrograde barium enema than on an antegrade upper gastrointestinal examination. With the latter, care must be taken not to miss a fistula by suggesting that the early colon filling by contrast is secondary to fast small bowel transit.

f. Miscellaneous lesions

Any mass adjacent to the colon, if large enough, can either narrow or obstruct the colon. As an example, a distended bladder can partially obstruct the rectosigmoid (27). The radiographic findings on a barium enema are characteristic. The colon is compressed in the anterior–posterior dimension and pressed against the sacral promontory. The right-to-left dimension of the colon is increased. The overall appearance is that of a mass passively compressing the colon with no signs of colon invasion present. A pelvic neoplasm can produce similar changes although the bladder outline below the neoplasm can usually be identified (Fig. H.6). With an enlarged bladder, however, there is only one large mass filling the pelvis (Fig. H.7). If doubt about the origin of the mass exists, either post-voiding or postcatheterization radiographs should be obtained.

Retractile mesenteritis is a rare cause of colon obstruction. This condition consists of an acute inflammatory phase with subsequent fibrosis and

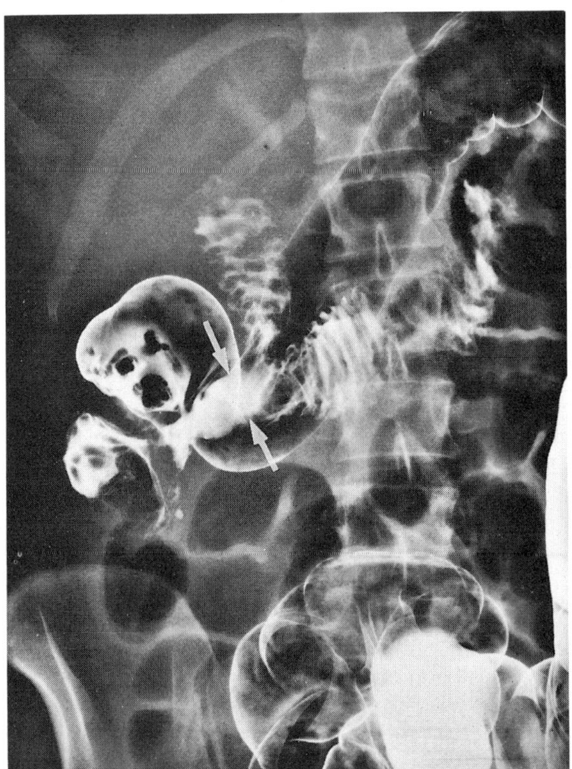

Fig. H.5. Duodenocolic fistula in a 30-year-old woman. She had known regional enteritis of the ascending colon. The fistula extends from the ascending colon to the junction of the second and third portions of the duodenum (arrows).

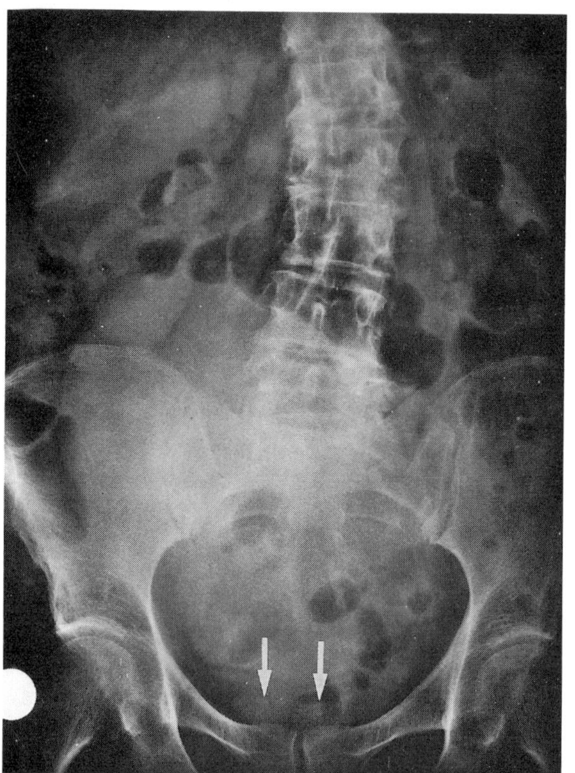

contraction from fibroblastic proliferation. Surgery generally reveals a large infiltrating fibrous mass. The ureters are involved most often, with occasional involvement of the small bowel; primary colon involvement is rare. When present, the narrowed segment mimics inflammation or colon ischemia. In one patient the stenosis cleared completely after bypass surgery and steroid therapy (28).

Adhesions are a rare cause of colon obstruction (29, 30). There is usually a sharp, circumferential narrowing with the colic folds compressed but not destroyed. The obstruction can be partial or complete. Adhesions occasionally appear as intramural masses, mimicking ischemia or a neoplasm (31).

Traumatic colon laceration usually manifests shortly after the accident, with many of these patients also sustaining injury to other intraabdom-

Fig. H.6. A large cystadenocarcinoma displaces the colon from the pelvis. The bladder outline (arrows) can be seen inferior to the tumor.

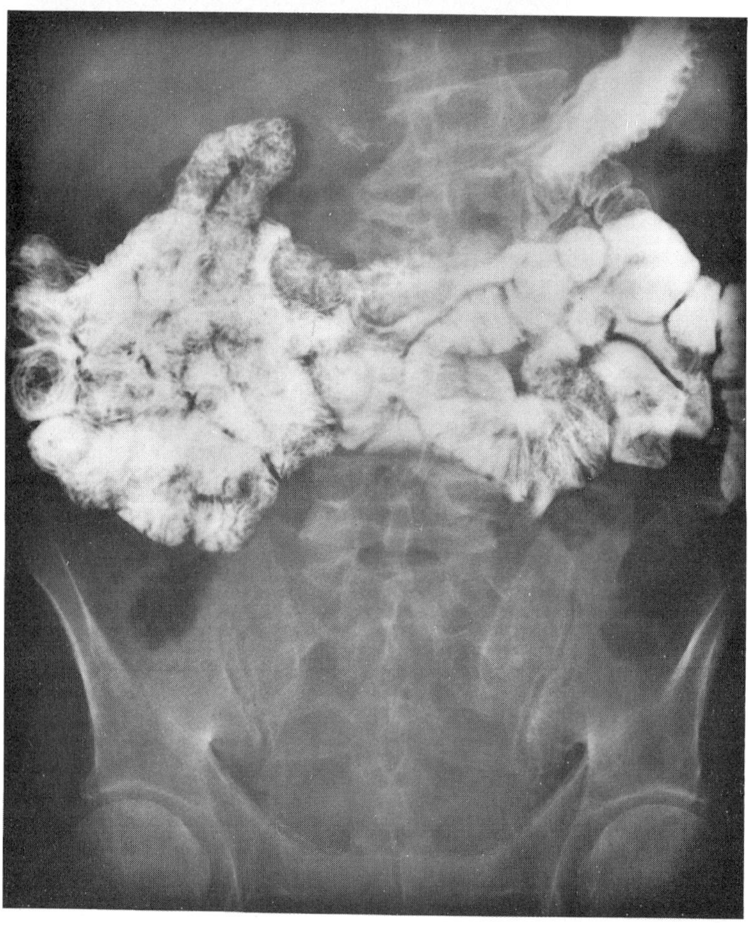

Fig. H.7. Enlarged bladder fills the pelvis and displaces bowel superiorly.

inal structures. If an extraperitoneal laceration occurs, however, the clinical signs of perforation can be masked for some time (Fig. H.8). Similar results are seen with enema catheter trauma to the rectum.

References

1. Ghahremani GG, Meyers MA: The cholecysto-colic relationships. A roentgen-anatomic study of the colonic manifestations of gallbladder disorders. AJR 125:21–33, 1975.
2. Balthazar EJ, Gurkin S: Cholecystoenteric fistulas: significance and radiographic diagnosis. Am J Gastroenterol 65:168–173, 1976.
3. Wise WS, Caldwell FT: Cholecystoduodenocolic fistula. Am J Surg 121:349–350, 1971.
4. Shocket E, Evans J, Jonas S: Cholecysto-duodeno-colic fistula with gallstone ileus. Arch Surg 101:523–526, 1970.
5. Sbihi H, Muntlak H, Kadiri R, Fathi K: Les malpositions coliques dans les agénésies rénales, les ectopies et les néphrectomies par voie antérieure. Ann Radiol 23:489–494, 1980.
6. Curtis JA, Sadhu V, Steiner RM: Malposition of the colon in right renal agenesis, ectopia and anterior nephrectomy. AJR 129:845–850, 1977.
7. Mascatello V, Lebowitz RL: Malposition of the colon in left renal agenesis and ectopia. Radiology 120:371–376, 1976.
8. Soulard JM, Chaulieu C, Colombel P, L'Hermite J, Régent D, Tréheux A: Expression colique des périnéphrites. J Radiol 60:503–508, 1979.
9. Meyers MA: Colonic changes secondary to left perinephritis: new observations. Radiology 111:525–528, 1974.
10. Meyers MA, Evans JA: Effects of pancreatitis on the small bowel and colon: spread along mesenteric planes. AJR 119:151–165, 1973.

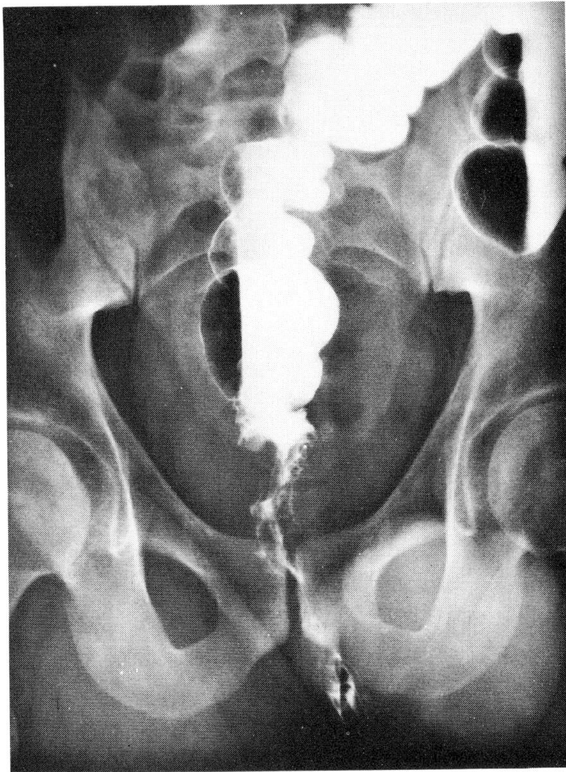

a

Fig. H.8. 35-year-old patient was involved in a motorcycle accident. (a) Frontal and (b) lateral radiographs show marked distortion and narrowing of the distal rectum. The presacral space is considerably widened. No rectal perforation could be identified at this time.

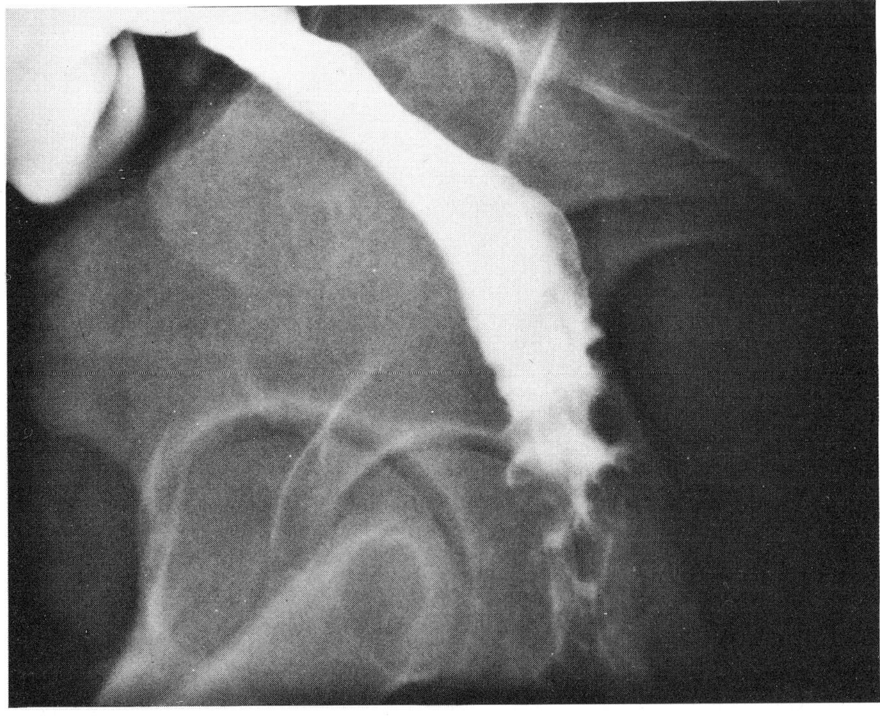

b

11. L'Herminé C, Pringot J, Monnier JP, Bret P, Roger J, Lemaitre L, Goncette L, Tubiana JM, Lescut J: Le retentissement colique des pancréatites. J Radiol 61:27–34, 1980.
12. Price CWR: The 'colon cut-off' sign in acute pancreatitis. Med J Aust 1:313–314, 1956.
13. Stuart C: Acute pancreatitis: Preliminary investigation of a new radiodiagnostic sign. Clin Radiol 8:50–58, 1956.
14. Thompson WM, Kelvin FM, Rice RP: Inflammation and necrosis of the transverse colon secondary to pancreatitis. AJR 128:943–948, 1977.
15. Dallemand S, Farman J, Stein D, Waxman M, Mitchell W: Colonic necrosis complicating pancreatitis. Gastrointest Radiol 2:27–30, 1977.
16. Thompson WM, Pizzo SV, Kelvin FM, Rice RP: Necrosis of the colon secondary to pancreatitis. Dig Dis Sci 23: 92S–96S, 1978.
17. Mason HDW, Forgash A, Balch HH: Intestinal fistula complicating pancreatic abscess. Surg Gynecol Obstet 140: 39–43, 1975.
18. Ravey M, Frish R, Reignier J: La sténose du colon, complication méconnue des pancréatites. Ann Chir 32: 291–294, 1978.
19. Mohuiddin S, Sakiyalak P, Gullick HD, Webb WR: Stenosing lesions of the colon secondary to pancreatitis. Arch Surg 102:229–231, 1971.
20. Hunt DR, Mildenhall P: Etiology of strictures of the colon associated with pancreatitis. Dig Dis Sci 20:941–946, 1975.
21. Farman J, Kutcher R, Dallemand S, Lane FC, Becker JA: Unusual pelvic complications of a pancreatic pseudocyst. Gastrointest Radiol 3:43–45, 1978.
22. Rosen RJ, Teplick SK, Shapiro JH: Spontaneous communication between a pancreatic pseudocyst and the colon: unusual clinical and radiographic presentation. Gastrointest Radiol 5:353–355, 1980.
23. Levitt RG, Sagel SS, Stanley RJ, Evens RG: Computed tomography of the pelvis. Semin Roentgenol 13:193–200, 1978.
24. Abbruzzese AA, Griffiths H: Colonic changes secondary to stomal ulcer. Am J Gastroenterol 55:447–450, 1971.
25. Laufer I, Thornley GD, Stolberg H: Gastrocolic fistula as a complication of benign gastric ulcer. Radiology 119:7–11 1976.
26. Yasui K, Tsukaguchi I, Ohara S, Sato K, Ono N, Sato T: Benign duodenocolic fistula due to duodenal diverticulum: report of two cases. Radiology 130:67–70, 1979.
27. Kleinhaus U, Kaftori J: Rectosigmoid pseudostenosis due to urinary retention. Radiology 127:645–647, 1978.
28. Williams RG, Nelson JA: Retractile mesenteritis: initial presentation as colonic obstruction. Radiology 126:35–37, 1978.
29. Twersky J, Himmelfarb E: Right colonic adhesions. Radiology 120:37–40, 1976.
30. Brodey PA, Schuldt DR, Magnuson A, Esterkyn S: Complete colonic obstruction secondary to adhesions. AJR 133:917–918, 1979.
31. Boulis ZF, Osborne DR: Pseudotumours of the colon due to adhesions. Br J Radiol 54:685–686, 1981.

III.4.I. Colon hernias

Hernias can be divided into two categories: external hernias resulting in bowel or omentum protruding through a defect beyond their usual abdominal location and internal hernias secondary to an anomaly in the mesentery or the peritoneum resulting in a portion of the colon being in an unnatural position in the abdomen. An example of the latter type of hernia is a herniation through the foramen of Winslow where a segment of the colon has herniated into the lesser sac.

a. Esophageal hiatal hernia

The esophageal hiatus is a common place for the stomach to herniate into the thorax. Because the colon is attached to the stomach by the gastrocolic ligament, the transverse colon can also be pulled up into the hernial sac. These patients present with one of two characteristic findings; if the gastrocolic ligament or the omentum only are herniated, a barium enema reveals sharp angulation of the transverse colon but the colon is essentially in a normal position. Or, a portion of the transverse colon is actually herniated into the thoracic cavity through the esophagal hiatus (Fig. I.1). The herniated soft tissues, generally composed of fat and associated bowel, can be readily identified by CT (1).

b. Pleuroperitoneal hernia

This congenital anomaly is caused by a failure of the postero-lateral portion of the diaphragm to develop normally. Most of these hernias through the diaphragm are large and a considerable portion of the usual intraabdominal content is within the chest. Because of the large size most of these hernias are generally picked up early in the pediatric age group. Rarely, a chest radiograph in the neonatal period is normal (2). It is unusual however to see an adult with a pleuroperitoneal hernia unless the hernia is small.

Commonly the colon is herniated into the chest. Most of these defects are on the left side. A lateral view shows the intrathoracic portion of the colon considerably more posterior than with a herniation through the esophageal hiatus. CT reveals a basal intrapulmonary soft tissue mass (3).

Although most of these hernias are readily diagnosable with noncontrast studies, if surgical intervention is being considered then a contrast study should be obtained in order to define which segment of the gastrointestinal tract is above the diaphragm. Usually a small bowel examination, with delayed radiographs to show the anatomic location of the colon, are all that is necessary.

The differential diagnosis of these hernias in the neonatal period includes pleural effusion, adenomatoid lung malformation, gastric herniation into the chest and diaphragmatic eventration.

c. Morgagni hernia

A hernia through the foramen of Morgagni is located anteriorly and medially. These foramina are congenital defects within the diaphragm, most have a small hiatus, and most occur on the right side. Noncontrast studies generally show a mass in the right cardiophrenic angle. Usually a contrast study is necessary to show that a loop of viscera is present within the herniation. Herniation of a portion of the transverse colon is not unusual. If herniation of only the omentum is present, contrast studies either show no abnormalities of the colon or there is a sharp angulation of a segment of the colon where the attached omentum has herniated into the chest.

d. Traumatic hernias

It is not unusual to see an elevated diaphragm secondary to trauma. If, in addition, there has been partial diaphragmatic rupture, viscera can herniate through the rupture into the chest. Most such hernias are on the left side; the liver tends to protect the right hemidiaphragm. The herniated viscera can include the colon, stomach, or portions of small bowel. Usually a history of trauma and a prior

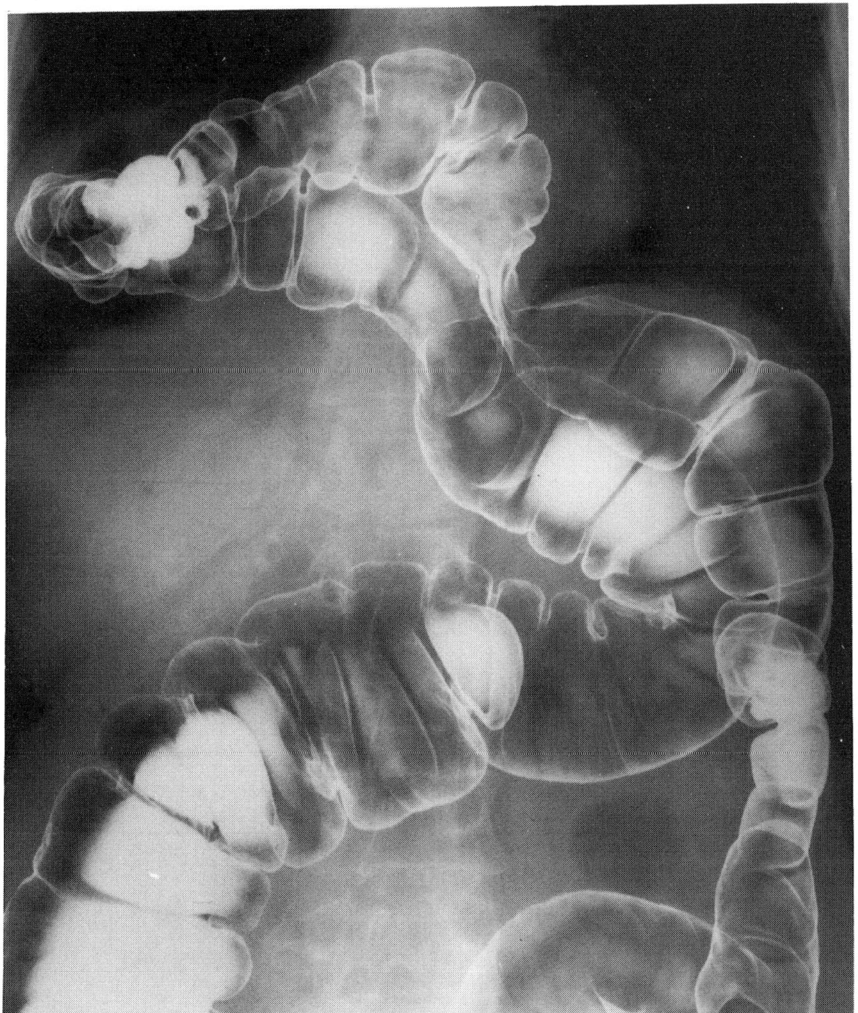

Fig. I.1. A portion of the transverse colon has herniated through the esophageal hiatus into the chest. Colon narrowing at the hiatus is evident. There was no obstruction.

normal examination allow ready differentiation from a congenital anomaly.

e. Inguinal hernias

Most of these hernias occur in men. If there is associated bowel herniation usually the small bowel is involved. Occasionally, the cecum is in an inguinal hernia on the right side and the sigmoid on the left side. Some of these patients present first with bowel obstruction.

Noncontrast radiographs of the abdomen are generally diagnostic if a loop of bowel is in the hernia (Fig. I.2). However, many of these hernias are missed because the radiologist simply did not include the area of interest on the radiograph. Within our department we insist that the inguinal regions routinely be included on the radiographs obtained for the acute abdominal examination. A barium enema is diagnostic (Fig. I.3).

Herniation through the femoral ring, seen primarily in women, usually does not involve the colon.

f. Umbilical hernias

Umbilical hernias are common in young pediatric patients, with many of these hernias regressing spontaneously. Most adults with an umbilical

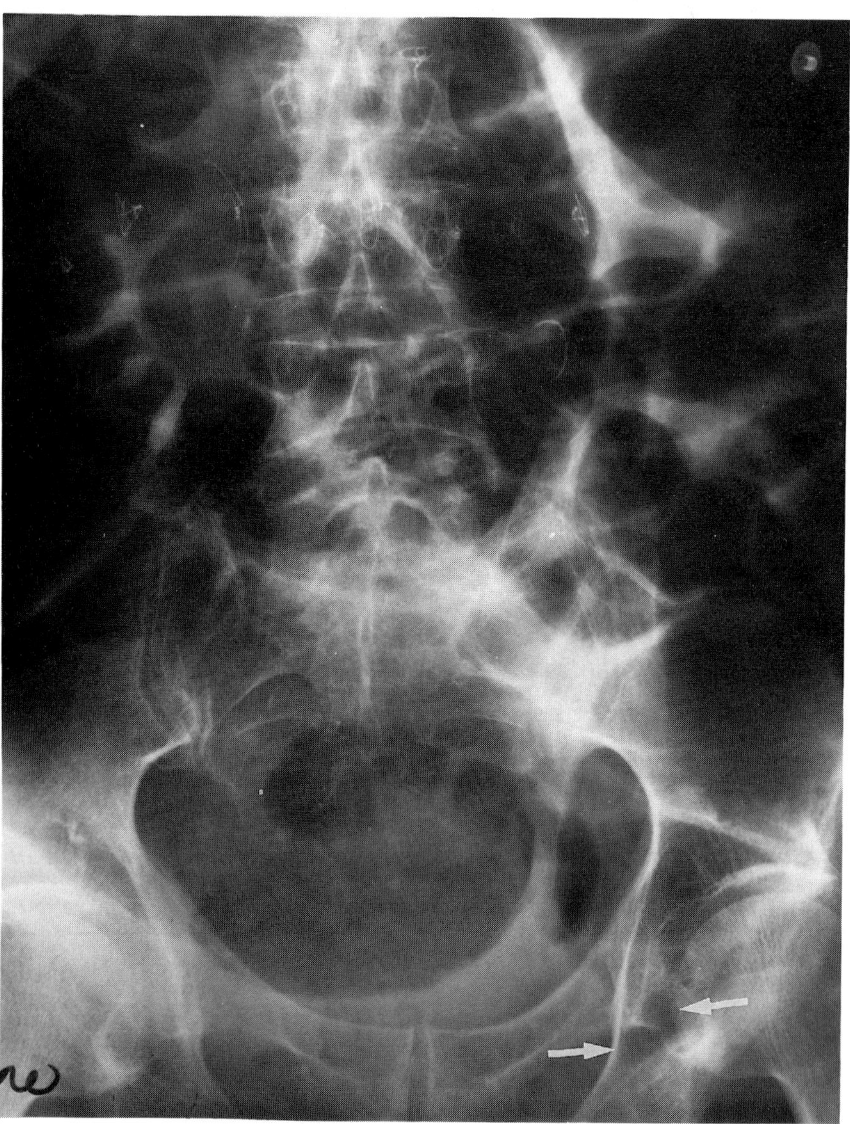

Fig I.2. Left inguinal hernia containing sigmoid colon (arrows). Partial obstruction was present (see also Fig. A.4, page 5).

hernia have increased intraabdominal pressure caused by some other underlying condition. These hernias can obstruct. Most of these hernias are palpable in the anterior abdominal wall and a lateral radiograph of the anterior portion of the abdomen during a barium enema will confirm the presence of colon with the hernia. The hernia can contain omentum, small bowel, or colon. The herniation can range from a single haustrum in the hernial sac to a large part of the transverse colon being herniated (4). At times the hernia can be manually reduced during fluoroscopy.

g. Spigelian hernia

This hernia is named after the 17th century Belgian anatomist Spiegel who initially described the linea

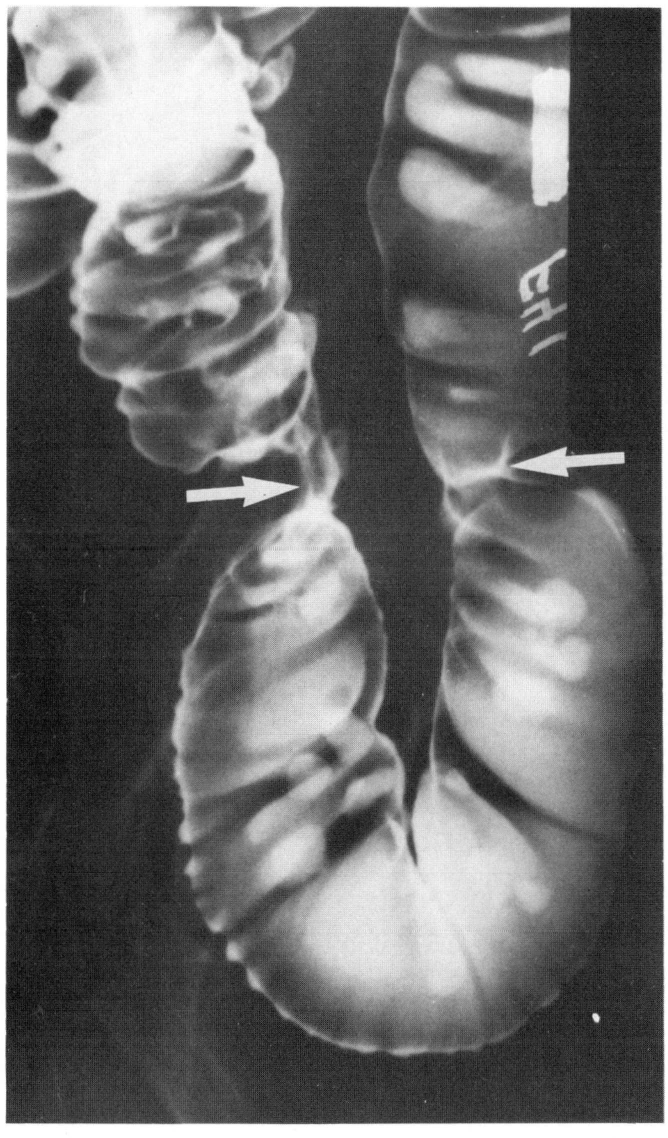

a

Fig. I.3. (a) Partially incarcerated sigmoid colon in an inguinal hernia. The neck of the hernia is readily identified (arrows). Numerous diverticula are scattered throughout. (b) Another patient with a loop of sigmoid in a left inguinal hernia. There is a polyp (arrow) and a diverticulum (arrowhead) within the herniated bowel.

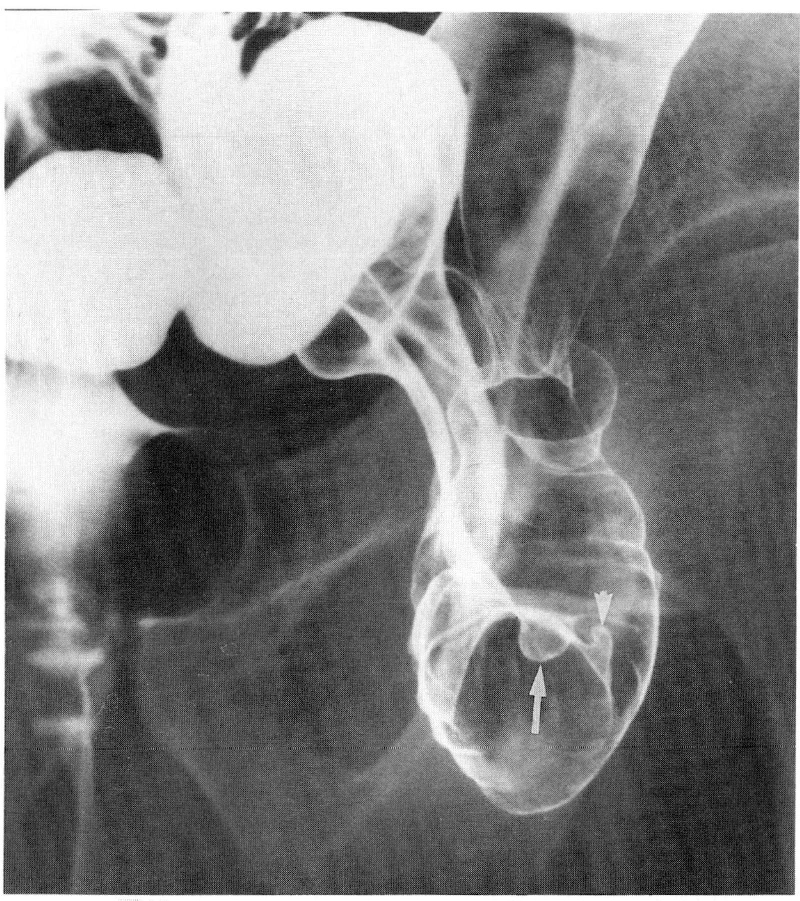

*Fig. I.3.***b.**

semilunaris. Because the lateral margin of the rectus sheath corresponds to the skin indentation known as the linea semilunaris (spigelian line), the name of this hernia is appropriate. Although these hernias are relatively rare, they can be readily diagnosed by the radiologist because of a characteristic appearance.

A spigelian hernia presents as a mass along the lateral margin of the rectus sheath. The hernia is located between the external and internal oblique muscles of the abdomen and is caused by weakness of the transverse abdominal and internal abdominal oblique muscle sheaths. Because the external abdominal oblique muscle is considerably stronger, herniation through the deeper muscle layers spreads out beneath the external oblique muscle (5). The herniation can consist of omentum, stomach, small intestine or colon (6). Depending upon the herniated organ and degree of obstruction the patient can be asymptomatic, have a palpable mass, or have signs of intestinal obstruction (7). If there is bowel within the hernia, occasionally the diagnosis can be suggested on abdominal radiographs. Usually, however, a contrast study of the appropriate bowel is necessary. These hernias generally have a narrow ring and the loop of bowel is constricted where it enters the hernia.

An extensive bibliography on Spigelian hernias has been presented by Holder and Schneider (5).

h. Incisional hernias

These usually are through the anterior abdominal wall and are the result of prior surgery. Depending upon location, the omentum, small bowel, or colon herniates through the abdominal wall defect.

i. Internal hernias

Internal hernias are considerably more important in the pediatric age group than in adults. In most instances the small bowel, rather than the colon, herniates and the result is small bowel obstruction. By far the most common such hernia is a paraduodenal hernia (8). The majority occur on the left side of the abdomen and radiographically appear as

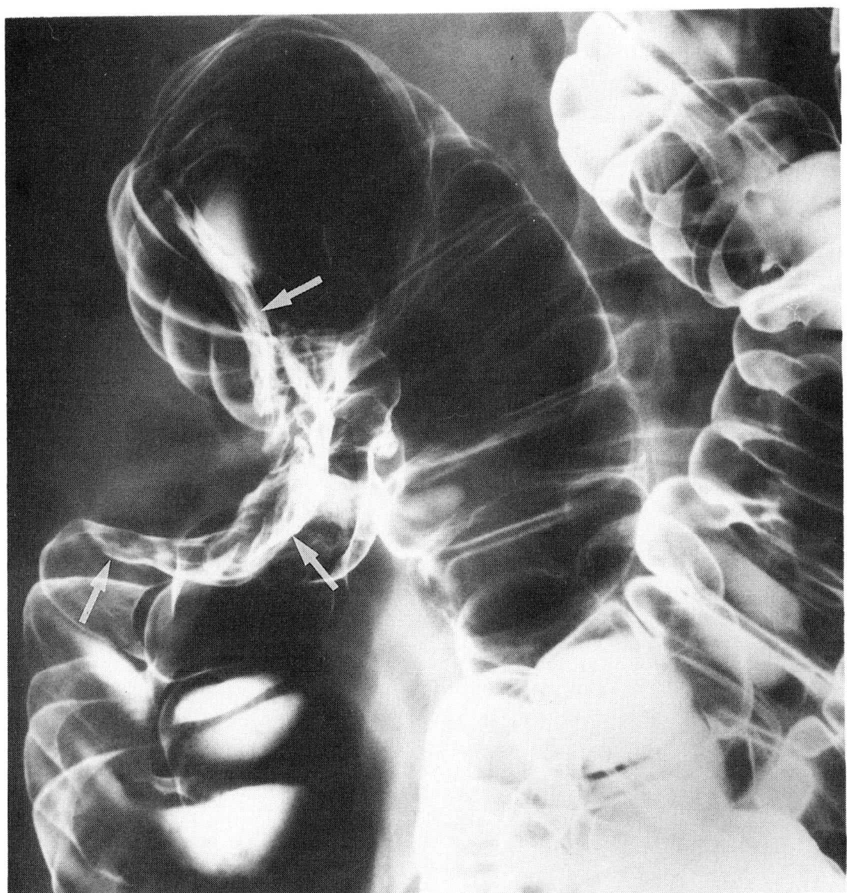

a

b

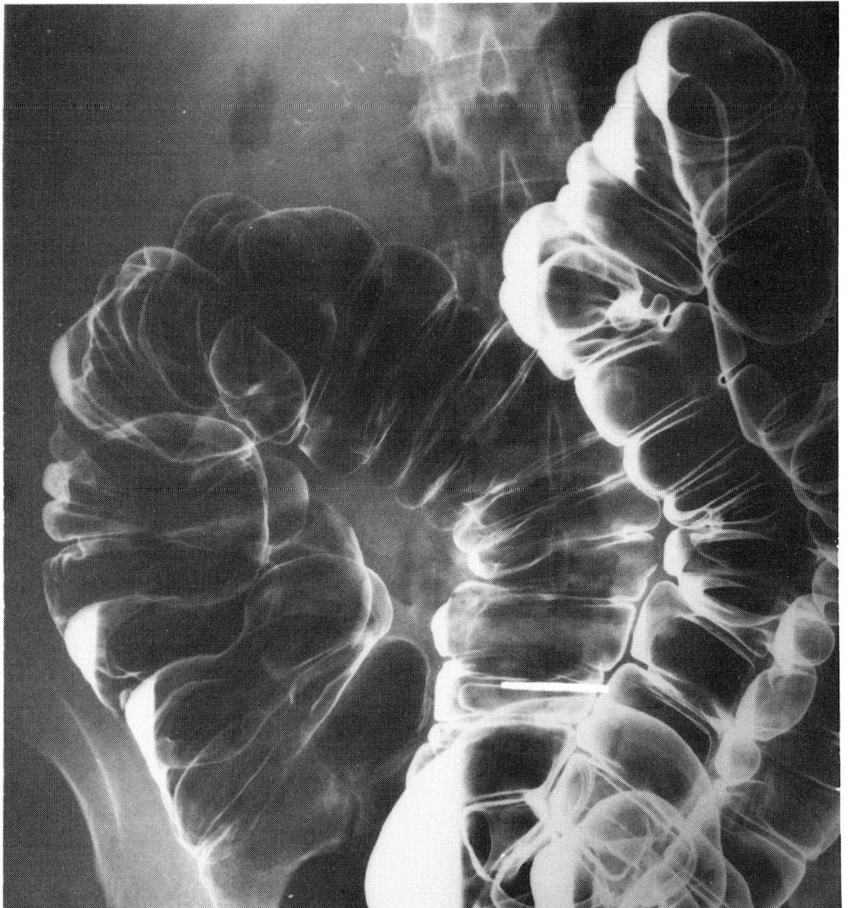

Fig. I.4. Right lateral paracolic hernia. (a) Loops of small bowel are localized by a 'sac' adjacent to the ascending colon (arrows). (b) The hernia reduces when the patient is in a right lateral decubitus position.

a well-defined collection of bowel adjacent to the fourth part of the duodenum. Colon herniation into a right paraduodenal hernia is less common but when present tends to be more massive. The radiographic appearance of loops of small bowel well localized by a 'sac' should suggest such an internal hernia.

Mesenteric hernias consist either of a hole through the mesentery or the mesentery simply acts as a pouch. There is a frequent association with malrotation. Aside from paraduodenal hernias, most others are around the cecum (8). Herniation through the mesentery between the ileocolic artery and the last ileal branch (Treves' field) has occasionally been reported (9).

Occasionally encountered is colon herniation through the foramen of Winslow (10–12). A predisposing cause is excessive mobility of the cecum. The radiographic appearance is that of centrally placed abnormal loops of bowel within the epigastrium. With cecal herniation, the cecum is not located in its usual position. The stomach is displaced anteriorly by a dilated loop of bowel and there is distal small bowel obstruction.

Other internal hernias are not common. Occasionally, as a congenital anomaly, either the ascending or descending portions of the colon are not retroperitoneal in location but have an associated mesocolon. Thus, this segment of the colon can be relatively mobile and result in a more medial location than usually encountered. Loops of small bowel can then herniate into the adjacent paracolic fossa, resulting in an internal hernia (Fig. I.4). If there is a defect in the mesocolon, small bowel

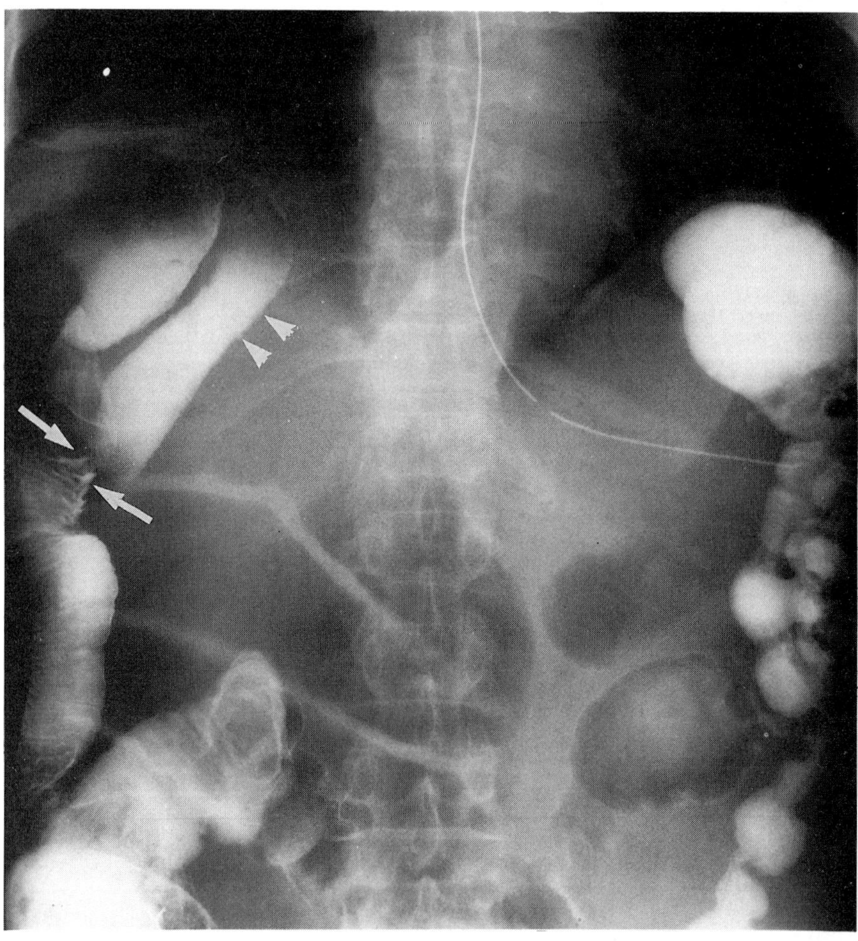

Fig. I.5. Small bowel herniation beneath adhesions. The patient presented with distal small bowel obstruction and a retrograde small bowel examination was performed to evaluate the obstruction. The postevacuation radiograph shows the distal ileum in the right upper quadrant. The ileum is narrowed at the neck of the hernia (arrows). Numerous shallow ulcers (arrowheads) are present in the herniated ileum, reflecting ischemia. Dilated small bowel is evident proximally.

or sigmoid colon can herniate through this defect and result in obstruction. The resultant radiographic picture will be bowel lateral or superior to the ascending or descending colon.

Postoperatively, herniation can take place beneath adhesions. These patients generally present with obstruction. Usually the small bowel is involved (Fig. I.5), although occasionally the sigmoid or cecum will herniate.

With a defect in the transverse mesocolon, bowel can herniate into the lesser sac posterior to the transverse colon. The radiographic appearance is very similar to herniation through the foramen of Winslow.

References

1. Coulomb M, Terraube P, Lebas JF, Chouteau H, Geindre M: Amas graisseux intra-thoraciques symptomatiques d'une hernie diaphragmatique chez l'adulte. J Radiol 62: 85–95, 1981.
2. Kozlowski K, Glasson MJ: 'Geometrical features' of the Bochdalek congenital diaphragmatic hernia. ROEFO 133: 155–157, 1980.
3. Kuckein D, Dobbelstein D: Bochdaleksche Zwerchfellhernie – ein computertomographischer Beitrag zur röntgenologischen Differentialdiagnose eines intrapulmonalen Rundherdes dorsobasal. ROEFO 131:327–328, 1979.
4. Forrest JV, Stanley RJ: Transverse colon in adult umbilical hernia. AJR 130:57–59, 1978.
5. Holder LE, Schneider HJ: Spigelian hernias: anatomy and roentgenographic manifestations. Radiology 112:309–313, 1974.
6. Hunter TB, Freudlich IM, Zukaski CF: Preoperative radiographic diagnosis of a Spigelian hernia containing large and small bowel. Gastrointest Radiol 1:379–381, 1977.
7. Arida EJ, Joh SK, Cucolo GF: The Spigelian hernia: radiographic manifestation. Br J Radiol 43:903–905, 1970.
8. Ghahremani GG, Meyers MA: Internal abdominal hernias. Curr Probl Radiol 5:1–30, 1975.
9. Harbin WP, Andres J, Kim SH, Borden S IV: Internal hernia into Treves' field pouch. Radiology 130:71–72, 1979.
10. Henisz A, Matesanz J, Westcott JL: Cecal herniation through the foramen of Winslow. Radiology 112:575–578, 1974.
11. Zinkin LD, Moore D: Herniation of the cecum through the foramen of Winslow. Dis Colon Rectum 23:276–279, 1980.
12. Goldberger LE, Berk RN: Cecal hernia into the lesser sac. Gastrointest Radiol 5:169–172, 1980.

II.4.J. Colon ileus

Colonic ileus, also known as adynamic ileus of the colon (1), pseudo-obstruction (2), Ogilvie's syndrome, and false colonic obstruction (3), results in marked bowel dilation, with no mechanical obstruction being present. In some patients the colon is primarily affected; in others, the small bowel is also involved. The condition can be chronic. Familial instances have been reported (4, 5).

It was believed by Ogilvie that colonic ileus results from interference with the colon's sympathetic innervation (6). Others believe that this condition exists because of an imbalance between the sympathetic and parasympathetic innervation and a resultant loss of colon coordination (7); the specific etiology is not known (8, 9). Colonic ileus can be encountered as an isoladed condition. Usually, however, it is associated with other systemic conditions ranging from infection, inflammation, metabolic derangement, and surgery not necessarily related to the colon (1, 10–12). Pelvic radiotherapy may also result in colonic ileus (13). These patients tend to have a diminished or absent gastrocolic response (14) and delayed intestinal transit. These findings are nonspecific, because an absent gastrocolic response is also seen in diabetics (15), a group that is prone to constipation.

The clinical picture is similar to that of colon obstruction. Symptoms generally develop over several days. The patients have crampy abdominal pain associated with distension. Bowel sounds are usually present and may be high-pitched. The abdominal distension can be striking, although the abdomen is soft. The colon gradually becomes more and more distended with gas, and if the distention is not relieved or the underlying condition not treated, perforation and peritonitis result.

Noncontrast radiographs of the abdomen reveal colon dilatation, especially prominent in the cecum (Fig. J.1). There is either a sharp 'cut-off' between a distended right colon and nondistended distal bowel or the entire colon is dilated. The rectum usually is not distended. The cecum can be massive, minicking cecal volvulus. The haustra are usually preserved and bowel wall edema is generally not seen (16). Associated small bowel distension is often present.

The law of Laplace explains why the cecum is so often markedly dilated. This law states that the pressure required to distend a structure is inversely proportional to the radius of that structure. Thus, the greater the original diameter, the less pressure is required to distend that organ. Because the cecum normally has the largest diameter in the colon, it is the cecum that distends the most.

Anatomically, the cecum is located uppermost in these sick patients, who usually lie supine. As a result, with poor peristalsis the cecum becomes distended with gas, the dependent ascending colon fills with fluid, and the cecum cannot empty properly. Often these patients can be managed medically simply by positioning them prone or in the decubitus position; changing the patient's position on an hourly basis can help relieve the 'pseudo-obstruction'.

Many of these patients are studied with a barium enema primarily to exclude colon obstruction. A single-contrast barium enema usually shows a non-dilated left colon, a transition in the transverse colon, and a considerably dilated right colon, but no anatomic abstruction can be demonstrated (Fig. J.2). With overdistension there is a possibility of cecal perforation; the examination should be terminated as soon as a colon obstruction has been excluded and before the entire colon is filled with barium. Such an approach also prevents excessive barium retention and impaction.

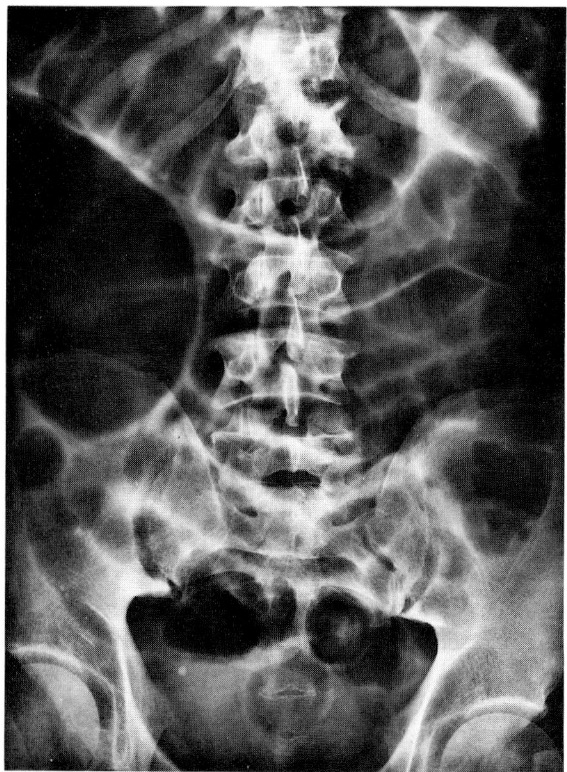

Fig. J.1. Colonic ileus. The cecum and transverse colon are moderately distended. The patient had major pelvic trauma and was essentially immobilized in the supine position. The ileus gradually cleared.

A post evacuation radiograph generally reveals collapse of the left side of the colon, with the right side of the colon still remaining dilated. Occasionally the barium enema stimulates colon contraction and the postevacuation radiograph shows decrease in caliber of the dilated right colon.

If the patient's condition does not improve on medical management, prompt cecostomy is necessary to relieve the distension (11, 17); a tube cecostomy can be performed under local anesthesia. Some investigators recommend colonoscopic decompression, thus avoiding surgery (18).

With significant bowel distension the intraluminal pressure increases, there is a decrease in venous blood flow, stasis, and eventual bowel wall ischemia. If there is rupture secondary to increased intraluminal pressure, the serosa ruptures first, followed by the muscle layers, then the mucosa herniates, with eventual rupture of the mucosa (19).

As long as the colon is not markedly distended most physicians treat these patients conservatively. With nonsurgical therapy, serial acute abdominal examinations should be obtained every 12 or 24 hours, depending upon the patient's condition. Perforation can occur with signs of peritoneal irritation (20) or these sick patients can show few clinical signs. With a perforation the colon distension can persist (21).

The differential diagnosis of this condition includes obstruction (mechanical ileus), volvulus, toxic dilation secondary to one of the colitides, pancreatitis and simply atonia because of lack of activity. Other conditions associated with a dilated colon include myxedema (22, 23), amyloidosis, collagen vascular diseases such as scleroderma (24), Chagas' disease, aganglionosis, celiac disease (25), congenital megacolon, myotonic dystrophy (26), idiopathic dilation as seen in psychiatric patients (27), post jejunoileal bypass for obesity (28), familial autonomic dysfunction, and Parkinson's disease. Some drugs, such as the anticholinergics, may likewise impair colon motility. An anticholinergic effect can be seen with the phenothiazines and the tricyclic antidepressants. Narcotics likewise can lead to an atonic colon (29); an often seen associated finding is considerable stool in the right side of the colon. Although unusual, prolonged laxative abuse can also eventually result in a dilated and hypotonic colon.

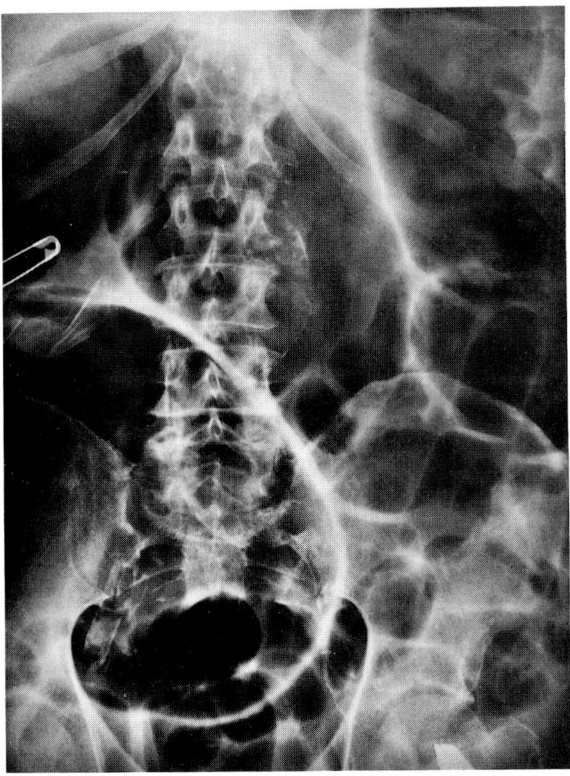

a

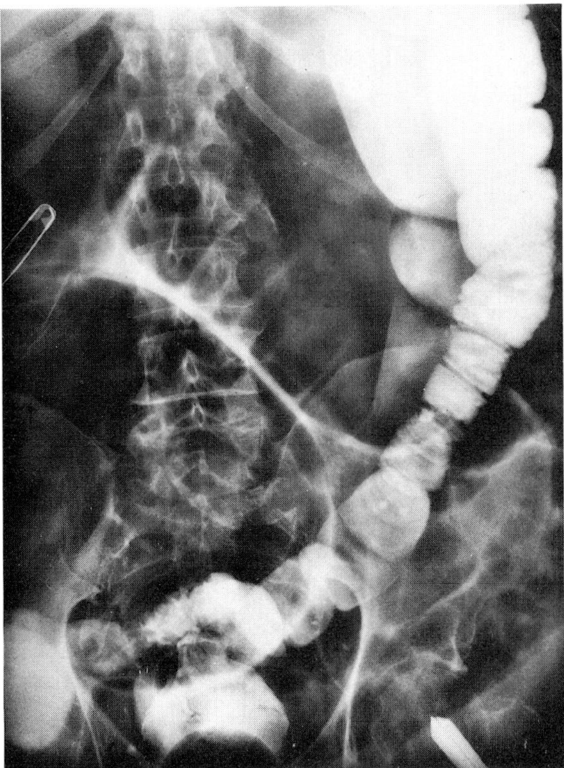

b

c

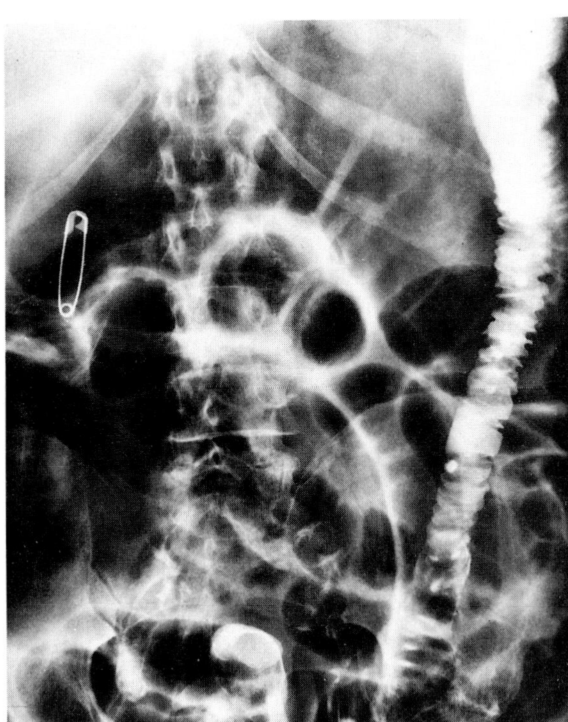

Fig. J.2. Postoperatively after right renal surgery this patient developed abdominal distension. (a) A supine radiograph reveals massive cecal and transverse colon dilation. Colon obstruction was suspected and a barium enema was performed. (b) The barium enema was terminated when barium reached the dilated transverse colon. No obstruction was identified on the study. (c) A postevacuation radiograph still shows the marked proximal colon dilation. The caliber of the descending colon is normal.

References

1. Morton JH, Schwartz SI, Gramiak R: Ileus of the colon. Arch Surg 81:425–434, 1960.
2. Wanebo H, Mathewson C, Conolly B: Pseudo-obstruction of the colon. Surg Gynecol Obstet 133:44–48, 1971.
3. Dunlop JA: Ogilvie's syndrome of false colonic obstruction: a case with post-mortem findings. Br Med J, I:890–891, 1949.
4. Schuffler MD, Lowe MC, Bill AH: Studies of idiopathic intestinal pseudo-obstruction. Hereditary hollow visceral myopathy: clinical and pathological studies. Gastroenterology 73:327–338, 1977.
5. Anuras S, Shirazi S, Faulk DL, Gardner GD, Christensen J: Surgical treatment in familial visceral myopathy. Ann Surg 189:306–310, 1979.
6. Ogilvie H: Large-intestine colic due to sympathetic deprivation. Br Med J 2:671–673, 1948.
7. Melamed M, Kubian E: Relationship of the autonomic nervous system to 'functional' obstruction of the intestinal tract. Radiology 80:22–29, 1963.
8. Attiyeh FF, Knapper WH: Pseudo-obstruction of the colon (Ogilvie's syndrome). Dis Colon Rectum 23:106–108, 1980.

9. Hanks JB, Meyers WC, Andersen DK, Woodard BH, Peete WPJ, Garbutt JT, Jones RS: Chronic primary intestinal pseudo-obstruction. Surgery 89:175–182, 1981.
10. Jensen HK: Spontaneous perforation of the caecum following caesarean section. Acta Obstet Gynec Scand 51:381–383, 1972.
11. Adams JT: Adynamic ileus of the colon: An indication for cecostomy. Surgery 109:503–507, 1974.
12. Søreide O, Bjerkeset T, Fossdal JE: Pseudo-obstruction of the colon (Ogilvie's syndrome), a genuine clinical condition? Review of the literature (1948–1975) and report of five cases. Dis Colon Rectum 20:487–491, 1977.
13. Lopez MJ, Memula N, Doss LL, Johnston WD: Pseudo-obstruction of the colon during pelvic radiotherapy. Dis Colon Rectum 24:201–204, 1981.
14. Snape WJ Jr, Sullivan MA, Cohen S: Abnormal gastro-colic response in patients with intestinal pseudo-obstruction. Arch Intern Med 140:386–387, 1980.
15. Battle WM, Snape WJ Jr, Alavi A, Cohen S, Braunstein S: Colonic dysfunction in diabetes mellitus. Gastroenterology 79:1217–1221, 1980.
16. Bryk D, Soong KY: Colonic ileus and its differential roentgen diagnosis. AJR 101:329–337, 1967.
17. Gierson ED, Storm FK, Shaw W, Coyne SK: Caecal rupture due to colonic ileus. Br J Surg 62:383–386, 1975.
18. Kukora JS, Dent TL: Colonoscopic decompression of massive nonobstructive cecal dilatation. Arch Surg 112:512–517, 1977.
19. Ravid JM: Diastasis and diastatic perforation of the gastrointestinal tract. A clinical, pathologic, and experimental study. Am J Path 27:33–52, 1951.
20. Macmanus Q, Krippaehne WW: Diastatic perforation of the cecum without distal obstruction. Arch Surg 112:1227–1230, 1977.
21. Meyers MA: Colonic ileus. Gastrointest Radiol 2:37–40, 1977.
22. Salerno N, Grey N: Myxedema pseudoobstruction. AJR 130:175–176, 1978.
23. Burrell M, Cronan J, Megna D, Toffler R: Myxedema megacolon. Gastrointest Radiol 5:181–186, 1980.
24. Ferrari BT, Ray JE, Robertson HD, Bonau RA, Gathright JB Jr: Colonic manifestations of collagen vascular diseases. Dis Colon Rectum 23:473–477, 1980.
25. Kappelman NB, Burrell M, Toffler R: Megacolon associated with celiac disease: report of four cases and review of the literature. AJR 128:65–68, 1977.
26. Weiner MJ: Myotonic megacolon in myotonic dystrophy. AJR 130:177–179, 1978.
27. Ehrentheil OF, Wells EP: Megacolon in psychotic patients. A clinical entity. Gastroenterology 29:285–294, 1955.
28. Wade DH, Richards V, Burhenne HJ: Radiographic changes after small bowel bypass for morbid obesity. Radiol Clin North Am 14:493–498, 1976.
29. Rubenstein RB, Wolff WI: Methadone ileus syndrome. Report of a fatal case. Dis Colon Rectum 19:357–359, 1976.

III.4.K. Colitis cystica profunda

Colitis cystica profunda is a rare condition consisting of mucinous cysts in the wall of the colon. The condition has also been called 'hamartomatous inverted polyp' (1), 'benign ulcer of the rectum' (2), and 'solitary ulcer syndrome' (3–7). The first description is attributed to Cruveilheir (8) in 1870, although the condition was probably described earlier (3).

Most of these patients have nonspecific symptoms of abdominal pain, bleeding or diarrhea, with bleeding being a prominent symptom. Anemia is not unusual. Only occasional pediatric patients have been described with this condition, with most patients being young adults (9). The adult distribution and associated complaints argue for colitis cystica profunda being an acquired condition.

The pathogenesis of this condition is not clear. Colitis cystica profunda is believed to represent malfunction of the puborectalis muscle, prolapse of a portion of the rectal mucosa, and possibly subsequent ischemia (7). Often there is associated rectal prolapse.

Most lesions are located on the anterior rectal wall close to one of the valves of Houston; they consist of nodules with an overlying erythematous mucosa (10). Microscopy reveals mucus-filled glands or cysts in the wall of the colon, with many located in the submucosa. The lamina propria is obliterated by fibroblasts and the mucularis mucosa is thickened (4, 6). Regenerating epithelium extends into the submucosa, with the glands distended by mucus. Biopsy should not reveal any neoplastic cells although there may be confusion clinically and histologically with carcinoma, which may lead to a mistaken diagnosis (11).

Because this condition is associated with inflammation, a superficial biopsy of the mucosa reveals inflammation or erosion of the mucosa. The true nature of the condition can be diagnosed with deeper biopsies extending into the submucosa.

A barium enema reveals nodularity, irregular polyps, possible stricture, and ulcers. The presacral space can be widened (9). Most of the lesions are centered along the anterior wall of the rectum; thus lateral radiographs are essential. The radiographic impression is similar to that of an infiltrating carcinoma or a localized colitis.

Colits cystica profunda should not be confused with stercoral ulcerations. The latter condition is generally associated with constipation, the ulcer is inflamed, and there can be subsequent colon perforation (12).

The differential diagnosis also includes urticaria or angioneurotic edema of the colon. Urticaria is generally associated with drugs (Table K.1), and cutaneous urticaria is present in many of these patients. A barium enema in patients with colon urticaria reveals focal areas of submucosal edema appearing as a mosaic of focal plaques with well-marginated blister-like imprints (Figs. K.1 and K.2).

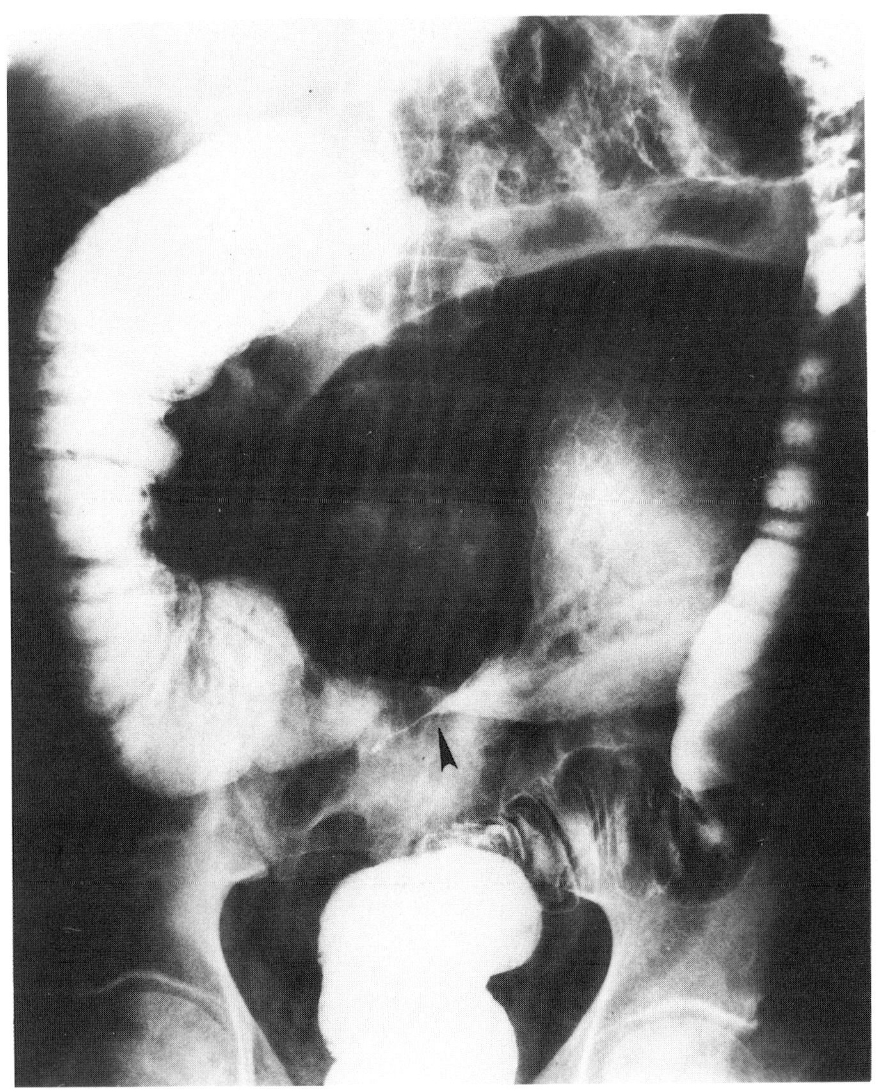

Fig. K.1. Colon urticaria associated with cecal volvulus. The volvulus is clearly seen (arrowhead). Numerous polygonal plaques are present in the cecum, compatible with urticaria. (Courtesy Drs. D.K. Yousefzadeh and J.G. Teplick (18); copyright, RSNA, 1979.)

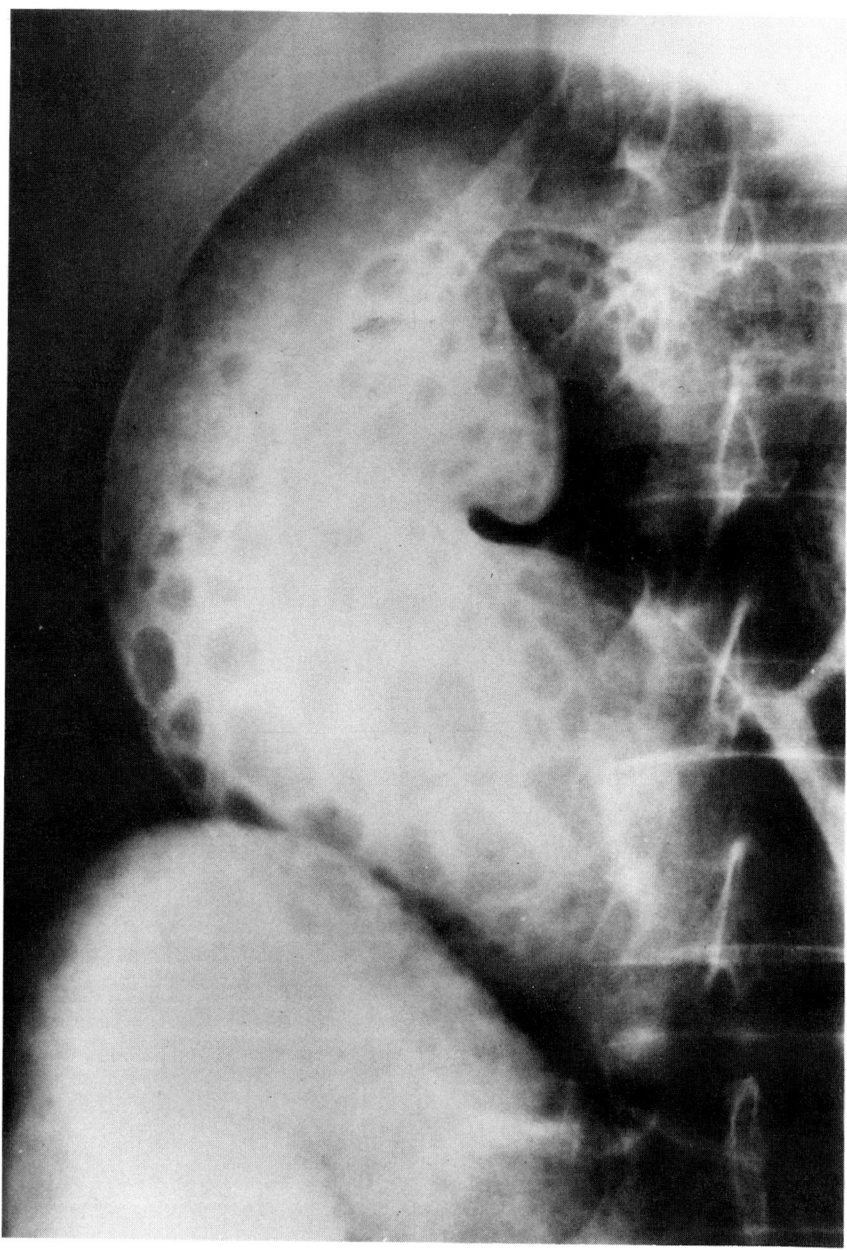

Fig. K.2. Colon urticaria occurring after patient received local anesthesia. Polygonal plaques are scattered in the ascending colon.

Table K.1. Urticaria of the colon.

Reference	Year	Associated conditions	Prior medications	Outcome
13	1968	Cutaneous urticaria	Penicillin	Recovery
14	1971	Colocolic intussusception	None	Recovery after resection
15	1971	None	Dulcolax	Anaphylactoid reaction and death
16	1973	Cutaneous urticaria	Multiple	Recovery
17	1977	Colitis	?	Recovery
18	1979	Cutaneous urticaria, cecal volvulus	Robaxin Mellaril	Recovery

References

1. Allen MS Jr: Hamartomatous inverted polyps of the rectum. Cancer 19:257–265, 1966.
2. Kennedy DK, Hughes ESR, Masterton JP: The natural history of benign ulcer of the rectum. Surg Gynecol Obstet 144:718–720, 1977.
3. Mulder H, TeVelde J: Colitis cystica profunda. Radiol Clin Biol 43:529–539, 1974.
4. Lewis FW, Mahoney MP, Heffernan CK: The solitary ulcer syndrome of the rectum: radiological features. Br J Radiol 50:227–228, 1977.
5. Fenzy A, Bogomoletz W, Puchelle JC: L'ulcère solitaire du rectum. Nouvelle Presse Méd 9:1297–1301, 1980.
6. Schweiger M, Alexander-Williams J: Solitary ulcer syndrome of the rectum. Its association with occult rectal prolapse. Lancet 1:170–171, 1977.
7. Feczko PJ, O'Connell DJ, Riddell RH, Frank PH: Solitary rectal ulcer syndrome: radiologic manifestations. AJR 135:499–506, 1980.
8. Cruveilhier J: Ulcere chronique du rectum. In: Anatomie Pathologique du Corps Humain, Tome 2, livre 25, Maladies du Rectum, 4 (J.B. Baillière, Paris), 1853.
9. Ledesma-Medina J, Reid BS, Girdany BR: Colitis cystica profunda. AJR 131:529–530, 1978.
10. Martin JK Jr, Culp CE, Weiland LH: Colitis cystica profunda. Dis Colon Rectum 23:488–491, 1980.
11. Morson BC, Dawson IMP: Gastrointestinal Pathology, 2nd Edn., pp 698–699. Blackwell Scientific, Oxford, 1979.
12. Gekas P, Schuster MM: Stercoral perforation of the colon: case report and review of the literature. Gastroenterology 80:1054–1058, 1981.
13. Clemett AR, Fishbone G, Levine RJ, James AE, Janower M: Gastrointestinal lesions in mastocytosis. AJR 103:405–412, 1968.
14. Johnson TH Jr, Caldwell KW: Angioneurotic edema of the colon. Radiology 99:61–63, 1971.
15. Berk RN, Millman SJ: Urticaria of the colon. Radiology 99:539–540, 1971.
16. Bléry M, Gaux JC, Ferrier JP, Bismuth V: Urticaire colique vraisemblable: manifestations radiologiques (présentation d'une observation). Arch Fr Mal App Dig 62:331–335, 1973.
17. Tubiana JM, Rouger P, Monnier JP, Levy VG, Chalut J: Un nouveau cas d'urticaire colique vraisemblable. Ann Radiol (Paris) 20:235–237, 1977.
18. Yousefzadeh DK, Teplick JG: Urticaria of the colon. Radiology 132:315–316, 1979.

SUBJECT INDEX